'An extraordinary achievement. Mukherjee's book has the vividness of an insider's account. It evokes what it feels like to be at the forefront of modern biomedicine and to bring new knowledge and technologies into the clinic. It's hard to think of many books for a general audience that have rendered any area of modern science and technology with such intelligence, accessibility, and compassion'
New Yorker

'Remarkable ... The reader devours this fascinating book. Mukherjee is a clear and determined writer ... An unusually humble, insightful book'
Los Angeles Times

'Magnificent, moving account of the history of cancer ... Drawing on Mukherjee's scientific clarity of thought for its compelling plot, and enhanced by his lightly worn profundity, it is a literary tour de force. At its heart are the questions that cancer has raised since first it appeared, about the role of doctors and science; about suffering, surviving. And, of course, about dying'
Herald

'Powerful and ambitious'
Scotsman

'Mukherjee brings an impressive balance of empathy and dispassion to this instantly essential piece of medical journalism'
Time

'Riveting and powerful'
San Francisco Chronicle

THE

EMPEROR

OF ALL

MALADIES

THE

EMPEROR

OF ALL

MALADIES

A BIOGRAPHY OF CANCER

SIDDHARTHA
MUKHERJEE

FOURTH ESTATE · London

Fourth Estate
An imprint of HarperCollins*Publishers*
77–85 Fulham Palace Road
London W6 8JB
www.4thestate.co.uk

This Fourth Estate paperback edition published 2011
2

First published in Great Britain by Fourth Estate in 2011

A catalogue record for this book
is available from the British Library

ISBN 978-0-00-725092-9

To
ROBERT SANDLER (1945–1948),
and to those who came before
and after him.

Illness is the night-side of life, a more onerous citizenship. Everyone who is born holds dual citizenship, in the kingdom of the well and in the kingdom of the sick. Although we all prefer to use only the good passport, sooner or later each of us is obliged, at least for a spell, to identify ourselves as citizens of that other place.

—Susan Sontag

Contents

In 2010, about six hundred thousand Americans, and more than 7 million humans around the world, will die of cancer. In the United States, one in three women and one in two men will develop cancer during their lifetime. A quarter of all American deaths, and about 15 percent of all deaths worldwide, will be attributed to cancer. In some nations, cancer will surpass heart disease to become the most common cause of death.

Author's Note

This book is a history of cancer. It is a chronicle of an ancient disease—once a clandestine, "whispered-about" illness—that has metamorphosed into a lethal shape-shifting entity imbued with such penetrating metaphorical, medical, scientific, and political potency that cancer is often described as the defining plague of our generation. This book is a "biography" in the truest sense of the word—an attempt to enter the *mind* of this immortal illness, to understand its personality, to demystify its behavior. But my ultimate aim is to raise a question beyond biography: Is cancer's end conceivable in the future? Is it possible to eradicate this disease from our bodies and societies forever?

Cancer is not one disease but many diseases. We call them all "cancer" because they share a fundamental feature: the abnormal growth of cells. And beyond the biological commonality, there are deep cultural and political themes that run through the various incarnations of cancer to justify a unifying narrative. It is not possible to consider the stories of every variant of cancer, but I have attempted to highlight the large themes that run through this 4,000-year history.

The project, evidently vast, began as a more modest enterprise. In the summer of 2003, having completed a residency in medicine and graduate work in cancer immunology, I began advanced training in cancer medicine (medical oncology) at the Dana-Farber Cancer Institute and Massachusetts General Hospital in Boston. I had initially envisioned writing a journal of that year—a view-from-the-trenches of cancer treatment. But that quest soon grew into a larger exploratory journey that carried me into the depths not only of science and medicine, but of culture, history, literature, and politics, into cancer's past and into its future.

Two characters stand at the epicenter of this story—both contemporaries, both idealists, both children of the boom in postwar science and technology in America, and both caught in the swirl of a hypnotic, obsessive quest to launch a national "War on Cancer." The first is Sidney Farber, the father of modern chemotherapy, who accidentally discovers a powerful anti-cancer chemical in a vitamin analogue and begins to dream of a universal cure for cancer. The second is Mary Lasker, the Manhattan socialite of legendary social and political energy, who joins Farber in his decades-long journey. But Lasker and Farber only exemplify the grit, imagination, inventiveness, and optimism of generations of men and women who have waged a battle against cancer for four thousand years. In a sense, this is a military history—one in which the adversary is formless, timeless, and pervasive. Here, too, there are victories and losses, campaigns upon campaigns, heroes and hubris, survival and resilience—and inevitably, the wounded, the condemned, the forgotten, the dead. In the end, cancer truly emerges, as a nineteenth-century surgeon once wrote in a book's frontispiece, as "the emperor of all maladies, the king of terrors."

A disclaimer: in science and medicine, where the primacy of a discovery carries supreme weight, the mantle of inventor or discoverer is assigned by a community of scientists and researchers. Although there are many stories of discovery and invention in this book, none of these establishes any legal claims of primacy.

This work rests heavily on the shoulders of other books, studies, journal articles, memoirs, and interviews. It rests also on the vast contributions of individuals, libraries, collections, archives, and papers acknowledged at the end of the book.

One acknowledgment, though, cannot be left to the end. This book is not just a journey into the past of cancer, but also a personal journey of my coming-of-age as an oncologist. That second journey would be impossible without patients, who, above and beyond all contributors, continued to teach and inspire me as I wrote. It is in their debt that I stand forever.

This debt comes with dues. The stories in this book present an important challenge in maintaining the privacy and dignity of these patients. In cases where the knowledge of the illness was already public (as with prior interviews or articles) I have used real names. In cases where there was no prior public knowledge, or when interviewees requested privacy, I have used a false name, and deliberately confounded dates and identities to make it difficult to track them. However, these are real patients and real encounters. I urge all my readers to respect their identities and boundaries.

THE

EMPEROR

OF ALL

MALADIES

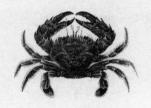

Prologue

On the morning of May 19, 2004, Carla Reed, a thirty-year-old kinder-garten teacher from Ipswich, Massachusetts, a mother of three young children, woke up in bed with a headache. "Not just any headache," she would recall later, "but a sort of numbness in my head. The kind of numbness that instantly tells you that something is terribly wrong."

Something had been terribly wrong for nearly a month. Late in April, Carla had discovered a few bruises on her back. They had suddenly appeared one morning, like strange stigmata, then grown and vanished over the next month, leaving large map-shaped marks on her back. Almost indiscernibly, her gums had begun to turn white. By early May, Carla, a vivacious, energetic woman accustomed to spending hours in the class-room chasing down five- and six-year-olds, could barely walk up a flight of stairs. Some mornings, exhausted and unable to stand up, she crawled down the hallways of her house on all fours to get from one room to another. She slept fitfully for twelve or fourteen hours a day, then woke up

1

feeling so overwhelmingly tired that she needed to haul herself back to the couch again to sleep.

Carla and her husband saw a general physician and a nurse twice during those four weeks, but she returned each time with no tests and without a diagnosis. Ghostly pains appeared and disappeared in her bones. The doctor fumbled about for some explanation. Perhaps it was a migraine, she suggested, and asked Carla to try some aspirin. The aspirin simply worsened the bleeding in Carla's white gums.

Outgoing, gregarious, and ebullient, Carla was more puzzled than worried about her waxing and waning illness. She had never been seriously ill in her life. The hospital was an abstract place for her; she had never met or consulted a medical specialist, let alone an oncologist. She imagined and concocted various causes to explain her symptoms—overwork, depression, dyspepsia, neuroses, insomnia. But in the end, something visceral arose inside her—a seventh sense—that told Carla something acute and catastrophic was brewing within her body.

On the afternoon of May 19, Carla dropped her three children with a neighbor and drove herself back to the clinic, demanding to have some blood tests. Her doctor ordered a routine test to check her blood counts. As the technician drew a tube of blood from her vein, he looked closely at the blood's color, obviously intrigued. Watery, pale, and dilute, the liquid that welled out of Carla's veins hardly resembled blood.

Carla waited the rest of the day without any news. At a fish market the next morning, she received a call.

"We need to draw some blood again," the nurse from the clinic said.

"When should I come?" Carla asked, planning her hectic day. She remembers looking up at the clock on the wall. A half-pound steak of salmon was warming in her shopping basket, threatening to spoil if she left it out too long.

In the end, commonplace particulars make up Carla's memories of illness: the clock, the car pool, the children, a tube of pale blood, a missed shower, the fish in the sun, the tightening tone of a voice on the phone. Carla cannot recall much of what the nurse said, only a general sense of urgency. "Come now," she thinks the nurse said. "Come now."

*

I heard about Carla's case at seven o'clock on the morning of May 21, on a train speeding between Kendall Square and Charles Street in Boston. The sentence that flickered on my beeper had the staccato and deadpan force of a true medical emergency: *Carla Reed/New patient with leukemia/14th Floor/Please see as soon as you arrive.* As the train shot out of a long, dark tunnel, the glass towers of the Massachusetts General Hospital suddenly loomed into view, and I could see the windows of the fourteenth floor rooms.

Carla, I guessed, was sitting in one of those rooms by herself, terrifyingly alone. Outside the room, a buzz of frantic activity had probably begun. Tubes of blood were shuttling between the ward and the laboratories on the second floor. Nurses were moving about with specimens, interns collecting data for morning reports, alarms beeping, pages being sent out. Somewhere in the depths of the hospital, a microscope was flickering on, with the cells in Carla's blood coming into focus under its lens.

I can feel relatively certain about all of this because the arrival of a patient with acute leukemia still sends a shiver down the hospital's spine—all the way from the cancer wards on its upper floors to the clinical laboratories buried deep in the basement. Leukemia is cancer of the white blood cells—cancer in one of its most explosive, violent incarnations. As one nurse on the wards often liked to remind her patients, with this disease "even a paper cut is an emergency."

For an oncologist in training, too, leukemia represents a special incarnation of cancer. Its pace, its acuity, its breathtaking, inexorable arc of growth forces rapid, often drastic decisions; it is terrifying to experience, terrifying to observe, and terrifying to treat. The body invaded by leukemia is pushed to its brittle physiological limit—every system, heart, lung, blood, working at the knife-edge of its performance. The nurses filled me in on the gaps in the story. Blood tests performed by Carla's doctor had revealed that her red cell count was critically low, less than a third of normal. Instead of normal white cells, her blood was packed with millions of large, malignant white cells—*blasts,* in the vocabulary of cancer. Her doctor, having finally stumbled upon the real diagnosis, had sent her to the Massachusetts General Hospital.

✑

In the long, bare hall outside Carla's room, in the antiseptic gleam of the floor just mopped with diluted bleach, I ran through the list of tests that would be needed on her blood and mentally rehearsed the conversation I would have with her. There was, I noted ruefully, something rehearsed and robotic even about my sympathy. This was the tenth month of my "fellowship" in oncology—a two-year immersive medical program to train cancer specialists—and I felt as if I had gravitated to my lowest point. In those ten indescribably poignant and difficult months, dozens of patients in my care had died. I felt I was slowly becoming inured to the deaths and the desolation—vaccinated against the constant emotional brunt.

There were seven such cancer fellows at this hospital. On paper, we seemed like a formidable force: graduates of five medical schools and four teaching hospitals, sixty-six years of medical and scientific training, and twelve postgraduate degrees among us. But none of those years or degrees could possibly have prepared us for this training program. Medical school, internship, and residency had been physically and emotionally grueling, but the first months of the fellowship flicked away those memories as if all of that had been child's play, the kindergarten of medical training.

Cancer was an all-consuming presence in our lives. It invaded our imaginations; it occupied our memories; it infiltrated every conversation, every thought. And if we, as physicians, found ourselves immersed in cancer, then our patients found their lives virtually obliterated by the disease. In Aleksandr Solzhenitsyn's novel *Cancer Ward,* Pavel Nikolayevich Rusanov, a youthful Russian in his midforties, discovers that he has a tumor in his neck and is immediately whisked away into a cancer ward in some nameless hospital in the frigid north. The diagnosis of cancer—not the disease, but the mere stigma of its presence—becomes a death sentence for Rusanov. The illness strips him of his identity. It dresses him in a patient's smock (a tragicomically cruel costume, no less blighting than a prisoner's jumpsuit) and assumes absolute control of his actions. To be diagnosed with cancer, Rusanov discovers, is to enter a borderless medical gulag, a state even more invasive and paralyzing than the one that he has left behind. (Solzhenitsyn may have intended his absurdly totalitarian cancer hospital to parallel the absurdly totalitarian state outside it, yet when I once asked a woman with invasive cervical cancer about the parallel, she said sardonically, "Unfortunately, I did not need any metaphors to read the book. The cancer ward *was* my confining state, my prison.")

As a doctor learning to tend cancer patients, I had only a partial glimpse of this confinement. But even skirting its periphery, I could still feel its power—the dense, insistent gravitational tug that pulls everything and everyone into the orbit of cancer. A colleague, freshly out of his fellowship, pulled me aside on my first week to offer some advice. "It's called an immersive training program," he said, lowering his voice. "But by immersive, they really mean drowning. Don't let it work its way into everything you do. Have a life outside the hospital. You'll need it, or you'll get swallowed."

But it was impossible not to be swallowed. In the parking lot of the hospital, a chilly, concrete box lit by neon floodlights, I spent the end of every evening after rounds in stunned incoherence, the car radio crackling vacantly in the background, as I compulsively tried to reconstruct the events of the day. The stories of my patients consumed me, and the decisions that I made haunted me. *Was it worthwhile continuing yet another round of chemotherapy on a sixty-six-year-old pharmacist with lung cancer who had failed all other drugs? Was is better to try a tested and potent combination of drugs on a twenty-six-year-old woman with Hodgkin's disease and risk losing her fertility, or to choose a more experimental combination that might spare it? Should a Spanish-speaking mother of three with colon cancer be enrolled in a new clinical trial when she can barely read the formal and inscrutable language of the consent forms?*

Immersed in the day-to-day management of cancer, I could only see the lives and fates of my patients played out in color-saturated detail, like a television with the contrast turned too high. I could not pan back from the screen. I knew instinctively that these experiences were part of a much larger battle against cancer, but its contours lay far outside my reach. I had a novice's hunger for history, but also a novice's inability to envision it.

❧

But as I emerged from the strange desolation of those two fellowship years, the questions about the larger story of cancer emerged with urgency: How old is cancer? What are the roots of our battle against this disease? Or, as patients often asked me: Where are we in the "war" on cancer? How did we get here? Is there an end? Can this war even be won?

This book grew out of the attempt to answer these questions. I delved into the history of cancer to give shape to the shape-shifting illness that I was confronting. I used the past to explain the present. The isolation and rage of a thirty-six-year-old woman with stage III breast cancer had ancient echoes in Atossa, the Persian queen who swaddled her diseased breast in cloth to hide it and then, in a fit of nihilistic and prescient fury, possibly had a slave cut it off with a knife. A patient's desire to amputate her stomach, ridden with cancer—"sparing nothing," as she put it to me—

5

carried the memory of the perfection-obsessed nineteenth-century surgeon William Halsted, who had chiseled away at cancer with larger and more disfiguring surgeries, all in the hopes that cutting more would mean curing more.

Roiling underneath these medical, cultural, and metaphorical interceptions of cancer over the centuries was the biological understanding of the illness—an understanding that had morphed, often radically, from decade to decade. Cancer, we now know, is a disease caused by the uncontrolled growth of a single cell. This growth is unleashed by mutations—changes in DNA that specifically affect genes that incite unlimited cell growth. In a normal cell, powerful genetic circuits regulate cell division and cell death. In a cancer cell, these circuits have been broken, unleashing a cell that cannot stop growing.

That this seemingly simple mechanism—cell growth without barriers—can lie at the heart of this grotesque and multifaceted illness is a testament to the unfathomable power of cell growth. Cell division allows us as organisms to grow, to adapt, to recover, to repair—to live. And distorted and unleashed, it allows cancer cells to grow, to flourish, to adapt, to recover, and to repair—to live at the cost of our living. Cancer cells can grow faster, adapt better. They are more perfect versions of ourselves.

The secret to battling cancer, then, is to find means to prevent these mutations from occurring in susceptible cells, or to find means to eliminate the mutated cells without compromising normal growth. The conciseness of that statement belies the enormity of the task. Malignant growth and normal growth are so genetically intertwined that unbraiding the two might be one of the most significant scientific challenges faced by our species. Cancer is built into our genomes: the genes that unmoor normal cell division are not foreign to our bodies, but rather mutated, distorted versions of the very genes that perform vital cellular functions. And cancer is imprinted in our society: as we extend our life span as a species, we inevitably unleash malignant growth (mutations in cancer genes accumulate with aging; cancer is thus intrinsically related to age). If we seek immortality, then so, too, in a rather perverse sense, does the cancer cell.

How, precisely, a future generation might learn to separate the entwined strands of normal growth from malignant growth remains a mystery. ("The universe," the twentieth-century biologist J. B. S. Haldane liked to say, "is not only queerer than we suppose, but queerer than we *can* suppose"—and so is the trajectory of science.) But this much is certain: the story, however it plays out, will contain indelible kernels of the past. It will be a story of inventiveness, resilience, and perseverance against what one writer called the most "relentless and insidious enemy" among human diseases. But it will also be a story of hubris, arrogance, paternalism, misperception, false hope, and hype, all leveraged against an illness that was just three decades ago widely touted as being "curable" within a few years.

ᴄᴘ

In the bare hospital room ventilated by sterilized air, Carla was fighting her own war on cancer. When I arrived, she was sitting with peculiar calm on her bed, a schoolteacher jotting notes. ("But what notes?" she would later recall. "I just wrote and rewrote the same thoughts.") Her mother, red-eyed and tearful, just off an overnight flight, burst into the room and then sat silently in a chair by the window, rocking forcefully. The din of activity around Carla had become almost a blur: nurses shuttling fluids in and out, interns donning masks and gowns, antibiotics being hung on IV poles to be dripped into her veins.

I explained the situation as best I could. Her day ahead would be full of tests, a hurtle from one lab to another. I would draw a bone marrow sample. More tests would be run by pathologists. But the preliminary tests suggested that Carla had acute lymphoblastic leukemia. It is one of the most common forms of cancer in children, but rare in adults. And it is—I paused here for emphasis, lifting my eyes up—often curable.

Curable. Carla nodded at that word, her eyes sharpening. Inevitable questions hung in the room: How curable? What were the chances that she would survive? How long would the treatment take? I laid out the odds. Once the diagnosis had been confirmed, chemotherapy would begin immediately and last more than one year. Her chances of being cured were about 30 percent, a little less than one in three.

We spoke for an hour, perhaps longer. It was now nine thirty in the morning. The city below us had stirred fully awake. The door shut behind me as I left, and a whoosh of air blew me outward and sealed Carla in.

———

PART ONE

"OF BLACKE CHOLOR, WITHOUT BOYLING"

In solving a problem of this sort, the grand thing is to be able to reason backwards. That is a very useful accomplishment, and a very easy one, but people do not practice it much.

—Sherlock Holmes, in Sir Arthur Conan Doyle's
A Study in Scarlet

"A suppuration of blood"

Physicians of the Utmost Fame
Were called at once; but when they came
They answered, as they took their Fees,
"There is no Cure for this Disease."
—Hilaire Belloc

Its palliation is a daily task, its cure a fervent hope.
—William Castle,
describing leukemia in 1950

In a damp fourteen-by-twenty-foot laboratory in Boston on a December morning in 1947, a man named Sidney Farber waited impatiently for the arrival of a parcel from New York. The "laboratory" was little more than a chemist's closet, a poorly ventilated room buried in a half-basement of the Children's Hospital, almost thrust into its back alley. A few hundred feet away, the hospital's medical wards were slowly thrumming to work. Children in white smocks moved restlessly on small wrought-iron cots. Doctors and nurses shuttled busily between the rooms, checking charts, writing orders, and dispensing medicines. But Farber's lab was listless and empty, a bare warren of chemicals and glass jars connected to the main hospital through a series of icy corridors. The sharp stench of embalming formalin wafted through the air. There were no patients in the rooms here, just the bodies and tissues of patients brought down through the tunnels for autopsies and examinations. Farber was a pathologist. His job involved dissecting specimens, performing autopsies, identifying cells, and diagnosing diseases, but never treating patients.

Farber's specialty was pediatric pathology, the study of children's diseases. He had spent nearly twenty years in these subterranean rooms star-

11

ing obsessively down his microscope and climbing through the academic ranks to become chief of pathology at Children's. But for Farber, pathology was becoming a disjunctive form of medicine, a discipline more preoccupied with the dead than with the living. Farber now felt impatient watching illness from its sidelines, never touching or treating a live patient. He was tired of tissues and cells. He felt trapped, embalmed in his own glassy cabinet.

And so, Farber had decided to make a drastic professional switch. Instead of squinting at inert specimens under his lens, he would try to leap into the life of the clinics upstairs—from the microscopic world that he knew so well into the magnified real world of patients and illnesses. He would try to use the knowledge he had gathered from his pathological specimens to devise new therapeutic interventions. The parcel from New York contained a few vials of a yellow crystalline chemical named aminopterin. It had been shipped to his laboratory in Boston on the slim hope that it might halt the growth of leukemia in children.

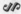

Had Farber asked any of the pediatricians circulating in the wards above him about the likelihood of developing an antileukemic drug, they would have advised him not to bother trying. Childhood leukemia had fascinated, confused, and frustrated doctors for more than a century. The disease had been analyzed, classified, subclassified, and subdivided meticulously; in the musty, leatherbound books on the library shelves at Children's—Anderson's *Pathology* or Boyd's *Pathology of Internal Diseases*—page upon page was plastered with images of leukemia cells and appended with elaborate taxonomies to describe the cells. Yet all this knowledge only amplified the sense of medical helplessness. The disease had turned into an object of empty fascination—a wax-museum doll—studied and photographed in exquisite detail but without any therapeutic or practical advances. "It gave physicians plenty to wrangle over at medical meetings," an oncologist recalled, "but it did not help their patients at all." A patient with acute leukemia was brought to the hospital in a flurry of excitement, discussed on medical rounds with professorial grandiosity, and then, as a medical magazine drily noted, "diagnosed, transfused—and sent home to die."

The study of leukemia had been mired in confusion and despair ever since its discovery. On March 19, 1845, a Scottish physician, John Bennett, had described an unusual case, a twenty-eight-year-old slate-layer with a mysterious swelling in his spleen. "He is of dark complexion," Bennett wrote of his patient, "usually healthy and temperate; [he] states that twenty months ago, he was affected with great listlessness on exertion, which has continued to this time. In June last he noticed a tumor in the left side of his abdomen which has gradually increased in size till four months since, when it became stationary."

The slate-layer's tumor might have reached its final, stationary point, but his constitutional troubles only accelerated. Over the next few weeks, Bennett's patient spiraled from symptom to symptom—fevers, flashes of bleeding, sudden fits of abdominal pain—gradually at first, then on a tighter, faster arc, careening from one bout to another. Soon the slate-layer was on the verge of death with more swollen tumors sprouting in his armpits, his groin, and his neck. He was treated with the customary leeches and purging, but to no avail. At the autopsy a few weeks later, Bennett was convinced that he had found the reason behind the symptoms. His patient's blood was chock-full of white blood cells. (White blood cells, the principal constituent of pus, typically signal the response to an infection, and Bennett reasoned that the slate-layer had succumbed to one.) "The following case seems to me particularly valuable," he wrote self-assuredly, "as it will serve to demonstrate the existence of true pus, formed universally within the vascular system."*

It would have been a perfectly satisfactory explanation except that Bennett could not find a source for the pus. During the necropsy, he pored carefully through the body, combing the tissues and organs for signs of an abscess or wound. But no other stigmata of infection were to be found. The blood had apparently spoiled—suppurated—of its own will, combusted spontaneously into true pus. "A suppuration of blood," Bennett called his case. And he left it at that.

Bennett was wrong, of course, about his spontaneous "suppuration" of blood. A little over four months after Bennett had described the slater's illness, a twenty-four-year-old German researcher, Rudolf Virchow, independently published a case report with striking similarities to Bennett's case. Virchow's patient was a cook in her midfifties. White cells had explo-

---

*Although the link between microorganisms and infection was yet to be established, the connection between pus—purulence—and sepsis, fever, and death, often arising from an abscess or wound, was well known to Bennett.

sively overgrown her blood, forming dense and pulpy pools in her spleen. At her autopsy, pathologists had likely not even needed a microscope to distinguish the thick, milky layer of white cells floating above the red.

Virchow, who knew of Bennett's case, couldn't bring himself to believe Bennett's theory. Blood, Virchow argued, had no reason to transform impetuously into anything. Moreover, the unusual symptoms bothered him: What of the massively enlarged spleen? Or the absence of any wound or source of pus in the body? Virchow began to wonder if the blood itself was abnormal. Unable to find a unifying explanation for it, and seeking a name for this condition, Virchow ultimately settled for *weisses Blut*— white blood—no more than a literal description of the millions of white cells he had seen under his microscope. In 1847, he changed the name to the more academic-sounding "leukemia"—from *leukos,* the Greek word for "white."

ּ֍

Renaming the disease—from the florid "suppuration of blood" to the flat *weisses Blut*—hardly seems like an act of scientific genius, but it had a profound impact on the understanding of leukemia. An illness, at the moment of its discovery, is a fragile idea, a hothouse flower—deeply, disproportionately influenced by names and classifications. (More than a century later, in the early 1980s, another change in name—from *gay related immune disease* (GRID) to *acquired immuno deficiency syndrome* (AIDS)—would signal an epic shift in the understanding of that disease.*) Like Bennett, Virchow didn't understand leukemia. But unlike Bennett, he didn't pretend to understand it. His insight lay entirely in the negative. By wiping the slate clean of all preconceptions, he cleared the field for thought.

The humility of the name (and the underlying humility about his understanding of cause) epitomized Virchow's approach to medicine. As a young professor at the University of Würzburg, Virchow's work soon extended far beyond naming leukemia. A pathologist by training, he launched a project that would occupy him for his life: describing human diseases in simple cellular terms.

---

* The identification of HIV as the pathogen, and the rapid spread of the virus across the globe, soon laid to rest the initially observed—and culturally loaded—"predeliction" for gay men.

It was a project born of frustration. Virchow entered medicine in the early 1840s, when nearly every disease was attributed to the workings of some invisible force: miasmas, neuroses, bad humors, and hysterias. Perplexed by what he couldn't see, Virchow turned with revolutionary zeal to what he could see: cells under the microscope. In 1838, Matthias Schleiden, a botanist, and Theodor Schwann, a physiologist, both working in Germany, had claimed that all living organisms were built out of fundamental building blocks called cells. Borrowing and extending this idea, Virchow set out to create a "cellular theory" of human biology, basing it on two fundamental tenets. First, that human bodies (like the bodies of all animals and plants) were made up of cells. Second, that cells only arose from other cells—*omnis cellula e cellula,* as he put it.

The two tenets might have seemed simplistic, but they allowed Virchow to propose a crucially important hypothesis about the nature of human growth. If cells only arose from other cells, then growth could occur in only two ways: either by increasing cell numbers or by increasing cell size. Virchow called these two modes hyperplasia and hypertrophy. In hypertrophy, the *number* of cells did not change; instead, each individual cell merely grew in size—like a balloon being blown up. Hyper*plasia,* in contrast, was growth by virtue of cells increasing in *number*. Every growing human tissue could be described in terms of hypertrophy and hyperplasia. In adult animals, fat and muscle usually grow by hypertrophy. In contrast, the liver, blood, the gut, and the skin all grow through hyperplasia—cells becoming cells becoming more cells, *omnis cellula e cellula e cellula*.

That explanation was persuasive, and it provoked a new understanding not just of normal growth, but of pathological growth as well. Like normal growth, pathological growth could also be achieved through hypertrophy and hyperplasia. When the heart muscle is forced to push against a blocked aortic outlet, it often adapts by making every muscle cell bigger to generate more force, eventually resulting in a heart so overgrown that it may be unable to function normally—pathological hypertrophy.

Conversely, and importantly for this story, Virchow soon stumbled upon the quintessential disease of pathological hyperplasia—cancer. Looking at cancerous growths through his microscope, Virchow discovered an uncontrolled growth of cells—hyperplasia in its extreme form. As Virchow examined the architecture of cancers, the growth often seemed to have acquired a life of its own, as if the cells had become possessed by a new and mysterious drive to grow. This was not just ordinary growth, but growth redefined, growth in a new form. Presciently (although oblivious of the mechanism) Virchow called it *neo*plasia—novel, inexplicable, distorted growth, a word that would ring through the history of cancer.*

By the time Virchow died in 1902, a new theory of cancer had slowly coalesced out of all these observations. Cancer was a disease of pathological hyperplasia in which cells acquired an autonomous will to divide. This aberrant, uncontrolled cell division created masses of tissue (tumors) that invaded organs and destroyed normal tissues. These tumors could also spread from one site to another, causing outcroppings of the disease—called metastases—in distant sites, such as the bones, the brain, or the lungs. Cancer came in diverse forms—breast, stomach, skin, and cervical cancer, leukemias and lymphomas. But all these diseases were deeply connected at the cellular level. In every case, cells had all acquired the same characteristic: uncontrollable pathological cell division.

With this understanding, pathologists who studied leukemia in the late 1880s now circled back to Virchow's work. Leukemia, then, was not a suppuration of blood, but *neoplasia* of blood. Bennett's earlier fantasy had germinated an entire field of fantasies among scientists, who had gone searching (and dutifully found) all sorts of invisible parasites and bacteria bursting out of leukemia cells. But once pathologists stopped looking for infectious causes and refocused their lenses on the disease, they discovered the obvious analogies between leukemia cells and cells of other forms of cancer. Leukemia was a malignant proliferation of white cells in the blood. It was cancer in a molten, liquid form.

With that seminal observation, the study of leukemias suddenly found clarity and spurted forward. By the early 1900s, it was clear that the disease came in several forms. It could be chronic and indolent, slowly choking the bone marrow and spleen, as in Virchow's original case (later termed chronic leukemia). Or it could be acute and violent, almost a different illness in its personality, with flashes of fever, paroxysmal fits of bleeding, and a dazzlingly rapid overgrowth of cells—as in Bennett's patient.

This second version of the disease, called acute leukemia, came in two further subtypes, based on the type of cancer cell involved. Normal white cells in the blood can be broadly divided into two types of cells—myeloid cells or lymphoid cells. Acute myeloid leukemia (AML) was a cancer of the

---

*Virchow did not coin the word, although he offered a comprehensive description of neoplasia.

myeloid cells. Acute lymphoblastic leukemia (ALL) was cancer of imma-ture *lymphoid* cells. (Cancers of more mature lymphoid cells are called lymphomas.)

In children, leukemia was most commonly ALL—lymphoblastic leuke-mia—and was almost always swiftly lethal. In 1860, a student of Virchow's, Michael Anton Biermer, described the first known case of this form of childhood leukemia. Maria Speyer, an energetic, vivacious, and playful five-year-old daughter of a Würzburg carpenter, was initially seen at the clinic because she had become lethargic in school and developed bloody bruises on her skin. The next morning, she developed a stiff neck and a fever, pre-cipitating a call to Biermer for a home visit. That night, Biermer drew a drop of blood from Maria's veins, looked at the smear using a candlelit bedside microscope, and found millions of leukemia cells in the blood. Maria slept fitfully late into the evening. Late the next afternoon, as Biermer was excit-edly showing his colleagues the specimens of *"exquisit Fall von Leukämie"* (an exquisite case of leukemia), Maria vomited bright red blood and lapsed into a coma. By the time Biermer returned to her house that evening, the child had been dead for several hours. From its first symptom to diagnosis to death, her galloping, relentless illness had lasted no more than three days.

Although nowhere as aggressive as Maria Speyer's leukemia, Carla's ill-ness was astonishing in its own right. Adults, on average, have about five thousand white blood cells circulating per microliter of blood. Carla's blood contained ninety thousand cells per microliter—nearly twentyfold the normal level. Ninety-five percent of these cells were blasts—malig-nant lymphoid cells produced at a frenetic pace but unable to mature into fully developed lymphocytes. In acute lymphoblastic leukemia, as in some other cancers, the overproduction of cancer cells is combined with a mysterious arrest in the normal maturation of cells. Lymphoid cells are thus produced in vast excess, but, unable to mature, they cannot ful-fill their normal function in fighting microbes. Carla had immunological poverty in the face of plenty.

White blood cells are produced in the bone marrow. Carla's bone mar-row biopsy, which I saw under the microscope the morning after I first met her, was deeply abnormal. Although superficially amorphous, bone marrow is a highly organized tissue—an organ, in truth—that generates blood in adults. Typically, bone marrow biopsies contain spicules of bone and, within these spicules, islands of growing blood cells—nurseries for the genesis of new blood. In Carla's marrow, this organization had been fully destroyed. Sheet upon sheet of malignant blasts packed the marrow space, obliterating all anatomy and architecture, leaving no space for any production of blood.

Carla was at the edge of a physiological abyss. Her red cell count had dipped so low that her blood was unable to carry its full supply of oxygen (her headaches, in retrospect, were the first sign of oxygen deprivation). Her platelets, the cells responsible for clotting blood, had collapsed to nearly zero, causing her bruises.

Her treatment would require extraordinary finesse. She would need chemotherapy to kill her leukemia, but the chemotherapy would collaterally decimate any remnant normal blood cells. We would push her deeper into the abyss to try to rescue her. For Carla, the only way out would be the way through.

❧

Sidney Farber was born in Buffalo, New York, in 1903, one year after Virchow's death in Berlin. His father, Simon Farber, a former bargeman in Poland, had immigrated to America in the late nineteenth century and worked in an insurance agency. The family lived in modest circumstances at the eastern edge of town, in a tight-knit, insular, and often economically precarious Jewish community of shop owners, factory workers, bookkeepers, and peddlers. Pushed relentlessly to succeed, the Farber children were held to high academic standards. Yiddish was spoken upstairs, but only German and English were allowed downstairs. The elder Farber often brought home textbooks and scattered them across the dinner table, expecting each child to select and master one book, then provide a detailed report for him.

Sidney, the third of fourteen children, thrived in this environment of high aspirations. He studied both biology and philosophy in college and graduated from the University of Buffalo in 1923, playing the violin at music halls to support his college education. Fluent in German, he trained in medicine at Heidelberg and Freiburg, then, having excelled in Germany, found a spot as a second-year medical student at Harvard Medical School in Boston. (The circular journey from New York to Boston via Heidelberg was not unusual. In the mid-1920s, Jewish students often found it impossible to secure medical-school spots in America—often succeeding in European, even German, medical schools before returning to study medicine in their native country.) Farber thus arrived at Harvard as an outsider. His colleagues found him arrogant and insufferable, but, he too, relearning lessons that he had already learned, seemed to be suffering through it all. He was formal, precise, and meticulous, starched in his appearance and his mannerisms and commanding in presence. He was promptly nicknamed Four-Button Sid for his propensity for wearing formal suits to his classes.

Farber completed his advanced training in pathology in the late 1920s and became the first full-time pathologist at the Children's Hospital in Boston. He wrote a marvelous study on the classification of children's tumors and a textbook, *The Postmortem Examination,* widely considered a classic in the field. By the mid-1930s, he was firmly ensconced in the back alleys of the hospital as a preeminent pathologist—a "doctor of the dead."

Yet the hunger to treat patients still drove Farber. And sitting in his basement laboratory in the summer of 1947, Farber had a single inspired idea: he chose, among all cancers, to focus his attention on one of its oddest and most hopeless variants—childhood leukemia. To understand cancer as a whole, he reasoned, you needed to start at the bottom of its complexity, in *its* basement. And despite its many idiosyncrasies, leukemia possessed a singularly attractive feature: it could be measured.

Science begins with counting. To understand a phenomenon, a scientist must first describe it; to describe it objectively, he must first measure it. If cancer medicine was to be transformed into a rigorous science, then cancer would need to be counted somehow—measured in some reliable, reproducible way.

In this, leukemia was different from nearly every other type of cancer. In a world before CT scans and MRIs, quantifying the change in size of an internal solid tumor in the lung or the breast was virtually impossible without surgery: you could not measure what you could not see. But leukemia, floating freely in the blood, could be measured as easily as blood cells—by drawing a sample of blood or bone marrow and looking at it under a microscope.

If leukemia could be counted, Farber reasoned, then any intervention—a chemical sent circulating through the blood, say—could be evaluated for its potency in living patients. He could watch cells grow or die in the blood and use that to measure the success or failure of a drug. He could perform an "experiment" on cancer.

The idea mesmerized Farber. In the 1940s and '50s, young biologists were galvanized by the idea of using simple models to understand complex phenomena. Complexity was best understood by building from the ground up. Single-celled organisms such as bacteria would reveal the workings of massive, multicellular animals such as humans. What is true for *E. coli* [a microscopic bacterium], the French biochemist Jacques Monod would grandly declare in 1954, must also be true for elephants.

For Farber, leukemia epitomized this biological paradigm. From this simple, atypical beast he would extrapolate into the vastly more complex world of other cancers; the bacterium would teach him to think about the elephant. He was, by nature, a quick and often impulsive thinker. And here, too, he made a quick, instinctual leap. The package from New York was waiting in his laboratory that December morning. As he tore it open, pulling out the glass vials of chemicals, he scarcely realized that he was throwing open an entirely new way of thinking about cancer.

"A monster more insatiable
than the guillotine"

*The medical importance of leukemia has always been
disproportionate to its actual incidence. . . . Indeed,
the problems encountered in the systemic treatment of
leukemia were indicative of the general directions in
which cancer research as a whole was headed.*
— Jonathan Tucker,
Ellie: A Child's Fight Against Leukemia

*There were few successes in the treatment of disseminated
cancer. . . . It was usually a matter of watching the tumor
get bigger, and the patient, progressively smaller.*
— John Laszlo, *The Cure of Childhood Leukemia:
Into the Age of Miracles*

Sidney Farber's package of chemicals happened to arrive at a particularly
pivotal moment in the history of medicine. In the late 1940s, a cornucopia of pharmaceutical discoveries was tumbling open in labs and clinics
around the nation. The most iconic of these new drugs were the antibiotics. Penicillin, that precious chemical that had to be milked to its last
droplet during World War II (in 1939, the drug was reextracted from the
urine of patients who had been treated with it to conserve every last molecule), was by the early fifties being produced in thousand-gallon vats. In
1942, when Merck had shipped out its first batch of penicillin—a mere
five and a half grams of the drug—that amount had represented half of
the entire stock of the antibiotic in America. A decade later, penicillin was

21

being mass-produced so effectively that its price had sunk to four cents for a dose, one-eighth the cost of a half gallon of milk.

New antibiotics followed in the footsteps of penicillin: chloramphenicol in 1947, tetracycline in 1948. In the winter of 1949, when yet another miraculous antibiotic, streptomycin, was purified out of a clod of mold from a chicken farmer's barnyard, *Time* magazine splashed the phrase "*The remedies are in our own backyard,*" prominently across its cover. In a brick building on the far corner of Children's Hospital, in Farber's own backyard, a microbiologist named John Enders was culturing poliovirus in rolling plastic flasks, the first step that culminated in the development of the Sabin and Salk polio vaccines. New drugs appeared at an astonishing rate: by 1950, more than half the medicines in common medical use had been unknown merely a decade earlier.

Perhaps even more significant than these miracle drugs, shifts in public health and hygiene also drastically altered the national physiognomy of illness. Typhoid fever, a contagion whose deadly swirl could decimate entire districts in weeks, melted away as the putrid water supplies of several cities were cleansed by massive municipal efforts. Even tuberculosis, the infamous "white plague" of the nineteenth century, was vanishing, its incidence plummeting by more than half between 1910 and 1940, largely due to better sanitation and public hygiene efforts. The life expectancy of Americans rose from forty-seven to sixty-eight in half a century, a greater leap in longevity than had been achieved over several previous centuries.

The sweeping victories of postwar medicine illustrated the potent and transformative capacity of science and technology in American life. Hospitals proliferated—between 1945 and 1960, nearly one thousand new hospitals were launched nationwide; between 1935 and 1952, the number of patients admitted more than doubled from 7 million to 17 million per year. And with the rise in medical *care* came the concomitant expectation of medical *cure*. As one student observed, "When a doctor has to tell a patient that there is no specific remedy for his condition, [the patient] is apt to feel affronted, or to wonder whether the doctor is keeping abreast of the times."

In new and sanitized suburban towns, a young generation thus dreamed of cures—of a death-free, disease-free existence. Lulled by the idea of the durability of life, they threw themselves into consuming durables: boat-size Studebakers, rayon leisure suits, televisions, radios, vacation homes, golf clubs, barbecue grills, washing machines. In Levittown, a sprawling suburban settlement built in a potato field on Long Island—a symbolic utopia—"illness" now ranked third in a list of "worries," falling behind "finances" and "child-rearing." In fact, rearing children was becoming a national preoccupation at an unprecedented level. Fertility rose steadily—by 1957, a baby was being born every seven seconds in America. The "affluent society," as the economist John Galbraith described it, also imagined itself as eternally young, with an accompanying guarantee of eternal health—the invincible society.

ॐ

But of all diseases, cancer had refused to fall into step in this march of progress. If a tumor was strictly local (i.e., confined to a single organ or site so that it could be removed by a surgeon), the cancer stood a chance of being cured. Extirpations, as these procedures came to be called, were a legacy of the dramatic advances of nineteenth-century surgery. A solitary malignant lump in the breast, say, could be removed via a radical mastectomy pioneered by the great surgeon William Halsted at Johns Hopkins in the 1890s. With the discovery of X-rays in the early 1900s, radiation could also be used to kill tumor cells at local sites.

But scientifically, cancer still remained a black box, a mysterious entity that was best cut away en bloc rather than treated by some deeper medical insight. To cure cancer (if it could be cured at all), doctors had only two strategies: excising the tumor surgically or incinerating it with radiation—a choice between the hot ray and the cold knife.

In May 1937, almost exactly a decade before Farber began his experiments with chemicals, *Fortune* magazine published what it called a "panoramic survey" of cancer medicine. The report was far from comforting: "The startling fact is that no new *principle* of treatment, whether for cure or prevention, has been introduced. . . . The *methods* of treatment have become more efficient and more humane. Crude surgery without anesthesia or asepsis has been replaced by modern painless surgery with its exquisite technical refinement. Biting caustics that ate into the flesh of past generations of cancer patients have been obsolesced by radiation with X-ray and radium. . . . But the fact remains that the cancer 'cure' still includes only two principles—the removal and destruction of diseased tissue [the former by surgery; the latter by X-rays]. No other means have been proved."

The *Fortune* article was titled "Cancer: The Great Darkness," and the "darkness," the authors suggested, was as much political as medical. Cancer medicine was stuck in a rut not only because of the depth of medical mysteries that surrounded it, but because of the systematic neglect of cancer research: "There are not over two dozen funds in the U.S. devoted to fundamental cancer research. They range in capital from about $500 up to about $2,000,000, but their aggregate capitalization is certainly not much more than $5,000,000. . . . The public willingly spends a third of that sum in an afternoon to watch a major football game."

This stagnation of research funds stood in stark contrast to the swift rise to prominence of the disease itself. Cancer had certainly been present and noticeable in nineteenth-century America, but it had largely lurked in the shadow of vastly more common illnesses. In 1899, when Roswell Park, a well-known Buffalo surgeon, had argued that cancer would some-day overtake smallpox, typhoid fever, and tuberculosis to become the leading cause of death in the nation, his remarks had been perceived as a rather "startling prophecy," the hyperbolic speculations of a man who, after all, spent his days and nights operating on cancer. But by the end of the decade, Park's remarks were becoming less and less startling, and more and more prophetic by the day. Typhoid, aside from a few scattered outbreaks, was becoming increasingly rare. Smallpox was on the decline; by 1949, it would disappear from America altogether. Meanwhile cancer was already outgrowing other diseases, ratcheting its way up the ladder of killers. Between 1900 and 1916, cancer-related mortality grew by 29.8 percent, edging out tuberculosis as a cause of death. By 1926, cancer had become the nation's second most common killer, just behind heart disease.

"Cancer: The Great Darkness" wasn't alone in building a case for a coor-dinated national response to cancer. In May that year, *Life* carried its own dispatch on cancer research, which conveyed the same sense of urgency. The *New York Times* published two reports on rising cancer rates, in April and June. When cancer appeared in the pages of *Time* in July 1937, inter-est in what was called the "cancer problem" was like a fierce contagion in the media.

∂∫∂

Proposals to mount a systematic national response against cancer had risen and ebbed rhythmically in America since the early 1900s. In 1907, a group of cancer surgeons had congregated at the New Willard Hotel in Washington to create an organization to lobby Congress for more funds for cancer research. By 1910, this organization, the American Association for Cancer Research, had convinced President Taft to propose to Congress a national laboratory dedicated to cancer research. But despite initial interest in the plan, the efforts had stalled in Washington after a few fitful attempts, largely because of a lack of political support.

In the late 1920s, a decade after Taft's proposal had been tabled, cancer research found a new and unexpected champion—Matthew Neely, a dogged and ebullient former lawyer from Fairmont, West Virginia, serving his first term in the Senate. Although Neely had relatively little experience in the politics of science, he had noted the marked increase in cancer mortality in the previous decade—from 70,000 men and women in 1911 to 115,000 in 1927. Neely asked Congress to advertise a reward of $5 million for any "information leading to the arrest of human cancer."

It was a lowbrow strategy—the scientific equivalent of hanging a mug shot in a sheriff's office—and it generated a reflexively lowbrow response. Within a few weeks, Neely's office in Washington was flooded with thousands of letters from quacks and faith healers purporting every conceivable remedy for cancer: rubs, tonics, ointments, anointed handkerchiefs, salves, and blessed water. Congress, exasperated with the response, finally authorized $50,000 for Neely's Cancer Control Bill, almost comically cutting its budget back to just 1 percent of the requested amount.

In 1937, the indefatigable Neely, reelected to the Senate, launched yet another effort to launch a national attack on cancer, this time jointly with Senator Homer Bone and Representative Warren Magnuson. By now, cancer had considerably magnified in the public eye. The *Fortune* and *Time* articles had fanned anxiety and discontent, and politicians were eager to demonstrate a concrete response. In June, a joint Senate-House conference was held to craft legislation to address the issue. After initial hearings, the bill raced through Congress and was passed unanimously by a joint session on July 23, 1937. Two weeks later, on August 5, President Roosevelt signed the National Cancer Institute Act.

The act created a new scientific unit called the National Cancer Institute (NCI), designed to coordinate cancer research and education.* An advisory council of scientists for the institute was assembled from universities and hospitals. A state-of-the-art laboratory space, with gleaming halls and conference rooms, was built among leafy arcades and gardens in suburban

---

* In 1944, the NCI would become a subsidiary component of the National Institutes of Health (NIH). This foreshadowed the creation of other disease-focused institutes over the next decades.

Bethesda, a few miles from the nation's capital. "The nation is marshaling its forces to conquer cancer, the greatest scourge that has ever assailed the human race," Senator Bone announced reassuringly while breaking ground for the building on October 3, 1938. After nearly two decades of largely fruitless efforts, a coordinated national response to cancer seemed to be on its way at last.

All of this was a bold, brave step in the right direction—except for its timing. By the early winter of 1938, just months after the inauguration of the NCI campus in Bethesda, the battle against cancer was overshadowed by the tremors of a different kind of war. In November, Nazi troops embarked on a nationwide pogrom against Jews in Germany, forcing thousands into concentration camps. By late winter, military conflicts had broken out all over Asia and Europe, setting the stage for World War II. By 1939, those skirmishes had fully ignited, and in December 1941, America was drawn inextricably into the global conflagration.

The war necessitated a dramatic reordering of priorities. The U.S. Marine Hospital in Baltimore, which the NCI had once hoped to convert into a clinical cancer center, was now swiftly reconfigured into a war hospital. Scientific research funding stagnated and was shunted into projects directly relevant to the war. Scientists, lobbyists, physicians, and surgeons fell off the public radar screen—"mostly silent," as one researcher recalled, "their contributions usually summarized in obituaries."

An obituary might as well have been written for the National Cancer Institute. Congress's promised funds for a "programmatic response to cancer" never materialized, and the NCI languished in neglect. Outfitted with every modern facility imaginable in the 1940s, the institute's sparkling campus turned into a scientific ghost town. One scientist jokingly called it "a nice quiet place out here in the country. In those days," the author continued, "it was pleasant to drowse under the large, sunny windows."*

The social outcry about cancer also drifted into silence. After the brief flurry of attention in the press, cancer again became the great unmentionable, the whispered-about disease that no one spoke about publicly. In the early 1950s, Fanny Rosenow, a breast cancer survivor and cancer advocate, called the *New York Times* to post an advertisement for a support group for women with breast cancer. Rosenow was put through, puzzlingly, to

---

*In 1946–47, Neely and Senator Claude Pepper launched a third national cancer bill. This was defeated in Congress by a small margin in 1947.

the society editor of the newspaper. When she asked about placing her announcement, a long pause followed. "I'm sorry, Ms. Rosenow, but the *Times* cannot publish the word *breast* or the word *cancer* in its pages.

"Perhaps," the editor continued, "you could say there will be a meeting about diseases of the chest wall."

Rosenow hung up, disgusted.

ℐℐℐ

When Farber entered the world of cancer in 1947, the public outcry of the past decade had dissipated. Cancer had again become a politically silent illness. In the airy wards of the Children's Hospital, doctors and patients fought their private battles against cancer. In the tunnels downstairs, Farber fought an even more private battle with his chemicals and experiments.

This isolation was key to Farber's early success. Insulated from the spotlights of public scrutiny, he worked on a small, obscure piece of the puzzle. Leukemia was an orphan disease, abandoned by internists, who had no drugs to offer for it, and by surgeons, who could not possibly operate on blood. "Leukemia," as one physician put it, "in some senses, had not [even] been cancer before World War II." The illness lived on the borderlands of illnesses, a pariah lurking between disciplines and departments—not unlike Farber himself.

If leukemia "belonged" anywhere, it was within hematology, the study of normal blood. If a cure for it was to be found, Farber reasoned, it would be found by studying blood. If he could uncover how *normal* blood cells were generated, he might stumble backward into a way to block the growth of abnormal leukemic cells. His strategy, then, was to approach the disease from the normal to the abnormal—to confront cancer in reverse.

Much of what Farber knew about normal blood he had learned from George Minot. A thin, balding aristocrat with pale, intense eyes, Minot ran a laboratory in a colonnaded, brick-and-stone structure off Harrison Avenue in Boston, just a few miles down the road from the sprawling hospital complex on Longwood Avenue that included Children's Hospital. Like many hematologists at Harvard, Farber had trained briefly with Minot in the 1920s before joining the staff at Children's.

Every decade has a unique hematological riddle, and for Minot's era, that riddle was pernicious anemia. Anemia is the deficiency of red blood cells—and its most common form arises from a lack of iron, a crucial nutrient used to build red blood cells. But pernicious anemia, the rare variant that Minot studied, was not caused by iron deficiency (indeed, its name derives from its intransigence to the standard treatment of anemia with iron). By feeding patients increasingly macabre concoctions—half a pound of chicken liver, half-cooked hamburgers, raw hog stomach, and even once the regurgitated gastric juices of one of his students (spiced up with butter, lemon, and parsley)—Minot and his team of researchers conclusively demonstrated in 1926 that pernicious anemia was caused by the lack of a critical micronutrient, a single molecule later identified as vitamin B_{12}. In 1934, Minot and two of his colleagues won the Nobel Prize for this pathbreaking work. Minot had shown that replacing a single molecule could restore the normalcy of blood in this complex hematological disease. Blood was an organ whose activity could be turned on and off by molecular switches.

There was another form of nutritional anemia that Minot's group had not tackled, an anemia just as "pernicious"—although in the moral sense of that word. Eight thousand miles away, in the cloth mills of Bombay (owned by English traders and managed by their cutthroat local middlemen), wages had been driven to such low levels that the mill workers lived in abject poverty, malnourished and without medical care. When English physicians tested these mill workers in the 1920s to study the effects of this chronic malnutrition, they discovered that many of them, particularly women after childbirth, were severely anemic. (This was yet another colonial fascination: to create the conditions of misery in a population, then subject it to social or medical experimentation.)

In 1928, a young English physician named Lucy Wills, freshly out of the London School of Medicine for Women, traveled on a grant to Bombay to study this anemia. Wills was an exotic among hematologists, an adventurous woman driven by a powerful curiosity about blood willing to travel to a faraway country to solve a mysterious anemia on a whim. She knew of Minot's work. But unlike Minot's anemia, she found that the anemia in Bombay couldn't be reversed by Minot's concoctions or by vitamin B_{12}. Astonishingly, she found she could cure it with Marmite, the dark, yeasty spread then popular among health fanatics in England and Australia. Wills could not determine the key chemical nutrient of Marmite. She called it the Wills factor.

Wills factor turned out to be folic acid, or folate, a vitamin-like substance found in fruits and vegetables (and amply in Marmite). When cells divide, they need to make copies of DNA—the chemical that carries all the genetic information in a cell. Folic acid is a crucial building block for

DNA and is thus vital for cell division. Since blood cells are produced by arguably the most fearsome rate of cell division in the human body—more than 300 billion cells a day—the genesis of blood is particularly dependent on folic acid. In its absence (in men and women starved of vegetables, as in Bombay) the production of new blood cells in the bone marrow halts. Millions of half-matured cells spew out, piling up like half-finished goods bottlenecked in an assembly line. The bone marrow becomes a dysfunctional mill, a malnourished biological factory oddly reminiscent of the cloth factories of Bombay.

∂∫∂

These links—between vitamins, bone marrow, and normal blood—kept Farber preoccupied in the early summer of 1946. In fact, his first clinical experiment, inspired by this very connection, turned into a horrific mistake. Lucy Wills had observed that folic acid, if administered to nutrient-deprived patients, could restore the normal genesis of blood. Farber wondered whether administering folic acid to children with leukemia might also restore normalcy to their blood. Following that tenuous trail, he obtained some synthetic folic acid, recruited a cohort of leukemic children, and started injecting folic acid into them.

In the months that passed, Farber found that folic acid, far from stopping the progression of leukemia, actually accelerated it. In one patient, the white cell count nearly doubled. In another, the leukemia cells exploded into the bloodstream and sent fingerlings of malignant cells to infiltrate the skin. Farber stopped the experiment in a hurry. He called this phenomenon acceleration, evoking some dangerous object in free fall careering toward its end.

Pediatricians at Children's Hospital were furious about Farber's trial. The folate analogues had not just accelerated the leukemia; they had likely hastened the death of the children. But Farber was intrigued. If folic acid accelerated the leukemia cells in children, what if he could cut off its supply with some other drug—an *anti*folate? Could a chemical that blocked the growth of white blood cells stop leukemia?

The observations of Minot and Wills began to fit into a foggy picture. If the bone marrow was a busy cellular factory to begin with, then a marrow occupied with leukemia was that factory in overdrive, a deranged manufacturing unit for cancer cells. Minot and Wills had turned the production lines of the bone marrow *on* by adding nutrients to the body. But could the malignant marrow be shut *off* by choking the supply of nutrients? Could the anemia of the mill workers in Bombay be re-created therapeutically in the medical units of Boston?

In his long walks from his laboratory under Children's Hospital to his house on Amory Street in Brookline, Farber wondered relentlessly about such a drug. Dinner, in the dark-wood-paneled rooms of the house, was usually a sparse, perfunctory affair. His wife, Norma, a musician and writer, talked about the opera and poetry; Sidney, of autopsies, trials, and patients. As he walked back to the hospital at night, Norma's piano tinkling practice scales in his wake, the prospect of an anticancer chemical haunted him. He imagined it palpably, visibly, with a fanatic's enthusiasm. But he didn't know what it was or what to call it. The word *chemotherapy*, in the sense we understand it today, had never been used for anticancer medicines.* The elaborate armamentarium of "antivitamins" that Farber had dreamed up so vividly in his fantasies did not exist.

⚬⚬

Farber's supply of folic acid for his disastrous first trial had come from the laboratory of an old friend, a chemist, Yellapragada Subbarao (SubbaRow)—or Yella, as most of his colleagues called him. Yella was a pioneer in many ways, a physician turned cellular physiologist, a chemist who had accidentally wandered into biology. His scientific meanderings had been presaged by more desperate and adventuresome physical meanderings. He had arrived in Boston in 1923, penniless and unprepared, having finished his medical training in India and secured a scholarship for a diploma at the School of Tropical Health at Harvard. The weather in Boston, Yella discovered, was far from tropical. Unable to find a medical job in the frigid, stormy winter (he had no license to practice medicine in the United States), he started as a night porter at the Brigham and Women's Hospital, opening doors, changing sheets, and cleaning urinals.

The proximity to medicine paid off. Subbarao made friends and connections at the hospital and switched to a day job as a researcher in the Division of Biochemistry. His initial project involved purifying molecules out of living cells, dissecting them chemically to determine their compositions—in

---

*In New York in the 1910s, William B. Coley, James Ewing, and Ernest Codman had treated bone sarcomas with a mixture of bacterial toxins—the so-called Coley's toxin. Coley had observed occasional responses, but the unpredictable responses, likely caused by immune stimulation, never fully captured the attention of oncologists or surgeons.

essence, performing a biochemical "autopsy" on cells. The approach required more persistence than imagination, but it produced remarkable dividends. Subbarao purified a molecule called ATP, the source of energy in all living beings (ATP carries chemical "energy" in the cell), and another molecule called creatine, the energy carrier in muscle cells. Any one of these achievements should have been enough to guarantee him a professorship at Harvard. But Subbarao was a foreigner, a reclusive, nocturnal, heavily accented vegetarian who lived in a one-room apartment downtown, befriended only by other nocturnal recluses such as Farber. In 1940, denied tenure and recognition, Yella huffed off to join Lederle Labs, a pharmaceutical laboratory in upstate New York, owned by the American Cyanamid Corporation, where he had been asked to run a group on chemical synthesis.

At Lederle, Yella Subbarao quickly reformulated his old strategy and focused on making synthetic versions of the natural chemicals that he had found within cells, hoping to use them as nutritional supplements. In the 1920s, another drug company, Eli Lilly, had made a fortune selling a concentrated form of vitamin B_{12}, the missing nutrient in pernicious anemia. Subbarao decided to focus his attention on the other anemia, the neglected anemia of folate deficiency. But in 1946, after many failed attempts to extract the chemical from pigs' livers, he switched tactics and started to synthesize folic acid from scratch, with the help of a team of scientists.

The chemical reactions to make folic acid brought a serendipitous bonus. Since the reactions had several intermediate steps, Subbarao's team* could create variants of folic acid through slight alterations in the recipe. These variants of folic acid—closely related molecular mimics—possessed counterintuitive properties. Enzymes and receptors in cells typically work by recognizing molecules using their chemical structure. But a "decoy" molecular structure—one that nearly mimics the natural molecule—can bind to the receptor or enzyme and block its action, like a false key jamming a lock. Some of Yella's molecular mimics could thus behave like *antagonists* to folic acid.

These were precisely the antivitamins that Farber had been fantasizing about. Farber wrote to Subbarao asking him if he could use their folate antagonists on patients with leukemia. Subbarao consented. In the late summer of 1947, the first package of antifolate left Lederle's labs in New York and arrived in Farber's laboratory.

---

* D. R. Seeger and B. Hutchings were other key members of the team.

Farber's Gauntlet

Throughout the centuries the sufferer from this disease has been the subject of almost every conceivable form of experimentation. The fields and forests, the apothecary shop and the temple, have been ransacked for some successful means of relief from this intractable malady. Hardly any animal has escaped making its contribution, in hair or hide, tooth or toenail, thymus or thyroid, liver or spleen, in the vain search by man for a means of relief.
> —William Bainbridge

The search for a way to eradicate this scourge . . . is left to incidental dabbling and uncoordinated research.
> —The Washington Post, 1946

Seven miles south of the Longwood hospitals in Boston, the town of Dorchester is a typical sprawling New England suburb, a triangle wedged between the sooty industrial settlements to the west and the gray-green bays of the Atlantic to its east. In the late 1940s, waves of Jewish and Irish immigrants—shipbuilders, iron casters, railway engineers, fishermen, and factory workers—settled in Dorchester, occupying rows of brick-and-clapboard houses that snaked their way up Blue Hill Avenue. Dorchester reinvented itself as the quintessential suburban family town, with parks and playgrounds along the river, a golf course, a church, and a synagogue. On Sunday afternoons, families converged at Franklin Park to walk through its leafy pathways or to watch ostriches, polar bears, and tigers at its zoo.

On August 16, 1947, in a house across from the zoo, the child of a ship worker in the Boston yards fell mysteriously ill with a low-grade fever that waxed and waned over two weeks without pattern, followed by increasing lethargy and pallor. Robert Sandler was two years old. His twin, Elliott, was an active, cherubic toddler in perfect health.

Ten days after his first fever, Robert's condition worsened significantly. His temperature climbed higher. His complexion turned from rosy to a spectral milky white. He was brought to Children's Hospital in Boston. His spleen, a fist-size organ that stores and makes blood (usually barely palpable underneath the rib cage), was visibly enlarged, heaving down like an overfilled bag. A drop of blood under Farber's microscope revealed the identity of his illness; thousands of immature lymphoid leukemic blasts were dividing in a frenzy, their chromosomes condensing and uncondensing, like tiny clenched and unclenched fists.

Sandler arrived at Children's Hospital just a few weeks after Farber had received his first package from Lederle. On September 6, 1947, Farber began to inject Sandler with pteroylaspartic acid or PAA, the first of Lederle's antifolates. (Consent to run a clinical trial for a drug—even a toxic drug—was not typically required. Parents were occasionally cursorily informed about the trial; children were almost never informed or consulted. The Nuremberg code for human experimentation, requiring explicit voluntary consent from patients, was drafted on August 9, 1947, less than a month before the PAA trial. It is doubtful that Farber in Boston had even heard of any such required consent code.)

PAA had little effect. Over the next month Sandler turned increasingly lethargic. He developed a limp, the result of leukemia pressing down on his spinal cord. Joint aches appeared, and violent, migrating pains. Then the leukemia burst through one of the bones in his thigh, causing a fracture and unleashing a blindingly intense, indescribable pain. By December, the case seemed hopeless. The tip of Sandler's spleen, more dense than ever with leukemia cells, dropped down to his pelvis. He was withdrawn, listless, swollen, and pale, on the verge of death.

On December 28, however, Farber received a new version of antifolate from Subbarao and Kiltie, aminopterin, a chemical with a small change from the structure of PAA. Farber snatched the drug as soon as it arrived and began to inject the boy with it, hoping, at best, for a minor reprieve in his cancer.

The response was marked. The white cell count, which had been climbing astronomically—ten thousand in September, twenty thousand in November, and nearly seventy thousand in December—suddenly stopped rising and hovered at a plateau. Then, even more remarkably, the count actually started to drop, the leukemic blasts gradually flickering out in the blood and then all but disappearing. By New Year's Eve, the count had dropped to nearly one-sixth of its peak value, bottoming out at a nearly normal level. The cancer hadn't vanished—under the microscope, there were still malignant white cells—but it had temporarily abated, frozen into a hematologic stalemate in the frozen Boston winter.

On January 13, 1948, Sandler returned to the clinic, walking on his own for the first time in two months. His spleen and liver had shrunk so dramatically that his clothes, Farber noted, had become "loose around the abdomen." His bleeding had stopped. His appetite turned ravenous, as if he were trying to catch up on six months of lost meals. By February, Farber noted, the child's alertness, nutrition, and activity were equal to his twin's. For a brief month or so, Robert Sandler and Elliott Sandler seemed identical again.

◈

Sandler's remission—unprecedented in the history of leukemia—set off a flurry of activity for Farber. By the early winter of 1948, more children were at his clinic: a three-year-old boy brought with a sore throat, a two-and-a-half-year-old girl with lumps in her head and neck, all eventually diagnosed with childhood ALL. Deluged with antifolates from Yella and with patients who desperately needed them, Farber recruited additional doctors to help him: a hematologist named Louis Diamond, and a group of assistants, James Wolff, Robert Mercer, and Robert Sylvester.

Farber had infuriated the authorities at Children's Hospital with his first clinical trial. With this, the second, he pushed them over the edge. The hospital staff voted to take all the pediatric interns off the leukemia chemotherapy unit (the atmosphere in the leukemia wards, it was felt, was far too desperate and experimental and thus not conducive to medical education)—in essence, leaving Farber and his assistants to perform all the patient care themselves. Children with cancer, as one surgeon noted, were typically "tucked in the farthest recesses of the hospital wards." They were on their deathbeds anyway, the pediatricians argued; wouldn't it be kinder and gentler, some insisted, to just "let them die in peace"? When one clinician suggested that Farber's novel "chemicals" be reserved only as a last resort for leukemic children, Farber, recalling his prior life as a pathologist, shot back, "By that time, the only chemical that you will need will be embalming fluid."

Farber outfitted a back room of a ward near the bathrooms into a makeshift clinic. His small staff was housed in various unused spaces in the Department of Pathology—in back rooms, stairwell shafts, and empty offices. Institutional support was minimal. Farber's assistants sharpened their own bone marrow needles, a practice as antiquated as a surgeon whetting his knives on a wheel. Farber's staff tracked the disease in patients with meticulous attention to detail: every blood count, every transfusion, every fever, was to be recorded. If leukemia was going to be beaten, Farber wanted every minute of that battle recorded for posterity—even if no one else was willing to watch it happen.

∽

That winter of 1948, a severe and dismal chill descended on Boston. Snowstorms broke out, bringing Farber's clinic to a standstill. The narrow asphalt road out to Longwood Avenue was piled with heaps of muddy sleet, and the basement tunnels, poorly heated even in the fall, were now freezing. Daily injections of antifolates became impossible, and Farber's team backed down to three times a week. In February, when the storms abated, the daily injections started again.

Meanwhile, news of Farber's experience with childhood leukemia was beginning to spread, and a slow train of children began to arrive at his clinic. And case by case, an incredible pattern emerged: the antifolates could drive leukemia cell counts down, occasionally even resulting in their complete disappearance—at least for a while. There were other remissions as dramatic as Sandler's. Two boys treated with aminopterin returned to school. Another child, a two-and-a-half-year-old girl, started to "play and run about" after seven months of lying in bed. The normalcy of blood almost restored a flickering, momentary normalcy to the childhood.

But there was always the same catch. After a few months of remission, the cancer would inevitably relapse, ultimately flinging aside even the most potent of Yella's drugs. The cells would return in the bone marrow, then burst out into the blood, and even the most active antifolates would not keep their growth down. Robert Sandler died in 1948, having responded for a few months.

Yet the remissions, even if temporary, were still genuine remissions—and historic. By April 1948, there was just enough data to put together a preliminary paper for the *New England Journal of Medicine*. The team had treated sixteen patients. Of the sixteen, ten had responded. And five children—about one-third of the initial group—remained alive four or even six months after their diagnosis. In leukemia, six months of survival was an eternity.

⳹⳹

Farber's paper, published on June 3, 1948, was seven pages long, jam-packed with tables, figures, microscope photographs, laboratory values, and blood counts. Its language was starched, formal, detached, and scientific. Yet, like all great medical papers, it was a page-turner. And like all good novels, it was timeless: to read it today is to be pitched behind the scenes into the tumultuous life of the Boston clinic, its patients hanging on for life as Farber and his assistants scrambled to find new drugs for a dreadful disease that kept flickering away and returning. It was a plot with a beginning, a middle, and, unfortunately, an end.

The paper was received, as one scientist recalls, "with skepticism, disbelief, and outrage." But for Farber, the study carried a tantalizing message: cancer, even in its most aggressive form, had been treated with a medicine, a chemical. In six months between 1947 and 1948, Farber thus saw a door open—briefly, seductively—then close tightly shut again. And through that doorway, he glimpsed an incandescent possibility. The disappearance of an aggressive systemic cancer via a chemical drug was virtually unprecedented in the history of cancer. In the summer of 1948, when one of Farber's assistants performed a bone marrow biopsy on a leukemic child after treatment with aminopterin, the assistant could not believe the results. "The bone marrow looked so normal," he wrote, "that one could dream of a cure."

And so Farber did dream. He dreamed of malignant cells being killed by specific anticancer drugs, and of normal cells regenerating and reclaiming their physiological spaces; of a whole gamut of such systemic antagonists to decimate malignant cells; of curing leukemia with chemicals, then applying his experience with chemicals and leukemia to more common cancers. He was throwing down a gauntlet for cancer medicine. It was then up to an entire generation of doctors and scientists to pick it up.

A Private Plague

We tend to think of cancer as a "modern" illness because its metaphors are so modern. It is a disease of overproduction, of fulminant growth—growth unstoppable, growth tipped into the abyss of no control. Modern biology encourages us to imagine the cell as a molecular machine. Cancer is that machine unable to quench its initial command (to grow) and thus transformed into an indestructible, self-propelled automaton.

The notion of cancer as an affliction that belongs paradigmatically to the twentieth century is reminiscent, as Susan Sontag argued so powerfully in her book *Illness as Metaphor,* of another disease once considered emblematic of another era: tuberculosis in the nineteenth century. Both diseases, as Sontag pointedly noted, were similarly "obscene—in the original meaning of that word: ill-omened, abominable, repugnant to the senses." Both drain vitality; both stretch out the encounter with death; in both cases, *dying*, even more than death, defines the illness.

But despite such parallels, tuberculosis belongs to another century. TB (or consumption) was Victorian romanticism brought to its pathological extreme—febrile, unrelenting, breathless, and obsessive. It was a disease of poets: John Keats involuting silently toward death in a small room overlooking the Spanish Steps in Rome, or Byron, an obsessive romantic, who fantasized about dying of the disease to impress his mistresses. "Death and disease are often beautiful, like . . . the hectic glow of consumption," Thoreau wrote in 1852. In Thomas Mann's *The Magic Mountain*, this "hectic glow" releases a feverish creative force in its victims—a clarifying, edifying, cathartic force that, too, appears to be charged with the essence of its era.

Cancer, in contrast, is riddled with more contemporary images. The cancer cell is a desperate individualist, "in every possible sense, a nonconformist," as the surgeon-writer Sherwin Nuland wrote. The word *metastasis*, used to describe the migration of cancer from one site to another, is a curious mix of *meta* and *stasis*—"beyond stillness" in Latin—an unmoored, partially unstable state that captures the peculiar instability of modernity. If consumption once killed its victims by pathological evisceration (the tuberculosis bacillus gradually hollows out the lung), then cancer asphyxiates us by filling bodies with too many cells; it is consumption in its alternate meaning—the pathology of excess. Cancer is an expansionist disease; it invades through tissues, sets up colonies in hostile landscapes, seeking "sanctuary" in one organ and then immigrating to another. It lives desperately, inventively, fiercely, territorially, cannily, and defensively—at times, as if teaching *us* how to survive. To confront cancer is to encounter a parallel species, one perhaps more adapted to survival than even we are.

This image—of cancer as our desperate, malevolent, contemporary doppelgänger—is so haunting because it is at least partly true. A cancer cell is an astonishing perversion of the normal cell. Cancer is a phenomenally successful invader and colonizer in part because it exploits the very features that make *us* successful as a species or as an organism.

Like the normal cell, the cancer cell relies on growth in the most basic, elemental sense: the division of one cell to form two. In normal tissues, this process is exquisitely regulated, such that growth is stimulated by specific signals and arrested by other signals. In cancer, unbridled growth gives rise to generation upon generation of cells. Biologists use the term *clone* to describe cells that share a common genetic ancestor. Cancer, we now know, is a clonal disease. Nearly every known cancer originates from one ancestral cell that, having acquired the capacity of limitless cell division and survival, gives rise to limitless numbers of descendants—Virchow's *omnis cellula e cellula e cellula* repeated ad infinitum.

But cancer is not simply a clonal disease; it is a clonally *evolving* disease. If growth occurred without evolution, cancer cells would not be imbued with their potent capacity to invade, survive, and metastasize. Every generation of cancer cells creates a small number of cells that is genetically different from its parents. When a chemotherapeutic drug or the immune system attacks cancer, mutant clones that can resist the attack grow out. The fittest cancer cell survives. This mirthless, relentless cycle of mutation, selection, and overgrowth generates cells that are more and more adapted to survival and growth. In some cases, the mutations speed up the acquisition of other mutations. The genetic instability, like a perfect madness, only provides more impetus to generate mutant clones. Cancer thus exploits the fundamental logic of evolution unlike any other illness. If we, as a species, are the ultimate product of Darwinian selection, then so, too, is this incredible disease that lurks inside us.

Such metaphorical seductions can carry us away, but they are unavoidable with a subject like cancer. In writing this book, I started off by imagining my project as a "history" of cancer. But it felt, inescapably, as if I were writing not about some*thing* but about some*one*. My subject daily morphed into something that resembled an individual—an enigmatic, if somewhat deranged, image in a mirror. This was not so much a medical history of an illness, but something more personal, more visceral: its biography.

❦

So to begin again, for every biographer must confront the birth of his subject: Where was cancer "born"? How old is cancer? Who was the first to record it as an illness?

In 1862, Edwin Smith—an unusual character: part scholar and part huckster, an antique forger and self-made Egyptologist—bought (or, some say, stole) a fifteen-foot-long papyrus from an antiques seller in Luxor in Egypt. The papyrus was in dreadful condition, with crumbling, yellow pages filled with cursive Egyptian script. It is now thought to have been written in the seventeenth century BC, a transcription of a manuscript dating back to 2500 BC. The copier—a plagiarist in a terrible hurry—had made errors as he had scribbled, often noting corrections in red ink in the margins.

Translated in 1930, the papyrus is now thought to contain the collected teachings of Imhotep, a great Egyptian physician who lived around 2625 BC. Imhotep, among the few nonroyal Egyptians known to us from the Old Kingdom, was a Renaissance man at the center of a sweeping Egyptian renaissance. As a vizier in the court of King Djozer, he dabbled in neurosurgery, tried his hand at architecture, and made early forays into astrology and astronomy. Even the Greeks, encountering the fierce, hot blast of his intellect as they marched through Egypt centuries later, cast him as an ancient magician and fused him to their own medical god, Asclepius.

But the surprising feature of the Smith papyrus is not magic and religion but the absence of magic and religion. In a world immersed in spells, incantations, and charms, Imhotep wrote about broken bones and dislocated vertebrae with a detached, sterile scientific vocabulary, as if he were writing a modern surgical textbook. The forty-eight cases in the papyrus—fractures of the hand, gaping abscesses of the skin, or shattered skull bones—are treated as medical conditions rather than occult phenomena, each with its own anatomical glossary, diagnosis, summary, and prognosis.

And it is under these clarifying headlamps of an ancient surgeon that cancer first emerges as a distinct disease. Describing case forty-five, Imhotep advises, "If you examine [a case] having bulging masses on [the] breast and you find that they have spread over his breast; if you place your hand upon [the] breast [and] find them to be cool, there being no fever at all therein when your hand feels him; they have no granulations, contain no fluid, give rise to no liquid discharge, yet they feel protuberant to your touch, you should say concerning him: 'This is a case of bulging masses I have to contend with. . . . Bulging tumors of the breast mean the existence of swellings on the breast, large, spreading, and hard; touching them is like touching a ball of wrappings, or they may be compared to the unripe hemat fruit, which is hard and cool to the touch.' "

A "bulging mass in the breast"—cool, hard, dense as a hemat fruit, and spreading insidiously under the skin—could hardly be a more vivid description of breast cancer. Every case in the papyrus was followed by a concise discussion of treatments, even if only palliative: milk poured through the ears of neurosurgical patients, poultices for wounds, balms for burns. But with case forty-five, Imhotep fell atypically silent. Under the section titled "Therapy," he offered only a single sentence: "There is none."

With that admission of impotence, cancer virtually disappeared from ancient medical history. Other diseases cycled violently through the globe, leaving behind their cryptic footprints in legends and documents. A furious plague—typhus, perhaps—blazed through the port city of Avaris in 1715 BC, decimating its population. Smallpox erupted volcanically in pockets, leaving its telltale pockmarks on the face of Ramses V in the twelfth century BC. Tuberculosis rose and ebbed through the Indus valley like its seasonal floods. But if cancer existed in the interstices of these massive epidemics, it existed in silence, leaving no easily identifiable trace in the medical literature—or in any other literature.

∂♪

More than two millennia pass after Imhotep's description until we once more hear of cancer. And again, it is an illness cloaked in silence, a private shame. In his sprawling *Histories,* written around 440 BC, the Greek historian Herodotus records the story of Atossa, the queen of Persia, who was suddenly struck by an unusual illness. Atossa was the daughter of Cyrus, and the wife of Darius, successive Achaemenid emperors of legendary brutality who ruled over a vast stretch of land from Lydia on the Mediterranean Sea to Babylonia on the Persian Gulf. In the middle of her reign, Atossa noticed a bleeding lump in her breast that may have arisen from a particularly malevolent form of breast cancer labeled inflammatory (in inflammatory breast cancer, malignant cells invade the lymph glands of the breast, causing a red, swollen mass).

If Atossa had desired it, an entire retinue of physicians from Babylonia to Greece would have flocked to her bedside to treat her. Instead, she descended into a fierce and impenetrable loneliness. She wrapped herself in sheets, in a self-imposed quarantine. Darius' doctors may have tried to treat her, but to no avail. Ultimately, a Greek slave named Democedes persuaded her to allow him to excise the tumor.

Soon after that operation, Atossa mysteriously vanishes from Herodotus' text. For him, she is merely a minor plot twist. We don't know whether the tumor recurred, or how or when she died, but the procedure was at least a temporary success. Atossa lived, and she had Democedes to thank for it. And that reprieve from pain and illness whipped her into a frenzy of gratitude and territorial ambition. Darius had been planning a campaign against Scythia, on the eastern border of his empire. Goaded by Democedes, who wanted to return to his native Greece, Atossa pleaded with her husband to turn his campaign westward—to invade Greece. That turn of the Persian empire from east to west, and the series of Greco-Persian wars that followed, would mark one of the definitive moments in the early history of the West. It was Atossa's tumor, then, that quietly launched a thousand ships. Cancer, even as a clandestine illness, left its fingerprints on the ancient world.

ॐ

But Herodotus and Imhotep are storytellers, and like all stories, theirs have gaps and inconsistencies. The "cancers" described by them may have been true neoplasms, or perhaps they were hazily describing abscesses, ulcers, warts, or moles. The only incontrovertible cases of cancer in history are those in which the malignant tissue has somehow been preserved. And to encounter one such cancer face-to-face—to actually stare the ancient illness in its eye—one needs to journey to a thousand-year-old gravesite in a remote, sand-swept plain in the southern tip of Peru.

The plain lies at the northern edge of the Atacama Desert, a parched, desolate six-hundred-mile strip caught in the leeward shadow of the giant furl of the Andes that stretches from southern Peru into Chile. Brushed continuously by a warm, desiccating wind, the terrain hasn't seen rain in recorded history. It is hard to imagine that human life once flourished here, but it did. The plain is strewn with hundreds of graves—small, shallow pits dug out of the clay, then lined carefully with rock. Over the centuries, dogs, storms, and grave robbers have dug out these shallow graves, exhuming history.

The graves contain the mummified remains of members of the Chiribaya tribe. The Chiribaya made no effort to preserve their dead, but the climate is almost providentially perfect for mummification. The clay leaches water and fluids out of the body from below, and the wind dries the tissues from above. The bodies, often placed seated, are thus swiftly frozen in time and space.

In 1990, one such large desiccated gravesite containing about 140 bodies caught the attention of Arthur Aufderheide, a professor at the University of Minnesota in Duluth. Aufderheide is a pathologist by training but his specialty is *paleo*pathology, a study of ancient specimens. His autopsies, unlike Farber's, are not performed on recently living patients, but on the mummified remains found on archaeological sites. He stores these human specimens in small, sterile milk containers in a vaultlike chamber in Minnesota. There are nearly five thousand pieces of tissue, scores of biopsies, and hundreds of broken skeletons in his closet.

At the Chiribaya site, Aufderheide rigged up a makeshift dissecting table and performed 140 autopsies over several weeks. One body revealed an extraordinary finding. The mummy was of a young woman in her midthirties, found sitting, with her feet curled up, in a shallow clay grave. When Aufderheide examined her, his fingers found a hard "bulbous mass" in her left upper arm. The papery folds of skin, remarkably preserved, gave way to that mass, which was intact and studded with spicules of bone. This, without question, was a malignant bone tumor, an osteosarcoma, a thousand-year-old cancer preserved inside of a mummy. Aufderheide suspects that the tumor had broken through the skin while she was still alive. Even small osteosarcomas can be unimaginably painful. The woman's pain, he suggests, must have been blindingly intense.

Aufderheide isn't the only paleopathologist to have found cancers in mummified specimens. (Bone tumors, because they form hardened and calcified tissue, are vastly more likely to survive over centuries and are best preserved.) "There are other cancers found in mummies where the malignant tissue has been preserved. The oldest of these is an abdominal cancer from Dakhleh in Egypt from about four hundred AD," he said. In other cases, paleopathologists have not found the actual tumors, but rather signs left by the tumors in the body. Some skeletons were riddled with tiny holes created by cancer in the skull or the shoulder bones, all arising from metastatic skin or breast cancer. In 1914, a team of archaeologists found a two-thousand-year old Egyptian mummy in the Alexandrian catacombs with a tumor invading the pelvic bone. Louis Leakey, the anthropologist who dug up some of the earliest known human skeletons, also discovered a jawbone dating from two million years ago from a nearby site that carried the signs of a peculiar form of lymphoma found endemically in southeastern Africa (although the origin of that tumor was never confirmed pathologically). If that finding does represent an ancient mark of malignancy, then cancer, far from being a "modern" disease, is one of the oldest diseases ever seen in a human specimen—quite possibly *the* oldest.

ॐ

The most striking finding, though, is not that cancer existed in the distant past, but that it was fleetingly rare. When I asked Aufderheide about this, he laughed. "The early history of cancer," he said, "is that there is very little early history of cancer." The Mesopotamians knew their migraines; the Egyptians had a word for seizures. A leprosy-like illness, *tsara'at*, is mentioned in the book of Leviticus. The Hindu Vedas have a medical term for dropsy and a goddess specifically dedicated to smallpox. Tuberculosis was so omnipresent and familiar to the ancients that—as with ice and the Eskimos—distinct words exist for each incarnation of it. But even common cancers, such as breast, lung, and prostate, are conspicuously absent. With a few notable exceptions, in the vast stretch of medical history there is no book or god for cancer.

There are several reasons behind this absence. Cancer is an age-related disease—sometimes exponentially so. The risk of breast cancer, for instance, is about 1 in 400 for a thirty-year-old woman and increases to 1 in 9 for a seventy-year-old. In most ancient societies, people didn't live long enough to get cancer. Men and women were long consumed by tuberculosis, dropsy, cholera, smallpox, leprosy, plague, or pneumonia. If cancer existed, it remained submerged under the sea of other illnesses. Indeed, cancer's emergence in the world is the product of a double negative: it becomes common only when all other killers themselves have been killed. Nineteenth-century doctors often linked cancer to civilization: cancer, they imagined, was caused by the rush and whirl of modern life, which somehow incited pathological growth in the body. The link was correct, but the causality was not: civilization did not cause cancer, but by extending human life spans—civilization *unveiled* it.

Longevity, although certainly the most important contributor to the prevalence of cancer in the early twentieth century, is probably not the only contributor. Our capacity to detect cancer earlier and earlier, and to attribute deaths accurately to it, has also dramatically increased in the last century. The death of a child with leukemia in the 1850s would have been attributed to an abscess or infection (or, as Bennett would have it, to a "suppuration of blood"). And surgery, biopsy, and autopsy techniques have further sharpened our ability to diagnose cancer. The introduction of mammography to detect breast cancer early in its course sharply increased its incidence—a seemingly paradoxical result that makes perfect sense when we realize that the X-rays allow earlier tumors to be diagnosed.

Finally, changes in the structure of modern life have radically shifted the spectrum of cancers—increasing the incidence of some, decreasing the incidence of others. Stomach cancer, for instance, was highly prevalent in certain populations until the late nineteenth century, likely the result of several carcinogens found in pickling reagents and preservatives and exacerbated by endemic and contagious infection with a bacterium that causes stomach cancer. With the introduction of modern refrigeration (and possibly changes in public hygiene that have diminished the rate of endemic infection), the stomach cancer epidemic seems to have abated. In contrast, lung cancer incidence in men increased dramatically in the 1950s as a result of an increase in cigarette smoking during the early twentieth century. In women, a cohort that began to smoke in the 1950s, lung cancer incidence has yet to reach its peak.

The consequence of these demographic and epidemiological shifts was, and is, enormous. In 1900, as Roswell Park noted, tuberculosis was by far the most common cause of death in America. Behind tuberculosis came pneumonia (William Osler, the famous physician from Johns Hopkins University, called it "captain of the men of death"), diarrhea, and gastroenteritis. Cancer still lagged at a distant seventh. By the early 1940s, cancer had ratcheted its way to second on the list, immediately behind heart disease. In that same span, life expectancy among Americans had increased by about twenty-six years. The proportion of persons above sixty years—the age when most cancers begin to strike—nearly doubled.

But the rarity of ancient cancers notwithstanding, it is impossible to forget the tumor growing in the bone of Aufderheide's mummy of a thirty-five-year-old. The woman must have wondered about the insolent gnaw of pain in her bone, and the bulge slowly emerging from her arm. It is hard to look at the tumor and not come away with the feeling that one has encountered a powerful monster in its infancy.

Onkos

Black bile without boiling causes cancers.
—Galen, AD 130

*We have learned nothing, therefore, about the real cause
of cancer or its actual nature. We are where the Greeks
were.*

—Francis Carter Wood in 1914

It's bad bile. It's bad habits. It's bad bosses. It's bad genes.
—Mel Greaves, *Cancer:
The Evolutionary Legacy*, 2000

*In some ways disease does not exist until we have agreed
that it does—by perceiving, naming, and responding to it.*
—C. E. Rosenberg

Even an ancient monster needs a name. To name an illness is to describe a certain condition of suffering—a literary act before it becomes a medical one. A patient, long before he becomes the subject of medical scrutiny, is, at first, simply a storyteller, a narrator of suffering—a traveler who has visited the kingdom of the ill. To relieve an illness, one must begin, then, by unburdening its story.

The names of ancient illnesses are condensed stories in their own right. Typhus, a stormy disease, with erratic, vaporous fevers, arose from the Greek *tuphon,* the father of winds—a word that also gives rise to the modern *typhoon. Influenza* emerged from the Latin *influentia* because medieval doctors imagined that the cyclical epidemics of flu were influenced by stars and planets revolving toward and away from the earth. *Tuberculosis* coagulated out of the Latin *tuber*, referring to the swollen lumps of glands that looked like small vegetables. Lymphatic tuberculosis, TB of the lymph glands, was called *scrofula*, from the Latin word for "piglet," evoking the rather morbid image of a chain of swollen glands arranged in a line like a group of suckling pigs.

It was in the time of Hippocrates, around 400 BC, that a word for cancer first appeared in the medical literature: *karkinos*, from the Greek word for "crab." The tumor, with its clutch of swollen blood vessels around it, reminded Hippocrates of a crab dug in the sand with its legs spread in a circle. The image was peculiar (few cancers truly resemble crabs), but also vivid. Later writers, both doctors and patients, added embellishments. For some, the hardened, matted surface of the tumor was reminiscent of the tough carapace of a crab's body. Others felt a crab moving under the flesh as the disease spread stealthily throughout the body. For yet others, the sudden stab of pain produced by the disease was like being caught in the grip of a crab's pincers.

Another Greek word would intersect with the history of cancer—*onkos*, a word used occasionally to describe tumors, from which the discipline of oncology would take its modern name. *Onkos* was the Greek term for a mass or a load, or more commonly a burden; cancer was imagined as a burden carried by the body. In Greek theater, the same word, *onkos*, would be used to denote a tragic mask that was often "burdened" with an unwieldy conical weight on its head to denote the psychic load carried by its wearer.

But while these vivid metaphors might resonate with our contemporary understanding of cancer, what Hippocrates called *karkinos* and the disease that we now know as cancer were, in fact, vastly different creatures. Hippocrates' *karkinos* were mostly large, superficial tumors that were easily visible to the eye: cancers of the breast, skin, jaw, neck, and tongue. Even the distinction between malignant and nonmalignant tumors likely escaped Hippocrates: his *karkinos* included every conceivable form of swelling—nodes, carbuncles, polyps, protrusions, tubercles, pustules, and glands—lumps lumped indiscriminately into the same category of pathology.

The Greeks had no microscopes. They had never imagined an entity called a cell, let alone seen one, and the idea that *karkinos* was the uncontrolled growth of cells could not possibly have occurred to them. They were, however, preoccupied with fluid mechanics—with waterwheels, pistons, valves, chambers, and sluices—a revolution in hydraulic science originating with irrigation and canal-digging and culminating with Archaemedes discovering his eponymous laws in his bathtub. This preoccupation with hydraulics also flowed into Greek medicine and pathology. To explain illness—all illness—Hippocrates fashioned an elaborate doctrine based on fluids and volumes, which he freely applied to pneumonia, boils, dysentery, and hemorrhoids. The human body, Hippocrates proposed, was composed of four cardinal fluids called humors: blood, black bile, yellow bile, and phlegm. Each of these fluids had a unique color (red, black, yellow, and white), viscosity, and essential character. In the normal body, these four fluids were held in perfect, if somewhat precarious, balance. In illness, this balance was upset by the excess of one fluid.

The physician Claudius Galen, a prolific writer and influential Greek doctor who practiced among the Romans around AD 160, brought Hippocrates' humoral theory to its apogee. Like Hippocrates, Galen set about classifying all illnesses in terms of excesses of various fluids. Inflammation—a red, hot, painful distension—was attributed to an overabundance of blood. Tubercles, pustules, catarrh, and nodules of lymph—all cool, boggy, and white—were excesses of phlegm. Jaundice was the overflow of yellow bile. For cancer, Galen reserved the most malevolent and disquieting of the four humors: black bile. (Only one other disease, replete with metaphors, would be attributed to an excess of this oily, viscous humor: depression. Indeed, *melancholia,* the medieval name for "depression," would draw its name from the Greek *melas,* "black," and *khole,* "bile." Depression and cancer, the psychic and physical diseases of black bile, were thus intrinsically intertwined.) Galen proposed that cancer was "trapped" black bile—static bile unable to escape from a site and thus congealed into a matted mass. "Of blacke cholor [bile], without boyling cometh cancer," Thomas Gale, the English surgeon, wrote of Galen's theory in the sixteenth century, "and if the humor be sharpe, it maketh ulceration, and for this cause, these tumors are more blacker in color."

That short, vivid description would have a profound impact on the future of oncology—much broader than Galen (or Gale) may have intended. Cancer, Galenic theory suggested, was the result of a *systemic* malignant state, an internal overdose of black bile. Tumors were just local outcroppings of a deep-seated bodily dysfunction, an imbalance of physiology that had pervaded the entire corpus. Hippocrates had once abstrusely opined that cancer was "best left untreated, since patients live longer that way." Five centuries later, Galen had explained his teacher's gnomic musings in a fantastical swoop of physiological conjecture. The problem with treating cancer surgically, Galen suggested, was that black bile was everywhere, as inevitable and pervasive as any fluid. You could cut cancer out, but the bile would flow right back, like sap seeping through the limbs of a tree.

Galen died in Rome in 199 AD, but his influence on medicine stretched over the centuries. The black-bile theory of cancer was so metaphorically seductive that it clung on tenaciously in the minds of doctors. The surgical removal of tumors—a local solution to a systemic problem—was thus perceived as a fool's operation. Generations of surgeons layered their own observations on Galen's, solidifying the theory even further. "Do not be led away and offer to operate," John of Arderne wrote in the mid-1300s. "It will only be a disgrace to you." Leonard Bertipaglia, perhaps the most influential surgeon of the fifteenth century, added his own admonishment: "Those who pretend to cure cancer by incising, lifting, and extirpating it only transform a nonulcerous cancer into an ulcerous one. . . . In all my practice, I have never seen a cancer cured by incision, nor known anyone who has."

Unwittingly, Galen may actually have done the future victims of cancer a favor—at least a temporary one. In the absence of anesthesia and antibiotics, most surgical operations performed in the dank chamber of a medieval clinic—or more typically in the back room of a barbershop with a rusty knife and leather straps for restraints—were disastrous, life-threatening affairs. The sixteenth-century surgeon Ambroise Paré described charring tumors with a soldering iron heated on coals, or chemically searing them with a paste of sulfuric acid. Even a small nick in the skin, treated thus, could quickly suppurate into a lethal infection. The tumors would often profusely bleed at the slightest provocation.

Lorenz Heister, an eighteenth-century German physician, once described a mastectomy in his clinic as if it were a sacrificial ritual: "Many females can stand the operation with the greatest courage and without hardly moaning at all. Others, however, make such a clamor that they may dishearten even the most undaunted surgeon and hinder the operation. To perform the operation, the surgeon should be steadfast and not allow himself to become discomforted by the cries of the patient."

Unsurprisingly, rather than take their chances with such "undaunted" surgeons, most patients chose to hang their fates with Galen and try systemic medicines to purge the black bile. The apothecary thus soon filled up with an enormous list of remedies for cancer: tincture of lead, extracts of arsenic, boar's tooth, fox lungs, rasped ivory, hulled castor, ground white-coral, ipecac, senna, and a smattering of purgatives and laxatives. There was alcohol and the tincture of opium for intractable pain. In the seventeenth century, a paste of crab's eyes, at five shillings a pound, was popular—using fire to treat fire. The ointments and salves grew increasingly bizarre by the century: goat's dung, frogs, crow's feet, dog fennel, tortoise liver, the laying of hands, blessed waters, or the compression of the tumor with lead plates.

Despite Galen's advice, an occasional small tumor was still surgically excised. (Even Galen had reportedly performed such surgeries, possibly for cosmetic or palliative reasons.) But the idea of surgical removal of cancer as a curative treatment was entertained only in the most extreme circumstances. When medicines and operations failed, doctors resorted to the only established treatment for cancer, borrowed from Galen's teachings: an intricate series of bleeding and purging rituals to squeeze the humors out of the body, as if it were an overfilled, heavy sponge.

Vanishing Humors

In the winter of 1533, a nineteen-year-old student from Brussels, Andreas Vesalius, arrived at the University of Paris hoping to learn Galenic anatomy and pathology and to start a practice in surgery. To Vesalius's shock and disappointment, the anatomy lessons at the university were in a preposterous state of disarray. The school lacked a specific space for performing dissections. The basement of the Hospital Dieu, where anatomy demonstrations were held, was a theatrically macabre space where instructors hacked their way through decaying cadavers while dogs gnawed on bones and drippings below. "Aside from the eight muscles of the abdomen, badly mangled and in the wrong order, no one had ever shown a muscle to me, nor any bone, much less the succession of nerves, veins, and arteries," Vesalius wrote in a letter. Without a map of human organs to guide them, surgeons were left to hack their way through the body like sailors sent to sea without a map—the blind leading the ill.

Frustrated with these ad hoc dissections, Vesalius decided to create his own anatomical map. He needed his own specimens, and he began to scour the graveyards around Paris for bones and bodies. At Montfaucon, he stumbled upon the massive gibbet of the city of Paris, where the bodies of petty prisoners were often left dangling. A few miles away, at the Cemetery of the Innocents, the skeletons of victims of the Great Plague lay half-exposed in their graves, eroded down to the bone.

The gibbet and the graveyard—the convenience stores for the medieval anatomist—yielded specimen after specimen for Vesalius, and he compulsively raided them, often returning twice a day to cut pieces dangling from the chains and smuggle them off to his dissection chamber. Anatomy came alive for him in this grisly world of the dead. In 1538, collaborating with artists in Titian's studio, Vesalius began to publish his detailed drawings in plates and books—elaborate and delicate etchings charting the courses of arteries and veins, mapping nerves and lymph nodes. In some plates, he pulled away layers of tissue, exposing the delicate surgical planes underneath. In another drawing, he sliced through the brain in deft horizontal sections—a human CT scanner, centuries before its time—to demonstrate the relationship between the cisterns and the ventricles.

Vesalius's anatomical project had started as a purely intellectual exercise but was soon propelled toward a pragmatic need. Galen's humoral theory of disease—that all diseases were pathological accumulations of the four cardinal fluids—required that patients be bled and purged to squeeze the culprit humors out of the body. But for the bleedings to be successful, they had to be performed at specific sites in the body. If the patient was to be bled prophylactically (that is, to *prevent* disease), then the purging was to be performed far away from the possible disease site, so that the humors could be diverted from it. But if the patient was being bled therapeutically—to *cure* an established disease—then the bleeding had to be done from nearby vessels leading *into* the site.

To clarify this already foggy theory, Galen had borrowed an equally foggy Hippocratic expression, κατ' ι'ξιυ—Greek for "straight into"—to describe isolating the vessels that led "straight into" tumors. But Galen's terminology had pitched physicians into further confusion. What on earth, they wondered, had Galen meant by "straight into"? Which vessels led "straight into" a tumor or an organ, and which led the way out? The instructions became a maze of misunderstanding. In the absence of a systematic anatomical map—without the establishment of normality—abnormal anatomy was impossible to fathom.

Vesalius decided to solve the problem by systematically sketching out every blood vessel and nerve in the body, producing an anatomical atlas for surgeons. "In the course of explaining the opinion of the divine Hippocrates and Galen," he wrote in a letter, "I happened to delineate the veins on a chart, thinking that thus I might be able easily to demonstrate what Hippocrates understood by the expression κατ' ι'ξιυ, for you know how much dissension and controversy on venesection was stirred up, even among the learned."

But having started this project, Vesalius found that he could not stop. "My drawing of the veins pleased the professors of medicine and all the students so much that they earnestly sought from me a diagram of the arteries and also one of the nerves. . . . I could not disappoint them." The body was endlessly interconnected: veins ran parallel to nerves, the nerves were connected to the spinal cord, the cord to the brain, and so forth. Anatomy could only be captured in its totality, and soon the project became so gargantuan and complex that it had to be outsourced to yet other illustrators to complete.

But no matter how diligently Vesalius pored through the body, he could not find Galen's black bile. The word *autopsy* comes from the Greek "to see for oneself"; as Vesalius learned to see for himself, he could no longer force Galen's mystical visions to fit his own. The lymphatic system carried a pale, watery fluid; the blood vessels were filled, as expected, with blood. Yellow bile was in the liver. But black bile—Galen's oozing carrier of cancer and depression—could not be found anywhere.

Vesalius now found himself in a strange position. He had emerged from a tradition steeped in Galenic scholarship; he had studied, edited, and republished Galen's books. But black bile—that glistening centerpiece of Galen's physiology—was nowhere to be found. Vesalius hedged about his discovery. Guiltily, he heaped even more praise on the long-dead Galen. But, an empiricist to the core, Vesalius left his drawings just as he saw things, leaving others to draw their own conclusions. There was no black bile. Vesalius had started his anatomical project to save Galen's theory, but, in the end, he quietly buried it.

⁂

In 1793, Matthew Baillie, an anatomist in London, published a textbook called *The Morbid Anatomy of Some of the Most Important Parts of the Human Body*. Baillie's book, written for surgeons and anatomists, was the obverse of Vesalius's project: if Vesalius had mapped out "normal" anatomy, Baillie mapped the body in its diseased, abnormal state. It was Vesalius's study read through an inverted lens. Galen's fantastical speculations about illnesses were even more at stake here. Black bile may not have existed discernably in normal tissue, but tumors should have been chock-full of it. But none was to be found. Baillie described cancers of the lung ("as large as an orange"), stomach ("a fungous appearance"), and the testicles ("a foul deep ulcer") and provided vivid engravings of these tumors. But he could not find the channels of bile anywhere—not even in his orange-size tumors, nor in the deepest cavities of his "foul deep ulcers." If Galen's web of invisible fluids existed, then it existed outside tumors, outside the pathological world, outside the boundaries of normal anatomical inquiry—in short, outside medical science. Like Vesalius, Baillie drew anatomy and cancer the way he actually saw it. At long last, the vivid channels of black bile, the humors in the tumors, that had so gripped the minds of doctors and patients for centuries, vanished from the picture.

"Remote Sympathy"

> *In treating of cancer, we shall remark, that little or*
> *no confidence should be placed either in internal . . .*
> *remedies, and that there is nothing, except the total*
> *separation of the part affected.*
> —*A Dictionary of Practical Surgery*, 1836

Matthew Baillie's *Morbid Anatomy* laid the intellectual foundation for the surgical extractions of tumors. If black bile did not exist, as Baillie had discovered, then removing cancer surgically might indeed rid the body of the disease. But surgery, as a discipline, was not yet ready for such operations. In the 1760s, a Scottish surgeon, John Hunter, Baillie's maternal uncle, had started to remove tumors from his patients in a clinic in London in quiet defiance of Galen's teachings. But Hunter's elaborate studies—initially performed on animals and cadavers in a shadowy menagerie in his own house—were stuck at a critical bottleneck. He could nimbly reach down into the tumors and, if they were "movable" (as he called superficial cancers), pull them out without disturbing the tender architecture of tissues underneath. "If a tumor is not only movable but the part naturally so," Hunter wrote, "they may be safely removed also. But it requires great caution to know if any of these consequent tumors are within proper reach, for we are apt to be deceived."

That last sentence was crucial. Albeit crudely, Hunter had begun to classify tumors into "stages." *Movable* tumors were typically early-stage, local cancers. *Immovable* tumors were advanced, invasive, and even metastatic. Hunter concluded that only movable cancers were worth removing surgically. For more advanced forms of cancer, he advised an honest, if chilling, remedy reminiscent of Imhotep's: "remote sympathy."*

---

*Hunter used this term both to describe metastatic—remotely disseminated—cancer and to argue that therapy was useless.

Hunter was an immaculate anatomist, but his surgical mind was far ahead of his hand. A reckless and restless man with nearly maniacal energy who slept only four hours a night, Hunter had practiced his surgical skills endlessly on cadavers from every nook of the animal kingdom—on monkeys, sharks, walruses, pheasants, bears, and ducks. But with live human patients, he found himself at a standstill. Even if he worked at breakneck speed, having drugged his patient with alcohol and opium to near oblivion, the leap from cool, bloodless corpses to live patients was fraught with danger. As if the pain *during* surgery were not bad enough, the threat of infections *after* surgery loomed. Those who survived the terrifying crucible of the operating table often died even more miserable deaths in their own beds soon afterward.

ॐ

In the brief span between 1846 and 1867, two discoveries swept away these two quandaries that had haunted surgery, thus allowing cancer surgeons to revisit the bold procedures that Hunter had tried to perfect in London.

The first of these discoveries, anesthesia, was publicly demonstrated in 1846 in a packed surgical amphitheater at Massachusetts General Hospital, less than ten miles from where Sidney Farber's basement laboratory would be located a century later. At about ten o'clock on the morning of October 16, a group of doctors gathered in a pitlike room at the center of the hospital. A Boston dentist, William Morton, unveiled a small glass vaporizer, containing about a quart of ether, fitted with an inhaler. He opened the nozzle and asked the patient, Edward Abbott, a printer, to take a few whiffs of the vapor. As Abbott lolled into a deep sleep, a surgeon stepped into the center of the amphitheater and, with a few brisk strokes, deftly made a small incision in Abbott's neck and closed a swollen, malformed blood vessel (referred to as a "tumor," conflating malignant and benign swellings) with a quick stitch. When Abbott awoke a few minutes later, he said, "I did not experience pain at any time, though I knew that the operation was proceeding."

Anesthesia—the dissociation of pain from surgery—allowed surgeons to perform prolonged operations, often lasting several hours. But the hurdle of postsurgical infection remained. Until the mid-nineteenth century, such infections were common and lethal, but their cause remained a mystery. "It must be some subtle principle contained [in the wound]," one surgeon concluded in 1819, "which eludes the sight."

In 1865, a Scottish surgeon named Joseph Lister made an unusual conjecture on how to neutralize that "subtle principle" lurking elusively in the wound. Lister began with an old clinical observation: wounds left open to the air would quickly turn gangrenous, while closed wounds would often remain clean and uninfected. In the postsurgical wards of the Glasgow infirmary, Lister had again and again seen an angry red margin begin to spread out from the wound and then the skin seemed to rot from inside out, often followed by fever, pus, and a swift death (a bona fide "suppuration").

Lister thought of a distant, seemingly unrelated experiment. In Paris, Louis Pasteur, the great French chemist, had shown that meat broth left exposed to the air would soon turn turbid and begin to ferment, while meat broth sealed in a sterilized vacuum jar would remain clear. Based on these observations, Pasteur had made a bold claim: the turbidity was caused by the growth of invisible microorganisms—bacteria—that had fallen out of the air into the broth. Lister took Pasteur's reasoning further. An open wound— a mixture of clotted blood and denuded flesh—was, after all, a human variant of Pasteur's meat broth, a natural petri dish for bacterial growth. Could the bacteria that had dropped into Pasteur's cultures in France also be dropping out of the air into Lister's patients' wounds in Scotland?

Lister then made another inspired leap of logic. If postsurgical infections were being caused by bacteria, then perhaps an antibacterial process or chemical could curb these infections. It "occurred to me," he wrote in his clinical notes, "that the decomposition in the injured part might be avoided without excluding the air, by applying as a dressing some material capable of destroying the life of the floating particles."

In the neighboring town of Carlisle, Lister had observed sewage disposers cleanse their waste with a cheap, sweet-smelling liquid containing carbolic acid. Lister began to apply carbolic acid paste to wounds after surgery. (That he was applying a sewage cleanser to his patients appears not to have struck him as even the slightest bit unusual.)

In August 1867, a thirteen-year-old boy who had severely cut his arm while operating a machine at a fair in Glasgow was admitted to Lister's infirmary. The boy's wound was open and smeared with grime—a setup for gangrene. But rather than amputating the arm, Lister tried a salve of carbolic acid, hoping to keep the arm alive and uninfected. The wound teetered on the edge of a terrifying infection, threatening to become an abscess. But Lister persisted, intensifying his application of carbolic acid paste. For a few weeks, the whole effort seemed hopeless. But then, like a fire running to the end of a rope, the wound began to dry up. A month later, when the poultices were removed, the skin had completely healed underneath.

It was not long before Lister's invention was joined to the advancing front of cancer surgery. In 1869, Lister removed a breast tumor from his sister, Isabella Pim, using a dining table as his operating table, ether for anesthesia, and carbolic acid as his antiseptic. She survived without an infection (although she would eventually die of liver metastasis three years later). A few months later, Lister performed an extensive amputation on another patient with cancer, likely a sarcoma in a thigh. By the mid-1870s, Lister was routinely operating on breast cancer and had extended his surgery to the cancer-afflicted lymph nodes under the breast.

৶৶

Antisepsis and anesthesia were twin technological breakthroughs that released surgery from its constraining medieval chrysalis. Armed with ether and carbolic soap, a new generation of surgeons lunged toward the forbiddingly complex anatomical procedures that Hunter and his colleagues had once concocted on cadavers. An incandescent century of cancer surgery emerged; between 1850 to 1950, surgeons brazenly attacked cancer by cutting open the body and removing tumors.

Emblematic of this era was the prolific Viennese surgeon Theodor Billroth. Born in 1821, Billroth studied music and surgery with almost equal verve. (The professions still often go hand in hand. Both push manual skill to its limit; both mature with practice and age; both depend on immediacy, precision, and opposable thumbs.) In 1867, as a professor in Berlin, Billroth launched a systematic study of methods to open the human abdomen to remove malignant masses. Until Billroth's time, the mortality following abdominal surgery had been forbidding. Billroth's approach to the problem was meticulous and formal: for nearly a decade, he spent surgery after surgery simply opening and closing abdomens of animals and human cadavers, defining clear and safe *routes* to the inside. By the early 1880s, he had established the routes: "The course so far is already sufficient proof that the operation is possible," he wrote. "Our next care, and the subject of our next studies, must be to determine the indications, and to develop the technique to suit all kinds of cases. I hope we have taken another good step forward towards securing unfortunate people hitherto regarded as incurable."

At the Allgemeines Krankenhaus, the teaching hospital in Vienna where he was appointed a professor, Billroth and his students now began to master and use a variety of techniques to remove tumors from the stomach, colon, ovaries, and esophagus, hoping to cure the body of cancer. The switch from exploration to cure produced an unanticipated challenge. A cancer surgeon's task was to remove malignant tissue while leaving normal tissues and organs intact. But this task, Billroth soon discovered, demanded a nearly godlike creative spirit.

Since the time of Vesalius, surgery had been immersed in the study of natural anatomy. But cancer so often disobeyed and distorted natural anatomical boundaries that unnatural boundaries had to be invented to constrain it. To remove the distal end of a stomach filled with cancer, for instance, Billroth had to hook up the pouch remaining after surgery to a nearby piece of the small intestine. To remove the entire bottom half of the stomach, he had to attach the remainder to a piece of distant jejunum. By the mid-1890s, Billroth had operated on forty-one patients with gastric carcinoma using these novel anatomical reconfigurations. Nineteen of these patients had survived the surgery.

These procedures represented pivotal advances in the treatment of cancer. By the early twentieth century, many locally restricted cancers (i.e., primary tumors without metastatic lesions) could be removed by surgery. These included uterine and ovarian cancer, breast and prostate cancer, colon cancer, and lung cancer. If these tumors were removed before they had invaded other organs, these operations produced cures in a significant fraction of patients. Surgery remains the mainstay in the treatment of localized tumors.

But despite these remarkable advances, some cancers—even seemingly locally restricted ones—still relapsed after surgery, prompting second and often third attempts to resect tumors. Surgeons returned to the operating table and cut and cut again, as if caught in a cat-and-mouse game, as cancer was slowly excavated out of the human body piece by piece.

But what if the whole of cancer could be uprooted at its earliest stage using the most definitive surgery conceivable? What if cancer, incurable by means of conventional local surgery, could be cured by a radical, aggressive operation that would dig out its roots so completely, so exhaustively, that no possible trace was left behind? In an era captivated by the potency and creativity of surgeons, the idea of a surgeon's knife extracting cancer by its roots was imbued with promise and wonder. It would land on the already brittle and combustible world of oncology like a firecracker thrown into gunpowder.

A Radical Idea

William Stewart Halsted, whose name was to be inseparably attached to the concept of "radical" surgery, did not ask for that distinction. Instead, it was handed to him almost without any asking, like a scalpel delivered wordlessly into the outstretched hand of a surgeon. Halsted didn't invent radical surgery. He inherited the idea from his predecessors and brought it to its extreme and logical perfection—only to find it inextricably attached to his name.

Halsted was born in 1852, the son of a well-to-do clothing merchant in New York. He finished high school at the Phillips Academy in Andover and attended Yale College, where his athletic prowess, rather than academic achievement, drew the attention of his teachers and mentors. He wandered into the world of surgery almost by accident, attending medical school not because he was driven to become a surgeon but because he could not imagine himself apprenticed as a merchant in his father's business. In 1874, Halsted matriculated at the College of Physicians and Surgeons at Columbia. He was immediately fascinated by anatomy. This fascination, like many of Halsted's other interests in his later years—purebred dogs, horses, starched tablecloths, linen shirts, Parisian leather shoes, and immaculate surgical sutures—soon grew into an obsessive quest. He swallowed textbooks of anatomy whole and, when the books were exhausted, moved on to real patients with an equally insatiable hunger.

In the mid-1870s, Halsted passed an entrance examination to be a surgical intern at Bellevue, a New York City hospital swarming with surgical patients. He split his time between the medical school and the surgical clinic, traveling several miles across New York between Bellevue and Columbia. Understandably, by the time he had finished medical school, he had already suffered a nervous breakdown. He recuperated for a few weeks on Block Island, then, dusting himself off, resumed his studies with just as much energy and verve. This pattern—heroic, Olympian exertion to the brink of physical impossibility, often followed by a near collapse—was to become a hallmark of Halsted's approach to nearly every challenge. It would leave an equally distinct mark on his approach to surgery, surgical education—and cancer.

Halsted entered surgery at a transitional moment in its history. Bloodletting, cupping, leaching, and purging were common procedures. One woman with convulsions and fever from a postsurgical infection was treated with even more barbaric attempts at surgery: "I opened a large orifice in each arm," her surgeon wrote with self-congratulatory enthusiasm in the 1850s, "and cut both temporal arteries and had her blood flowing freely from all at the same time, determined to bleed her until the convulsions ceased." Another doctor, prescribing a remedy for lung cancer, wrote, "Small bleedings give temporary relief, although, of course, they cannot often be repeated." At Bellevue, the "internes" ran about in corridors with "pus-pails," the bodily drippings of patients spilling out of them. Surgical sutures were made of catgut, sharpened with spit, and left to hang from incisions into the open air. Surgeons walked around with their scalpels dangling from their pockets. If a tool fell on the blood-soiled floor, it was dusted off and inserted back into the pocket—or into the body of the patient on the operating table.

In October 1877, leaving behind this gruesome medical world of purgers, bleeders, pus-pails, and quacks, Halsted traveled to Europe to visit the clinics of London, Paris, Berlin, Vienna, or Leipzig, where young American surgeons were typically sent to learn refined European surgical techniques. The timing was fortuitous: Halsted arrived in Europe when cancer surgery was just emerging from its chrysalis. In the high-baroque surgical amphitheaters of the Allgemeines Krankenhaus in Vienna, Theodor Billroth was teaching his students novel techniques to dissect the stomach (the complete surgical removal of cancer, Billroth told his students, was merely an "audacious step" away). At Halle, a few hundred miles from Vienna, the German surgeon Richard von Volkmann was working on a technique to operate on breast cancer. Halsted met the giants of European surgery: Hans Chiari, who had meticulously deconstructed the anatomy of the liver; Anton Wolfler, who had studied with Billroth and was learning to dissect the thyroid gland.

For Halsted, this whirlwind tour through Berlin, Halle, Zurich, London, and Vienna was an intellectual baptism. When he returned to practice in New York in the early 1880s, his mind was spinning with the ideas he had encountered in his journey: Lister's carbolic sprays, Volkmann's early attempts at cancer surgery, and Billroth's miraculous abdominal operations. Energized and inspired, Halsted threw himself to work, operating on patients at Roosevelt Hospital, at the College of Physicians and Surgeons at Columbia, at Bellevue, and at Chambers Hospital. Bold, inventive, and daring, his confidence in his handiwork boomed. In 1882, he removed an infected gallbladder from his mother on a kitchen table, successfully performing one of the first such operations in America. Called urgently to see his sister, who was bleeding heavily after childbirth, he withdrew his own blood and transfused her with it. (He had no knowledge of blood types; but fortunately Halsted and his sister were a perfect match.)

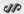

In 1884, at the prime of his career in New York, Halsted read a paper describing the use of a new surgical anesthetic called cocaine. At Halle, in Volkmann's clinic, he had watched German surgeons perform operations using this drug; it was cheap, accessible, foolproof, and easy to dose— the fast food of surgical anesthesia. His experimental curiosity aroused,

Halsted began to inject himself with the drug, testing it before using it to numb patients for his ambitious surgeries. He found that it produced much more than a transitory numbness: it amplified his instinct for tirelessness; it synergized with his already manic energy. His mind became, as one observer put it, "clearer and clearer, with no sense of fatigue and no desire or ability to sleep." He had, it would seem, conquered all his mortal imperfections: the need to sleep, exhaustion, and nihilism. His restive personality had met its perfect pharmacological match.

For the next five years, Halsted sustained an incredible career as a young surgeon in New York despite a fierce and growing addiction to cocaine. He wrested some control over his addiction by heroic self-denial and discipline. (At night, he reportedly left a sealed vial of cocaine by his bedside, thus testing himself by constantly having the drug within arm's reach.) But he relapsed often and fiercely, unable to ever fully overcome his habit. He voluntarily entered the Butler sanatorium in Providence, where he was treated with morphine to treat his cocaine habit—in essence, exchanging one addiction for another. In 1889, still oscillating between the two highly addictive drugs (yet still astonishingly productive in his surgical clinic in New York), he was recruited to the newly built Johns Hopkins Hospital by the renowned physician William Welch—in part to start a new surgical department and in equal part to wrest him out of his New York world of isolation, overwork, and drug addiction.

Hopkins was meant to change Halsted, and it did. Gregarious and outgoing in his former life, he withdrew sharply into a cocooned and private empire where things were controlled, clean, and perfect. He launched an awe-inspiring training program for young surgical residents that would build them in his own image—a superhuman initiation into a superhuman profession that emphasized heroism, self-denial, diligence, and tirelessness. ("It will be objected that this apprenticeship is too long, that the young surgeon will be stale," he wrote in 1904, but "these positions are not for those who so soon weary of the study of their profession.") He married Caroline Hampton, formerly his chief nurse, and lived in a sprawling three-story mansion on the top of a hill ("cold as stone and most unlivable," as one of his students described it), each residing on a separate floor. Childless, socially awkward, formal, and notoriously reclusive, the Halsteds raised thoroughbred horses and purebred dachshunds. Halsted was still deeply addicted to morphine, but he took the drug in such controlled doses and on such a strict schedule that not even his closest students suspected it. The couple diligently avoided Baltimore society. When visitors came unannounced to their mansion on the hill, the maid was told to inform them that the Halsteds were not home.

With the world around him erased and silenced by this routine and rhythm, Halsted now attacked breast cancer with relentless energy. At Volkmann's clinic in Halle, Halsted had witnessed the German surgeon performing increasingly meticulous and aggressive surgeries to remove tumors from the breast. But Volkmann, Halsted knew, had run into a wall. Even though the surgeries had grown extensive and exhaustive, breast cancer had still relapsed, eventually recurring months or even years after the operation.

What caused this relapse? At St. Luke's Hospital in London in the 1860s, the English surgeon Charles Moore had also noted these vexing local recurrences. Frustrated by repeated failures, Moore had begun to record the anatomy of each relapse, denoting the area of the original tumor, the precise margin of the surgery, and the site of cancer recurrence by drawing tiny black dots on a diagram of a breast—creating a sort of historical dartboard of cancer recurrence. And to Moore's surprise, dot by dot, a pattern had emerged. The recurrences had accumulated precisely around the margins of the original surgery, as if minute remnants of cancer had been left behind by incomplete surgery and grown back. "Mammary cancer requires the careful extirpation of the entire organ," Moore concluded. "Local recurrence of cancer after operations is due to the continuous growth of fragments of the principal tumor."

Moore's hypothesis had an obvious corollary. If breast cancer relapsed due to the inadequacy of the original surgical excisions, then even more breast tissue should be removed during the initial operation. Since the *margins* of extirpation were the problem, then why not extend the margins? Moore argued that surgeons, attempting to spare women the disfiguring (and often life-threatening) surgery were exercising "mistaken kindness"—letting cancer get the better of their knives. In Germany, Halsted had seen Volkmann remove not just the breast, but a thin, fanlike muscle spread out under the breast called the pectoralis minor, in the hopes of cleaning out the minor fragments of leftover cancer.

Halsted took this line of reasoning to its next inevitable step. Volkmann may have run into a wall; Halsted would excavate his way past it. Instead of stripping away the thin pectoralis minor, which had little function, Halsted decided to dig even deeper into the breast cavity, cutting through the pectoralis *major*, the large, prominent muscle responsible for moving the shoulder and the hand. Halsted was not alone in this innovation: Willy Meyer, a surgeon operating in New York, independently arrived at the same operation in the 1890s. Halsted called this procedure the "radical mastectomy," using the word *radical* in the original Latin sense to mean "root"; he was uprooting cancer from its very source.

But Halsted, evidently scornful of "mistaken kindness," did not stop his surgery at the pectoralis major. When cancer still recurred despite his radical mastectomy, he began to cut even farther into the chest. By 1898, Halsted's mastectomy had taken what he called "an even more radical" turn. Now he began to slice through the collarbone, reaching for a small cluster of lymph nodes that lay just underneath it. "We clean out or strip the supraclavicular fossa with very few exceptions," he announced at a surgical conference, reinforcing the notion that conservative, nonradical surgery left the breast somehow "unclean."

At Hopkins, Halsted's diligent students now raced to outpace their master with their own scalpels. Joseph Bloodgood, one of Halsted's first surgical residents, had started to cut farther into the neck to evacuate a chain of glands that lay above the collarbone. Harvey Cushing, another star apprentice, even "cleaned out the anterior mediastinum," the deep lymph nodes buried inside the chest. "It is likely," Halsted noted, "that we shall, in the near future, remove the mediastinal contents at some of our primary operations." A macabre marathon was in progress. Halsted and his disciples would rather evacuate the entire contents of the body than be faced with cancer recurrences. In Europe, one surgeon evacuated three ribs and other parts of the rib cage and amputated a shoulder and a collarbone from a woman with breast cancer.

Halsted acknowledged the "physical penalty" of his operation; the mammoth mastectomies permanently disfigured the bodies of his patients. With the pectoralis major cut off, the shoulders caved inward as if in a perpetual shrug, making it impossible to move the arm forward or sideways. Removing the lymph nodes under the armpit often disrupted the flow of lymph, causing the arm to swell up with accumulated fluid like an elephant's leg, a condition he vividly called "surgical elephantiasis." Recuperation from surgery often took patients months, even years. Yet Halsted accepted all these consequences as if they were the inevitable war wounds in an all-out battle. "The patient was a young lady whom I was loath to disfigure," he wrote with genuine concern, describing an operation extending all the way into the neck that he had performed in the 1890s. Something tender, almost paternal, appears in his surgical notes, with outcomes scribbled alongside personal reminiscences. "Good use of arm. Chops wood with it . . . no swelling," he wrote at the end of one case. "Married, Four Children," he scribbled in the margins of another.

But did the Halsted mastectomy save lives? Did radical surgery *cure* breast cancer? Did the young woman that he was so "loath to disfigure" benefit from the surgery that had disfigured her?

Before answering those questions, it's worthwhile understanding the milieu in which the radical mastectomy flourished. In the 1870s, when Halsted had left for Europe to learn from the great masters of the art, surgery was a discipline emerging from its adolescence. By 1898, it had transformed into a profession booming with self-confidence, a discipline so swooningly self-impressed with its technical abilities that great surgeons unabashedly imagined themselves as showmen. The operating room was called an operating theater, and surgery was an elaborate performance often watched by a tense, hushed audience of observers from an oculus above the theater. To watch Halsted operate, one observer wrote in 1898, was to watch the "performance of an artist close akin to the patient and minute labor of a Venetian or Florentine intaglio cutter or a master worker in mosaic." Halsted welcomed the technical challenges of his operation, often conflating the most difficult cases with the most curable: "I find myself inclined to welcome largeness [of a tumor]," he wrote—challenging cancer to duel with his knife.

But the immediate technical success of surgery was not a predictor of its long-term success, its ability to decrease the relapse of cancer. Halsted's mastectomy may have been a Florentine mosaic worker's operation, but if cancer was a chronic relapsing disease, then perhaps cutting it away, even with Halsted's intaglio precision, was not enough. To determine whether Halsted had truly cured breast cancer, one needed to track not immediate survival, or even survival over five or ten months, but survival over five or ten *years*.

The procedure had to be put to a test by following patients longitudinally in time. So, in the mid-1890s, at the peak of his surgical career, Halsted began to collect long-term statistics to show that his operation was the superior choice. By then, the radical mastectomy was more than a decade old. Halsted had operated on enough women and extracted enough tumors to create what he called an entire "cancer storehouse" at Hopkins.

৶৹

Halsted would almost certainly have been right in his theory of radical surgery: that attacking even small cancers with aggressive local surgery was the best way to achieve a cure. But there was a deep conceptual error. Imagine a population in which breast cancer occurs at a fixed incidence, say 1 percent per year. The tumors, however, demonstrate a spectrum of behavior right from their inception. In some women, by the time the disease has been diagnosed the tumor has already spread beyond the breast: there is metastatic cancer in the bones, lungs, and liver. In other women, the cancer is confined to the breast, or to the breast and a few nodes; it is truly a local disease.

Position Halsted now, with his scalpel and sutures, in the middle of this population, ready to perform his radical mastectomy on any woman with breast cancer. Halsted's ability to cure patients with breast cancer obviously depends on the sort of cancer—the stage of breast cancer—that he confronts. The woman with the metastatic cancer is not going to be cured by a radical mastectomy, no matter how aggressively and meticulously Halsted extirpates the tumor in her breast: her cancer is no longer a local problem. In contrast, the woman with the small, confined cancer *does* benefit from the operation—but for her, a far less aggressive procedure, a local mastectomy, would have done just as well. Halsted's mastectomy is thus a peculiar misfit in both cases; it underestimates its target in the first case and overestimates it in the second. In both cases, women are forced to undergo indiscriminate, disfiguring, and morbid operations—too much, too early for the woman with local breast cancer, and too little, too late, for the woman with metastatic cancer.

On April 19, 1898, Halsted attended the annual conference of the American Surgical Association in New Orleans. On the second day, before a hushed and eager audience of surgeons, he rose to the podium armed with figures and tables showcasing his highly anticipated data. At first glance, his observations were astounding: his mastectomy had outperformed every other surgeon's operation in terms of local recurrence. At Baltimore, Halsted had slashed the rate of local recurrence to a bare few percent, a drastic improvement on Volkmann's or Billroth's numbers. Just as Halsted had promised, he had seemingly exterminated cancer at its root.

But if one looked closely, the roots had persisted. The evidence for a true cure of breast cancer was much more disappointing. Of the seventy-six patients with breast cancer treated with the "radical method," only forty had survived for more than three years. Thirty-six, or nearly half the original number, had died within three years of the surgery—consumed by a disease supposedly "uprooted" from the body.

But Halsted and his students remained unfazed. Rather than address the real question raised by the data—did radical mastectomy truly extend lives?—they clutched to their theories even more adamantly. A surgeon should "operate on the neck in every case," Halsted emphasized in New Orleans. Where others might have seen reason for caution, Halsted only saw opportunity: "I fail to see why the neck involvement in itself is more serious than the axillary [area]. The neck can be cleaned out as thoroughly as the axilla."

In the summer of 1907, Halsted presented more data to the American Surgical Association in Washington, D.C. He divided his patients into three groups based on whether the cancer had spread before surgery to lymph nodes in the axilla or the neck. When he put up his survival tables, a pattern became apparent. Of the sixty patients with no cancer-afflicted nodes in the axilla or the neck, the substantial number of forty-five had been cured of breast cancer at five years. Of the forty patients *with* such nodes, only three had survived.

The ultimate survival from breast cancer, in short, had little to do with how extensively a surgeon operated on the breast; it depended on how extensively the cancer had spread before surgery. As George Crile, one of the most fervent critics of radical surgery, later put it, "If the disease was so advanced that one had to get rid of the muscles in order to get rid of the tumor, then it had already spread through the system"—making the whole operation moot.

But if Halsted came to the brink of this realization in 1907, he just as emphatically shied away from it. He relapsed to stale aphorisms. "But even without the proof which we offer, it is, I think, incumbent upon the surgeon to perform in many cases the supraclavicular operation," he advised in one paper. By now the perpetually changing landscape of breast cancer was beginning to tire him out. Trials, tables, and charts had never been his forte; he was a surgeon, not a bookkeeper. "It is especially true of mammary cancer," he wrote, "that the surgeon interested in furnishing the best statistics may in perfectly honorable ways provide them." That statement—almost vulgar by Halsted's standards—exemplified his growing skepticism about putting his own operation to a test. He instinctively knew that he had come to the far edge of his understanding of this amorphous illness that was constantly slipping out of his reach.

The 1907 paper was to be Halsted's last and most comprehensive discussion on breast cancer. He wanted new and open anatomical vistas where he could practice his technically brilliant procedures in peace, not debates about the measurement and remeasurement of end points of surgery. Never having commanded a particularly good bedside manner, he retreated fully into his cloistered operating room and into the vast, cold library of his mansion. He had already moved on to other organs—the thorax, the thyroid, the great arteries—where he continued to make brilliant surgical innovations. But he never wrote another scholarly analysis of the majestic and flawed operation that bore his name.

∂∤ß

Between 1891 and 1907—in the sixteen hectic years that stretched from the tenuous debut of the radical mastectomy in Baltimore to its center-stage appearances at vast surgical conferences around the nation—the quest for a cure for cancer took a great leap forward and an equally great step back. Halsted proved beyond any doubt that massive, meticulous surgeries were technically possible in breast cancer. These operations could drastically reduce the risk for the local recurrence of a deadly disease. But what Halsted could not prove, despite his most strenuous efforts, was far more revealing. After nearly two decades of data gathering, having been levitated, praised, analyzed, and reanalyzed in conference after conference, the superiority of radical surgery in "curing" cancer still stood on shaky ground. More surgery had just not translated into more effective therapy.

Yet all this uncertainty did little to stop other surgeons from operating just as aggressively. "Radicalism" became a psychological obsession, burrowing its way deeply into cancer surgery. Even the word *radical* was a seductive conceptual trap. Halsted had used it in the Latin sense of "root" because his operation was meant to dig out the buried, subterranean roots of cancer. But *radical* also meant "aggressive," "innovative," and "brazen," and it was this meaning that left its mark on the imaginations of patients.

What man or woman, confronting cancer, would willingly choose *non*-radical, or "conservative," surgery?

Indeed, radicalism became central not only to how surgeons saw cancer, but also in how they imagined themselves. "With no protest from any other quarter and nothing to stand in its way, the practice of radical surgery," one historian wrote, "soon fossilized into dogma." When heroic surgery failed to match its expectations, some surgeons began to shrug off the responsibility of a cure altogether. "Undoubtedly, if operated upon properly the condition may be cured locally, and that is the only point for which the surgeon must hold himself responsible," one of Halsted's disciples announced at a conference in Baltimore in 1931. The best a surgeon could do, in other words, was to deliver the most technically perfect operation. Curing cancer was someone else's problem.

This trajectory toward more and more brazenly aggressive operations—"the more radical the better"—mirrored the overall path of surgical thinking of the early 1930s. In New York, the surgeon Alexander Brunschwig devised an operation for cervical cancer, called a "complete pelvic exenteration," so strenuous and exhaustive that even the most Halstedian surgeon needed to break midprocedure to rest and change positions. The New York surgeon George Pack was nicknamed Pack the Knife (after the popular song "Mack the Knife"), as if the surgeon and his favorite instrument had, like some sort of ghoulish centaur, somehow fused into the same creature.

Cure was a possibility now flung far into the future. "Even in its widest sense," an English surgeon wrote in 1929, "the measure of operability depend[s] on the question: 'Is the lesion removable?' and not on the question: 'Is the removal of the lesion going to *cure* the patient?'" Surgeons often counted themselves lucky if their patients merely survived these operations. "There is an old Arabian proverb," a group of surgeons wrote at the end of a particularly chilling discussion of stomach cancer in 1933, "that he is no physician who has not slain many patients, and the surgeon who operates for carcinoma of the stomach must remember that often."

To arrive at that sort of logic—the Hippocratic oath turned upside down—demands either a terminal desperation or a terminal optimism. In the 1930s, the pendulum of cancer surgery swung desperately between those two points. Halsted, Brunschwig, and Pack persisted with their mammoth operations because they genuinely believed that they could relieve the dreaded symptoms of cancer. But they lacked formal proof, and as they went further up the isolated promontories of their own beliefs, proof became irrelevant and trials impossible to run. The more fervently surgeons believed in the inherent good of their operations, the more untenable it became to put these to a formal scientific trial. Radical surgery thus drew the blinds of circular logic around itself for nearly a century.

∂∕ρ

The allure and glamour of radical surgery overshadowed crucial developments in less radical surgical procedures for cancer that were evolving in its penumbra. Halsted's students fanned out to invent new procedures to extirpate cancers. Each was "assigned" an organ. Halsted's confidence in his heroic surgical training program was so supreme that he imagined his students capable of confronting and annihilating cancer in any organ system. In 1897, having intercepted a young surgical resident, Hugh Hampton Young, in a corridor at Hopkins, Halsted asked him to become the head of the new department of urological surgery. Young protested that he knew nothing about urological surgery. "I know you didn't know anything," Halsted replied curtly, "but we believe that you can learn"—and walked on.

Inspired by Halsted's confidence, Young delved into surgery for urological cancers—cancers of the prostate, kidney, and bladder. In 1904, with Halsted as his assistant, Young successfully devised an operation for prostate cancer by excising the entire gland. Although called the radical prostatectomy in the tradition of Halsted, Hampton's surgery was rather conservative by comparison. He did not remove muscles, lymph nodes, or bone. He retained the notion of the en bloc removal of the organ from radical surgery, but stopped short of evacuating the entire pelvis or extirpating the urethra or the bladder. (A modification of this procedure is still used to remove localized prostate cancer, and it cures a substantial portion of patients with such tumors.)

Harvey Cushing, Halsted's student and chief surgical resident, concentrated on the brain. By the early 1900s, Cushing had found ingenious ways to surgically extract brain tumors, including the notorious glioblastomas—tumors so heavily crisscrossed with blood vessels that they could hemorrhage any minute, and meningiomas wrapped like sheaths around delicate and vital structures in the brain. Like Young, Cushing inherited Haslted's intaglio surgical technique—"the slow separation of brain from tumor, working now here, now there, leaving small, flattened pads of hot, wrung-out cotton to control oozing"—but not Halsted's penchant for radical surgery. Indeed Cushing found radical operations on brain tumors not just difficult, but inconceivable: even if he desired it, a surgeon could not extirpate the entire organ.

In 1933, at the Barnes Hospital in St. Louis, yet another surgical innovator, Evarts Graham, pioneered an operation to remove a lung afflicted with cancer by piecing together prior operations that had been used to remove tubercular lungs. Graham, too, retained the essential spirit of Halstedian surgery: the meticulous excision of the organ en bloc and the cutting of wide margins around the tumor to prevent local recurrences. But he tried to sidestep its pitfalls. Resisting the temptation to excise more and more tissue—lymph nodes throughout the thorax, major blood vessels, or the adjacent fascia around the trachea and esophagus—he removed just the lung, keeping the specimen as intact as possible.

Even so, obsessed with Halstedian theory and unable to see beyond its realm, surgeons sharply berated such attempts at nonradical surgery. A surgical procedure that did not attempt to obliterate cancer from the body was pooh-poohed as a "makeshift operation." To indulge in such makeshift operations was to succumb to the old flaw of "mistaken kindness" that a generation of surgeons had tried so diligently to banish.

The Hard Tube and the Weak Light

We have found in [X-rays] a cure for the malady.
—Los Angeles Times, April 6, 1902

By way of illustration [of the destructive power of X-rays]
let us recall that nearly all pioneers in the medical X-ray
laboratories in the United States died of cancers induced
by the burns.

—The Washington Post, 1945

In late October 1895, a few months after Halsted had unveiled the radical mastectomy in Baltimore, Wilhelm Röntgen, a lecturer at the Würzburg Institute in Germany, was working with an electron tube—a vacuum tube that shot electrons from one electrode to another—when he noticed a strange leakage. The radiant energy was powerful and invisible, capable of penetrating layers of blackened cardboard and producing a white phosphorescent glow on a barium screen accidentally left on a bench in the room.

Röntgen whisked his wife, Anna, into the lab and placed her hand between the source of his rays and a photographic plate. The rays penetrated through her hand and left a silhouette of her finger bones and her metallic wedding ring on the photographic plate—the inner anatomy of a hand seen as if through a magical lens. "I have seen my death," Anna said—but her husband saw something else: a form of energy so powerful that it could pass through most living tissues. Röntgen called his form of light X-rays.

At first, X-rays were thought to be an artificial quirk of energy produced by electron tubes. But in 1896, just a few months after Röntgen's discovery, Henri Becquerel, the French chemist, who knew of Röntgen's work, discovered that certain natural materials—uranium among them—autonomously emitted their own invisible rays with properties similar to those of X-rays. In Paris, friends of Becquerel's, a young physicist-chemist couple named Pierre and Marie Curie, began to scour the natural world for even more powerful chemical sources of X-rays. Pierre and Marie (then Maria Skłodowska, a penniless Polish immigrant living in a garret in Paris) had met at the Sorbonne and been drawn to each other because of a common interest in magnetism. In the mid-1880s, Pierre Curie had used minuscule quartz crystals to craft an instrument called an electrometer, capable of measuring exquisitely small doses of energy. Using this device, Marie had shown that even tiny amounts of radiation emitted by uranium ores could be quantified. With their new measuring instrument for radioactivity, Marie and Pierre began hunting for new sources of X-rays. Another monumental journey of scientific discovery was thus launched with measurement.

In a waste ore called pitchblende, a black sludge that came from the peaty forests of Joachimsthal in what is now the Czech Republic, the Curies found the first signal of a new element—an element many times more radioactive than uranium. The Curies set about distilling the boggy sludge to trap that potent radioactive source in its purest form. From several tons of pitchblende, four hundred tons of washing water, and hundreds of buckets of distilled sludge waste, they finally fished out one-tenth of a gram of the new element in 1902. The metal lay on the far edge of the periodic table, emitting X-rays with such feverish intensity that it glowered with a hypnotic blue light in the dark, consuming itself. Unstable, it was a strange chimera between matter and energy—matter decomposing into energy. Marie Curie called the new element radium, from the Greek word for "light."

Radium, by virtue of its potency, revealed a new and unexpected property of X-rays: they could not only carry radiant energy through human tissues, but also deposit energy deep *inside* tissues. Röntgen had been able to photograph his wife's hand because of the first property: his X-rays had traversed through flesh and bone and left a shadow of the tissue on the film. Marie Curie's hands, in contrast, bore the painful legacy of the second effect: having distilled pitchblende into a millionth part for week after week in the hunt for purer and purer radioactivity, the skin in her palm had begun to chafe and peel off in blackened layers, as if the tissue had been burnt from the inside. A few milligrams of radium left in a vial in Pierre's pocket scorched through the heavy tweed of his waistcoat and left a permanent scar on his chest. One man who gave "magical" demonstrations at a public fair with a leaky, unshielded radium machine developed swollen and blistered lips, and his cheeks and nails fell out. Radiation would eventually burn into Marie Curie's bone marrow, leaving her permanently anemic.

It would take biologists decades to fully decipher the mechanism that lay behind these effects, but the spectrum of damaged tissues—skin, lips, blood, gums, and nails—already provided an important clue: radium was attacking DNA. DNA is an inert molecule, exquisitely resistant to most chemical reactions, for its job is to maintain the stability of genetic information. But X-rays can shatter strands of DNA or generate toxic chemicals that corrode DNA. Cells respond to this damage by dying or, more often, by ceasing to divide. X-rays thus preferentially kill the most rapidly proliferating cells in the body, cells in the skin, nails, gums, and blood.

This ability of X-rays to selectively kill rapidly dividing cells did not go unnoticed—especially by cancer researchers. In 1896, barely a year after Röntgen had discovered his X-rays, a twenty-one-year-old Chicago medical student, Emil Grubbe, had the inspired notion of using X-rays to treat cancer. Flamboyant, adventurous, and fiercely inventive, Grubbe had worked in a factory in Chicago that produced vacuum X-ray tubes, and he had built a crude version of a tube for his own experiments. Having encountered X-ray-exposed factory workers with peeling skin and nails—his own hands had also become chapped and swollen from repeated exposures—Grubbe quickly extended the logic of this cell death to tumors.

On March 29, 1896, in a tube factory on Halsted Street (the name bears no connection to Halsted the surgeon) in Chicago, Grubbe began to bombard Rose Lee, an elderly woman with breast cancer, with radiation using an improvised X-ray tube. Lee's cancer had relapsed after a mastectomy, and the tumor had exploded into a painful mass in her breast. She had been referred to Grubbe as a last-ditch measure, more to satisfy his experimental curiosity than to provide any clinical benefit. Grubbe looked through the factory for something to cover the rest of the breast, and finding no sheet of metal, wrapped Lee's chest in some tinfoil that he found in the bottom of a Chinese tea box. He irradiated her cancer every night for eighteen consecutive days. The treatment was painful—but somewhat successful. The tumor in Lee's breast ulcerated, tightened, and shrank, producing the first documented local response in the history of X-ray therapy. A few months after the initial treatment, though, Lee became dizzy and nauseated. The cancer had metastasized to her spine, brain, and liver, and she died shortly after. Grubbe had stumbled on another important observation: X-rays could only be used to treat cancer locally, with little effect on tumors that had already metastasized.*

Inspired by the response, even if it had been temporary, Grubbe began using X-ray therapy to treat scores of other patients with local tumors. A new branch of cancer medicine, radiation oncology, was born, with X-ray clinics mushrooming up in Europe and America. By the early 1900s, less than a decade after Röntgen's discovery, doctors waxed ecstatic about the possibility of curing cancer with radiation. "I believe this treatment is an absolute cure for all forms of cancer," a Chicago physician noted in 1901. "I do not know what its limitations are."

With the Curies' discovery of radium in 1902, surgeons could beam thousandfold more powerful bursts of energy on tumors. Conferences and societies on high-dose radiation therapy were organized in a flurry of excitement. Radium was infused into gold wires and stitched directly into tumors, to produce even higher local doses of X-rays. Surgeons implanted radon pellets into abdominal tumors. By the 1930s and '40s, America had a national *surplus* of radium, so much so that it was being advertised for sale to laypeople in the back pages of journals. Vacuum-tube technology advanced in parallel; by the mid-1950s variants of these tubes could deliver blisteringly high doses of X-ray energy into cancerous tissues.

Radiation therapy catapulted cancer medicine into its atomic age—an age replete with both promise and peril. Certainly, the vocabulary, the images, and the metaphors bore the potent symbolism of atomic power unleashed on cancer. There were "cyclotrons" and "supervoltage rays" and "linear accelerators" and "neutron beams." One man was asked to think of his X-ray therapy as "millions of tiny bullets of energy." Another account of a radiation treatment is imbued with the thrill and horror of a space journey: "The patient is put on a stretcher that is placed in the oxygen chamber. As a team of six doctors, nurses, and technicians hover at chamber-side, the radiologist maneuvers a betatron into position. After slamming shut a hatch at the end of the chamber, technicians force oxygen in. After fifteen

---

* Metastatic sites of cancer can occasionally be treated with X-rays, although with limited success.

minutes under full pressure . . . the radiologist turns on the betatron and shoots radiation at the tumor. Following treatment, the patient is decompressed in deep-sea-diver fashion and taken to the recovery room."

Stuffed into chambers, herded in and out of hatches, hovered upon, monitored through closed-circuit television, pressurized, oxygenated, decompressed, and sent back to a room to recover, patients weathered the onslaught of radiation therapy as if it were an invisible benediction.

And for certain forms of cancer, it was a benediction. Like surgery, radiation was remarkably effective at obliterating locally confined cancers. Breast tumors were pulverized with X-rays. Lymphoma lumps melted away. One woman with a brain tumor woke up from her yearlong coma to watch a basketball game in her hospital room.

But like surgery, radiation medicine also struggled against its inherent limits. Emil Grubbe had already encountered the first of these limits with his earliest experimental treatments: since X-rays could only be directed locally, radiation was of limited use for cancers that had metastasized.* One could double and quadruple the doses of radiant energy, but this did not translate into more cures. Instead, indiscriminate irradiation left patients scarred, blinded, and scalded by doses that had far exceeded tolerability.

The second limit was far more insidious: radiation *produced* cancers. The very effect of X-rays killing rapidly dividing cells—DNA damage—also created cancer-causing mutations in genes. In the 1910s, soon after the Curies had discovered radium, a New Jersey corporation called U.S. Radium began to mix radium with paint to create a product called Undark—radium-infused paint that emitted a greenish white light at night. Although aware of the many injurious effects of radium, U.S. Radium promoted Undark for clock dials, boasting of glow-in-the-dark watches. Watch painting was a precise and artisanal craft, and young women with nimble, steady hands were commonly employed. These women were encouraged to use the paint without precautions, and to frequently lick the brushes with their tongues to produce sharp lettering on watches.

Radium workers soon began to complain of jaw pain, fatigue, and skin and tooth problems. In the late 1920s, medical investigations revealed that

---

* Radiation can be used to control or palliate metastatic tumors in selected cases, but is rarely curative in these circumstances.

the bones in their jaws had necrosed, their tongues had been scarred by irradiation, and many had become chronically anemic (a sign of severe bone marrow damage). Some women, tested with radioactivity counters, were found to be glowing with radioactivity. Over the next decades, dozens of radium-induced tumors sprouted in these radium-exposed workers—sarcomas and leukemias, and bone, tongue, neck, and jaw tumors. In 1927, a group of five severely afflicted women in New Jersey—collectively termed "Radium girls" by the media—sued U.S. Radium. None of them had yet developed cancers; they were suffering from the more acute effects of radium toxicity—jaw, skin, and tooth necrosis. A year later, the case was settled out of court with a compensation of $10,000 each to the girls, and $600 per year to cover living and medical expenses. The "compensation" was not widely collected. Many of the Radium girls, too weak even to raise their hands to take an oath in court, died of leukemia and other cancers soon after their case was settled.

Marie Curie died of leukemia in July 1934. Emil Grubbe, who had been exposed to somewhat weaker X-rays, also succumbed to the deadly late effects of chronic radiation. By the mid-1940s, Grubbe's fingers had been amputated one by one to remove necrotic and gangrenous bones, and his face was cut up in repeated operations to remove radiation-induced tumors and premalignant warts. In 1960, at the age of eighty-five, he died in Chicago, with multiple forms of cancer that had spread throughout his body.

⁂

The complex intersection of radiation with cancer—cancer-curing at times, cancer-causing at others—dampened the initial enthusiasm of cancer scientists. Radiation was a powerful invisible knife—but still a knife. And a knife, no matter how deft or penetrating, could only reach so far in the battle against cancer. A more discriminating therapy was needed, especially for cancers that were nonlocalized.

In 1932, Willy Meyer, the New York surgeon who had invented the radical mastectomy contemporaneously with Halsted, was asked to address the annual meeting of the American Surgical Association. Gravely ill and bedridden, Meyer knew he would be unable to attend the meeting, but he forwarded a brief, six-paragraph speech to be presented. On May 31, six weeks after Meyer's death, his letter was read aloud to the roomful of surgeons. There is, in that letter, an unfailing recognition that cancer medicine had reached some terminus, that a new direction was needed. "If a biological systemic after-treatment were added in every instance," Meyer wrote, "we believe the majority of such patients would remain cured after a properly conducted radical operation."

Meyer had grasped a deep principle about cancer. Cancer, even when it begins locally, is inevitably waiting to explode out of its confinement. By the time many patients come to their doctor, the illness has often spread beyond surgical control and spilled into the body exactly like the black bile that Galen had envisioned so vividly nearly two thousand years ago.

In fact, Galen seemed to have been right after all—in the accidental, aphoristic way that Democritus had been right about the atom or Erasmus had made a conjecture about the Big Bang centuries before the discovery of galaxies. Galen had, of course, missed the actual cause of cancer. There was no black bile clogging up the body and bubbling out into tumors in frustration. But he had uncannily captured something essential about cancer in his dreamy and visceral metaphor. Cancer *was* often a humoral disease. Crablike and constantly mobile, it could burrow through invisible channels from one organ to another. It was a "systemic" illness, just as Galen had once made it out to be.

Dyeing and Dying

> *Those who have not been trained in chemistry or medicine may not realize how difficult the problem of cancer treatment really is. It is almost—not quite, but almost—as hard as finding some agent that will dissolve away the left ear, say, and leave the right ear unharmed. So slight is the difference between the cancer cell and its normal ancestor.*
>
> —William Woglom

> *Life is . . . a chemical incident.*
> —Paul Ehrlich
> as a schoolboy, 1870

A systemic disease demands a systemic cure—but what kind of systemic therapy could possibly cure cancer? Could a drug, like a microscopic surgeon, perform an ultimate pharmacological mastectomy—sparing normal tissue while excising cancer cells? Willy Meyer wasn't alone in fantasizing about such a magical therapy—generations of doctors before him had also fantasized about such a medicine. But how might a drug coursing through the whole body specifically attack a diseased organ?

Specificity refers to the ability of any medicine to discriminate between its intended target and its host. Killing a cancer cell in a test tube is not a particularly difficult task: the chemical world is packed with malevolent poisons that, even in infinitesimal quantities, can dispatch a cancer cell within minutes. The trouble lies in finding a *selective* poison—a drug that will kill cancer without annihilating the patient. Systemic therapy without specificity is an indiscriminate bomb. For an anticancer poison to become a useful drug, Meyer knew, it needed to be a fantastically nimble knife: sharp enough to kill cancer yet selective enough to spare the patient.

The hunt for such specific, systemic poisons for cancer was precipitated by the search for a very different sort of chemical. The story begins with colonialism and its chief loot: cotton. In the mid-1850s, as ships from India and Egypt laden with bales of cotton unloaded their goods in English ports, cloth milling boomed into a spectacularly successful business in England, an industry large enough to sustain an entire gamut of subsidiary industries. A vast network of mills sprouted up in the industrial basin of the Midlands, stretching through Glasgow, Lancashire, and Manchester. Textile exports dominated the British economy. Between 1851 and 1857, the export of printed goods from England more than quadrupled—from 6 million to 27 million pieces per year. In 1784, cotton products had represented a mere 6 percent of total British exports. By the 1850s, that proportion had peaked at 50 percent.

The cloth-milling boom set off a boom in cloth dyeing, but the two industries—cloth and color—were oddly out of technological step. Dyeing, unlike milling, was still a preindustrial occupation. Cloth dyes had to be extracted from perishable vegetable sources—rusty carmines from Turkish madder root, or deep blues from the indigo plant—using antiquated processes that required patience, expertise, and constant supervision. Printing on textiles with colored dyes (to produce the ever-popular calico prints, for instance) was even more challenging—requiring thickeners, mordants, and solvents in multiple steps—and often took the dyers weeks to complete. The textile industry thus needed professional chemists to dissolve its bleaches and cleansers, to supervise the extraction of dyes, and to find ways to fasten the dyes on cloth. A new discipline called practical chemistry, focused on synthesizing products for textile dyeing, was soon flourishing in polytechnics and institutes all over London.

In 1856, William Perkin, an eighteen-year-old student at one of these institutes, stumbled on what would soon become a Holy Grail of this industry: an inexpensive chemical dye that could be made entirely from scratch. In a makeshift one-room laboratory in his apartment in the East End of London ("half of a small but long-shaped room with a few shelves for bottles and a table") Perkin was boiling nitric acid and benzene in smuggled glass flasks and precipitated an unexpected reaction. A chemical had formed inside the tubes with the color of pale, crushed violets. In an era obsessed with dye-making, any colored chemical was considered a potential dye—and a quick dip of a piece of cotton into the flask revealed the new chemical could color cotton. Moreover, this new chemical did not bleach or bleed. Perkin called it aniline mauve.

Perkin's discovery was a godsend for the textile industry. Aniline mauve was cheap and imperishable—vastly easier to produce and store than vegetable dyes. As Perkin soon discovered, its parent compound could act as a molecular building block for other dyes, a chemical skeleton on which a variety of side chains could be hung to produce a vast spectrum of vivid colors. By the mid-1860s, a glut of new synthetic dyes, in shades of lilac, blue, magenta, aquamarine, red, and purple flooded the cloth factories of Europe. In 1857, Perkin, barely nineteen years old, was inducted into the Chemical Society of London as a full fellow, one of the youngest in its history to be thus honored.

Aniline mauve was discovered in England, but dye making reached its chemical zenith in Germany. In the late 1850s, Germany, a rapidly industrializing nation, had been itching to compete in the cloth markets of Europe and America. But unlike England, Germany had scarcely any access to natural dyes: by the time it had entered the scramble to capture colonies, the world had already been sliced up into so many parts, with little left to divide. German cloth millers thus threw themselves into the development of artificial dyes, hoping to rejoin an industry that they had once almost given up as a lost cause.

Dye making in England had rapidly become an intricate chemical business. In Germany—goaded by the textile industry, cosseted by national subsidies, and driven by expansive economic growth—synthetic chemistry underwent an even more colossal boom. In 1883, the German output of alizarin, the brilliant red chemical that imitated natural carmine, reached twelve thousand tons, dwarfing the amount being produced by Perkin's factory in London. German chemists rushed to produce brighter, stronger, cheaper chemicals and muscled their way into textile factories all around Europe. By the mid-1880s, Germany had emerged as the champion of the chemical arms race (which presaged a much uglier military one) to become the "dye basket" of Europe.

Initially, the German textile chemists lived entirely in the shadow of the dye industry. But emboldened by their successes, the chemists began to synthesize not just dyes and solvents, but an entire universe of new molecules: phenols, alcohols, bromides, alkaloids, alizarins, and amides, chemicals never encountered in nature. By the late 1870s, synthetic chemists in

Germany had created more molecules than they knew what to do with. "Practical chemistry" had become almost a caricature of itself: an industry seeking a practical purpose for the products that it had so frantically raced to invent.

⁂

Early interactions between synthetic chemistry and medicine had largely been disappointing. Gideon Harvey, a seventeenth-century physician, had once called chemists the "most impudent, ignorant, flatulent, fleshy, and vainly boasting sort of mankind." The mutual scorn and animosity between the two disciplines had persisted. In 1849, August Hofmann, William Perkin's teacher at the Royal College, gloomily acknowledged the chasm between medicine and chemistry: "None of these compounds have, as yet, found their way into any of the appliances of life. We have not been able to use them . . . for curing disease."

But even Hofmann knew that the boundary between the synthetic world and the natural world was inevitably collapsing. In 1828, a Berlin scientist named Friedrich Wöhler had sparked a metaphysical storm in science by boiling ammonium cyanate, a plain, inorganic salt, and creating urea, a chemical typically produced by the kidneys. The Wöhler experiment—seemingly trivial—had enormous implications. Urea was a "natural" chemical, while its precursor was an inorganic salt. That a chemical produced by natural organisms could be derived so easily in a flask threatened to overturn the entire conception of living organisms: for centuries, the chemistry of living organisms was thought to be imbued with some mystical property, a vital essence that could not be duplicated in a laboratory—a theory called vitalism. Wöhler's experiment demolished vitalism. Organic and inorganic chemicals, he proved, were interchangeable. Biology was chemistry: perhaps even a human body was no different from a bag of busily reacting chemicals—a beaker with arms, legs, eyes, brain, and soul.

With vitalism dead, the extension of this logic to medicine was inevitable. If the chemicals of life could be synthesized in a laboratory, could they work on living systems? If biology and chemistry were so interchangeable, could a molecule concocted in a flask affect the inner workings of a biological organism?

Wöhler was a physician himself, and with his students and collaborators he tried to backpedal from the chemical world into the medical one. But his synthetic molecules were still much too simple—mere stick figures of chemistry where vastly more complex molecules were needed to intervene on living cells.

But such multifaceted chemicals already existed: the laboratories of the dye factories of Frankfurt were full of them. To build his interdisciplinary bridge between biology and chemistry, Wöhler only needed to take a short day-trip from his laboratory in Göttingen to the labs of Frankfurt. But neither Wöhler nor his students could make that last connection. The vast panel of molecules sitting idly on the shelves of the German textile chemists, the precursors of a revolution in medicine, may as well have been a continent away.

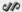

It took a full fifty years after Wöhler's urea experiment for the products of the dye industry to finally make physical contact with living cells. In 1878, in Leipzig, a twenty-four-year-old medical student, Paul Ehrlich, hunting for a thesis project, proposed using cloth dyes—aniline and its colored derivatives—to stain animal tissues. At best, Ehrlich hoped that the dyes might stain the tissues to make microscopy easier. But to his astonishment, the dyes were far from indiscriminate darkening agents. Aniline derivatives stained only parts of the cell, silhouetting certain structures and leaving others untouched. The dyes seemed able to discriminate among chemicals hidden inside cells—binding some and sparing others.

This molecular specificity, encapsulated so vividly in that reaction between a dye and a cell, began to haunt Ehrlich. In 1882, working with Robert Koch, he discovered yet another novel chemical stain, this time for mycobacteria, the organisms that Koch had discovered as the cause of tuberculosis. A few years later, Ehrlich found that certain toxins, injected into animals, could generate "antitoxins," which bound and inactivated poisons with extraordinary specificity (these antitoxins would later be identified as antibodies). He purified a potent serum against diphtheria toxin from the blood of horses, then moved to the Institute for Sera Research and Serum Testing in Steglitz to prepare this serum in gallon buckets, and then to Frankfurt to set up his own laboratory.

But the more widely Ehrlich explored the biological world, the more he spiraled back to his original idea. The biological universe was full of molecules picking out their partners like clever locks designed to fit a key: toxins clinging inseparably to antitoxins, dyes that highlighted only particular parts of cells, chemical stains that could nimbly pick out one class of germs from a mixture of microbes. If biology was an elaborate mix-and-match game of chemicals, Ehrlich reasoned, what if some chemical could discriminate bacterial cells from animal cells—and kill the former without touching the host?

Returning from a conference late one evening, in the cramped compartment of a night train from Berlin to Frankfurt, Ehrlich animatedly described his idea to two fellow scientists, "It has occurred to me that . . . it should be possible to find artificial substances which are really and specifically curative for certain diseases, not merely palliatives acting favorably on one or another symptom. . . . Such curative substances—*a priori*—must directly destroy the microbes responsible for the disease; not by 'action from a distance,' but only when the chemical compound is fixed by the parasites. The parasites can only be killed if the chemical compound has a particular relation, a specific affinity for them."

By then, the other inhabitants of Ehrlich's train compartment had dozed off to sleep. But this rant in a train compartment was one of medicine's most important ideas in its distilled, primordial form. "Chemotherapy," the use of specific chemicals to heal the diseased body, was conceptually born in the middle of the night.

◌◌

Ehrlich began looking for his "curative substances" in a familiar place: the treasure trove of dye-industry chemicals that had proved so crucial to his earlier biological experiments. His laboratory was now physically situated near the booming dye factories of Frankfurt—the Frankfurter Anilinfarben-Fabrik and the Leopold Cassella Company—and he could easily procure dye chemicals and derivatives via a short walk across the valley. With thousands of compounds available to him, Ehrlich embarked on a series of experiments to test their biological effects in animals.

He began with a hunt for antimicrobial chemicals, in part because he already knew that chemical dyes could specifically bind microbial cells. He infected mice and rabbits with *Trypanosoma brucei,* the parasite responsible for the dreaded sleeping sickness, then injected the animals with chemical derivatives to determine if any of them could halt the infection. After several hundred chemicals, Ehrlich and his collaborators had their first antibiotic hit: a brilliant ruby-colored dye derivative that Ehrlich called Trypan Red. It was a name—a disease juxtaposed with a dye color—that captured nearly a century of medical history.

Galvanized by his discovery, Ehrlich unleashed volleys of chemical experiments. A universe of biological chemistry opened up before him: molecules with peculiar properties, a cosmos governed by idiosyncratic rules. Some compounds switched from precursors into active drugs in the bloodstream; others transformed backward from active drugs to inactive molecules. Some were excreted in the urine; others condensed in the bile or fell apart immediately in the blood. One molecule might survive for days in an animal, but its chemical cousin—a variant by just a few critical atoms—might vanish from the body in minutes.

On April 19, 1910, at the densely packed Congress for Internal Medicine in Wiesbaden, Ehrlich announced that he had discovered yet another molecule with "specific affinity"—this one a blockbuster. The new drug, cryptically called compound 606, was active against a notorious microbe, *Treponema pallidum,* which caused syphilis. In Ehrlich's era, syphilis—the "secret malady" of eighteenth-century Europe—was a sensational illness, a tabloid pestilence. Ehrlich knew that an antisyphilitic drug would be an instant sensation and he was prepared. Compound 606 had secretly been tested in patients in the hospital wards of St. Petersburg, then retested in patients with neurosyphilis at the Magdeburg Hospital—each time with remarkable success. A gigantic factory, funded by Hoechst Chemical Works, was already being built to manufacture it for commercial use.

Ehrlich's successes with Trypan Red and compound 606 (which he named Salvarsan, from the word *salvation*) proved that diseases were just pathological locks waiting to be picked by the right molecules. The line of potentially curable illnesses now stretched endlessly before him. Ehrlich called his drugs "magic bullets"—*bullets* for their capacity to kill and *magic* for their specificity. It was a phrase with an ancient, alchemic ring that would sound insistently through the future of oncology.

❧

Ehrlich's magic bullets had one last target to fell: cancer. Syphilis and trypanosomiasis are microbial diseases. Ehrlich was slowly inching toward his ultimate goal: the malignant *human* cell. Between 1904 and 1908, he rigged several elaborate schemes to find an anticancer drug using his vast arsenal of chemicals. He tried amides, anilines, sulfa derivatives, arsenics, bromides, and alcohols to kill cancer cells. None of them worked. What was poison to cancer cells, he found, was inevitably poison to normal cells as well. Discouraged, he tried even more fantastical strategies. He thought of starving sarcoma cells of metabolites, or tricking them into death by using decoy molecules (a strategy that would presage Subbarao's antifolate derivatives by nearly fifty years). But the search for the ultimate, discriminating anticancer drug proved fruitless. His pharmacological bullets, far from magical, were either too indiscriminate or too weak.

In 1908, soon after Ehrlich won the Nobel Prize for his discovery of the principle of specific affinity, Kaiser Wilhelm of Germany invited him to a private audience in his palace. The Kaiser was seeking counsel: a noted hypochondriac afflicted by various real and imagined ailments, he wanted to know whether Ehrlich had an anticancer drug within reach.

Ehrlich hedged. The cancer cell, he explained, was a fundamentally different target from a bacterial cell. Specific affinity relied, paradoxically, not on "affinity," but on its opposite—on difference. Ehrlich's chemicals had successfully targeted bacteria because bacterial enzymes were so radically dissimilar to human enzymes. With cancer, it was the *similarity* of the cancer cell to the normal human cell that made it nearly impossible to target.

Ehrlich went on in this vein, almost musing to himself. He was circling around something profound, an idea in its infancy: to target the abnormal cell, one would need to decipher the biology of the normal cell. He had returned, decades after his first encounter with aniline, to specificity again, to the bar codes of biology hidden inside every living cell.

Ehrlich's thinking was lost on the Kaiser. Having little interest in this cheerless disquisition with no obvious end, he cut the audience short.

In 1915, Ehrlich fell ill with tuberculosis, a disease that he had likely acquired from his days in Koch's laboratory. He went to recuperate in Bad Homburg, a spa town famous for its healing carbonic-salt baths. From his room, overlooking the distant plains below, he watched bitterly as his country pitched itself into the First World War. The dye factories that had once supplied his therapeutic chemicals—Bayer and Hoechst among them—were converted to massive producers of chemicals that would be turned into precursors for war gases. One particularly toxic gas was a colorless, blistering liquid produced by reacting the solvent thiodiglycol (a dye intermediate) with boiling hydrochloric acid. The gas's smell was unmistakable, described alternatively as reminiscent of mustard, burnt garlic, or horseradishes ground on a fire. It came to be known as mustard gas.

On the foggy night of July 12, 1917, two years after Ehrlich's death, a volley of artillery shells marked with small, yellow crosses rained down on British troops stationed near the small Belgian town of Ypres. The liquid in the bombs quickly vaporized, a "thick, yellowish green cloud veiling the sky," as a soldier recalled, then diffused through the cool night air. The men in their barracks and trenches, asleep for the night, awoke to a nauseatingly sharp smell that they would remember for decades to come: the acrid whiff of horseradishes spreading through the chalk fields. Within seconds, soldiers ran for cover, coughing and sneezing in the mud, the blind scrambling among the dead. Mustard gas diffused through leather and rubber, and soaked through layers of cloth. It hung like a toxic mist over the battlefield for days until the dead smelled of mustard. On that night alone, mustard gas injured or killed two thousand soldiers. In a single year, it left thousands dead in its wake.

The acute, short-term effects of nitrogen mustard—the respiratory complications, the burnt skin, the blisters, the blindness—were so amply monstrous that its long-term effects were overlooked. In 1919, a pair of American pathologists, Edward and Helen Krumbhaar, analyzed the effects of the Ypres bombing on the few men who had survived it. They found that the survivors had an unusual condition of the bone marrow. The normal blood-forming cells had dried up; the bone marrow, in a bizarre mimicry of the scorched and blasted battlefield, was markedly depleted. The men were anemic and needed transfusions of blood, often up to once a month. They were prone to infections. Their white cell counts often hovered persistently below normal.

In a world less preoccupied with other horrors, this news might have caused a small sensation among cancer doctors. Although evidently poisonous, this chemical had, after all, targeted the bone marrow and wiped out only certain populations of cells—a chemical with specific affinity. But Europe was full of horror stories in 1919, and this seemed no more remarkable than any other. The Krumbhaars published their paper in a second-tier medical journal and it was quickly forgotten in the amnesia of war.

The wartime chemists went back to their labs to devise new chemicals for other battles, and the inheritors of Ehrlich's legacy went hunting elsewhere for his specific chemicals. They were looking for a magic bullet that would rid the body of cancer, not a toxic gas that would leave its victims half-dead, blind, blistered, and permanently anemic. That their bullet would eventually appear out of that very chemical weapon seemed like a perversion of specific affinity, a ghoulish distortion of Ehrlich's dream.

Poisoning the Atmosphere

> *What if this mixture do not work at all? . . .*
> *What if it be a poison . . . ?*
> —Romeo and Juliet

> *We shall so poison the atmosphere of the first act that no*
> *one of decency shall want to see the play through to the*
> *end.*
> —James Watson, speaking about
> chemotherapy, 1977

Every drug, the sixteenth-century physician Paracelsus once opined, is a poison in disguise. Cancer chemotherapy, consumed by its fiery obsession to obliterate the cancer cell, found its roots in the obverse logic: every poison might be a drug in disguise.

On December 2, 1943, more than twenty-five years after the yellow-crossed bombs had descended on Ypres, a fleet of Luftwaffe planes flew by a group of American ships huddled in a harbor just outside Bari in southern Italy and released a volley of shells. The ships were instantly on fire. Unbeknown even to its own crew, one of the ships in the fleet, the *John Harvey*, was stockpiled with seventy tons of mustard gas stowed away for possible use. As the *Harvey* blew up, so did its toxic payload. The Allies had, in effect, bombed themselves.

The German raid was unexpected and a terrifying success. Fishermen and residents around the Bari harbor began to complain of the whiff of burnt garlic and horseradishes in the breeze. Grimy, oil-soaked men, mostly young American sailors, were dragged out from the water seizing with pain and terror, their eyes swollen shut. They were given tea and wrapped in blankets, which only trapped the gas closer to their bodies. Of the 617 men rescued, 83 died within the first week. The gas spread quickly over the Bari harbor, leaving an arc of devastation. Nearly a thousand men and women died of complications over the next months.

The Bari "incident," as the media called it, was a terrible political embarrassment for the Allies. The injured soldiers and sailors were swiftly relocated to the States, and medical examiners were secretly flown in to perform autopsies on the dead civilians. The autopsies revealed what the Krumbhaars had noted earlier. In the men and women who had initially survived the bombing but succumbed later to injuries, white blood cells had virtually vanished in their blood, and the bone marrow was scorched and depleted. The gas had specifically targeted bone marrow cells—a grotesque molecular parody of Ehrlich's healing chemicals.

The Bari incident accelerated the effort to investigate war gases and their effects on soldiers. An undercover unit, called the Chemical Warfare Unit (housed within the wartime Office of Scientific Research and Development) was created to study war gases. Contracts for research on various toxic compounds were spread across research institutions around the nation. The contract for investigating nitrogen mustard was issued to two scientists, Louis Goodman and Alfred Gilman, at Yale University.

Goodman and Gilman weren't interested in the "vesicant" properties of mustard gas—its capacity to burn skin and membranes. They were captivated by the Krumbhaar effect—the gas's capacity to decimate white blood cells. Could this effect, or some etiolated cousin of it, be harnessed in a controlled setting, in a hospital, in tiny, monitored doses, to target *malignant* white cells?

To test this concept, Gilman and Goodman began with animal studies. Injected intravenously into rabbits and mice, the mustards made the normal white cells of the blood and bone marrow almost disappear, without producing all the nasty vesicant actions, dissociating the two pharmacological effects. Encouraged, Gilman and Goodman moved on to human studies, focusing on lymphomas—cancers of the lymph glands. In 1942, they persuaded a thoracic surgeon, Gustaf Lindskog, to treat a forty-eight-year-old New York silversmith with lymphoma with ten continuous doses of intravenous mustard. It was a one-off experiment but it worked. In men, as in mice, the drug produced miraculous remissions. The swollen glands disappeared. Clinicians described the phenomenon as an eerie "softening" of the cancer, as if the hard carapace of cancer that Galen had so vividly described nearly two thousand years ago had melted away.

But the responses were followed, inevitably, by relapses. The softened tumors would harden again and recur—just as Farber's leukemias had vanished then reappeared violently. Bound by secrecy during the war years, Goodman and Gilman eventually published their findings in 1946, several months before Farber's paper on antifolates appeared in the press.

ఎౕ

Just a few hundred miles south of Yale, at the Burroughs Wellcome laboratory in New York, the biochemist George Hitchings had also turned to Ehrlich's method to find molecules with a specific ability to kill cancer cells. Inspired by Yella Subbarao's anti-folates, Hitchings focused on synthesizing decoy molecules that when taken up by cells killed them. His first targets were precursors of DNA and RNA. Hitchings's approach was broadly disdained by academic scientists as a "fishing expedition." "Scientists in academia stood disdainfully apart from this kind of activity," a colleague of Hitchings's recalled. "[They] argued that it would be premature to attempt chemotherapy without sufficient basic knowledge about biochemistry, physiology, and pharmacology. In truth, the field had been sterile for thirty-five years or so since Ehrlich's work."

By 1944, Hitchings's fishing expedition had yet to yield a single chemical fish. Mounds of bacterial plates had grown around him like a molding, decrepit garden with still no sign of a promised drug. Almost on instinct, he hired a young assistant named Gertrude Elion, whose future seemed even more precarious than Hitchings's. The daughter of Lithuanian immigrants, born with a precocious scientific intellect and a thirst for chemical knowledge, Elion had completed a master's degree in chemistry from New York University in 1941 while teaching high school science during the day and performing her research for her thesis at night and on weekends. Although highly qualified, talented, and driven, she had been unable to find a job in an academic laboratory. Frustrated by repeated rejections, she had found a position as a supermarket product supervisor. When Hitchings found Trudy Elion, who would soon become one of the most innovative synthetic chemists of her generation (and a future Nobel laureate), she was working for a food lab in New York, testing the acidity of pickles and the color of egg yolk going into mayonnaise.

Rescued from a life of pickles and mayonnaise, Gertrude Elion leapt into synthetic chemistry. Like Hitchings, she started off by hunting for chemicals that could block bacterial growth by inhibiting DNA—but then added her own strategic twist. Instead of sifting through mounds of unknown chemicals at random, Elion focused on one class of compounds, called purines. Purines were ringlike molecules with a central core of six carbon atoms that were known to be involved in the building of DNA. She thought she would add various chemical side chains to each of the six carbon atoms, producing dozens of new variants of purine.

Elion's collection of new molecules was a strange merry-go-round of beasts. One molecule—2,6-diaminopurine—was too toxic at even low doses to give the drug to animals. Another molecule smelled like garlic purified a thousand times. Many were unstable, or useless, or both. But in 1951, Elion found a variant molecule called 6-mercaptopurine, or 6-MP.

6-MP failed some preliminary toxicological tests on animals (the drug is strangely toxic to dogs), and was nearly abandoned. But the success of mustard gas in killing cancer cells had boosted the confidence of early chemotherapists. In 1948, Cornelius "Dusty" Rhoads, a former army officer, left his position as chief of the army's Chemical Warfare Unit to become the director of the Memorial Hospital (and its attached research institute), thus sealing the connection between the chemical warfare of the battlefields and chemical warfare in the body. Intrigued by the cancer-killing properties of poisonous chemicals, Rhoads actively pursued a collaboration between Hitchings and Elion's lab at Burroughs Wellcome and Memorial Hospital. Within months of having been tested on cells in a petri dish, 6-MP was packaged off to be tested in human patients.

Predictably, the first target was acute lymphoblastic leukemia—the rare tumor that now occupied the limelight of oncology. In the early 1950s, two physician-scientists, Joseph Burchenal and Mary Lois Murphy, launched a clinical trial at Memorial to use 6-MP on children with ALL.

Burchenal and Murphy were astonished by the speedy remissions produced by 6-MP. Leukemia cells flickered and vanished in the bone marrow and the blood, often within a few days of treatment. But, like the remissions in Boston, these were disappointingly temporary, lasting only a few weeks. As with the anti-folates, there was only a fleeting glimpse of a cure.

The Goodness of Show Business

The name "Jimmy" is a household word in New England
. . . a nickname for the boy next door.
                         —The House That "Jimmy" Built

I've made a long voyage and been to a strange country,
and I've seen the dark man very close.
                         —Thomas Wolfe

Flickering and feeble, the leukemia remissions in Boston and New York nevertheless mesmerized Farber. If lymphoblastic leukemia, one of the most lethal forms of cancer, could be thwarted by two distinct chemicals (even if only for a month or two), then perhaps a deeper principle was at stake. Perhaps a series of such poisons was hidden in the chemical world, perfectly designed to obliterate cancer cells but spare normal cells. The fingerling of that idea kept knocking in his mind as he paced up and down the wards every evening, writing notes and examining smears late into the night. Perhaps he had stumbled upon an even more provocative principle—that cancer could be cured by chemicals alone.

But how might he jump-start the discovery of these incredible chemicals? His operation in Boston was clearly far too small. How might he create a more powerful platform to propel him toward the cure for childhood leukemia—and then for cancer at large?

Scientists often study the past as obsessively as historians because few other professions depend so acutely on it. Every experiment is a conversation with a prior experiment, every new theory a refutation of the old. Farber, too, studied the past compulsively—and the episode that pivotally fascinated him was the story of the national polio campaign. As a student at Harvard in the 1920s, Farber had witnessed polio epidemics sweeping through the city, leaving waves of paralyzed children in their wake. In the acute phase of polio, the virus can paralyze the diaphragm, making it nearly impossible to breathe. Even a decade later, in the mid-1930s, the only treatment available for this paralysis was an artificial respirator known as the iron lung. As Farber had rounded on the wards of Children's Hospital as a resident, iron lungs had continuously huffed in the background, with children suspended within these dreaded contraptions often for weeks on end. The suspension of patients inside these iron lungs symbolized the limbolike, paralytic state of polio research. Little was known about the nature of the virus or the biology of the infection, and campaigns to control the spread of polio were poorly advertised and generally ignored by the public.

Polio research was shaken out of its torpor by Franklin Roosevelt in 1937. A victim of a prior epidemic, paralyzed from the waist down, Roosevelt had launched a polio hospital and research center, called the Warm Springs Foundation, in Georgia in 1927. At first, his political advisers tried to distance his image from the disease. (A paralyzed president trying to march a nation out of a depression was considered a disastrous image; Roosevelt's public appearances were thus elaborately orchestrated to show him only from the waist up.) But reelected by a staggering margin in 1936, a defiant and resurgent Roosevelt returned to his original cause and launched the National Foundation for Infantile Paralysis, an advocacy group to advance research on and publicize polio.

The foundation, the largest disease-focused association in American history, galvanized polio research. Within one year of its launch, the actor Eddie Cantor created the March of Dimes campaign for the foundation—a massive and highly coordinated national fund-raising effort that asked every citizen to send Roosevelt a dime to support polio education and research. Hollywood celebrities, Broadway stars, and radio personalities soon joined the bandwagon, and the response was dazzling. Within a few weeks, 2,680,000 dimes had poured into the White House. Posters were widely circulated, and money and public attention flooded into polio research. By the late 1940s, funded in part by these campaigns, John Enders had nearly succeeded in culturing poliovirus in his lab, and Sabin and Salk, building on Enders's work, were well on their way to preparing the first polio vaccines.

Farber fantasized about a similar campaign for leukemia, perhaps for cancer in general. He envisioned a foundation for children's cancer that would spearhead the effort. But he needed an ally to help launch the foundation, preferably an ally outside the hospital, where he had few allies.

പ

Farber did not need to look far. In early May 1947, while Farber was still in the middle of his aminopterin trial, a group of men from the Variety Club of New England, led by Bill Koster, toured his laboratory.

Founded in 1927 in Philadelphia by a group of men in show business—producers, directors, actors, entertainers, and film-theater owners—the Variety Club had initially been modeled after the dining clubs of New York and London. But in 1928, just a year after its inception, the club had unwittingly acquired a more active social agenda. In the winter of 1928, with the city teetering on the abyss of the Depression, a woman had abandoned her child at the doorstep of the Sheridan Square Film Theater. A note pinned on the child read:

> *Please take care of my baby. Her name is Catherine. I can no longer take care of her. I have eight others. My husband is out of work. She was born on Thanksgiving Day. I have always heard of the goodness of show business and I pray to God that you will look out for her.*

The cinematic melodrama of the episode, and the heartfelt appeal to the "goodness of show business," made a deep impression on the members of the fledgling club. Adopting the orphan girl, the club paid for her upbringing and education. She was given the name Catherine Variety Sheridan—her middle name for the club and her last name for the theater outside which she had been found.

The Catherine Sheridan story was widely reported in the press and brought more media exposure to the club than its members had ever envisioned. Thrust into the public eye as a philanthropic organization, the club now made children's welfare its project. In the late 1940s, as the boom in postwar moviemaking brought even more money into the club's coffers, new chapters of the club sprouted in cities throughout the nation. Catherine Sheridan's story and her photograph were printed and publicized in club offices throughout the nation. Sheridan became the club's unofficial mascot.

The influx of money and public attention also brought a search for other children's charity projects. Koster's visit to the Children's Hospital in Boston was a scouting mission to find another such project. He was escorted around the hospital to the labs and clinics of prominent doctors. When Koster asked the chief of hematology at Children's for suggestions for donations to the hospital, the chief was characteristically cautious: "Well, I need a new microscope," he said.

In contrast, when Koster stopped by Farber's office, he found an excitable, articulate scientist with a larger-than-life vision—a messiah in a box. Farber didn't want a microscope; he had an audacious telescopic plan that captivated Koster. Farber asked the club to help him create a new fund to build a massive research hospital dedicated to children's cancer.

Farber and Koster got started immediately. In early 1948, they launched an organization called the Children's Cancer Research Fund to jump-start research and advocacy around children's cancers. In March 1948, they organized a raffle to raise money and netted $45,456—an impressive amount to start, but still short of what Farber and Koster hoped for. Cancer research, they felt, needed a more effective message, a strategy to catapult it into public fame. Sometime that spring, Koster, remembering the success with Sheridan, had the inspired idea of finding a "mascot" for Farber's research fund—a Catherine Sheridan for cancer. Koster and Farber searched Children's wards and Farber's clinic for a poster child to pitch the fund to the public.

It was not a promising quest. Farber was treating several children with aminopterin, and the beds in the wards upstairs were filled with miserable patients—dehydrated and nauseated from chemotherapy, children barely able to hold their heads and bodies upright, let alone be paraded publicly as optimistic mascots for cancer treatment. Looking frantically through the patient lists, Farber and Koster found a single child healthy enough to carry the message—a lanky, cherubic, blue-eyed, blond child named Einar Gustafson, who did not have leukemia but was being treated for a rare kind of lymphoma in his intestines.

Gustafson was quiet and serious, a precociously self-assured boy from New Sweden, Maine. His grandparents were Swedish immigrants, and he lived on a potato farm and attended a single-room schoolhouse. In the late summer of 1947, just after blueberry season, he had complained of a gnawing, wrenching pain in his stomach. Doctors in Lewiston, suspecting appendicitis, had operated on his appendix, but found the lymphoma instead. Survival rates for the disease were low at 10 percent. Thinking that chemotherapy had a slight chance to save him, his doctors sent Gustafson to Farber's care in Boston.

Einar Gustafson, though, was a mouthful of a name. Farber and Koster, in a flash of inspiration, rechristened him Jimmy.

♂♀

Koster now moved quickly to market Jimmy. On May 22, 1948, on a warm Saturday night in the Northeast, Ralph Edwards, the host of the radio show *Truth or Consequences,* interrupted his usual broadcast from California and linked to a radio station in Boston. "Part of the function of *Truth or Consequences,*" Edwards began, "is to bring this old parlor game to people who are unable to come to the show. . . . Tonight we take you to a little fellow named Jimmy.

"We are not going to give you his last name because he's just like thousands of other young fellows and girls in private homes and hospitals all over the country. Jimmy is suffering from cancer. He's a swell little guy, and although he cannot figure out why he isn't out with the other kids, he does love his baseball and follows every move of his favorite team, the Boston Braves. Now, by the magic of radio, we're going to span the breadth of the United States and take you right up to the bedside of Jimmy, in one of America's great cities, Boston, Massachusetts, and into one of America's great hospitals, the Children's Hospital in Boston, whose staff is doing such an outstanding job of cancer research. Up to now, Jimmy has not heard us. . . . Give us Jimmy please."

Then, over a crackle of static, Jimmy could be heard.

Jimmy: Hi.
Edwards: Hi, Jimmy! This is Ralph Edwards of the *Truth or Consequences* radio program. I've heard you like baseball. Is that right?
Jimmy: Yeah, it's my favorite sport.
Edwards: It's your favorite sport! Who do you think is going to win the pennant this year?
Jimmy: The Boston Braves, I hope.

After more banter, Edwards sprung the "parlor trick" that he had promised.

Edwards: Have you ever met Phil Masi?
Jimmy: No.
Phil Masi (walking in): Hi, Jimmy. My name is Phil Masi.

Edwards: What? Who's that, Jimmy?

Jimmy (gasping): *Phil Masi!*

Edwards: And where is he?

Jimmy: In my room!

Edwards: Well, what do you know? Right here in your hospital room—Phil Masi from Berlin, Illinois! Who's the best home-run hitter on the team, Jimmy?

Jimmy: Jeff Heath.

(Heath entered the room.)

Edwards: Who's that, Jimmy?

Jimmy: Jeff . . . Heath.

As Jimmy gasped, player after player filed into his room bearing T-shirts, signed baseballs, game tickets, and caps: Eddie Stanky, Bob Elliott, Earl Torgeson, Johnny Sain, Alvin Dark, Jim Russell, Tommy Holmes. A piano was wheeled in. The Braves struck up the song, accompanied by Jimmy, who sang loudly and enthusiastically off-key:

> *Take me out to the ball game,*
> *Take me out with the crowd.*
> *Buy me some peanuts and Cracker Jack,*
> *I don't care if I never get back*

The crowd in Edwards's studio cheered, some noting the poignancy of the last line, many nearly moved to tears. At the end of the broadcast, the remote link from Boston was disconnected. Edwards paused and lowered his voice.

"Now listen, folks. Jimmy can't hear this, can he? . . . We're not using any photographs of him, or using his full name, or he will know about this. Let's make Jimmy and thousands of boys and girls who are suffering from cancer happy by aiding the research to help find a cure for cancer in children. Because by researching children's cancer, we automatically help the adults and stop it at the outset.

"Now we know that one thing little Jimmy wants most is a television set to watch the baseball games as well as hear them. If you and your friends send in your quarters, dollars, and tens of dollars tonight to Jimmy for the Children's Cancer Research Fund, and over two hundred thousand dollars is contributed to this worthy cause, we'll see to it that Jimmy gets his television set."

The Edwards broadcast lasted eight minutes. Jimmy spoke twelve sentences and sang one song. The word *swell* was used five times. Little was said of Jimmy's cancer: it lurked unmentionably in the background, the ghost in the hospital room. The public response was staggering. Even before the Braves had left Jimmy's room that evening, donors had begun to line up outside the lobby of the Children's Hospital. Jimmy's mailbox was inundated with postcards and letters, some of them addressed simply to "Jimmy, Boston, Massachusetts." Some sent dollar bills with their letters or wrote checks; children mailed in pocket money, in quarters and dimes. The Braves pitched in with their own contributions. By May 1948, the $20,000 mark set by Koster had long been surpassed; more than $231,000 had rolled in. Hundreds of red-and-white tin cans for donations for the Jimmy Fund were posted outside baseball games. Cans were passed around in film theaters to collect dimes and quarters. Little League players in baseball uniforms went door-to-door with collection cans on sweltering summer nights. Jimmy Days were held in the small towns throughout New England. Jimmy's promised television—a black-and-white set with a twelve-inch screen set into a wooden box—arrived and was set up on a white bench between hospital beds.

In the fast-growing, fast-consuming world of medical research in 1948, the $231,000 raised by the Jimmy Fund was an impressive, but still modest sum—enough to build a few floors of a new building in Boston, but far from enough to build a national scientific edifice against cancer. In comparison, in 1944, the Manhattan Project spent $100 million every month at the Oak Ridge site. In 1948, Americans spent more than $126 million on Coca-Cola alone.

But to measure the genius of the Jimmy campaign in dollars and cents is to miss its point. For Farber, the Jimmy Fund campaign was an early experiment—the building of another model. The campaign against cancer, Farber learned, was much like a political campaign: it needed icons, mascots, images, slogans—the strategies of advertising as much as the tools of science. For any illness to rise to political prominence, it needed to be marketed, just as a political campaign needed marketing. A disease needed to be transformed politically before it could be transformed scientifically.

If Farber's antifolates were his first discovery in oncology, then this critical truth was his second. It set off a seismic transformation in his career that would far outstrip his transformation from a pathologist to a leukemia doctor. This second transformation—from a clinician into an advocate for cancer research—reflected the transformation of cancer itself. The emergence of cancer from *its* basement into the glaring light of publicity would change the trajectory of this story. It is a metamorphosis that lies at the heart of this book.

The House That Jimmy Built

Etymologically, patient means sufferer. It is not suffering as such that is most deeply feared but suffering that degrades.

—Susan Sontag, *Illness as Metaphor*

Sidney Farber's entire purpose consists only of "hopeless cases."

—*Medical World News*,
November 25, 1966

There was a time when Sidney Farber had joked about the smallness of his laboratory. "One assistant and ten thousand mice," he had called it. In fact, his entire medical life could have been measured in single digits. One room, the size of a chemist's closet, stuffed into the basement of a hospital. One drug, aminopterin, which sometimes briefly extended the life of a child with leukemia. One remission in five, the longest lasting no longer than one year.

By the early months of 1951, however, Farber's work was growing exponentially, moving far beyond the reaches of his old laboratory. His outpatient clinic, thronged by parents and their children, had to be moved outside the hospital to larger quarters in a residential apartment building on the corner of Binney Street and Longwood Avenue. But even the new clinic was soon overloaded. The inpatient wards at Children's had also filled up quickly. Since Farber was considered an intruder by many of the pediatricians at Children's, increasing ward space within the hospital was out of the question. "Most of the doctors thought him conceited and inflexible," a hospital volunteer recalled. At Children's, even if there was space for a few of his bodies, there was no more space for his ego.

Isolated and angry, Farber now threw himself into fund-raising. He needed an entire building to house all his patients. Frustrated in his efforts to galvanize the medical school into building a new cancer center for children, he launched his own effort. He would build a hospital in the face of a hospital.

Emboldened by his early fund-raising success, Farber devised ever-larger drives for research money, relying on his glitzy retinue of Hollywood stars, political barons, sports celebrities, and moneymakers. In 1953, when the Braves franchise left Boston for Milwaukee, Farber and Koster successfully approached the Boston Red Sox to make the Jimmy Fund their official charity.

Farber soon found yet another famous recruit: Ted Williams—a young ballplayer of celluloid glamour—who had just returned after serving in the Korean War. In August 1953, the Jimmy Fund planned a "Welcome Home, Ted" party for Williams, a massive fund-raising bash with a dinner billed at $100 per plate that raised $150,000. By the end of that year, Williams was a regular visitor at Farber's clinic, often trailing a retinue of tabloid photographers seeking pictures of the great ballplayer with a young cancer patient.

The Jimmy Fund became a household name and a household cause. A large, white "piggy bank" for donations (shaped like an enormous baseball) was placed outside the Statler Hotel. Advertisements for the Children's Cancer Research Fund were plastered across billboards throughout Boston. Countless red-and-white collection canisters—called "Jimmy's cans"—sprouted up outside movie theaters. Funds poured in from sources large and small: $100,000 from the NCI, $5,000 from a bean supper in Boston, $111 from a lemonade stand, a few dollars from a children's circus in New Hampshire.

By the early summer of 1952, Farber's new building, a large, solid cube perched on the edge of Binney Street, just off Longwood Avenue, was almost ready. It was lean, functional, and modern—self-consciously distinct from the marbled columns and gargoyles of the hospitals around it. One could see the obsessive hand of Farber in the details. A product of the 1930s, Farber was instinctively frugal ("You can take the child out of the Depression, but you can't take the Depression out of the child," Leonard Lauder liked to say about his generation), but with Jimmy's Clinic, Farber pulled out all the stops. The wide cement steps leading up to the front foyer—graded by only an inch, so that children could easily climb them—

were steam-heated against the brutal Boston blizzards that had nearly stopped Farber's work five winters before.

Upstairs, the clean, well-lit waiting room had whirring carousels and boxes full of toys. A toy electric train, set into a stone "mountain," chugged on its tracks. A television set was embedded on the face of the model mountain. "If a little girl got attached to a doll," *Time* reported in 1952, "she could keep it; there were more where it came from." A library was filled with hundreds of books, three rocking horses, and two bicycles. Instead of the usual portraits of dead professors that haunted the corridors of the neighboring hospitals, Farber commissioned an artist to paint full-size pictures of fairy-book characters—Snow White, Pinocchio, and Jiminy Cricket. It was Disney World fused with Cancerland.

The fanfare and pomp might have led a casual viewer to assume that Farber had almost found his cure for leukemia, and the brand-new clinic was his victory lap. But in truth his goal—a cure for leukemia—still eluded him. His Boston group had now added another drug, a steroid, to their antileukemia regimen, and by assiduously combining steroids and antifolates, the remissions had been stretched out by several months. But despite the most aggressive therapy, the leukemia cells eventually grew resistant and recurred, often furiously. The children who played with the dolls and toy trains in the bright rooms downstairs were inevitably brought back to the glum wards in the hospital, delirious or comatose and in terminal agony.

One woman whose child was treated for cancer in Farber's clinic in the early fifties wrote, "Once I discover that almost all the children I see are doomed to die within a few months, I never cease to be astonished by the cheerful atmosphere that generally prevails. True, upon closer examination, the parents' eyes look suspiciously bright with tears shed and unshed. Some of the children's robust looks, I find, are owing to one of the antileukemia drugs that produces a swelling of the body. And there are children with scars, children with horrible swellings on different parts of their bodies, children missing a limb, children with shaven heads, looking pale and wan, clearly as a result of recent surgery, children limping or in wheelchairs, children coughing, and children emaciated."

Indeed, the closer one looked, the more sharply the reality hit. Ensconced in his new, airy building, with dozens of assistants swirling around him, Farber must have been haunted by that inescapable fact. He was trapped in his own waiting room, still looking for yet another drug to eke out a few more months of remission in his children. His patients—having walked up the fancy steamed stairs to his office, having pranced around on the musical carousel and immersed themselves in the cartoonish gleam of happiness—would die, just as inexorably, of the same kinds of cancer that had killed them in 1947.

But for Farber, the lengthening, deepening remissions bore quite another message: he needed to expand his efforts even further to launch a concerted battle against leukemia. "Acute leukemia," he wrote in 1953, has "responded to a more marked degree than any other form of cancer . . . to the new chemicals that have been developed within the last few years. Prolongation of life, amelioration of symptoms, and a return to a far happier and even a normal life for weeks and many months have been produced by their use."

Farber needed a means to stimulate and fund the effort to find even more powerful antileukemia drugs. "We are pushing ahead as fast as possible," he wrote in another letter—but it was not quite fast enough for him. The money that he had raised in Boston "has dwindled to a disturbingly small amount," he noted. He needed a larger drive, a larger platform, and perhaps a larger vision for cancer. He had outgrown the house that Jimmy had built.

PART TWO

———

AN IMPATIENT WAR

Perhaps there is only one cardinal sin: impatience. Because of impatience we were driven out of Paradise, because of impatience we cannot return.

—Franz Kafka

The 325,000 patients with cancer who are going to die this year cannot wait; nor is it necessary, in order to make great progress in the cure of cancer, for us to have the full solution of all the problems of basic research . . . the history of Medicine is replete with examples of cures obtained years, decades, and even centuries before the mechanism of action was understood for these cures.

—Sidney Farber

Why don't we try to conquer cancer by America's 200th birthday? What a holiday that would be!

—Advertisement published in
the *New York Times* by the Laskerites,
December 1969

"They form a society"

All of this demonstrates why few research scientists are in policy-making positions of public trust. Their training for detail produces tunnel vision, and men of broader perspective are required for useful application of scientific progress.

—Michael Shimkin

I am aware of some alarm in the scientific community that singling out cancer for . . . a direct presidential initiative will somehow lead to the eventual dismantling of the National Institutes of Health. I do not share these feelings. . . . We are at war with an insidious, relentless foe. [We] rightly demand clear decisive action—not endless committee meetings, interminable reviews and tired justifications of the status quo.

—Lister Hill

In 1831, Alexis de Tocqueville, the French aristocrat, toured the United States and was astonished by the obsessive organizational energy of its citizens. "Americans of all ages, all conditions, and all dispositions constantly form associations . . . of a thousand other kinds—religious, moral, serious, futile, general or restricted, enormous or diminutive," Tocqueville wrote. "Americans make associations to give entertainments, to found seminaries, to build inns, to construct churches, to diffuse books, to send missionaries to the antipodes. . . . If it is proposed to inculcate some truth or to foster some feeling by the encouragement of a great example, they form a society."

More than a century after Tocqueville toured the States, as Farber sought to transform the landscape of cancer, he instinctively grasped the truth behind Tocqueville's observation. If visionary changes were best forged by groups of private citizens forming societies, then Farber needed such a coalition to launch a national attack on cancer. This was a journey that he could not begin or finish alone. He needed a colossal force behind him—a force that would far exceed the Jimmy Fund in influence, organization, and money. Real money, and the real power to transform, still lay under congressional control. But prying open vast federal coffers meant deploying the enormous force of a society of private citizens. And Farber knew that this scale of lobbying was beyond him.

There was, he knew, one person who possessed the energy, resources, and passion for this project: a pugnacious New Yorker who had declared it her personal mission to transform the geography of American health through group-building, lobbying, and political action. Wealthy, politically savvy, and well connected, she lunched with the Rockefellers, danced with the Trumans, dined with the Kennedys, and called Lady Bird Johnson by her first name. Farber had heard of her from his friends and donors in Boston. He had run into her during his early political forays in Washington. Her disarming smile and frozen bouffant were as recognizable in the political circles in Washington as in the salons of New York. Just as recognizable was her name: Mary Woodard Lasker.

ℐℛ

Mary Woodard was born in Watertown, Wisconsin, in 1900. Her father, Frank Woodard, was a successful small-town banker. Her mother, Sara Johnson, had emigrated from Ireland in the 1880s, worked as a saleswoman at the Carson's department store in Chicago, and ascended briskly through professional ranks to become one of the highest-paid saleswomen at the store. Salesmanship, as Lasker would later write, was "a natural talent" for Johnson. Johnson had later turned from her work at the department store to lobbying for philanthropic ventures and public projects—selling ideas instead of clothes. She was, as Lasker once put it, a woman who "could sell . . . anything that she wanted to."

Mary Lasker's own instruction in sales began in the early 1920s, when, having graduated from Radcliffe College, she found her first job selling European paintings on commission for a gallery in New York—a cutthroat profession that involved as much social maneuvering as canny business sense. In the mid-1930s, Lasker left the gallery to start an entrepreneurial venture called Hollywood Patterns, which sold simple prefab dress designs to chain stores. Once again, good instincts crisscrossed with good timing. As women joined the workforce in increasing numbers in the 1940s, Lasker's mass-produced professional clothes found a wide market. Lasker emerged from the Depression and the war financially rejuvenated. By the late 1940s, she had grown into an extraordinarily powerful businesswoman, a permanent fixture in the firmament of New York society, a rising social star.

In 1939, Mary Woodard met Albert Lasker, the sixty-year-old president of Lord and Thomas, an advertising firm based in Chicago. Albert Lasker, like Mary Woodard, was considered an intuitive genius in his profession. At Lord and Thomas, he had invented and perfected a new strategy of advertising that he called "salesmanship in print." A successful advertisement, Lasker contended, was not merely a conglomeration of jingles and images designed to seduce consumers into buying an object; rather, it was a masterwork of copywriting that would tell a consumer *why* to buy a product. Advertising was merely a carrier for information and reason, and for the public to grasp its impact, information had to be distilled into its essential elemental form. Each of Lasker's widely successful ad campaigns—for Sunkist oranges, Pepsodent toothpaste, and Lucky Strike cigarettes among many others—highlighted this strategy. In time, a variant of this idea, of advertising as a lubricant of information and of the need to distill information into elemental iconography would leave a deep and lasting impact on the cancer campaign.

Mary and Albert had a brisk romance and a whirlwind courtship, and they were married just fifteen months after they met—Mary for the second time, Albert for the third. Mary Lasker was now forty years old. Wealthy, gracious, and enterprising, she now launched a search for her own philanthropic cause—retracing her mother's conversion from a businesswoman into a public activist.

For Mary Lasker, this search soon turned inward, into her personal life. Three memories from her childhood and adolescence haunted her. In one, she awakes from a terrifying illness—likely a near-fatal bout of bacterial dysentery or pneumonia—febrile and confused, and overhears a family friend say to her mother that she will likely not survive: "Sara, I don't think that you will ever raise her."

In another, she has accompanied her mother to visit her family's laundress in Watertown, Wisconsin. The woman is recovering from surgery for breast cancer—radical mastectomies performed on both breasts. Lasker enters a dark shack with a low, small cot with seven children running around and she is struck by the desolation and misery of the scene. The notion of breasts being excised to stave cancer—"Cut off?" Lasker asks her mother searchingly—puzzles and grips her. The laundress survives; "cancer," Lasker realizes, "can be cruel but it does not need to be fatal."

In the third, she is a teenager in college, and is confined to an influenza ward during the epidemic of 1918. The lethal Spanish flu rages outside, decimating towns and cities. Lasker survives—but the flu will kill six hundred thousand Americans that year, and take nearly fifty million lives worldwide, becoming the deadliest pandemic in history.

A common thread ran through these memories: the devastation of illness—so proximal and threatening at all times—and the occasional capacity, still unrealized, of medicine to transform lives. Lasker imagined unleashing the power of medical research to combat diseases—a power that, she felt, was still largely untapped. In 1939, the year that she met Albert, her life collided with illness again: in Wisconsin, her mother suffered a heart attack and then a stroke, leaving her paralyzed and incapacitated. Lasker wrote to the head of the American Medical Association to inquire about treatment. She was amazed—and infuriated, again—at the lack of knowledge and the unrealized potential of medicine: "I thought that was ridiculous. Other diseases could be treated . . . the sulfa drugs had come into existence. Vitamin deficiencies could be corrected, such as scurvy and pellagra. And I thought there was no good reason why you couldn't do something about stroke, because people didn't universally die of stroke . . . there must be some element that was influential."

In 1940, after a prolonged and unsuccessful convalescence, Lasker's mother died in Watertown. For Lasker, her mother's death brought to a boil the fury and indignation that had been building within her for decades. She had found her mission. "I am opposed to heart attacks and cancer," she would later tell a reporter, "the way one is opposed to sin." Mary Lasker chose to eradicate diseases as some might eradicate sin—through evangelism. If people did not believe in the importance of a national strategy against diseases, she would *convert* them, using every means at her disposal.

Her first convert was her husband. Grasping Mary's commitment to the idea, Albert Lasker became her partner, her adviser, her strategist, her coconspirator. "There are unlimited funds," he told her. "I will show you how to get them." This idea—of transforming the landscape of American medical research using political lobbying and fund-raising at an unprecedented scale—electrified her. The Laskers were professional socialites, in the same way that one can be a professional scientist or a professional athlete; they were extraordinary networkers, lobbyists, minglers, conversers, persuaders, letter writers, cocktail party–throwers, negotiators, name-droppers, deal makers. Fund-raising—and, more important, *friend*-raising—was instilled in their blood, and the depth and breadth of their social connections allowed them to reach deeply into the minds—and pockets—of private donors and of the government.

"If a toothpaste . . . deserved advertising at the rate of two or three or four million dollars a year," Mary Lasker reasoned, "then research against diseases maiming and crippling people in the United States and in the rest of the world deserved hundreds of millions of dollars." Within just a few years, she transformed, as *BusinessWeek* magazine once put it, into "the fairy godmother of medical research."

⁂

The "fairy godmother" blew into the world of cancer research one morning with the force of an unexpected typhoon. In April 1943, Mary Lasker visited the office of Dr. Clarence Cook Little, the director of the American Society for the Control of Cancer in New York. Lasker was interested in finding out what exactly his society was doing to advance cancer research, and how her foundation could help.

The visit left her cold. The society, a professional organization of doctors and a few scientists, was self-contained and moribund, an ossifying Manhattan social club. Of its small annual budget of about $250,000, it spent an even smaller smattering on research programs. Fund-raising was outsourced to an organization called the Women's Field Army, whose volunteers were not represented on the ASCC board. To the Laskers, who were accustomed to massive advertising blitzes and saturated media attention—to "salesmanship in print"—the whole effort seemed haphazard, ineffectual, stodgy, and unprofessional. Lasker was bitingly critical: "Doctors," she wrote, "are not administrators of large amounts of money. They're usually really small businessmen . . . small professional men"—men who clearly lacked a systematic vision for cancer. She made a $5,000 donation to the ASCC and promised to be back.

Lasker quickly got to work on her own. Her first priority was to make a vast public issue out of cancer. Sidestepping major newspapers and prominent magazines, she began with the one outlet of the media that she knew would reach furthest into the trenches of the American psyche: *Reader's Digest*. In October 1943, Lasker persuaded a friend at the *Digest* to run a series of articles on the screening and detection of cancer. Within weeks, the articles set off a deluge of postcards, telegrams, and handwritten notes to the magazine's office, often accompanied by small amounts of pocket money, personal stories, and photographs. A soldier grieving the death of his mother sent in a small contribution: "My mother died from cancer a few years ago. . . . We are living in foxholes in the Pacific theater of war, but would like to help out." A schoolgirl whose grandfather had died of cancer enclosed a dollar bill. Over the next months, the *Digest* received thousands of letters and $300,000 in donations, exceeding the ASCC's entire annual budget.

Energized by the response, Lasker now set about thoroughly overhauling the flailing ASCC in the larger hopes of reviving the flailing effort against cancer. In 1949, a friend wrote to her, "A two-pronged attack on the nation's ignorance of the facts of its health could well be undertaken: a long-range program of joint professional-lay cooperation . . . and a shorter-range pressure group." The ASCC, then, had to be refashioned into this "shorter-range pressure group." Albert Lasker, who joined the ASCC board, recruited Emerson Foote, an advertising executive, to join the society to streamline its organization. Foote, just as horrified by the mildewy workings of the agency as the Laskers, drafted an immediate action plan: he would transform the moribund social club into a highly organized lobbying group. The mandate demanded men of action: businessmen, movie producers, admen, pharmaceutical executives, lawyers—friends and contacts culled from the Laskers' extensive network—rather than biologists, epidemiologists, medical researchers, and doctors. By 1945, the nonmedical representation in the ASCC governing board had vastly increased, edging out its former members. The "Lay Group," as it was called, rechristened the organization the American Cancer Society, or the ACS.

Subtly, although discernibly, the tone of the society changed as well. Under Little, the ASCC had spent its energies drafting insufferably detailed memorandums on standards of cancer care for medical practitioners. (Since there was little treatment to offer, these memoranda were not particularly useful.) Under the Laskers, predictably, advertising and fund-raising efforts began to dominate its agenda. In a single year, it printed 9 million "educational" pieces, 50,000 posters, 1.5 million window stickers, 165,000 coin boxes, 12,000 car cards, and 3,000 window exhibits. The Women's Field Army—the "Ladies' Garden Club," as one Lasker associate scathingly described it—was slowly edged out and replaced by an intense, well-oiled fund-raising machine. Donations shot through the roof: $832,000 in 1944, $4,292,000 in 1945, $12,045,000 in 1947.

Money, and the shift in public visibility, brought inevitable conflicts between the former members and the new ones. Clarence Little, the ASCC president who had once welcomed Lasker into the group, found himself increasingly marginalized by the Lay Group. He complained that the lob-byists and fund-raisers were "unjustified, troublesome and aggressive"— but it was too late. At the society's annual meeting in 1945, after a bitter showdown with the "laymen," he was forced to resign.

With Little deposed and the board replaced, Foote and Lasker were unstoppable. The society's bylaws and constitution were rewritten with nearly vengeful swiftness to accommodate the takeover, once again emphasizing its lobbying and fund-raising activities. In a telegram to Mary Lasker, Jim Adams, the president of the Standard Corporation (and one of the chief instigators of the Lay Group), laid out the new rules, arguably among the more unusual set of stipulations to be adopted by a scientific organization: "The Committee should not include more than four profes-sional and scientific members. The Chief Executive should be a layman."

In those two sentences, Adams epitomized the extraordinary change that had swept through the ACS. The society was now a high-stakes jug-gernaut spearheaded by a band of fiery "laymen" activists to raise money and publicity for a medical campaign. Lasker was the center of this col-lective, its nucleating force, its queen bee. Collectively, the activists began to be known as the "Laskerites" in the media. It was a name that they embraced with pride.

ぷ

In five years, Mary Lasker had raised the cancer society from the dead. Her "shorter-range pressure group" was working in full force. The Laskerites now had their long-range target: Congress. If they could obtain *federal* backing for a War on Cancer, then the scale and scope of their campaign would be astronomically multiplied.

"You were probably the first person to realize that the War against Cancer has to be fought first on the floor of Congress—in order to continue the fight in laboratories and hospitals," the breast cancer patient and activist Rose Kushner once wrote admiringly to Mary Lasker. But cannily, Lasker grasped an even more essential truth: that the fight had to *begin* in the lab before being brought to Congress. She needed yet another ally— someone from the world of science to initiate a fight for science funding. The War on Cancer needed a bona fide scientific sponsor among all the advertisers and lobbyists—a real doctor to legitimize the spin doctors. The person in question would need to understand the Laskerites' political priorities almost instinctually, then back them up with unquestionable and unimpeachable scientific authority. Ideally, he or she would be immersed in cancer research, yet willing to emerge out of that immersion to occupy a much larger national arena. The one man—and perhaps the only man— who could possibly fit the role was Sidney Farber.

In fact, their needs were perfectly congruent: Farber needed a political lobbyist as urgently as the Laskerites needed a scientific strategist. It was like the meeting of two stranded travelers, each carrying one-half of a map.

&

Farber and Mary Lasker met in Washington in late 1940s, not long after Farber had shot to national fame with his antifolates. In the winter of 1948, barely a few months after Farber's paper on antifolates had been published, John Heller, the director of the NCI, wrote to Lasker introducing her to the idea of chemotherapy and to the doctor who had dreamed up the notion in Boston. The idea of chemotherapy—a chemical that could cure cancer outright ("a penicillin for cancer," as the oncologist Dusty Rhoads at Memorial Hospital liked to describe it)—fascinated Lasker. By the early 1950s, she was regularly corresponding with Farber about such drugs. Farber wrote back long, detailed, meandering letters—"scientific treatises," he called them—educating her on his progress in Boston.

For Farber, the burgeoning relationship with Lasker had a cleansing, clarifying quality—"a catharsis," as he called it. He unloaded his scientific knowledge on her, but more important, he also unloaded his scientific and political ambition, an ambition he found easily reflected, even magnified, in her eyes. By the mid-1950s, the scope of their letters had considerably broadened: Farber and Lasker openly broached the possibility of launching an all-out, coordinated attack on cancer. "An organizational pattern is developing at a much more rapid rate than I could have hoped," Farber wrote.

He spoke about his visits to Washington to try to reorganize the National Cancer Institute into a more potent and directed force against cancer.

Lasker was already a "regular on the Hill," as one doctor described her—her face, with its shellacked frieze of hair, and her hallmark gray suit and pearls omnipresent on every committee and focus group related to health care. Farber, too, was now becoming a "regular." Dressed perfectly for his part in a crisp, dark suit, his egghead reading-glasses often perched at the edge of his nose, he was a congressman's spitting image of a physician-scientist. He possessed an "evangelistic pizzazz" for medical science, an observer recalled. "Put a tambourine in [his] hands" and he would immediately "go to work."

To Farber's evangelistic tambourine, Lasker added her own drumbeats of enthusiasm. She spoke and wrote passionately and confidently about her cause, emphasizing her points with quotes and questions. Back in New York, she employed a retinue of assistants to scour newspapers and magazines and clip out articles containing even a passing reference to cancer—all of which she read, annotated on the margins with questions in small, precise script, and distributed to the other Laskerites every week.

"I have written to you so many times in what is becoming a favorite technique—mental telepathy," Farber wrote affectionately to Lasker, "but such letters are never mailed." As acquaintance bloomed into familiarity, and familiarity into friendship, Farber and Lasker struck up a synergistic partnership that would stretch over decades. In the 1950s, Farber began to use the word *crusade* to describe their campaign against cancer. The word was deeply symbolic. For Sidney Farber, as for Mary Lasker, the cancer campaign was indeed turning into a "crusade," a scientific battle imbued with such fanatical intensity that only a religious metaphor could capture its essence. It was as if they had stumbled upon an unshakable, fixed vision of a cure—and they would stop at nothing to drag even a reluctant nation toward it.

"These new friends of chemotherapy"

> The death of a man is like the fall of a mighty nation
> That had valiant armies, captains, and prophets,
> And wealthy ports and ships all over the seas
> But now it will not relieve any besieged city
> It will not enter into an alliance
> —Czeslaw Milosz, "The Fall"

> I had recently begun to notice that events outside science,
> such as Mary Lasker's cocktail parties or Sidney Farber's
> Jimmy Fund, had something to do with the setting of
> science policy.
> —Robert Morison

In 1951, as Farber and Lasker were communicating with "telepathic" intensity about a campaign against cancer, a seminal event drastically altered the tone and urgency of their efforts. Albert Lasker was diagnosed with colon cancer. Surgeons in New York heroically tried to remove the tumor, but the lymph nodes around the intestines were widely involved, and there was little that could be done surgically. By February 1952, Albert was confined to the hospital, numb with the shock of diagnosis and awaiting death.

The sardonic twist of this event could not have escaped the Laskerites. In their advertisements in the late 1940s to raise awareness of cancer, the Laskerites had often pointed out that one in four Americans would succumb to cancer. Albert was now the "one in four"—struck by the very disease that he had once sought to conquer. "It seems a little unfair," one of his close friends from Chicago wrote (with vast understatement), "for someone who has done as much as you have to forward the work in this field to have to suffer personally."

In her voluminous collection of papers—in nearly eight hundred boxes filled with memoirs, letters, notes, and interviews—Mary Lasker left few signs of her response to this terrifying tragedy. Although obsessed with illness, she was peculiarly silent about its corporality, about the vulgarity of dying. There are occasional glimpses of interiority and grief: her visits to the Harkness Pavilion in New York to watch Albert deteriorate into a coma, or letters to various oncologists—including Farber—inquiring about yet another last-ditch drug. In the months before Albert's death, these letters acquired a manic, insistent tone. He had seeded metastasis into the liver, and she searched discreetly, but insistently, for any possible therapy, however far-fetched, that might stay his illness. But for the vast part, there was silence—impenetrable, dense, and impossibly lonely. Mary Lasker chose to descend into melancholy alone.

Albert Lasker died at eight o'clock on the morning of May 30, 1952. A small private funeral was held in the Lasker residence in New York. In his obituary, the *Times* noted, "He was more than a philanthropist, for he gave not only of his substance, but of his experience, ability and strength."

Mary Lasker gradually forged her way back to public life after her husband's death. She returned to her routine of fund-raisers, balls, and benefits. Her social calendar filled up: dances for various medical foundations, a farewell party for Harry Truman, a fund-raiser for arthritis. She seemed self-composed, fiery, and energetic—blazing meteorically into the rarefied atmosphere of New York.

But the person who charged her way back into New York's society in 1953 was fundamentally different from the woman who had left it a year before. Something had broken and annealed within her. In the shadow of Albert's death, Mary Lasker's cancer campaign took on a more urgent and insistent tone. She no longer sought a strategy to *publicize* a crusade against cancer; she sought a strategy to *run* it. "We are at war with an insidious, relentless foe," as her friend Senator Lister Hill would later put it—and a war of this magnitude demanded a relentless, total, unflinching commitment. Expediency must not merely inspire science; it must invade science. To fight cancer, the Laskerites wanted a radically restructured cancer agency, an NCI rebuilt from the ground up, stripped of its bureaucratic excesses, intensely funded, closely supervised—a goal-driven institute that would decisively move toward finding a cancer cure. The national effort against cancer, Mary Lasker believed, had become ad hoc, diffuse, and abstract. To rejuvenate it, it needed the disembodied legacy of Albert

Lasker: a targeted, directed strategy borrowed from the world of business and advertising.

Farber's life also collided with cancer—a collision that he had perhaps presaged for a decade. In the late 1940s, he had developed a mysterious and chronic inflammatory disease of the intestines—likely ulcerative colitis, a debilitating precancerous illness that predisposes the colon and bile duct to cancer. In the mid-1950s (we do not know the precise date), Farber underwent surgery to remove his inflamed colon at Mount Auburn Hospital in Boston, likely choosing the small and private Cambridge hospital across the Charles River to keep his diagnosis and surgery hidden from his colleagues and friends on the Longwood campus. It is also likely that more than just "precancer" was discovered upon surgery—for in later years, Mary Lasker would refer to Farber as a "cancer survivor," without ever divulging the nature of his cancer. Proud, guarded, and secretive—reluctant to conflate his battle against cancer with *the* battle—Farber also pointedly refused to discuss his personal case publicly. (Thomas Farber, his son, would also not discuss it. "I will neither confirm nor deny it," he said, although he admitted that his father lived "in the shadow of illness in his last years"—an ambiguity that I choose to respect.) The only remnant of the colon surgery was a colostomy bag; Farber hid it expertly under his white cuffed shirt and his four-button suit during his hospital rounds.

Although cloaked in secrecy and discretion, Farber's personal confrontation with cancer also fundamentally altered the tone and urgency of his campaign. As with Lasker, cancer was no longer an abstraction for him; he had sensed its shadow flitting darkly over himself. "[It is not] necessary," he wrote, "in order to make great progress in the cure of cancer, for us to have the full solution of all the problems of basic research . . . the history of Medicine is replete with examples of cures obtained years, decades, and even centuries before the mechanism of action was understood for these cures."

"Patients with cancer who are going to die this year cannot wait," Farber insisted. Neither could he or Mary Lasker.

ঔ৲

Mary Lasker knew that the stakes of this effort were enormous: the Laskerites' proposed strategy for cancer ran directly against the grain of the dominant model for biomedical research in the 1950s. The chief architect of the prevailing model was a tall, gaunt, MIT-trained engineer named

Vannevar Bush, who had served as the director of the Office of Scientific Research and Development (OSRD). Created in 1941, the OSRD had played a crucial role during the war years, in large part by channeling American scientific ingenuity toward the invention of novel military technologies for the war. To achieve this, the agency had recruited scientists performing basic research into projects that emphasized "programmatic research." Basic research—diffuse and open-ended inquiry on fundamental questions—was a luxury of peacetime. The war demanded something more urgent and goal-directed. New weapons needed to be manufactured, and new technologies invented to aid soldiers in the battlefield. This was a battle progressively suffused with military technology—a "wizard's war," as newspapers called it—and a cadre of scientific wizards was needed to help America win it.

The "wizards" had wrought astonishing technological magic. Physicists had created sonar, radar, radio-sensing bombs, and amphibious tanks. Chemists had produced intensely efficient and lethal chemical weapons, including the infamous war gases. Biologists had studied the effects of high-altitude survival and seawater ingestion. Even mathematicians, the archbishops of the arcane, had been packed off to crack secret codes for the military.

The undisputed crown jewel of this targeted effort, of course, was the atomic bomb, the product of the OSRD-led Manhattan Project. On August 7, 1945, the morning after the Hiroshima bombing, the New York Times gushed about the extraordinary success of the project: "University professors who are opposed to organizing, planning and directing research after the manner of industrial laboratories . . . have something to think about now. A most important piece of research was conducted on behalf of the Army in precisely the means adopted in industrial laboratories. End result: an invention was given to the world in three years, which it would have taken perhaps half-a-century to develop if we had to rely on primadonna research scientists who work alone. . . . A problem was stated, it was solved by teamwork, by planning, by competent direction, and not by the mere desire to satisfy curiosity."

The congratulatory tone of that editorial captured a general sentiment about science that had swept through the nation. The Manhattan Project had overturned the prevailing model of scientific discovery. The bomb had been designed, as the Times scoffingly put it, not by tweedy "primadonna" university professors wandering about in search of obscure truths (driven by the "mere desire to satisfy curiosity"), but by a focused SWAT team of researchers sent off to accomplish a concrete mission. A new model of scientific governance emerged from the project—research driven by specific mandates, timelines, and goals ("frontal attack" science, to use one scientist's description)—which had produced the remarkable technological boom during the war.

But Vannevar Bush was not convinced. In a deeply influential report to President Truman entitled *Science the Endless Frontier*, first published in 1945, Bush had laid out a view of postwar research that had turned his own model of wartime research on its head: "Basic research," Bush wrote, "is performed without thought of practical ends. It results in general knowledge and an understanding of nature and its laws. This general knowledge provides the means of answering a large number of important practical problems, though it may not give a complete specific answer to any one of them. . . .

"Basic research leads to new knowledge. It provides scientific capital. It creates the fund from which the practical applications of knowledge must be drawn. . . . Basic research is the pacemaker of technological progress. In the nineteenth century, Yankee mechanical ingenuity, building largely upon the basic discoveries of European scientists, could greatly advance the technical arts. Now the situation is different. A nation which depends upon others for its new basic scientific knowledge will be slow in its industrial progress and weak in its competitive position in world trade, regardless of its mechanical skill."

Directed, targeted research—"programmatic" science—the cause célèbre during the war years, Bush argued, was not a sustainable model for the future of American science. As Bush perceived it, even the widely lauded Manhattan Project epitomized the virtues of basic inquiry. True, the bomb was the product of Yankee "mechanical ingenuity." But that mechanical ingenuity stood on the shoulders of scientific discoveries about the fundamental nature of the atom and the energy locked inside it—research performed, notably, with no driving mandate to produce anything resembling the atomic bomb. While the bomb might have come to life physically in Los Alamos, intellectually speaking it was the product of prewar physics and chemistry rooted deeply in Europe. The iconic homegrown product of wartime American science was, at least philosophically speaking, an import.

A lesson Bush had learned from all of this was that goal-directed strategies, so useful in wartime, would be of limited use during periods of peace. "Frontal attacks" were useful on the war front, but postwar science could not be produced by fiat. So Bush had pushed for a radically inverted model of scientific development, in which researchers were allowed full autonomy over their explorations and open-ended inquiry was prioritized.

The plan had a deep and lasting influence in Washington. The National Science Foundation (NSF), founded in 1950, was explicitly created to encourage scientific autonomy, turning in time, as one historian put it, into a veritable "embodiment [of Bush's] grand design for reconciling government money and scientific independence." A new culture of research—"long-term, basic scientific research rather than sharply focused quests for treatment and disease prevention"—rapidly proliferated at the NSF and subsequently at the NIH.

*

For the Laskerites, this augured a profound conflict. A War on Cancer, they felt, demanded precisely the sort of focus and undiluted commitment that had been achieved so effectively at Los Alamos. World War II had clearly surcharged medical research with new problems and new solutions; it had prompted the development of novel resuscitation techniques, research on blood and frozen plasma, on the role of adrenal steroids in shock and on cerebral and cardiac blood flow. Never in the history of medicine, as A. N. Richards, the chairman of the Committee on Medical Research, put it, had there been "so great a coordination of medical scientific labor."

This sense of common purpose and coordination galvanized the Laskerites: they wanted a Manhattan Project for cancer. Increasingly, they felt that it was no longer necessary to wait for fundamental questions about cancer to be solved before launching an all-out attack on the problem. Farber had, after all, forged his way through the early leukemia trials with scarcely any foreknowledge of how aminopterin worked even in *normal* cells, let alone cancer cells. Oliver Heaviside, an English mathematician from the 1920s, once wrote jokingly about a scientist musing at a dinner table, "Should I refuse my dinner because I don't understand the digestive system?" To Heaviside's question, Farber might have added his own: should I refuse to attack cancer because I have not solved its basic cellular mechanisms?

Other scientists echoed this frustration. The outspoken Philadelphia pathologist Stanley Reimann wrote, "Workers in cancer must make every effort to organize their work with goals in view not just because they are 'interesting' but because they will help in the solution of the cancer problem." Bush's cult of open-ended, curiosity-driven inquiry—"interesting" science—had ossified into dogma. To battle cancer, that dogma needed to be overturned.

The first, and most seminal, step in this direction was the creation of a focused drug-discovery unit for anticancer drugs. In 1954, after a furious bout of political lobbying by Laskerites, the Senate authorized the NCI to build a program to find chemotherapeutic drugs in a more directed, targeted manner. By 1955, this effort, called the Cancer Chemotherapy National Service Center (CCNSC), was in full swing. Between 1954 and 1964, this unit would test 82,700 synthetic chemicals, 115,000 fermentation products, and 17,200 plant derivatives and treat nearly 1 million mice every year with various chemicals to find an ideal drug.

Farber was ecstatic, but impatient. "The enthusiasm . . . of these new friends of chemotherapy is refreshing and seems to be on a genuine foundation," he wrote to Lasker in 1955. "It nevertheless seems frightfully slow. It sometimes becomes monotonous to see more and more men brought into the program go through the joys of discovering America."

જ

Farber had, meanwhile, stepped up his own drug-discovery efforts in Boston. In the 1940s, the soil microbiologist Selman Waksman had systematically scoured the world of soil bacteria and purified a diverse series of antibiotics. (Like the *Penicillium* mold, which produces penicillin, bacteria also produce antibiotics to wage chemical warfare on other microbes.) One such antibiotic came from a rod-shaped microbe called *Actinomyces*. Waksman called it actinomycin D. An enormous molecule shaped like an ancient Greek statue, with a small, headless torso and two extended wings, actinomycin D was later found to work by binding and damaging DNA. It potently killed bacterial cells—but unfortunately it also killed human cells, limiting its use as an antibacterial agent.

But a cellular poison could always excite an oncologist. In the summer of 1954, Farber persuaded Waksman to send him a number of antibiotics, including actinomycin D, to repurpose them as antitumor agents by testing the drugs on a series of mouse tumors. Actinomycin D, Farber found, was remarkably effective in mice. Just a few doses melted away many mouse cancers, including leukemias, lymphomas, and breast cancers. "One hesitates to call them 'cures,'" Farber wrote expectantly, "but it is hard to classify them otherwise."

Energized by the animal "cures," in 1955 he launched a series of trials to evaluate the efficacy of the drug in humans. Actinomycin D had no effect on leukemias in children. Undeterred, Farber unleashed the drug on 275 children with a diverse range of cancers: lymphomas, kidney sarcomas, muscle sarcomas, and neuroblastic tumors. The trial was a pharmacist's nightmare. Actinomycin D was so toxic that it had to be heavily diluted in saline; if even minute amounts leaked out of the veins, then the skin around the leak would necrose and turn black. In children with small veins, the drug was often given through an intravenous line inserted into the scalp.

The one form of cancer that responded in these early trials was Wilms' tumor, a rare variant of kidney cancer. Often detected in very young children, Wilms' tumor was typically treated by surgical removal of the affected kidney. Surgical removal was followed by X-ray radiation to the affected kidney bed. But not all Wilms' cases could be treated using local therapy. In a fraction of cases, by the time the tumor was detected, it had already metastasized, usually to the lungs. Recalcitrant to treatment there, Wilms' tumors were usually bombarded with X-rays and assorted drugs but with little hopes of a sustained response.

Farber found that actinomycin D, administered intravenously, potently inhibited the growth of these lung metastases, often producing remissions that lasted months. Intrigued, he pressed further. If X-rays and actinomycin D could both attack Wilms' metastases independently, what if the agents could be combined? In 1958, he set a young radiologist couple named Giulio D'Angio and Audrey Evans and an oncologist named Donald Pinkel to work on the project. Within months, the team had confirmed that X-rays and actinomycin D were remarkably synergistic, each multiplying the toxic effect of the other. Children with metastatic cancer treated with the combined regimen often responded briskly. "In about three weeks lungs previously riddled with Wilms' tumor metastasis cleared completely," D'Angio recalled. "Imagine the excitement of those days when one could say for the first time with justifiable confidence, 'We can fix that.'"

The enthusiasm generated by these findings was infectious. Although combination X-ray and chemotherapy did not always produce long-term cures, Wilms' tumor was the first metastatic solid tumor to respond to chemotherapy. Farber had achieved his long-sought leap from the world of liquid cancers to solid tumors.

∂∫∂

By the late 1950s, Farber was bristling with a fiery brand of optimism. Yet visitors to the Jimmy Fund clinic in the mid-1950s might have witnessed a more nuanced and complex reality. For Sonja Goldstein, whose two-year-old son, David, was treated with chemotherapy for Wilms' tumor in 1956, the clinic seemed perpetually suspended between two poles—both "wonderful and tragic . . . unspeakably depressing and indescribably hopeful." On entering the cancer ward, Goldstein would write later, "I sense an undercurrent of excitement, a feeling (persistent despite repeated frustrations) of being on the verge of discovery, which makes me almost hopeful.

"We enter a large hall decorated with a cardboard train along one wall. Half way down the ward is an authentic-looking stop sign, which can flash green, red, and amber lights. The train's engine can be climbed into and the bell pulled. At the other end of the ward is a life-size gasoline pump, registering amount sold and price. . . . My first impression is one of overweening activity, almost snake pit-like in its intensity."

It was a snake-pit—only of cancer, a seething, immersed box coiled with illness, hope, and desperation. A girl named Jenny, about four years old, played with a new set of crayons in the corner. Her mother, an attractive, easily excitable woman, kept Jenny in constant sight, holding her child with the clawlike intensity of her gaze as Jenny stooped to pick up the colors. No activity was innocent here; anything might be a sign, a symptom, a portent. Jenny, Goldstein realized, "has leukemia and is currently in the hospital because she developed jaundice. Her eyeballs are still yellow"—presaging fulminant liver failure. She, like many of the ward's inhabitants, was relatively oblivious to the meaning of her illness. Jenny's only concern was an aluminum teakettle to which she was deeply attached.

"Sitting in a go-cart in the hall is a little girl, who, I think at first, has been given a black eye. . . . Lucy, a 2-year old, suffers from a form of cancer that spreads to the area behind the eye and causes hemorrhaging there. She is not a very attractive child, and wails almost incessantly that first day. So does Debbie, an angelic-looking 4-year old whose face is white and frowning with suffering. She has the same type of tumor as Lucy—a neuroblastoma. Alone in a room lies Teddy. It takes many days before I venture inside it, for, skeleton-thin and blinded, Teddy has a monstrosity for a face. His tumor, starting behind the ear, has engulfed one side of his head and obliterated his normal features. He is fed through a tube in the nostril, and is fully conscious."

Throughout the ward were little inventions and improvisations, often devised by Farber himself. Since the children were usually too exhausted to walk, tiny wooden go-carts were scattered about the room so that the patients could move around with relative freedom. IV poles for chemotherapy were strung up on the carts to allow chemo to be given at all times during the day. "To me," Goldstein wrote, "one of the most pathetic sights of all that I have seen is the little go-cart, with the little child, leg or arm tightly bandaged to hold needle in vein, and a tall IV pole with its burette. The combined effect is that of a boat with mast but no sail, helplessly drifting alone in a rough, uncharted sea."

ঔ

Every evening, Farber came to the wards, forcefully driving his own sailless boat through this rough and uncharted sea. He paused at each bed, taking notes and discussing the case, often barking out characteristically brusque instructions. A retinue followed him: medical residents, nurses, social workers, psychiatrists, nutritionists, and pharmacists. Cancer, he insisted, was a total disease—an illness that gripped patients not just physically, but psychically, socially, and emotionally. Only a multipronged, multidisciplinary attack would stand any chance of battling this disease. He called the concept "total care."

But despite all efforts at providing "total care," death stalked the wards relentlessly. In the winter of 1956, a few weeks after David's visit, a volley of deaths hit Farber's clinic. Betty, a child with leukemia, was the first to die. Then it was Jenny, the four-year-old with the aluminum teakettle. Teddy, with retinoblastoma, was next. A week later, Axel, another child with leukemia, bled to death, with hemorrhages in his mouth. Goldstein observed, "Death assumes shape, form, and routine. Parents emerge from their child's room, as they have perhaps done periodically for days for short rests. A nurse takes them to the doctor's small office; the doctor comes in and shuts the door behind him. Later, a nurse brings coffee. Still later, she hands the parents a large brown paper bag, containing odds and ends of belongings. A few minutes later, back at our promenade, we note another empty bed. *Finish.*"

In the winter of 1956, after a prolonged and bruising battle, Sonja's son, three-year-old David Goldstein, died of metastatic Wilms' tumor at the Jimmy Fund clinic, having spent the last few hours of his life delirious and whimpering under an oxygen mask. Sonja Goldstein left the hospital carrying her own brown paper bag containing the remains of her child.

But Farber was unfazed. The arsenal of cancer chemotherapy, having been empty for centuries, had filled up with new drugs. The possibilities thrown open by these discoveries were enormous: permutations and combinations of medicines, variations in doses and schedules, trials containing two-, three-, and four-drug regimens. There was, at least in principle, the capacity to re-treat cancer with one drug if another had failed, or to try one combination followed by another. This, Farber kept telling himself with hypnotic conviction, was not the "*finish.*" This was just the beginning of an all-out attack.

ॐ

In her hospital bed on the fourteenth floor, Carla Reed was still in "isolation"—trapped in a cool, sterile room where even the molecules of air arrived filtered through dozens of sieves. The smell of antiseptic soap pervaded her clothes. A television occasionally flickered on and off. Food came on a tray labeled with brave, optimistic names—Chunky Potato Salad or Chicken Kiev—but everything tasted as if it had been boiled and seared almost to obliteration. (It had been; the food had to be sterilized before it could enter the room.) Carla's husband, a computer engineer, came in every afternoon to sit by her bed. Ginny, her mother, spent the days rocking mechanically in a chair, exactly as I had found her the first morning. When Carla's children stopped by, in masks and gloves, she wept quietly, turning her face toward the window.

For Carla, the physical isolation of those days became a barely concealed metaphor for a much deeper, fiercer loneliness, a psychological quarantine even more achingly painful than her actual confinement. "In those first two weeks, I withdrew into a different person," she said. "What went into the room and what came out were two different people.

"I thought over and over again about my chances of surviving through all this. Thirty percent. I would repeat that number to myself at night. Not even a third. I would stay up at night looking up at the ceiling and think: What *is* thirty percent? What happens thirty percent of the time? I am thirty years old—about thirty percent of ninety. If someone gave me thirty percent odds in a game, would I take the odds?"

The morning after Carla had arrived at the hospital, I walked into her room with sheaves of paper. They were consent forms for chemotherapy that would allow us to instantly start pumping poisons into her body to kill cancer cells.

Chemotherapy would come in three phases. The first phase would last about a month. The drugs—given in rapid-fire succession—would hopefully send the leukemia into a sustained remission. They would certainly kill her normal white blood cells as well. Her white cell count would drop in free fall, all the way to zero. For a few critical days, she would inhabit one of the most vulnerable states that modern medicine can produce: a body with no immune system, defenseless against the environment around it.

If the leukemia did go into remission, then we would "consolidate" and intensify that remission over several months. That would mean more chemotherapy, but at lower doses, given over longer intervals. She would be able to leave the hospital and return home, coming back every week for more chemotherapy. Consolidation and intensification would last for eight additional weeks, perhaps longer.

The worst part, perhaps, I kept for last. Acute lymphoblastic leukemia has an ugly propensity for hiding in the brain. The intravenous chemotherapy that we would give Carla, no matter how potent, simply couldn't break into the cisterns and ventricles that bathed her brain. The blood-brain barrier essentially made the brain into a "sanctuary" (an unfortunate word, implying that your own body could be abetting the cancer) for the leukemia cells. To send drugs directly into that sanctuary, the medicines would need to be injected directly into Carla's spinal fluid, through a series of spinal taps. Whole-brain radiation treatment—highly penetrant X-rays dosed directly through her skull—would also be used prophylactically against leukemia growth in her brain. And there would be even more chemotherapy to follow, spanning over two years, to "maintain" the remission if we achieved it.

Induction. Intensification. Maintenance. Cure. An arrow in pencil connecting the four points on a blank piece of paper. Carla nodded.

When I went through the avalanche of chemotherapy drugs that would be used over the next two years to treat her, she repeated the names softly after me under her breath, like a child discovering a new tongue twister: "Cyclophosphamide, cytarabine, prednisone, asparaginase, Adriamycin, thioguanine, vincristine, 6-mercaptopurine, methotrexate."

"The butcher shop"

Randomised screening trials are bothersome. It takes
ages to come to an answer, and these need to be large-
scale projects to be able to answer the questions. [But . . .]
there is no second-best option.
—H. J. de Koning,
Annals of Oncology, 2003

The best [doctors] seem to have a sixth sense about
disease. They feel its presence, know it to be there,
perceive its gravity before any intellectual process can
define, catalog, and put it into words. Patients sense
this about such a physician as well: that he is attentive,
alert, ready; that he cares. No student of medicine should
miss observing such an encounter. Of all the moments
in medicine, this one is most filled with drama, with
feeling, with history.
—Michael LaCombe,
Annals of Internal Medicine, 1993

It was in Bethesda, at the very institute that had been likened to a sub-urban golfing club in the 1940s, that the new arsenal of oncology was deployed on living patients.

In April 1955, in the midst of a humid spring in Maryland, a freshly recruited researcher at the National Cancer Institute named Emil Freireich walked up to his new office in the redbrick Clinical Center Building and found, to his exasperation, that his name had been misspelled on the door, with the last five letters lopped off. The plate on the door read EMIL FREI, MD. "My first thought, of course, was: Isn't it typical of the government?"

It wasn't a misspelling. When Freireich entered the office, he confronted a tall, thin young man who identified himself as Emil *Frei*. Freireich's office, with the name correctly spelled, was next door.

Their names notwithstanding, the two Emils were vastly different characters. Freireich—just thirty-five years old and fresh out of a hematology fellowship at Boston University—was flamboyant, hot-tempered, and adventurous. He spoke quickly, often explosively, with a booming voice followed often by an even more expressive boom of laughter. He had been a medical intern at the fast-paced "Ward 55" of the Cook County Hospital in Chicago—and such a nuisance to the authorities that he had been released from his contract earlier than usual. In Boston, Freireich had worked with Chester Keefer, one of Minot's colleagues who had subsequently spearheaded the production of penicillin during World War II. Antibiotics, folic acid, vitamins, and antifolates were stitched into Freireich's soul. He admired Farber intensely—not just the meticulous, academic scientist, but the irreverent, impulsive, larger-than-life Farber who could antagonize his enemies as quickly as he could seduce his benefactors. "I have never seen Freireich in a moderate mood," Frei would later say.

If Freireich had been a character in a film, he would have needed a cinematic foil, a Laurel to his Hardy or a Felix to his Oscar. The tall, thin man who confronted him at the door at the NCI that afternoon was that foil. Where Freireich was brusque and flamboyant, impulsive to a fault, and passionate about every detail, Frei was cool, composed, and cautious, a poised negotiator who preferred to work backstage. Emil Frei—known to most of his colleagues by his nickname, Tom—had been an art student in St. Louis in the thirties. He had attended medical school almost as an afterthought in the late 1940s, served in the navy in the Korean War, and returned to St. Louis as a resident in medicine. He was charming, soft-spoken, and careful—a man of few, chosen words. To watch him manage critically ill children and their testy, nervous parents was to watch a champion swimmer glide through water—so adept in the art that he made artistry vanish.

৵৸

The person responsible for bringing the two Emils to Bethesda was Gordon Zubrod, the new director of the NCI's Clinical Center. Intellectual, deliberate, and imposing, a clinician and scientist known for his regal composure, Zubrod had arrived at the NIH having spent nearly a decade developing antimalaria drugs during World War II, an experience that would deeply influence his early interests in clinical trials for cancer.

Zubrod's particular interest was children's leukemia—the cancer that Farber had plunged into the very forefront of clinical investigation. But to contend with leukemia, Zubrod knew, was to contend with its fieriness and brittleness, its moody, volcanic unpredictability. Drugs could be tested, but first, the children needed to be kept alive. A quintessential delegator—an "Eisenhower" of cancer research, as Freireich once called him—Zubrod quickly conscripted two young doctors to maintain the front lines of the wards: Freireich and Frei, fresh from their respective fellowships in Boston and St. Louis. Frei drove cross-country in a beat-up old Studebaker to join Zubrod. Freireich came just a few weeks later, in a ramshackle Oldsmobile containing all his belongings, his pregnant wife, and his nine-month-old daughter.

It could easily have been a formula for disaster—but it worked. Right from the start, the two Emils found that they shared a unique synergy. Their collaboration was symbolic of a deep intellectual divide that ran through the front lines of oncology: the rift between overmoderated caution and bold experimentation. Each time Freireich pushed too hard on one end of the experimental fulcrum—often bringing himself and his patients to the brink of disaster—Frei pushed back to ensure that the novel, quixotic, and often deeply toxic therapies were mitigated by caution. Frei and Freireich's battles soon became emblematic of the tussles within the NCI. "Frei's job," one researcher recalled, "in those days was to keep Freireich from getting in trouble."

ॐ

Zubrod had his own schemes to keep leukemia research out of trouble. As new drugs, combinations, and trials proliferated, Zubrod worried that institutions would be caught at cross-purposes, squabbling over patients and protocols when they should really be battling cancer. Burchenal in New York, Farber in Boston, James Holland at Roswell Park, and the two Emils at the NCI were all chomping at the bit to launch clinical trials. And since ALL was a rare disease, every patient was a precious resource for a leukemia trial. To avert conflicts, Zubrod proposed that a "consortium" of researchers be created to share patients, trials, data, and knowledge.

The proposal changed the field. "Zubrod's cooperative group model galvanized cancer medicine," Robert Mayer (who would later become the chair of one of these groups) recalls. "For the first time, an academic oncologist felt as if he had a community. The cancer doctor was not the outcast anymore, not the man who prescribed poisons from some underground chamber in the hospital." The first group meeting, chaired by Farber, was a resounding success. The researchers agreed to proceed with a series of common trials, called protocols, as soon as possible.

Zubrod next set about organizing the process by which trials could be run. Cancer trials, he argued, had thus far been embarrassingly chaotic and disorganized. Oncologists needed to emulate the best trials in medicine. And to learn how to run objective, unbiased, state-of-the-art clinical trials, they would need to study the history of the development of antibiotics.

In the 1940s, as new antibiotics had begun to appear on the horizon, physicians had encountered an important quandary: how might one objectively test the efficacy of any novel drug? At the Medical Research Council in Britain, the question had taken on a particularly urgent and rancorous note. The discovery of streptomycin, a new antimicrobial drug in the early forties, had set off a flurry of optimism that tuberculosis could be cured. Streptomycin killed tuberculosis-causing mycobacteria in petri dishes, but its efficacy in humans was unknown. The drug was in critically short supply, with doctors parrying to use even a few milligrams of it to treat a variety of other infections. To ration streptomycin, an objective experiment to determine its efficacy in human tuberculosis was needed.

But what sort of experiment? An English statistician named Bradford Hill (a former victim of TB himself) proposed an extraordinary solution. Hill began by recognizing that doctors, of all people, could not be entrusted to perform such an experiment without inherent biases. Every biological experiment requires a "control" arm—untreated subjects against whom the efficacy of a treatment can be judged. But left to their own devices, doctors were inevitably likely (even if unconsciously so) to select certain types of patients upfront, then judge the effects of a drug on this highly skewed population using subjective criteria, piling bias on top of bias.

Hill's proposed solution was to remove such biases by *randomly* assigning patients to treatment with streptomycin versus a placebo. By "randomizing" patients to each arm, any doctors' biases in patient assignment would be dispelled. Neutrality would be enforced—and thus a hypothesis could be strictly tested.

Hill's randomized trial was a success. The streptomycin arm of the trial clearly showed an improved response over the placebo arm, enshrining the antibiotic as a new anti-TB drug. But perhaps more important, it was Hill's methodological invention that was permanently enshrined. For medical scientists, the randomized trial became the most stringent means to evaluate the efficacy of any intervention in the most unbiased manner.

Zubrod was inspired by these early antimicrobial trials. He had used these principles in the late 1940s to test antimalarials, and he proposed using them to lay down the principles by which the NCI would test its new protocols. The NCI's trials would be systematic: every trial would test a crucial piece of logic or hypothesis and produce yes and no answers. The trials would be sequential: the lessons of one trial would lead to the next and so forth—a relentless march of progress until leukemia had been cured. The trials would be objective, randomized if possible, with clear, unbiased criteria to assign patients and measure responses.

✑

Trial methodology was not the only powerful lesson that Zubrod, Frei, and Freireich learned from the antimicrobial world. "The analogy of drug resistance to antibiotics was given deep thought," Freireich remembered. As Farber and Burchenal had discovered to their chagrin in Boston and New York, leukemia treated with a single drug would inevitably grow resistant to the drug, resulting in the flickering, transient responses followed by the devastating relapses.

The situation was reminiscent of TB. Like cancer cells, mycobacteria— the germs that cause tuberculosis—also became resistant to antibiotics if the drugs were used singly. Bacteria that survived a single-drug regimen divided, mutated, and acquired drug resistance, thus making that original drug useless. To thwart this resistance, doctors treating TB had used a blitzkrieg of antibiotics—two or three used together like a dense pharmaceutical blanket meant to smother all cell division and stave off bacterial resistance, thus extinguishing the infection as definitively as possible.

But could two or three drugs be tested simultaneously against cancer— or would the toxicities be so forbidding that they would instantly kill patients? As Freireich, Frei, and Zubrod studied the growing list of antileukemia drugs, the notion of combining drugs emerged with growing clarity: toxicities notwithstanding, annihilating leukemia might involve using a combination of two or more drugs.

The first protocol was launched to test different doses of Farber's methotrexate combined with Burchenal's 6-MP, the two most active antileukemia drugs. Three hospitals agreed to join: the NCI, Roswell Park, and the Children's Hospital in Buffalo, New York. The aims of the trial were kept intentionally simple. One group would be treated with intensive methotrexate dosing, while the other group would be treated with milder and less intensive dosing. Eighty-four patients enrolled. On arrival day, parents of the children were handed white envelopes with the randomized assignment sealed inside.

Despite the multiple centers and the many egos involved, the trial ran surprisingly smoothly. Toxicities multiplied; the two-drug regimen was barely tolerable. But the intensive group fared better, with longer and more durable responses. The regimen, though, was far from a cure: even the intensively treated children soon relapsed and died by the end of one year.

Protocol I set an important precedent. Zubrod's and Farber's cherished model of a cancer cooperative group was finally in action. Dozens of doctors, nurses, and patients in three independent hospitals had yoked themselves to follow a single formula to treat a group of patients—and each one, suspending its own idiosyncrasies, had followed the instructions perfectly. "This work is one of the first comparative studies in the chemotherapy of malignant neoplastic disease," Frei noted. In a world of ad hoc, often desperate strategies, conformity had finally come to cancer.

In the winter of 1957, the leukemia group launched yet another modification to the first experiment. This time, one group received a combined regimen, while the other two groups were given one drug each. And with the question even more starkly demarcated, the pattern of responses was even clearer. Given alone, either of the drugs performed poorly, with a response rate between 15 and 20 percent. But when methotrexate and 6-MP were administered together, the remission rate jumped to 45 percent.

The next chemotherapy protocol, launched just two years later in 1959, ventured into even riskier territory. Patients were treated with two drugs to send them into complete remission. Then half the group received several months of additional drugs, while the other group was given a placebo. Once again, the pattern was consistent. The more aggressively treated group had longer and more durable responses.

Trial by trial, the group crept forward, like a spring uncoiling to its end. In just six pivotal years, the leukemia study group had slowly worked itself to giving patients not one or two, but four chemotherapy drugs, often in succession. By the winter of 1962, the compass of leukemia medicine pointed unfailingly in one direction. If two drugs were better than one, and if three better than two, then what if four antileukemia drugs could be given *together*—in combination, as with TB?

Both Frei and Freireich sensed that this was the inevitable culmination of the NCI's trials. But even if they knew it subconsciously, they tiptoed around the notion for months. "The resistance would be fierce," Freireich knew. The leukemia ward was already being called a "butcher shop" by others at the NCI. "The idea of treating children with three or four highly cytotoxic drugs was considered cruel and insane," Freireich said. "Even Zubrod could not convince the consortium to try it. No one wanted to turn the NCI into a National Institute of Butchery."

An Early Victory

. . . But I do subscribe to the view that words have very powerful texts and subtexts. "War" has truly a unique status, "war" has a very special meaning. It means putting young men and women in situations where they might get killed or grievously wounded. It's inappropriate to retain that metaphor for a scholarly activity in these times of actual war. The NIH is a community of scholars focused on generating knowledge to improve the public health. That's a great activity. That's not a war.

—Samuel Broder, NCI director

In the midst of this nervy deliberation about the use of four-drug combination therapy, Frei and Freireich received an enormously exciting piece of news. Just a few doors down from Freireich's office at the NCI, two researchers, Min Chiu Li and Roy Hertz, had been experimenting with choriocarcinoma, a cancer of the placenta. Even rarer than leukemia, choriocarcinoma often grows out of the placental tissue surrounding an abnormal pregnancy, then metastasizes rapidly and fatally into the lung and the brain. When it occurs, choriocarcinoma is thus a double tragedy: an abnormal pregnancy compounded by a lethal malignancy, birth tipped into death.

If cancer chemotherapists were generally considered outsiders by the medical community in the 1950s, then Min Chiu Li was an outsider even among outsiders. He had come to the United States from Mukden University in China, then spent a brief stint at the Memorial Hospital in New York. In a scramble to dodge the draft during the Korean War, he had finagled a two-year position in Hertz's service as an assistant obstetrician. He was interested in research (or at least feigned interest), but Li was considered an intellectual fugitive, unable to commit to any one question or plan. His current plan was to lie low in Bethesda until the war blew over.

But what had started off as a decoy fellowship for Li turned, within a single evening in August 1956, into a full-time obsession. On call late one evening, he tried to medically stabilize a woman with metastatic chorio-carcinoma. The tumor was in its advanced stages and bled so profusely that the patient died in front of Li's eyes in three hours. Li had heard of Farber's antifolates. Almost instinctually, he had made a link between the rapidly dividing leukemia cells in the bone marrow of the children in Boston and the rapidly dividing placental cells in the women in Bethesda. Antifolates had never been tried in this disease, but if the drugs could stop aggressive leukemias from growing—even if temporarily—might they not at least partially relieve the eruptions of choriocarcinoma?

Li did not have to wait long. A few weeks after the first case, another patient, a young woman called Ethel Longoria, was just as terrifyingly ill as the first patient. Her tumors, growing in grapelike clusters in her lungs, had begun to bleed into the linings of her lungs—so fast that it had become nearly impossible to keep up with the blood loss. "She was bleed-ing so rapidly," a hematologist recalled, "that we thought we might trans-fuse her back with her own blood. So [the doctors] scrambled around and set up tubes to collect the blood that she had bled and put it right back into her, like an internal pump." (The solution bore the quintessen-tial mark of the NCI. Transfusing a person with blood leaking out from her own tumor would have been considered extraordinary, even repulsive, elsewhere, but at the NCI, this strategy—*any* strategy—was par for the course.) "They stabilized her and then started antifolates. After the first dose, when the doctors left for the night, they didn't expect that they'd find her in rounds the next morning. At the NCI, you didn't expect. You just waited and watched and took surprises as they came."

Ethel Longoria hung on. At rounds the next morning, she was still alive, breathing slowly but deeply. The bleeding had now abated to the point that a few more doses could be tried. At the end of four rounds of chemotherapy, Li and Hertz expected to see minor changes in the size of the tumors. What they found, instead, left them flabbergasted: "The tumor masses disappeared, the chest X-ray improved, and the patient looked normal," Freireich wrote. The level of choriogonadotropin, the hormone secreted by the cancer cells, rapidly plummeted toward zero. The tumors had actually vanished. No one had ever seen such a response. The X-rays, thought to have been mixed up, were sent down for reexamination. The response was real: a metastatic, solid cancer had vanished with chemotherapy. Jubilant, Li and Hertz rushed to publish their findings.

❧

But there was a glitch in all this—an observation so minor that it could easily have been brushed away. Choriocarcinoma cells secrete a marker, a hormone called choriogonadotropin, a protein that can be measured with an extremely sensitive test in the blood (a variant of this test is used to detect pregnancies). Early in his experiments, Li had decided that he would use that hormone level to track the course of the cancer as it responded to methotrexate. The hcg level, as it was called, would be a surrogate for the cancer, its fingerprint in the blood.

The trouble was, at the end of the scheduled chemotherapy, the hcg level had fallen to an almost negligible value, but to Li's annoyance, it hadn't gone all the way to normal. He measured and remeasured it in his laboratory weekly, but it persisted, a pip-squeak of a number that wouldn't go away.

Li became progressively obsessed with the number. The hormone in the blood, he reasoned, was the fingerprint of cancer, and if it was still present, then the cancer had to be present, too, hiding in the body somewhere even if the visible tumors had disappeared. So, despite every other indication that the tumors had vanished, Li reasoned that his patients had not been fully cured. In the end, he seemed almost to be treating a number rather than a patient; ignoring the added toxicity of additional rounds of the drug, Li doggedly administered dose upon dose until, at last, the hcg level sank to zero.

❧

When the Institutional Board at the NCI got wind of Li's decision, it responded with fury. These patients were women who had supposedly been "cured" of cancer. Their tumors were invisible, and giving them additional chemotherapy was tantamount to poisoning them with unpredictable doses of highly toxic drugs. Li was already known to be a renegade, an iconoclast. This time, the NCI felt, he had gone too far. In mid-July, the board summoned him to a meeting and promptly fired him.

"Li was accused of experimenting on people," Freireich said. "But of course, *all* of us were experimenting. Tom [Frei] and Zubrod and the rest of them—we were all experimenters. To *not* experiment would mean to follow the old rules—to do absolutely nothing. Li wasn't prepared to sit back and watch and do nothing. So he was fired for acting on his convictions, for doing something."

Freireich and Li had been medical residents together in Chicago. At the NCI, they had developed a kinship as two outcasts. When Freireich heard about Li's dismissal, he immediately went over to Li's house to console him, but Li was inconsolable. In a few months, he huffed off to New York, bound back for Memorial Sloan-Kettering. He never returned to the NCI.

But the story had a final plot twist. As Li had predicted, with several additional doses of methotrexate, the hormone level that he had so compulsively trailed did finally vanish to zero. His patients finished their additional cycles of chemotherapy. Then, slowly, a pattern began to emerge. While the patients who had stopped the drug early inevitably relapsed with cancer, the patients treated on Li's protocol remained free of disease—even months after the methotrexate had been stopped.

Li had stumbled on a deep and fundamental principle of oncology: cancer needed to be systemically treated long after every visible sign of it had vanished. The hcg level—the hormone secreted by choriocarcinoma—had turned out to be its real fingerprint, its marker. In the decades that followed, trial after trial would prove this principle. But in 1960, oncology was not yet ready for this proposal. Not until several years later did it strike the board that had fired Li so hastily that the patients he had treated with the prolonged maintenance strategy would *never* relapse. This strategy—which cost Min Chiu Li his job—resulted in the first chemotherapeutic cure of cancer in adults.

Mice and Men

A model is a lie that helps you see the truth.
—Howard Skipper

Min Chiu Li's experience with choriocarcinoma was a philosophical nudge for Frei and Freireich. "Clinical research is a matter of urgency," Freireich argued. For a child with leukemia, even a week's delay meant the difference between life and death. The academic stodginess of the leukemia consortium—its insistence on progressively and systematically testing one drug combination after another—was now driving Freireich progressively and systematically mad. To test three drugs, the group insisted on testing "all of the three possible combinations *and* then you've got to do all of the four combinations *and* with different doses and schedules for each." At the rate that the leukemia consortium was moving, he argued, it would take dozens of years before any significant advance in leukemia was made. "The wards were filling up with these terribly sick children. A boy or girl might be brought in with a white cell count of three hundred and be dead overnight. I was the one sent the next morning to speak with the parents. Try explaining Zubrod's strategy of sequential, systematic, and objective trials to a woman whose daughter has just slumped into a coma and died," Freireich recalled.

The permutations of possible drugs and doses were further increased when yet another new anticancer agent was introduced at the Clinical Center in 1960. The newcomer, vincristine, was a poisonous plant-alkaloid that came from the Madagascar periwinkle, a small, weedlike creeper with violet flowers and an entwined, coiled stem. (The name *vincristine* comes from *vinca*, the Latin word for "bind.") Vincristine had been discovered in 1958 at the Eli Lilly company through a drug-discovery program that involved grinding up thousands of pounds of plant material and testing the extracts in various biological assays. Although originally intended as an antidiabetic, vincristine at small doses was found to kill leukemia cells. Rapidly growing cells, such as those of leukemia, typically create a skeletal scaffold of proteins (called microtubules) that allows two daughter cells to separate from each other and thereby complete cell division. Vincristine works by binding to the end of these microtubules and then paralyzing the cellular skeleton in its grip—thus, quite literally, evoking the Latin word after which it was originally named.

With vincristine added to the pharmacopoeia, leukemia researchers found themselves facing the paradox of excess: how might one take four independently active drugs—methotrexate, prednisone, 6-MP, and vincristine—and stitch them together into an effective regimen? And since each drug was potentially severely toxic, could one ever find a combination that would kill the leukemia but not kill a child?

Two drugs had already spawned dozens of possibilities; with four drugs, the leukemia consortium would take not fifty, but a hundred and fifty years to finish its trials. David Nathan, then a new recruit at the NCI, recalled the near standstill created by the avalanche of new medicines: "Frei and Freireich were simply taking drugs that were available and adding them together in combinations. . . . The possible combinations, doses, and schedules of four or five drugs were infinite. Researchers could work for years on finding the right combination of drugs and schedules." Zubrod's sequential, systematic, objective trials had reached an impasse. What was needed was quite the opposite of a systematic approach—an intuitive and inspired leap of faith into the deadly abyss of deadly drugs.

A scientist from Alabama, Howard Skipper—a scholarly, soft-spoken man who liked to call himself a "mouse doctor"—provided Frei and Freireich a way out of the impasse. Skipper was an outsider to the NCI. If leukemia was a model form of cancer, then Skipper had been studying the disease by artificially inducing leukemias in animals—in effect, by building a model of a model. Skipper's model used a mouse cell line called L-1210, a lymphoid leukemia that could be grown in a petri dish. When laboratory mice were injected with these cells, they would acquire the leukemia—a process known as engraftment because it was akin to transferring a piece of normal tissue (a graft) from one animal to another.

Skipper liked to think about cancer not as a disease but as an abstract mathematical entity. In a mouse transplanted with L-1210 cells, the cells divided with nearly obscene fecundity—often twice a day, a rate startling even for cancer cells. A single leukemia cell engrafted into the mouse could thus take off in a terrifying arc of numbers: 1, 4, 16, 64, 256, 1,024, 4,096, 16,384, 65,536, 262,144, 1,048,576 . . . and so forth, all the way to infinity. In sixteen or seventeen days, more than 2 billion daughter cells could grow out of that single cell—more than the entire number of blood cells in the mouse.

Skipper learned that he could halt this effusive cell division by administering chemotherapy to the leukemia-engrafted mouse. By charting the life and death of leukemia cells as they responded to drugs in these mice, Skipper emerged with two pivotal findings. First, he found that chemotherapy typically killed a fixed *percentage* of cells at any given instance no matter what the total number of cancer cells was. This percentage was a unique, cardinal number particular to every drug. In other words, if you started off with 100,000 leukemia cells in a mouse and administered a drug that killed 99 percent of those cells in a single round, then every round would kill cells in a fractional manner, resulting in fewer and fewer cells after every round of chemotherapy: 100,000 . . . 1,000 . . . 10 . . . and so forth, until the number finally fell to zero after four rounds. Killing leukemia was an *iterative* process, like halving a monster's body, then halving the half, and halving the remnant half.

Second, Skipper found that by adding drugs in combination, he could often get synergistic effects on killing. Since different drugs elicited different resistance mechanisms, and produced different toxicities in cancer cells, using drugs in concert dramatically lowered the chance of resistance and increased cell killing. Two drugs were therefore typically better than one, and three drugs better than two. With several drugs and several iterative rounds of chemotherapy in rapid-fire succession, Skipper cured leukemias in his mouse model.

For Frei and Freireich, Skipper's observations had an inevitable, if frightening, conclusion. If human leukemias were like Skipper's mouse leukemias, then children would need to be treated with a regimen containing not one or two, but multiple drugs. Furthermore, a single treatment would not suffice. "Maximal, intermittent, intensive, up-front" chemotherapy would need to be administered with nearly ruthless, inexorable persistence, dose after dose after dose after dose, pushing the outermost limits of tolerability. There would be no stopping, not even after the leukemia cells had apparently disappeared in the blood and the children had apparently been "cured."

Freireich and Frei were now ready to take their pivotal and intuitive leap into the abyss. The next regimen they would try would be a combination of all four drugs: vincristine, amethopterin, mercaptopurine, and prednisone. The regimen would be known by a new acronym, with each letter standing for one of the drugs: VAMP.

The name had many intended and unintended resonances. *Vamp* is a word that means to improvise or patch up, to cobble something together from bits and pieces that might crumble apart any second. It can mean a seductress—one who promises but does not deliver. It also refers to the front of a boot, the part that carries the full brunt of force during a kick.

VAMP

Doctors are men who prescribe medicines of which they know little, to cure diseases of which they know less, in human beings of whom they know nothing.
—Voltaire

If we didn't kill the tumor, we killed the patient.
—William Moloney on the early days of chemotherapy

VAMP—high-dose, life-threatening, four-drug combination therapy for leukemia—might have made obvious sense to Skipper, Frei, and Freireich, but to many of their colleagues, it was a terrifying notion, an abomination. Freireich finally approached Zubrod with his idea: "I wanted to treat them with full doses of vincristine *and* amethopterin, combined with the 6-MP *and* prednisone." The *and*s in the sentence were italicized to catch Zubrod's attention.

Zubrod was stunned. "It is the dose that makes a poison," runs the old adage in medicine: all medicines were poisons in one form or another merely diluted to an appropriate dose. But chemotherapy was poison even at the *correct* dose.* A child with leukemia was already stretched to the brittle limits of survival, hanging on to life by a bare physiological thread. People at the NCI would often casually talk of chemotherapy as the "poison of the month." If four poisons of the month were simultaneously pumped

---

* Since most of the early anticancer drugs were cytotoxic—cell-killing—the threshold between a therapeutic (cancer-killing) dose and a toxic dose was extremely narrow. Many of the drugs had to be very carefully dosed to avoid the unwarranted but inextricably linked toxicity.

daily into a three- or six-year-old child, there was virtually no guarantee that he or she could survive even the first dose of this regimen, let alone survive week after week after week.

When Frei and Freireich presented their preliminary plan for VAMP at a national meeting on blood cancers, the audience balked. Farber, for one, favored giving one drug at a time and adding the second only after relapse and so forth, following the leukemia consortium's slow but steady method of adding drugs carefully and sequentially. "Oh, boy," Freireich recalled, "it was a terrible, catastrophic showdown. We were laughed at and then called insane, incompetent, and cruel." With limited patients and hundreds of drugs and combinations to try, every new leukemia trial had to wind its way through a complex approval process through the leukemia group. Frei and Freireich, it was felt, were making an unauthorized quantum leap. The group refused to sponsor VAMP—at least not until the many other trials had been completed.

But Frei wrangled a last-minute compromise: VAMP would be studied independently at the NCI, outside the purview of the ALGB. "The idea was preposterous," Freireich recalled. "To run the trial, we would need to split with the ALGB, the very group that we had been so instrumental in founding." Zubrod wasn't pleased with the compromise: it was a break from his cherished "cooperative" model. Worse still, if VAMP failed, it would be a political nightmare for him. "If the children had died, we'd be accused of experimenting on people at this federal installation of the National Cancer Institute," Freireich acknowledged. Everyone knew it was chancy territory. Embroiled in controversy, even if he had resolved it as best he could, Frei resigned as the chair of the ALGB. Years later, Freireich acknowledged the risks involved: "We could have killed all of those kids."

ॐ

The VAMP trial was finally launched in 1961. Almost instantly, it seemed like an abysmal mistake—precisely the sort of nightmare that Zubrod had been trying to avoid.

The first children to be treated "were already terribly, terribly ill," Freireich recalled. "We started VAMP, and by the end of the week, many of them were infinitely worse than before. It was a disaster." The four-drug chemo regimen raged through the body and wiped out all the normal cells. Some children slumped into near coma and were hooked to respirators. Freireich, desperate to save them, visited his patients obsessively in their hospital beds. "You can imagine the tension," he wrote. "I could just hear people saying, 'I told you so, this girl or boy is going to die.'" He hovered in the wards, pestering the staff with questions and suggestions. His paternal, possessive instincts were aroused: "These were my kids. I really tried to take care of them."

The NCI, as a whole, watched tensely—for *its* life, too, was on the line. "I did little things," Freireich wrote. "Maybe I could make them more comfortable, give them a little aspirin, lower their temperatures, get them a blanket." Thrown into the uncertain front lines of cancer medicine, juggling the most toxic and futuristic combinations of drugs, the NCI doctors fell back to their oldest principles. They provided comfort. They nurtured. They focused on caregiving and support. They fluffed pillows.

At the end of three excruciating weeks, a few of Freireich's patients somehow pulled through. Then, unexpectedly—at a time when it was almost unbearable to look for it—there was a payoff. The normal bone marrow cells began to recover gradually, but the leukemia went into remission. The bone marrow biopsies came back one after another—all without leukemia cells. Red blood cells and white blood cells and platelets sprouted up in an otherwise scorched field of bone marrow. But the leukemia did not return. Another set of biopsies, weeks later, confirmed the finding. Not a single leukemia cell was visible under the microscope. This—after near-complete devastation—was a remission so deep that it exceeded the expectations of everyone at the NCI.

A few weeks later, the NCI team drummed up enough courage to try VAMP on yet another small cohort of patients. Once again, after the nearly catastrophic dip in counts—"like a drop from a cliff with a thread tied to your ankles," as one researcher remembered it—the bone marrow recovered and the leukemia vanished. A few days later, the bone marrow began to regenerate, and Freireich performed a hesitant biopsy to look at the cells. The leukemia had vanished again. What it had left behind was full of promise: normal cobblestones of blood cells growing back in the marrow.

By 1962, Frei and Freireich had treated six patients with several doses of VAMP. Remissions were reliable and durable. The Clinical Center was now filled with the familiar chatter of children in wigs and scarves who had survived two or three seasons of chemotherapy—a strikingly anomalous phenomenon in the history of leukemia. Critics were slowly turning into converts. Other clinical centers around the nation joined Frei and Freireich's experimental regimen. The patient "is amazingly recovered," a hematologist in Boston treating an eleven-year-old wrote in 1964. Astonishment slowly gave way to buoyancy. Even William Dameshek, the opinionated Harvard-trained hematologist and one of the most prominent early opponents of VAMP, wrote, "The mood among pediatric oncologists changed virtually overnight from one of 'compassionate fatalism' to one of 'aggressive optimism.'"

⁂

The optimism was potent, but short-lived. In September 1963, not long after Frei and Freireich had returned from one of those triumphant conferences celebrating the unexpected success of VAMP, a few children in remission came back to the clinic with minor complaints: a headache, a seizure, an occasional tingling of a nerve in the face.

"Some of us didn't make much of it at first," a hematologist recalled. "We imagined the symptoms would go away." But Freireich, who had studied the spread of leukemia cells in the body for nearly a decade, knew that these were headaches that would not go away. By October, there were more children back at the clinic, this time with numbness, tingling, headaches, seizures, and facial paralysis. Frei and Freireich were both getting nervous.

In the 1880s, Virchow had observed that leukemia cells could occasionally colonize the brain. To investigate the possibility of a brain invasion by cancer cells, Frei and Freireich looked directly at the spinal fluid using a spinal tap, a method to withdraw a few milliliters of fluid from the spinal canal using a thin, straight needle. The fluid, a clear liquid that circulates in direct connection with the brain, is a surrogate for examining the brain.

In the folklore of science, there is the often-told story of the moment of discovery: the quickening of the pulse, the spectral luminosity of ordinary facts, the overheated, standstill second when observations crystallize and fall together into patterns, like pieces of a kaleidoscope. The apple drops from the tree. The man jumps up from a bathtub; the slippery equation balances itself.

But there is another moment of discovery—its antithesis—that is rarely recorded: the discovery of failure. It is a moment that a scientist often encounters alone. A patient's CT scan shows a relapsed lymphoma. A cell once killed by a drug begins to grow back. A child returns to the NCI with a headache.

What Frei and Freireich discovered in the spinal fluid left them cold:

leukemia cells were growing explosively in the spinal fluid by the millions, colonizing the brain. The headaches and the numbness were early signs of much more profound devastations to come. In the months that followed, one by one, all the children came back to the institute with a spectrum of neurological complaints—headaches, tinglings, abstract speckles of light—then slumped into coma. Bone marrow biopsies were clean. No cancer was found in the body. But the leukemia cells had invaded the nervous system, causing a quick, unexpected demise.

It was a consequence of the body's own defense system subverting cancer treatment. The brain and spinal cord are insulated by a tight cellular seal called the blood-brain barrier that prevents foreign chemicals from easily getting into the brain. It is an ancient biological system that has evolved to keep poisons from reaching the brain. But the same system had likely also kept VAMP out of the nervous system, creating a natural "sanctuary" for cancer within the body. The leukemia had grown out in that sanctuary, colonizing the one place that is fundamentally unreachable by chemotherapy. The children died one after the other—felled by virtue of the adaptation designed to protect them.

Frei and Freireich were hit hard by those relapses. For a clinical scientist, a trial is like a child, a deeply personal investment. To watch this sort of intense, intimate enterprise fold up and die is to suffer the loss of a child. One leukemia doctor wrote, "I know the patients, I know their brothers and sisters, I know their dogs and cats by name. . . . The pain is that a lot of love affairs end."

After seven exhilarating and intensive trials, the love affair at the NCI had indeed ended. The brain relapses after VAMP seemed to push morale at the institute to the breaking point. Frei, who had so furiously tried to keep VAMP alive through its most trying stages—twelve months of manipulating, coaxing, and wheedling—now found himself drained of his last stores of energy. Even the indefatigable Freireich was beginning to lose steam. He felt a growing hostility from others at the institute. At the peak of his career, he, too, felt tired of the interminable institutional scuffles that had once invigorated him.

In the winter of 1963, Frei left for a position at the MD Anderson Cancer Center in Houston, Texas. The trials were temporarily put on hold (although they would eventually be resurrected in Texas). Freireich soon left the NCI to join Frei in Houston. The fragile ecosystem that had sustained Freireich, Frei, and Zubrod dissolved in a few months.

But the story of leukemia—the story of cancer—isn't the story of doctors who struggle and survive, moving from one institution to another. It is the story of patients who struggle and survive, moving from one embankment of illness to another. Resilience, inventiveness, and survivorship—qualities often ascribed to great physicians—are reflected qualities, emanating first from those who struggle with illness and only then mirrored by those who treat them. If the history of medicine is told through the stories of doctors, it is because their contributions stand in place of the more substantive heroism of their patients.

I said that all the children had relapsed and died—but this is not quite true. A few, a small handful, for mysterious reasons, never relapsed with leukemia in the central nervous system. At the NCI and the few other hospitals brave enough to try VAMP, about 5 percent of the treated children finished their yearlong journey. They remained in remission not just for weeks or months, but for years. They came back, year after year, and sat nervously in waiting rooms at trial centers all around the nation. Their voices deepened. Their hair grew back. Biopsy after biopsy was performed. And there was no visible sign of cancer.

On a summer afternoon, I drove through western Maine to the small town of Waterboro. Against the foggy, overcast sky, the landscape was spectacular, with ancient pine and birch forests tipping into crystalline lakes. On the far edge of the town, I turned onto a dirt road leading away from the water. At the end of the road, surrounded by deep pine forests, was a tiny clapboard house. A fifty-six-year-old woman in a blue T-shirt answered the door. It had taken me seventeen months and innumerable phone calls, questions, interviews, and references to track her down. One afternoon, scouring the Internet, I had found a lead. I remember dialing the number, excited beyond words, and waiting for interminable rings before a woman answered. I had fixed up an appointment to meet her that week and driven rather recklessly to Maine to keep it. When I arrived, I realized that I was twenty minutes early.

I cannot remember what I said, or struggled to say, as a measure of introduction. But I felt awestruck. Standing before me against the door, smiling nervously, was one of the survivors of that original VAMP cohort cured of childhood leukemia.

The basement was flooded and the couch was growing mildew, so we sat outdoors in the shadows of the trees in a screened tent with deerflies and mosquitoes buzzing outside. The woman—Ella, I'll call her—had collected a pile of medical records and photographs for me to look through. As she handed them over, I sensed a shiver running through her body, as if even today, forty-five years after her ordeal, the memory haunts her viscerally.

Ella was diagnosed with leukemia in June 1964, about eighteen months after VAMP was first used at the NCI. She was eleven years old. In the photographs taken before her diagnosis, she was a typical preteen with bangs and braces. In the photograph taken just six months later (after chemotherapy), she was transformed—bald, sheet-white from anemia, and severely underweight, collapsed on a wheelchair and unable to walk.

Ella was treated with VAMP. (Her oncologists in Boston, having heard of the spectacular responses at the NCI, had rather bravely chosen to treat her—off trial—with the four-drug regimen.) It had seemed like a cataclysm at first. The high doses of vincristine caused such severe collateral nerve damage that she was left with a permanent burning sensation in her legs and fingers. Prednisone made her delirious. The nurses, unable to deal with a strong-willed, deranged preteen wandering through the corridors of the hospital screaming and howling at night, restrained her by tying her arms with ropes to the bedposts. Confined to her bed, she often crouched in a fetal position, her muscles wasting away, the neuropathy worsening. At twelve years of age, she became addicted to morphine, which was prescribed for her pain. (She "detoxed" herself by sheer force of will, she said, by "lasting it out through the spasms of withdrawal.") Her lower lip is still bruised from the time she bit herself in those awful months while waiting out the hour for the next dose of morphine.

Yet, remarkably, the main thing she remembers is the overwhelming feeling of being spared. "I feel as if I slipped through," she told me, arranging the records back into their envelopes. She looked away, as if to swat an imaginary fly, and I could see her eyes welling up with tears. She had met several other children with leukemia in the hospital wards; none had survived. "I don't know why I deserved the illness in the first place, but then I don't know why I deserved to be cured. Leukemia is like that. It mystifies you. It changes your life." My mind briefly flashed to the Chiribaya mummy, to Atossa, to Halsted's young woman awaiting her mastectomy.

Sidney Farber never met Ella, but he encountered patients just like her—long-term survivors of VAMP. In 1964, the year that Ella began her chemotherapy, he triumphantly brought photographs of a few such patients to Washington as a sort of show-and-tell for Congress, living proof that chemotherapy could cure cancer. The path was now becoming increasingly clear to him. Cancer research needed an additional thrust: more money, more research, more publicity, and a directed trajectory toward a cure. His testimony before Congress thus acquired a nearly devotional, messianic fervor. After the photographs and his testimony, one observer recalled, any further proof was "anticlimactic and unnecessary." Farber was now ready to leap out from the realm of leukemia into the vastly more common real cancers. "We are attempting to develop chemicals which might affect otherwise incurable tumors of the breast, the ovary, the uterus, the lung, the kidney, the intestine, and highly malignant tumors of the skin, such as the black cancer, or melanoma," he wrote. The cure of even one such solid cancer in adults, Farber knew, would singularly revolutionize oncology. It would provide the most concrete proof that this was a winnable war.

An Anatomist's Tumor

*It took plain old courage to be a chemotherapist in the
1960s and certainly the courage of the conviction that
cancer would eventually succumb to drugs.*
—Vincent DeVita, National Cancer Institute
investigator (and eventually NCI director)

On a chilly February morning in 2004, a twenty-four-year-old athlete, Ben
Orman, discovered a lump in his neck. He was in his apartment, reading
the newspaper, when, running his hand absentmindedly past his face, his
fingers brushed against a small swelling. The lump was about the size of a
small dried grape. If he took a deep breath, he could swallow it back into
the cavity of his chest. He dismissed it. It was a lump, he reasoned, and
athletes were used to lumps: calluses, swollen knees, boils, bumps, bruises
coming and going with no remembered cause. He returned to his newspaper and worry vanished from his mind. The lump in his neck, whatever
it was, would doubtless vanish in time as well.

But it grew instead, imperceptibly at first, then more assertively, turning from grape-size to prune-size in about a month. He could feel it on the
shallow dip of his collarbone. Worried, Orman went to the walk-in clinic
of the hospital, almost apologetic about his complaints. The triage nurse
scribbled in her notes: "Lump in his neck"—and added a question mark
at the end of the sentence.

With that sentence, Orman entered the unfamiliar world of oncology—swallowed, like his own lump, into the bizarre, cavitary universe of
cancer. The doors of the hospital opened and closed behind him. A doctor in a blue scrub suit stepped through the curtains and ran her hands
up and down his neck. He had blood tests and X-rays in rapid succession, followed by CT scans and more examinations. The scans revealed
that the lump in the neck was merely the tip of a much deeper iceberg

of lumps. Beneath that sentinel mass, a chain of masses coiled from his neck down into his chest, culminating in a fist-size tumor just behind his sternum. Large masses located in the anterior chest, as medical students learn, come in four *T*'s, almost like a macabre nursery rhyme for cancer: thyroid cancer, thymoma, teratoma, and terrible lymphoma. Orman's problem—given his age and the matted, dense appearance of the lumps—was almost certainly the last of these, a lymphoma—cancer of the lymph glands.

❧

I saw Ben Orman nearly two months after that visit to the hospital. He was sitting in the waiting room, reading a book (he read fiercely, athletically, almost competitively, often finishing one novel a week, as if in a race). In the eight weeks since his ER visit, he had undergone a PET scan, a visit with a surgeon, and a biopsy of the neck lump. As suspected, the mass was a lymphoma, a relatively rare variant called Hodgkin's disease.

More news followed: the scans revealed that Orman's cancer was confined entirely to one side of his upper torso. And he had none of the ghostly B symptoms—weight loss, fever, chills, or night sweats—that occasionally accompany Hodgkin's disease. In a staging system that ran from I to IV (with an *A* or *B* added to denote the absence or presence of the occult symptoms), he fell into stage IIA—relatively early in the progression of the disease. It was somber news, but of all the patients shuttling in and out of the waiting room that morning, Orman arguably carried the most benign prognosis. With an intensive course of chemotherapy, it was more than likely—85 percent likely—that he would be cured.

"By intensive," I told him, "I mean several months, perhaps even stretching out to half a year. The drugs will be given in cycles, and there will have to be visits in between to check blood counts." Every three weeks, just as his counts recovered, the whole cycle would begin all over again—Sisyphus on chemotherapy.

He would lose his hair with the first cycle. He would almost certainly become permanently infertile. There might be life-threatening infections during the times when his white counts would bottom out nearly to zero. Most ominously, the chemo might cause a second cancer in the future. He nodded. I watched the thought pick up velocity in his brain, until it had reached its full impact.

"It's going to be a long haul. A marathon," I stammered apologetically, groping for an analogy. "But we'll get to the end."

He nodded again silently, as if he already knew.

დ

On a Wednesday morning, not long after my meeting with Orman, I took a shuttle across Boston to see my patients at the Dana-Farber Cancer Institute. Most of us called the institute simply "the Farber." Large already in life, Sidney Farber had become even larger in death: the eponymous Farber was now a sprawling sixteen-story labyrinth of concrete crammed full of scientists and physicians, a comprehensive lab-cum-clinic-cum-pharmacy-cum-chemotherapy-unit. There were 2,934 employees, dozens of conference rooms, scores of laboratories, a laundry unit, four banks of elevators, and multiple libraries. The site of the original basement lab had long been dwarfed by the massive complex of buildings around it. Like a vast, overbuilt, and overwrought medieval temple, the Farber had long swallowed its shrine.

As you entered the new building, an oil painting of the man himself—with his characteristic half-scowling, half-smiling face—stared back at you in the foyer. Little bits and pieces of him, it seemed, were strewn every-where. The corridor on the way to the fellows' office was still hung with the cartoonish "portraits" that he had once commissioned for the Jimmy Fund: Snow White, Pinocchio, Jiminy Cricket, Dumbo. The bone marrow nee-dles with which we performed our biopsies looked and felt as if they came from another age; perhaps they had been sharpened by Farber or one of his trainees fifty years ago. Wandering through these labs and clinics, you often felt as if you could stumble onto cancer history at any minute. One morning I did: bolting to catch the elevator, I ran headlong into an old man in a wheelchair whom I first took to be a patient. It was Tom Frei, a profes-sor emeritus now, heading up to his office on the sixteenth floor.

დ

My patient that Wednesday morning was a seventy-six-year-old woman named Beatrice Sorenson. Bea, as she liked to be called, reminded me of one of those tiny insects or animals that you read about in natural-history textbooks that can carry ten times their weight or leap five times their height. She was almost preternaturally minuscule: about eighty-five pounds and four and a half feet tall, with birdlike features and delicate bones that seemed to hang together like twigs in winter. To this diminutive frame, however, she brought a fierce force of personality, the lightness of body counterbalanced by the heftiness of soul. She had been a marine and served in two wars. Even as I towered over her on the examination table, I felt awkward and humbled, as if she were towering over me in spirit.

Sorenson had pancreatic cancer. The tumor had been discovered almost accidentally in the late summer of 2003, when she had had a bout of abdominal pain and diarrhea and a CT scan had picked up a four-centimeter solid nodule hanging off the tail of her pancreas. (In retrospect, the diarrhea may have been unrelated.) A brave surgeon had attempted to resect it, but the margins of the resection still contained some tumor cells. Even in oncology, a dismal discipline to begin with, this—unresected pancreatic cancer—was considered the epitome of the dismal.

Sorenson's life had turned upside down. "I want to beat it to the end," she had told me at first. We had tried. Through the early fall, we blasted her pancreas with radiation to kill the tumor cells, then followed with chemotherapy, using the drug 5-fluorouracil. The tumor had grown right through all the treatments. In the winter, we had switched to a new drug called gemcitabine, or Gemzar. The tumor cells had shrugged the new drug off—instead mockingly sending a shower of painful metastases into her liver. At times, it felt as if we would have been better off with no drugs at all.

Sorenson was at the clinic that morning to see if we could offer anything else. She wore white pants and a white shirt. Her paper-thin skin was marked with dry lines. She may have been crying, but her face was a cipher that I could not read.

"She will try anything, anything," her husband pleaded. "She is stronger than she looks."

But strong or not, there was nothing left to try. I stared down at my feet, unable to confront the obvious questions. The attending physician shifted uncomfortably in his chair.

Beatrice finally broke the awkward silence. "I'm sorry." She shrugged her shoulders and looked vacantly past us. "I know we have reached an end."

We hung our heads, ashamed. It was, I suspected, not the first time that a patient had consoled a doctor about the ineffectuality of his discipline.

Two lumps seen on two different mornings. Two vastly different incarnations of cancer: one almost certainly curable, the second, an inevitable spiral into death. It felt—nearly twenty-five hundred years after Hippocrates had naively coined the overarching term *karkinos*—that modern oncology was hardly any more sophisticated in its taxonomy of cancer. Orman's lymphoma and Sorenson's pancreatic cancer were both, of course, "cancers," malignant proliferations of cells. But the diseases could not have been further apart in their trajectories and personalities. Even referring to them by the same name, *cancer,* felt like some sort of medical anachronism, like the medieval habit of using *apoplexy* to describe anything from a stroke to a hemorrhage to a seizure. Like Hippocrates, it was as if we, too, had naively lumped the lumps.

But naive or not, it was this lumping—this emphatic, unshakable faith in the underlying *singularity* of cancer more than its pluralities—that galvanized the Laskerites in the 1960s. Oncology was on a quest for cohesive truths—a "universal cure," as Farber put it in 1962. And if the oncologists of the 1960s imagined a common cure for all forms of cancer, it was because they imagined a common disease called cancer. Curing one form, the belief ran, would inevitably lead to the cure of another, and so forth like a chain reaction, until the whole malignant edifice had crumbled like a set of dominoes.

That assumption—that a monolithic hammer would eventually demolish a monolithic disease—surcharged physicians, scientists, and cancer lobbyists with vitality and energy. For the Laskerites, it was an organizing principle, a matter of faith, the only certain beacon toward which they all gravitated. Indeed, the *political* consolidation of cancer that the Laskerites sought in Washington (a single institute, a single source of funds, led by a single physician or scientist) relied on a deeper notion of a *medical* consolidation of cancer into a single disease, a monolith, a single, central narrative. Without this grand, embracing narrative, neither Mary Lasker nor Sidney Farber could have envisioned a systematic, targeted war.

ↀ

The illness that had brought Ben Orman to the clinic late that evening, Hodgkin's lymphoma, was itself announced late to the world of cancer. Its discoverer, Thomas Hodgkin, was a thin, short, nineteenth-century English anatomist with a spadelike beard and an astonishingly curved nose—a character who might have walked out of an Edward Lear poem.

Hodgkin was born in 1798 to a Quaker family in Pentonville, a small hamlet outside London. A precocious child, he grew quickly into an even more precocious young man, whose interests loped freely from geology to mathematics to chemistry. He apprenticed briefly as a geologist, then as an apothecary, and finally graduated from the University of Edinburgh with a degree in medicine.

A chance event enticed Hodgkin into the world of pathological anatomy and led him toward the disease that would bear his name. In 1825, a struggle within the faculty of St. Thomas' and Guy's hospital in London broke up the venerable institution into two bickering halves: Guy's hospital and its new rival, St. Thomas'. This divorce, like many marital spats, was almost immediately followed by a vicious argument over the partition of property. The "property" here was a macabre ensemble—the precious anatomical collection of the hospital: brains, hearts, stomachs, and skeletons in pickling jars of formalin that had been hoarded for use as teaching tools for the hospital's medical students. St. Thomas' hospital refused to part with its precious specimens, so Guy's scrambled to cobble together its own anatomical museum. Hodgkin had just returned from his second visit to Paris, where he had learned to prepare and dissect cadaveric specimens. He was promptly recruited to collect specimens for Guy's new museum. The job's most inventive academic perk, perhaps, was his new title: the Curator of the Museum and the Inspector of the Dead.

Hodgkin proved to be an extraordinary Inspector of the Dead, a compulsive anatomical curator who hoarded hundreds of samples within a few years. But collecting specimens was a rather mundane task; Hodgkin's particular genius lay in *organizing* them. He became a librarian as much as a pathologist; he devised his own systematics for pathology. The original building that housed his collection has been destroyed. But the new museum, where Hodgkin's original specimens are still on display, is a strange marvel. A four-chambered atrium located deep inside a larger building, it is an enormous walk-in casket-of-wonders constructed of wrought iron and glass. You enter a door and ascend a staircase, then find yourself on the top floor of a series of galleries that cascade downward. Along every wall are rows of formalin-filled jars: lungs in one gallery, hearts in another, brains, kidneys, bones, and so forth. This method of organizing pathological anatomy—by organ system rather than by date or disease—was a revelation. By thus "inhabiting" the body conceptually—by climbing in and out of the body at will, often noting the correlations between organs and systems—Hodgkin found that he could recognize patterns within patterns instinctually, sometimes without even consciously registering them.

In the early winter of 1832, Hodgkin announced that he had collected a series of cadavers, mostly of young men, who possessed a strange systemic disease. The illness was characterized, as he put it, by "a peculiar enlargement of lymph glands." To the undiscerning eye, this enlargement could easily have been from tuberculosis or syphilis—the more common sources of glandular swelling at that time. But Hodgkin was convinced that he had encountered an entirely new disease, an unknown pathology unique to these young men. He wrote up the case of seven such cadavers and had his paper, "On Some Morbid Appearances of the Absorbent Glands and Spleen," presented to the Medical and Chirurgical Society.

The story of a compulsive young doctor putting old swellings into new pathological bottles was received without much enthusiasm. Only eight members of the society reportedly attended the lecture. They filed out afterward in silence, not even bothering to record their names on the dusty attendance roster.

Hodgkin, too, was a little embarrassed by his discovery. "A pathological paper may perhaps be thought of little value if unaccompanied by suggestions designed to assist in the treatment, either curative or palliative," he wrote. Merely describing an illness, without offering any therapeutic suggestions, seemed like an empty academic exercise to him, a form of intellectual frittering. Soon after publishing his paper, he began to drift away from medicine altogether. In 1837, after a rather vicious political spat with his superiors, he resigned his post at Guy's. He had a brief stint at St. Thomas' hospital as its curator—a rebound affair that was doomed to fail. In 1844, he gave up his academic practice altogether. His anatomical studies slowly came to a halt.

In 1898, some thirty years after Hodgkin's death, an Austrian pathologist, Carl Sternberg, was looking through a microscope at a patient's glands when he found a peculiar series of cells staring back at him: giant, disorganized cells with cleaved, bilobed nuclei—"owl's eyes," as he described them, glaring sullenly out from the forests of lymph. Hodgkin's anatomy had reached its final cellular resolution. These owl's-eye cells were *malignant* lymphocytes, lymph cells that had turned cancerous. Hodgkin's disease was a cancer of the lymph glands—a lymphoma.

✧

Hodgkin may have been disappointed by what he thought was only a descriptive study of his disease. But he had underestimated the value of careful observation—by compulsively studying anatomy alone, he had stumbled upon the most critical revelation about this form of lymphoma: Hodgkin's disease had a peculiar propensity of infiltrating lymph nodes *locally* one by one. Other cancers could be more unpredictable—more "capricious," as one oncologist put it. Lung cancer, for instance, might start as a spicular nodule in the lung, then unmoor itself and ambulate unexpectedly into the brain. Pancreatic cancer was notoriously known to send sprays of malignant cells into faraway sites such as the bones and the liver. But Hodgkin's—an anatomist's discovery—was anatomically deferential: it moved, as if with a measured, ordered pace, from one contiguous node to another—from gland to gland and from region to region.

It was this propensity to spread *locally* from one node to the next that poised Hodgkin's uniquely in the history of cancer. Hodgkin's disease was yet another hybrid among malignant diseases. If Farber's leukemia had occupied the hazy border between liquid and solid tumors, then Hodgkin's disease inhabited yet another strange borderland: a local disease on the verge of transforming into a systemic one—Halsted's vision of cancer on its way to becoming Galen's.

✺

In the early 1950s, at a cocktail party in California, Henry Kaplan, a professor of radiology at Stanford, overheard a conversation about the plan to build a linear accelerator for use by physicists at Stanford. A linear accelerator is an X-ray tube taken to an extreme form. Like a conventional X-ray tube, a linear accelerator also fires electrons onto a target to generate high-intensity X-rays. Unlike a conventional tube, however, the "linac" imbues massive amounts of energy into the electrons, pushing them to dizzying velocities before smashing them against the metal surface. The X-rays that emerge from this are deeply penetrating—powerful enough not only to pass through tissue, but to scald cells to death.

Kaplan had trained at the NCI, where he had learned to use X-rays to treat leukemia in animals, but his interest had gradually shifted to solid tumors in humans—lung cancer, breast cancer, lymphomas. Solid tumors could be treated with radiation, he knew, but the outer shell of the cancer, like its eponymous crab's carapace, needed to be penetrated deeply to kill cancer cells. A linear accelerator with its sharp, dense, knifelike beam might allow him to reach tumor cells buried deep inside tissues. In 1953, he persuaded a team of physicists and engineers at Stanford to tailor-make an accelerator exclusively for the hospital. The accelerator was installed in a vaultlike warehouse in San Francisco in 1956. Dodging traffic between Fillmore Street and Mission Hill, Kaplan personally wheeled in its colossal block of lead shielding on an automobile jack borrowed from a neighboring garage owner.

Through a minuscule pinhole in that lead block, he could now direct tiny, controlled doses of a furiously potent beam of X-rays—millions of electron volts of energy in concentrated bursts—to lancinate any cancer cell to death. But what form of cancer? If Kaplan had learned one lesson at the NCI, it was that by focusing microscopically on a single disease, one could extrapolate into the entire universe of diseases. The characteristics that Kaplan sought in his target were relatively well defined. Since the linac could only focus its killer beam on local sites, it would have to be a local, not a systemic, cancer. Leukemia was out of the question. Breast and lung cancer were important targets, but both were unpredictable, mercurial diseases, with propensities for occult and systemic spread. The powerful oculus of Kaplan's intellect, swiveling about through the malignant world, ultimately landed on the most natural target for his investigation: Hodgkin's disease.

∂∫∂

"Henry Kaplan *was* Hodgkin's disease," George Canellos, a former senior clinician at the NCI told me, leaning back in his chair. We were sitting in his office while he rummaged through piles of manuscripts, monographs, articles, books, catalogs, and papers, pulling out occasional pictures of Kaplan from his files. Here was Kaplan, dressed in a bow tie, looking at sheaves of papers at the NCI. Or Kaplan in a white coat standing next to the linac at Stanford, its 5-million-volt probe just inches from his nose.

Kaplan wasn't the first doctor to treat Hodgkin's with X-rays, but he was certainly the most dogged, the most methodical, and the most single-minded. In the mid-1930s, a Swiss radiologist named Rene Gilbert had shown that the swollen lymph nodes of Hodgkin's disease could effectively and dramatically be reduced with radiation. But Gilbert's patients had typically relapsed after treatment, often in the lymph nodes immediately contiguous to the original radiated area. At the Toronto General Hospital, a Canadian surgeon named Vera Peters had furthered Gilbert's studies by broadening the radiation field even farther—delivering X-rays not to a single swollen node, but to an entire area of lymph nodes. Peters called her strategy "extended field radiation." In 1958, analyzing the cohort of patients that she had treated, Peters observed that broad-field radiation could significantly improve long-term survival for early-stage Hodgkin's patients. But Peters's data was retrospective—based on the historical analysis of prior-treated patients. What Peters needed was a more rigorous medical experiment, a randomized clinical trial. (Historical series can be biased by doctors' highly selective choices of patients for therapy, or by their counting only the ones that do the best.)

Independently of Peters, Kaplan had also realized that extended field radiation could improve relapse-free survival, perhaps even cure early-stage Hodgkin's disease. But he lacked formal proof. In 1962, challenged by one of his students, Henry Kaplan set out to prove the point.

The trials that Kaplan designed still rank among the classics of study design. In the first set, called the L1 trials, he assigned equal numbers of patients to either extended field radiation or to limited "involved field" radiation and plotted relapse-free survival curves. The answer was definitive. Extended field radiation—"meticulous radiotherapy" as one doctor described it—drastically diminished the relapse rate of Hodgkin's disease.

But Kaplan knew that a diminished relapse rate was not a cure. So he delved further. Two years later, the Stanford team carved out a larger field of radiation, involving nodes around the aorta, the large arch-shaped blood vessel that leads out of the heart. Here they introduced an innovation that would prove pivotal to their success. Kaplan knew that only patients that had localized Hodgkin's disease could possibly benefit from radiation therapy. To truly test the efficacy of radiation therapy, then, Kaplan realized that he would need a strictly limited cohort of patients whose Hodgkin's disease involved just a few contiguous lymph nodes. To exclude patients with more disseminated forms of lymphoma, Kaplan devised an intense battery of tests to stage his patients. There were blood tests, a detailed clinical exam, a procedure called lymphangiography (a primitive ancestor of a CT scan for the lymph nodes), and a bone marrow biopsy. Even so, Kaplan was unsatisfied: doubly careful, he began to perform exploratory abdominal surgery and biopsy internal nodes to ensure that only patients with locally confined disease were entering his trials.

The doses of radiation were now daringly high. But gratifyingly, the responses soared as well. Kaplan documented even greater relapse-free intervals, now stretching out into dozens of months—then years. When the first batch of patients had survived five years without relapses, he began to speculate that some may have been cured by extended field X-rays. Kaplan's experimental idea had finally made its way out of a San Francisco warehouse into the mainstream clinical world.

But hadn't Halsted wagered on the same horse and lost? Hadn't radical surgery become entangled in the same logic—carving out larger and larger areas for treatment—and then spiraled downward? Why did Kaplan succeed where others had failed?

First, because Kaplan meticulously restricted radiotherapy to patients with early-stage disease. He went to exhaustive lengths to stage patients before unleashing radiation on them. By strictly narrowing the group of patients treated, Kaplan markedly increased the likelihood of his success.

And second, he succeeded because he had picked the right disease. Hodgkin's was, for the most part, a regional illness. "Fundamental to all attempts at curative treatment of Hodgkin's disease," one reviewer commented memorably in the *New England Journal of Medicine* in 1968, "is the assumption that in the significant fraction of cases, [the disease] is localized." Kaplan treated the intrinsic biology of Hodgkin's disease with utmost seriousness. If Hodgkin's lymphoma had been more capricious in its movement through the body (and occult areas of spread more common, as in some forms of breast cancer), then Kaplan's staging strategy, for all his excruciatingly detailed workups, would inherently have been doomed to fail. Instead of trying to tailor the disease to fit his medicine, Kaplan learned to tailor his medicine to fit the right disease.

This simple principle—the meticulous matching of a particular therapy to a particular form and stage of cancer—would eventually be given its due merit in cancer therapy. Early-stage, local cancers, Kaplan realized, were often inherently different from widely spread, metastatic cancers—even within the same form of cancer. A hundred instances of Hodgkin's disease, even though pathologically classified as the same entity, were a hundred variants around a common theme. Cancers possessed temperaments, personalities—behaviors. And biological heterogeneity demanded therapeutic heterogeneity; the same treatment could not indiscriminately be applied to all. But even if Kaplan understood it fully in 1963 and made an example of it in treating Hodgkin's disease, it would take decades for a generation of oncologists to come to the same realization.

An Army on the March

Now we are an army on the march.
—Sidney Farber in 1963

The next step—the complete cure—is almost sure to follow.
—Kenneth Endicott,
NCI director, 1963

*The role of aggressive multiple drug therapy in the quest
for long-term survival [in cancer] is far from clear.*
—R. Stein, a scientist in 1969

One afternoon in the late summer of 1963, George Canellos, then a senior fellow at the NCI, walked into the Clinical Center to find Tom Frei scribbling furiously on one of the institute's blackboards. Frei, in his long white coat, was making lists of chemicals and drawing arrows. On one side of the board was a list of cytotoxic drugs—Cytoxan, vincristine, procarbazine, methotrexate. On the other side was a list of new cancers that Zubrod and Frei wanted to target: breast, ovarian, lung cancers, lymphomas. Connecting the two halves of the blackboard were chalky lines matching combinations of cytotoxic drugs to cancers. For a moment, it almost looked as if Frei had been deriving mathematical equations: A+B kills C; E+F eliminates G.

The drugs on Frei's list came largely from three sources. Some, such as aminopterin or methotrexate, were the products of inspired guesswork by scientists (Farber had discovered aminopterin by guessing that an antifolate might block the growth of leukemia cells). Others, such as nitrogen mustard or actinomycin D, came from serendipitous sources, such as mustard gas or soil bacteria, found accidentally to kill cancer cells. Yet others, such as 6-MP, came from drug-screening efforts in which thousands of molecules were tested to find the handful that possessed cancer-killing activity.

The notable common feature that linked all these drugs was that they were all rather indiscriminate inhibitors of cellular growth. Nitrogen mustard, for instance, damages DNA and kills nearly all dividing cells; it kills cancer cells somewhat preferentially because cancer cells divide most actively. To design an ideal anticancer drug, one would need to identify a specific molecular target in a cancer cell and create a chemical to attack that target. But the fundamental biology of cancer was so poorly understood that defining such molecular targets was virtually inconceivable in the 1960s. Yet, even lacking such targets, Frei and Freireich had cured leukemia in some children. Even generic cellular poisons, dosed with adequate brio, could thus eventually obliterate cancer.

The bravado of that logic was certainly hypnotic. Vincent DeVita, another fellow at the institute during that time, wrote, "A new breed of cancer investigators in the 1960s had been addressing the generic question of whether or not cytotoxic chemotherapy was ever capable of curing patients with any type of advanced malignancies." For Frei and Zubrod, the only way to answer that "generic question" was to direct the growing armamentarium of combination chemotherapy against another cancer—a solid tumor this time—which would retrace their steps with leukemia. If yet another kind of cancer responded to this strategy, then there could be little doubt that oncology had stumbled upon a generic solution to the generic problem. A cure would then be within reach for all cancers.

But which cancer would be used to test the principle? Like Kaplan, Zubrod, DeVita, and Canellos also focused on Hodgkin's disease—a cancer that lived on the ill-defined cusp between solid and liquid, a stepping-stone between leukemia and, say, lung cancer or breast cancer. At Stanford, Kaplan had already demonstrated that Hodgkin's lymphoma could be staged with exquisite precision and that local disease could be cured with high-dose extended field radiation. Kaplan had solved half the equation: he had used local therapy with radiation to cure localized forms of Hodgkin's disease. If metastatic Hodgkin's disease could be cured by systemic and aggressive combination chemotherapy, then Zubrod's "generic solution" would begin to sound plausible. The equation would be fully solved.

೨ಿ

Outspoken, pugnacious, and bold, a child of the rough-and-tumble Yonkers area of New York who had bulldozed his way through college and medical school, Vincent DeVita had come to the NCI in 1963 and fallen into the intoxicating orbit of Zubrod, Frei, and Freireich. The unorthodoxy of their approach—the "maniacs doing cancer research," as he called it—had instantly fascinated him. These were the daredevils of medical research, acrobats devising new drugs that nearly killed patients; these men played chicken with death. "Somebody had to show the skeptics that you could actually cure cancer with the right drugs," he believed. In the early months of 1964, he set out to prove the skeptics wrong.

The first test of intensive combination chemotherapy for advanced-stage Hodgkin's disease, led by DeVita, combined four drugs—methotrexate, vincristine (also called Oncovin), nitrogen mustard, and prednisone, a highly toxic cocktail called MOMP. Only fourteen patients were treated. All suffered the predictable consequences of combination chemotherapy; all were hospitalized and confined in isolation chambers to prevent infections during the life-threatening drop in blood counts. As expected, the regimen was sharply criticized at the NCI; this, again, was a quantum leap into a deadly world of mixed poisons. But Frei intervened, silencing the critics and allowing the program to continue.

In 1964, DeVita modified the regimen further. Methotrexate was substituted with a more powerful agent, procarbazine, and the duration of treatment was lengthened from two and a half months to six months. With a team of young, like-minded fellows at the NCI, DeVita began to enroll patients with advanced Hodgkin's disease in a trial of this new cocktail, called MOPP. Like lymphoblastic leukemia, Hodgkin's disease is a rare illness, but the researchers did not need to look hard to find patients. Advanced Hodgkin's disease, often accompanied by the spectral B symptoms, was uniformly fatal. Young men and women (the disease typically strikes men and women in their twenties and thirties) were often referred to the NCI as hopeless cases—and therefore ideal experimental subjects. In just three years, DeVita and Canellos thus accumulated cases at a furious clip, forty-three patients in all. Nine had been blasted with increasing fields of radiation, à la Kaplan, and still progressed inexorably to disseminated, widely metastatic disease. Others had been treated with an ad hoc mix of single agents. None had shown any durable response to prior drugs.

So, like the younger band of leukemics that had gone before them, a fresh new cohort appeared at the institute every two weeks, occupying the plastic chairs of the Clinical Center, lining up for the government-issued cookies and awaiting the terrifying onslaught of the experimental drugs. The youngest was twelve, not even a teenager yet, with lymphoma cells packed in her lungs and liver. A thirteen-year-old boy had Hodgkin's in his pleural cavity; malignant fluid had compressed itself into the lining between his chest wall and lung and made it hard to breathe. The oldest was a sixty-nine-year-old woman with Hodgkin's disease choking off the entrance to her intestine.

♌

If the terror of VAMP was death by infection—children slumped on ventilators with no white blood cells to speak of and bacteria streaming in their blood—then the terror of MOPP was more visceral: death by nausea. The nausea that accompanied the therapy was devastating. It appeared suddenly, then abated just as suddenly, almost capable of snapping the mind shut with its intensity. Many of the patients on the protocol were flown in from nearby cities every fortnight. The trip back home, with the drugs lurching in the blood and the plane lurching in the air, was, for many, a nightmare even worse than their disease.

The nausea was merely a harbinger. As DeVita charged ahead with combination chemotherapy, more complex and novel devastations were revealed. Chemotherapy caused permanent sterility in men and some women. The annihilation of the immune system by the cytotoxic drugs allowed peculiar infections to sprout up: the first adult case of a rare form of pneumonia, caused by an organism, *Pneumocystis carinii* (PCP), was observed in a patient receiving MOPP (the same pneumonia, arising spontaneously in immune-compromised gay men in 1981, would auger the arrival of the HIV epidemic in America). Perhaps the most disturbing side effect of chemotherapy would emerge nearly a decade later. Several young men and women, cured of Hodgkin's disease, would relapse with a second cancer—typically an aggressive, drug-resistant leukemia—caused by the prior treatment with MOPP chemotherapy. As with radiation, cytotoxic chemotherapy would thus turn out to be a double-edged sword: cancer-curing on one hand, and cancer-causing on the other.

But the evidently grim litany of side effects notwithstanding, even early in the course of treatment, there was payoff. In many of the young men and women, the palpable, swollen lymph nodes dissolved in weeks. A twelve-year-old boy from Illinois had been so ravaged by Hodgkin's that his weight had sunk to fifty pounds; within three months of treatment, he gained nearly half his body weight and shot up two feet in height. In others, the strangle-hold of Hodgkin's disease loosened on the organs. Pleural effusions gradually cleared and the nodes in the gut disappeared. As the months passed, it was clear that combination chemo had struck gold once again. At the end of half a year, thirty-five of the forty-three patients had achieved a complete remission. The MOPP trial did not have a control group, but one was not needed to discern the effect. The response and remission rate were unprecedented for advanced Hodgkin's disease. The success would continue in the long-term: more than half the initial cohort of patients would be cured.

Even Kaplan, not an early believer in chemotherapy, was astonished. "Some of the patients with advanced disease have now survived relapse free," he wrote. "The advent of multiple-drug chemotherapy has dramatically changed the prognosis of patients with previously untreated stage III or stage IV Hodgkin's disease."

✑

In May 1968, as the MOPP trial was ascending to its unexpected crescendo, there was equally unexpected news in the world of lymphoblastic leukemia.

Frei and Freireich's VAMP regimen had trailed off at a strange and bleak point. Combination chemo had cured most of the children of leukemia in their blood and bone marrow, but the cancer had explosively relapsed in the brain. In the months following VAMP in 1962, most of these children had hobbled back to the clinic with seemingly innocuous neurological complaints and then spiraled furiously toward their deaths just a week or two afterward. VAMP, once widely touted as the institute's success story, had turned, instead, into its progressive nightmare. Of the fifteen patients treated on the initial protocol, only two still survived. At the NCI, the ambition and bravado that had spurred the original studies was rapidly tipping toward a colder reality. Perhaps Farber's critics had been right. Perhaps lymphoblastic leukemia was a disease that could, at best, be sent into a flickering remission, but never cured. Perhaps palliative care was the best option after all.

But having tasted the success of high-dose chemotherapy, many oncologists could not scale back their optimism: What if even VAMP had not been intensive enough? What if a chemotherapy regimen could be muscled up further, pushed closer to the brink of tolerability?

The leader of this gladiatorial camp was a protégé of Farber's, a thirty-six-year-old oncologist, Donald Pinkel, who had been recruited from Boston to start a leukemia program in Memphis, Tennessee.* In many ways, Memphis was the antipode of Boston. Convulsing with bitter racial tensions and rock-and-roll music—gyrating between the gold and pink of the Graceland mansion in its south and the starkly segregated black neighborhoods in its north—Memphis was turbulent, unpredictable, colorful, perennially warm, and, medically speaking, virtually a no-man's-land. Pinkel's new hospital, called St. Jude's (named, aptly enough, after the patron saint of lost causes), rose like a marooned concrete starfish out of a concrete parking lot on a barren field. In 1961, when Pinkel arrived, the hospital was barely functional, with "no track record, uncertain finances, an unfinished building, no employees or faculty."

Still, Pinkel got a chemotherapy ward up and running, with nurses, residents, and fellows trained in administering the toxic, mercurial drugs. And flung far from the epicenters of leukemia research in New York and Boston, Pinkel's team was determined to outdo every other leukemia trial—the edge outmoding the center—to push the logic of high-dose combination chemotherapy to its extreme. Pinkel thus hammered away in trial after trial, edging his way toward the outer limit of tolerability. And Pinkel and his collaborators emerged with four crucial innovations to the prior regimens.†

First, Pinkel reasoned that while combinations of drugs were necessary to induce remissions, combinations were insufficient in themselves. Perhaps one needed *combinations of combinations*—six, seven, or even eight different chemical poisons mixed and matched together for maximum effect.

Second, since the nervous system relapses had likely occurred because even these highly potent chemicals could not breach the blood-brain barrier, perhaps one needed to instill chemotherapy directly into the nervous system by injecting it into the fluid that bathes the spinal cord.

---

*Although trained in Boston under Farber, Pinkel had spent several years at the Roswell Park Cancer Institute in Buffalo, New York, before moving to Memphis in 1961.

† The Roswell Park group, led by James Holland, and Joseph Burchenal at the Memorial Hospital in New York continued to collaborate with Pinkel in developing the leukemia protocols.

Third, perhaps even that instillation was not enough. Since X-rays could penetrate the brain regardless of the blood-brain barrier, perhaps one needed to add high-dose radiation to the skull to kill residual cells in the brain.

And finally, as Min Chiu Li had seen with choriocarcinoma, perhaps one needed to continue chemotherapy not just for weeks and months as Frei and Freireich had done, but for month after month, stretching into two or even three years.

The treatment protocol that emerged from these guiding principles could only be described as, as one of Pinkel's colleagues called it, "an all-out combat." To start with, the standard antileukemic drugs were given in rapid-fire succession. Then, at defined intervals, methotrexate was injected into the spinal canal using a spinal tap. The brain was irradiated with high doses of X-rays. Then, chemotherapy was bolstered even further with higher doses of drugs and alternating intervals, "in maximum tolerated doses." Antibiotics and transfusions were usually needed, often in succession, often for weeks on end. The treatment lasted up to two and a half years; it involved multiple exposures to radiation, scores of blood tests, dozens of spinal taps, and multiple intravenous drugs—a strategy so precise and demanding that one journal refused to publish it, concerned that it was impossible to even dose it and monitor it correctly without killing several patients in the trials. Even at St. Jude's, the regimen was considered so overwhelmingly toxic that the trial was assigned to relatively junior physicians under Pinkel's supervision because the senior researchers, knowing its risks, did not want to run it. Pinkel called it "total therapy."

As fellows, we called it "total hell."

❧

Carla Reed entered this form of hell in the summer of 2004. Chemotherapy and radiation came back-to-back, one dark tide after another. Some days she got home in the evening (her children already in bed, her husband waiting with dinner) only to turn around and come back the next morning. She lost sleep, her hair, and her appetite and then something more important and ineffable—her animus, her drive, her will. She walked around the hospital like a zombie, shuffling in small steps from the blue vinyl couch in the infusion room to the water dispenser in the central corridor, then back to the couch in those evenly measured steps. "The radiation treatment was the last straw," she recalled. "Lying on the treatment table as still as death, with the mask on my face, I often wondered whether I would even wake up." Even her mother, who had flown in and out of Boston regularly during Carla's first month of treatment, retreated to her own house in Florida, red-eyed and exhausted.

Carla withdrew even more deeply into her own world. Her melancholy hardened into something impenetrable, a carapace, and she pulled into it instinctually, shutting everything out. She lost her friends. During her first few visits, I noticed that she often brought a cheerful young woman as a companion. One morning, I noticed that the friend was missing.

"No company today?" I asked.

Carla looked away and shrugged her shoulders. "We had a falling-out." There was something steely, mechanical in her voice. "She needed to be needed, and I just couldn't fulfill that demand. Not now."

I found myself, embarrassingly enough, sympathizing with the missing friend. As Carla's doctor, I needed to be needed as well, to be acknowledged, even as a peripheral participant in her battle. But Carla had barely any emotional energy for her own recuperation—and certainly none to spare for the needs of others. For her, the struggle with leukemia had become so deeply personalized, so interiorized, that the rest of us were ghostly onlookers in the periphery: *we* were the zombies walking outside her head. Her clinic visits began and ended with awkward pauses. Walking across the hospital in the morning to draw yet another bone marrow biopsy, with the wintry light crosshatching the rooms, I felt a certain dread descend on me, a heaviness that bordered on sympathy but never quite achieved it.

Test came after test. Seven months into her course, Carla had now visited the clinic sixty-six times, had had fifty-eight blood tests, seven spinal taps, and several bone marrow biopsies. One writer, a former nurse, described the typical course of "total therapy" in terms of the tests involved: "From the time of his diagnosis, Eric's illness had lasted 628 days. He had spent one quarter of these days either in a hospital bed or visiting the doctors. He had received more than eight hundred blood tests, numerous spinal and bone marrow taps, 30 X-rays, 120 biochemical tests, and more than two hundred transfusions. No fewer than twenty doctors—hematologists, pulmonologists, neurologists, surgeons, specialists and so on—were involved in his treatment, not including the psychologist and a dozen nurses."

∾

How Pinkel and his team convinced four- and six-year-olds in Memphis to complete that typical routine remains a mystery in its own right. But he did. In July 1968, the St. Jude's team published its preliminary data on the results of the most advanced iteration of total therapy. (Pinkel's team would run eight consecutive trials between 1968 and 1979, each adding another modification to the regimen.) This particular trial, an early variant, was nonrandomized and small, a single hospital's experience with a single cohort of patients. But despite all the caveats, the result was electrifying. The Memphis team had treated thirty-one patients in all. Twenty-seven of them had attained a full remission. The median time to relapse (the time between diagnosis and relapse, a measure of the efficacy of treatment) had stretched out to nearly five years—more than twenty times the longest remissions achieved by most of Farber's first patients.

But most important, thirteen patients, about a third of the original cohort, had *never* relapsed. They were still alive, off chemotherapy. The children had come back to the clinic month after month. The longest remission was now in its sixth year, half the lifetime of that child.

In 1979, Pinkel's team revisited the entire cohort of patients treated over several years with total therapy. Overall, 278 patients in eight consecutive trials had completed their courses of medicines and stopped chemotherapy. Of those, about one-fifth had relapsed. The rest, 80 percent—remained disease free after chemotherapy—"cured," as far as anyone could tell. "ALL in children cannot be considered an incurable disease," Pinkel wrote in a review article. "Palliation is no longer an acceptable approach to its initial treatment."

He was writing to the future, of course, but in a more mystical sense he was writing back to the past, to the doctors who had been deeply nihilistic about therapy for leukemia and had once argued with Farber to let his children quietly "die in peace."

The Cart and the Horse

*I am not opposed to optimism, but I am fearful of the kind
that comes from self-delusion.*
  —Marvin Davis, in the *New England Journal
    of Medicine,* talking about the "cure" for cancer

*The iron is hot and this is the time to pound without
cessation.*
                        —Sidney Farber to Mary Lasker,
                          September 1965

One swallow is a coincidence, but two swallows make summer. By the
autumn of 1968, as the trials in Bethesda and in Memphis announced
their noteworthy successes, the landscape of cancer witnessed a seismic
shift. In the late fifties, as DeVita recalled, "it took plain old courage to be a
chemotherapist . . . and certainly the courage of the conviction that cancer
would eventually succumb to drugs. Clearly, proof was necessary."

Just a decade later, the burden of proof had begun to shift dramatically.
The cure of lymphoblastic leukemia with high-dose chemotherapy might
have been dismissed as a biological fluke, but the success of the same strategy in Hodgkin's disease made it seem like a general principle. "A revolution
[has been] set in motion," DeVita wrote. Kenneth Endicott, the NCI director, concurred: "The next step—the complete cure—is almost sure to follow."

In Boston, Farber greeted the news by celebrating the way he knew best—
by throwing a massive public party. The symbolic date for the party was not
hard to come by. In September 1968, the Jimmy Fund turned twenty-one.*

---

*The Jimmy Fund was launched in May 1948. September 1968 marked its twenty-first
year. The date of Jimmy's "birthday" was arbitrarily assigned by Farber.

Farber recast the occasion as the symbolic twenty-first birthday of Jimmy, a coming-of-age moment for his "child with cancer." The Imperial Ballroom of the Statler Hotel, outside which the Variety Club had once positioned its baseball-shaped donation box for Jimmy in the 1950s, was outfitted for a colossal celebration. The guest list included Farber's typically glitzy retinue of physicians, scientists, philanthropists, and politicians. Mary Lasker couldn't attend the event, but she sent Elmer Bobst from the ACS. Zubrod flew up from the NCI. Kenneth Endicott came from Bethesda.

Conspicuously missing from the list was the original Jimmy himself—Einar Gustafson. Farber knew of Jimmy's whereabouts (he was alive and well, Farber told the press opaquely) but deliberately chose to shroud the rest in anonymity. Jimmy, Farber insisted, was an icon, an abstraction. The real Jimmy had returned to a private, cloistered life on a farm in rural Maine where he now lived with his wife and three children—his restored *normalcy* a sign of victory against cancer. He was thirty-two years old. No one had seen or photographed him for nearly two decades.

At the end of the evening, as the demitasse cups were being wheeled away, Farber rose to the stage in the full glare of the lights. Jimmy's Clinic, he said, now stood at "the most fortunate time in the history of science and medicine." Institutions and individuals across the nation—"the Variety Club, the motion picture industry, the Boston Braves . . . the Red Sox, the world of sports, the press, the television, the radio"—had come together around cancer. What was being celebrated in the ballroom that evening, Farber announced, was not an individual's birthday, but the birth of a once-beleaguered community that had clustered around a disease.

That community now felt on the verge of a breakthrough. As DeVita described it, "The missing piece of the therapeutic puzzle, effective chemotherapy for systemic cancers," had been discovered. High-dose combination chemotherapy would cure *all* cancers—once the right combinations had been found. "The chemical arsenal," one writer noted, "now in the hands of prescribing physicians gives them every bit as much power . . . as the heroic surgeon wielding the knife at the turn of the century."

The prospect of a systematic solution to a cure intoxicated oncologists. It equally intoxicated the political forces that had converged around cancer. Potent, hungry, and expansive, the word *war* captured the essence of the anticancer campaign. Wars demand combatants, weapons, soldiers, the wounded, survivors, bystanders, collaborators, strategists, sentinels, victories—and it was not hard to find a metaphorical analogue to each of these for this war as well.

Wars also demand a clear definition of an enemy. They imbue even formless adversaries with forms. So cancer, a shape-shifting disease of colossal diversity, was recast as a single, monolithic entity. It was *one* disease. As Isaiah Fidler, the Houston oncologist, described it succinctly, cancer was thought to possess "one cause, one mechanism and one cure."

ॐ

If clinical oncologists had multidrug cytotoxic chemotherapy to offer as their unifying solution for cancer—"one cure"—then cancer scientists had their own theory to advance for its unifying cause: viruses. The grandfather of this theory was Peyton Rous, a stooping, white-haired chicken virologist who had been roosting quietly in a laboratory at the Rockefeller Institute in New York until he was dragged out of relative oblivion in the 1960s.

In 1909 (note that date: Halsted had just wrapped up his study of the mastectomy; Neely was yet to advertise his "reward" for the cure for cancer), then a thirty-year-old scientist freshly launching his lab at the Rockefeller Institute, Peyton Rous had been brought a tumor growing on the back of a hen of a black-and-white species of chicken called Plymouth Rock. A rare tumor in a chicken might have left others unimpressed, but the indefatigable Rous secured a $200 grant to study the chicken cancer. Soon, he had categorized the tumor as a sarcoma, a cancer of the connective tissues, with sheet upon sheet of rhomboid, fox-eyed cells invading the tendons and muscle.

Rous's initial work on the chicken sarcoma was thought to have little relevance to human cancers. In the 1920s, the only known causes of human cancer were environmental carcinogens such as radium (recall Marie Curie's leukemia) or organic chemicals, such as paraffin and dye by-products, that were known to cause solid tumors. In the late eighteenth century, an English surgeon named Percivall Pott had argued that cancer of the scrotum, endemic among chimney sweeps, was caused by chronic exposure to chimney soot and smoke. (We will meet Pott again in subsequent pages.)

These observations had led to a theory called the somatic mutation hypothesis of cancer. The somatic theory of cancer argued that environmental carcinogens such as soot or radium somehow permanently altered the structure of the cell and thus caused cancer. But the precise nature of the alteration was unknown. Clearly, soot, paraffin, and radium possessed the capacity to alter a cell in some fundamental way to generate a malignant cell. But how could such a diverse range of insults all converge on the same pathological insult? Perhaps a more systematic explanation was missing—a deeper, more fundamental theory of carcinogenesis.

In 1910, unwittingly, Rous threw the somatic theory into grave doubt. Experimenting with the spindle-cell sarcoma, Rous injected the tumor in one chicken into another chicken and found that the cancer could be transmitted from one bird to another. "I have propagated a spindle-cell sarcoma of the common fowl into its fourth generation," he wrote. "The neoplasm grows rapidly, infiltrates, metastasizes, and remains true to type."

This was curious, but nonetheless still understandable—cancer was a disease of cellular origin, and transferring cells from one organism to another might have been expected to transmit the cancer. But then Rous stumbled on an even more peculiar result. Shuttling tumors from one bird to another, he began to pass the cells through a set of filters, a series of finer and finer cellular sieves, until the cells had been eliminated from the mix and all that was left was the filtrate derived from the cells. Rous expected the tumor transmission to stop, but instead, the tumors continued propagating with a ghostly efficacy—at times even increasing in transmissibility as the cells had progressively vanished.

The agent responsible for carrying the cancer, Rous concluded, was not a cell or an environmental carcinogen, but some tiny particle lurking *within* a cell. The particle was so small that it could easily pass through most filters and keep producing cancer in animals. The only biological particle that had these properties was a virus. His virus was later called Rous sarcoma virus, or RSV for short.

ले

The discovery of RSV, the first cancer-causing virus, felled a deep blow to the somatic mutation theory and set off a frantic search for more cancer viruses. The causal agent for cancer, it seemed, had been found. In 1935, a colleague of Rous's named Richard Schope reported a papillomavirus that caused wartlike tumors in cottontail rabbits. Ten years later, in the mid-1940s, came news of a leukemia-causing virus in mice and then in cats—but still no sign of a bona fide cancer virus in humans.

In 1958, after nearly a three-decade effort, the hunt finally yielded an important prize. An Irish surgeon, Denis Burkitt, discovered an aggressive form of lymphoma—now called Burkitt's lymphoma—that occurred endemically among children in the malaria-ridden belt of sub-Saharan Africa. The pattern of distribution suggested an infectious cause. When two British virologists analyzed the lymphoma cells from Africa, they discovered an infectious agent lodged inside them—not malaria parasites, but a human cancer virus. The new virus was named Epstein-Barr virus or EBV. (EBV is more familiar to us as the virus that causes infectious mononucleosis, or mono.)

The grand total of cancer-causing viruses in humans now stood at one. But the modesty of that number aside, the cancer virus theory was in full spate now—in part because viruses were the new rage in all of medicine. Viral diseases, having been considered incurable for centuries, were now becoming potentially preventable: the polio vaccine, introduced in the summer of 1952, had been a phenomenal success, and the notion that cancer and infectious diseases could eventually collapse into a single pathological entity was simply too seductive to resist.

"Cancer may be infectious," a *Life* magazine cover piece asserted in 1962. Rous received hundreds of letters from anxious men and women asking about exposures to cancer-causing bacteria or viruses. Speculation soon inched toward hysteria and fear. If cancer was infectious, some wondered, why not quarantine patients to prevent its spread? Why not send cancer patients to sanitation wards or isolation facilities, where TB and smallpox victims had once been confined? One woman who believed that she had been exposed to a coughing lung cancer patient wrote, "Is there something I can do to kill the cancer germ? Can the rooms be fumigated . . . ? Should I give up my lease and move out?"

If the "cancer germ" had infected one space most acutely, it was the imagination of the public—and, equally, the imagination of researchers. Farber turned into a particularly fervent believer. In the early 1960s, goaded by his insistence, the NCI inaugurated a Special Virus Cancer Program, a systematic hunt for human cancer viruses patterned explicitly after the chemotherapy discovery program. The project snowballed into public prominence, gathering enormous support. Hundreds of monkeys at the NCI-funded lab were inoculated with human tumors with the hopes of turning the monkeys into viral incubators for vaccine development. Unfortunately, the monkeys failed to produce even a single cancer virus, but nothing dimmed the optimism. Over the next decade, the cancer virus program siphoned away more than 10 percent of the NCI contract budget—nearly $500 million. (In contrast, the institute's cancer nutrition program, meant to evaluate the role of diet in cancer—a question of at least equal import—received one-twentieth of that allocation.)

Peyton Rous was rehabilitated into the scientific mainstream and levitated into permanent scientific sainthood. In 1966, having been overlooked for a full fifty-five years, he was awarded the Nobel Prize for physiology and medicine. On the evening of December 10 at the ceremony in Stockholm, he rose to the podium like a resurrected messiah. Rous acknowledged in his talk that the virus theory of cancer still needed much more work and clarity. "Relatively few viruses have any connection with the production of neoplasms," Rous said. But bulldogish and unwilling to capitulate, Rous lambasted the idea that cancer could be caused by something inherent to the cells, such as a genetic mutation. "A favorite explanation has been that oncogenes cause alterations in the genes of the cells of the body, somatic mutations as these are termed. But numerous facts, when taken together, decisively exclude this supposition."

He groused elsewhere: "What have been [the fruits] of this somatic mutation hypothesis? . . . Most serious of all the results of the somatic mutation hypothesis has been its effect on research workers. It acts as a tranquilizer on those who believe it."

Rous had his own tranquilizer to offer: a unifying hypothesis that viruses caused cancer. And many in his audience, in no mood for caveats and complexities, were desperate to swallow his medicine. The somatic mutation theory of cancer was dead. The scientists who had studied environmental carcinogenesis needed to think of other explanations why radium or soot might cause cancer. (Perhaps, the virus theorists reasoned, these insults activated endogenous viruses.)

∂∫∂

Two superficial theories were thus stitched audaciously—and prematurely—into one comprehensive whole. One offered a cause: *viruses caused cancer* (although a vast majority of them were yet undiscovered). The second offered a cure: *particular combinations of cytotoxic poisons would cure cancer* (although specific combinations for the vast majority of cancers were yet undiscovered).

Viral carcinogenesis clearly demanded a deeper explanation: how might viruses—elemental microbes floating from cell to cell—cause so profound a change in a cell's physiology as to create a malignant cell? The success of cytotoxic chemotherapy provoked equally fundamental questions: why had a series of rather general poisons cured some forms of cancer, while leaving other forms completely unscathed?

Obviously, a more fundamental explanation lurked beneath all of this, an explanation that would *connect* cause and cure. So some researchers urged patience, diligence, and time. "The program directed by the National Cancer Institute has been derided as one that puts the cart before the horse by searching for a cure before knowing the cause," Kenneth Endicott, the NCI director, acknowledged in 1963. "We have certainly not found a cure for cancer. We have a dozen chemicals which are somewhat better than those known before the program began but none are dramatically better. They prolong the patient's life somewhat and make him more comfortable, but that is all."

But the Laskerites had little time for such nuanced descriptions of progress; this cart would have to drag the horse. "The iron is hot and this is the time to pound without cessation," Farber wrote to Lasker. The groundwork for an all-out battle had already been laid. All that was necessary was to put pressure on Congress to release funds. "No large mission or goal-directed effort [against cancer], supported with adequate funds has ever been organized," Mary Lasker announced in an open letter to Congress in 1969.

Lasker's thoughts were echoed by Solomon Garb, a little-known professor of pharmacology at the University of Missouri who shot to prominence by publishing the book *Cure for Cancer: A National Goal* in 1968. "The theme of this book," Garb began, "is that the time has come for a closer look at cancer research and for a new consolidation of effort aimed at cure or control of cancer. . . . A major hindrance to cancer effort has been a chronic, severe shortage of funds—a situation that is not generally recognized. It is not enough, however, to point this out or to repeat it; it is also necessary to explain how additional funds would be used, what projects they would pay for, why such projects deserve support, and where the skilled scientists and technicians to do the work would come from."

Garb's book was described as a "springboard to progress," and the Laskerites certainly sprang. As with Farber, a doctor's word was the ultimate prescription. That Garb had prescribed precisely the strategy advocated by the Laskerites instantly transformed him in their eyes into a messianic figure. His book became their bible.

Religious movements and cults are often founded on a tetrad of elements: a prophet, a prophecy, a book, and a revelation. By the summer of 1969, the cancer crusade had acquired three of these four essential elements. Its prophet was Mary Lasker, the woman who had guided it out of the dark wilderness of the 1950s into national prominence just two decades later. Its prophecy was the cure for childhood leukemia, inaugurated by Farber's experiments in Boston and ending with Pinkel's astonishing successes in Memphis. Its book was Garb's *Cure for Cancer*. The final missing element was a revelation—a sign that would auger the future and capture the imagination of the public. In the spirit of all great revelations, this one would also appear unexpectedly and mystically out of the blue. It would appear, quite literally, from the heavens.

ℐℓ

At 4:17 p.m. EDT on July 20, 1969, a fifteen-ton spacecraft moved silently through the cold, thin atmosphere above the moon and landed on a rocky basalt crater on the lunar surface. A vast barren landscape—a "magnificent desolation"—stretched out around the spacecraft. "It suddenly struck me," one of the two astronauts would recall, "that that tiny pea, pretty and blue, was the earth. I put up my thumb and shut one eye, and my thumb blotted out the planet."

On that pea-size blue planet glimmering on the horizon, this was a moment of reckoning. "It was a stunning scientific and intellectual accomplishment," *Time* reported in July 1969, "for a creature who, in the space of a few million years—an instant in evolutionary chronology—emerged from primeval forests to hurl himself at the stars. . . . It was, in any event, a shining reaffirmation of the optimistic premise that whatever man imagines he can bring to pass."

The cancer crusaders could not have asked for a more exuberant vindication for their own project. Here was another "programmatic" effort—planned, targeted, goal-oriented, and intensely focused—that had delivered its results in record time. When Max Faget, the famously taciturn engineer of the Apollo program, was later asked to comment on the principal scientific challenge of the moon landing, he could only come up with a single word: "Propulsion." The impression was that the moon walk had turned out to be a technological cakewalk—no more complicated than building a more powerful jet plane, magnifying it several dozenfold, and pointing it vertically at the moon.

The Laskerites, transfixed in front of their flickering television sets in Boston, Washington, and New York on the evening of the moon landing, were primed to pick up on all these analogies. Like Faget, they believed that the missing element in the cancer crusade was some sort of propulsion, a simple, internal vertical thrust that would transform the scale and scope of their efforts and catapult them toward the cure.

In fact, the missing propulsion, they believed, had finally been found. The success against childhood leukemia—and more recently, Hodgkin's disease—stood out as proofs of principle, the first hesitant explorations of a vast unexplored space. Cancer, like the moon, was also a landscape of magnificent desolation—but a landscape on the verge of discovery. In her letters, Mary Lasker began to refer to a programmatic War on Cancer as the conquest of "inner space" (as opposed to "outer space"), instantly unifying the two projects.

The moon landing thus marked a turning point in the life cycle of the cancer crusade. In the past, the Laskerites had concentrated much of their efforts on *political* lobbying in Washington. When advertisements or posters had been pitched directly to the public, they had been mainly educational. The Laskerites had preferred to maneuver backstage, preferring political advocacy to public advocacy.

But by 1969, politics had changed. Lister Hill, the Alabama senator and one of Mary Lasker's strongest supporters, was retiring after several decades in the Senate. Senator Edward Kennedy, Farber's ally from Boston, was so deeply embroiled in the Chappaquiddick scandal (in July 1969, a car carrying Kennedy and a campaign worker veered off a Martha's Vineyard bridge and sank underwater, drowning his passenger; Kennedy pleaded guilty for leaving the crime scene and received a suspended sentence) that he had virtually disappeared into legislative oblivion. The Laskerites were now doubly orphaned. "We're in the worst," Lasker recalled. "We're back to a phase that we were in the early fifties when . . . we had no friend in the Senate. We went on constantly—but no effective sympathy."

With their voices now muted in Washington, with little sympathy in the House and no friend in the Senate, the Laskerites were forced to revamp the strategy for their crusade—from backstage political maneuvering to front-stage public mobilization. In retrospect, that turn in their trajectory was well-timed. The success of *Apollo 11* may have dramatically affected the Laskerites' own view of their project, but, more important perhaps, it created an equally seismic shift in the public perception of science. That cancer could be conquered, just as the moon had been conquered, was scarcely a matter of doubt. The Laskerites coined a phrase to describe this analogy. They called it a "moon shot" for cancer.

"A moon shot for cancer"

> *The relationship of government to science in the post-*
> *war years is a case in point. Without very much visible*
> *deliberation, but with much solemnity, we have in*
> *little more than a decade elevated science to a level of*
> *extraordinary influence in national policy; and now that*
> *it is there, we are not very certain what to do with it.*
> —William Carey, 1963

> *What has Santa Nixon given us lately?*
> —*New York Times*, 1971

On December 9, 1969, on a chilly Sunday morning, a full-page advertisement appeared in the *Washington Post*:*

Mr. Nixon: You can cure cancer.

If prayers are heard in Heaven, this prayer is heard the most:
"Dear God, please. Not cancer."

Still, more than 318,000 Americans died of cancer last year.

This year, Mr. President, you have it in your power to begin to end this
curse.

As you agonize over the Budget, we beg you to remember the agony of
those 318,000 Americans. And their families.

. . . We ask a better perspective, a better way to allocate our money to
save hundreds of thousands of lives each year.

. . . Dr. Sidney Farber, Past President of the American Cancer Society,
believes: "We are so close to a cure for cancer. We lack only the will and

---

*It would run in the *New York Times* on December 17.

the kind of money and comprehensive planning that went into putting a
man on the moon."

. . . If you fail us, Mr. President, this will happen:

One in six Americans now alive, 34,000,000 people, will die of cancer
unless new cures are found.

One in four Americans now alive, 51,000,000 people, will have cancer
in the future.

We simply cannot afford this.

A powerful image accompanied the text. Across the bottom of the page,
a cluster of cancer cells was loosely grouped into a mass. Some of these
cells were crumbling off that mass, sending a shower of metastatic fingerlings through the text. The letters *e* and *r* in *cancer* had been eaten through
by these cells, like holes punched out in the bone by breast cancer.

It is an unforgettable picture, a confrontation. The cells move across the
page, almost tumbling over each other in their frenzy. They divide with
hypnotic intensity; they metastasize in the imagination. This is cancer in
its most elemental form—naked, ghoulish, and magnified.

The *Times* ad marked a seminal intersection in the history of cancer.
With it, cancer declared its final emergence from the shadowy interiors
of medicine into the full glare of public scrutiny, morphing into an illness of national and international prominence. This was a generation
that no longer whispered about cancer. There was cancer in newspapers
and cancer in books, cancer in theater and in films: in 450 articles in the
New York Times in 1971; in Aleksandr Solzhenitsyn's *Cancer Ward*, a blistering account of a cancer hospital in the Soviet Union; in *Love Story*, a
1970 film about a twenty-four-year-old woman who dies of leukemia; in
Bang the Drum Slowly, a 1973 release about a baseball catcher diagnosed
with Hodgkin's disease; in *Brian's Song*, the story of the Chicago Bears
star Brian Piccolo, who died of testicular cancer. A torrent of op-ed pieces
and letters appeared in newspapers and magazines. One man wrote to
the *Wall Street Journal* describing how his family had been "plunged into
numb agony" when his son was diagnosed with cancer. "Cancer changes
your life," a patient wrote after her mastectomy. "It alters your habits. . . .
Everything becomes magnified."

There is, in retrospect, something preformed in that magnification,
a deeper resonance—as if cancer had struck the raw strings of anxiety
already vibrating in the public psyche. When a disease insinuates itself so

potently into the imagination of an era, it is often because it impinges on an anxiety latent within that imagination. AIDS loomed so large on the 1980s in part because this was a generation inherently haunted by its sexuality and freedom; SARS set off a panic about global spread and contagion at a time when globalism and social contagion were issues simmering nervously in the West. Every era casts illness in its own image. Society, like the ultimate psychosomatic patient, matches its medical afflictions to its psychological crises; when a disease touches such a visceral chord, it is often because that chord is already resonating.

So it was with cancer. As the writer and philosopher Renata Salecl described it, "A radical change happened to the perception of the object of horror" in the 1970s, a progression from the external to the internal. In the 1950s, in the throes of the Cold War, Americans were preoccupied with the fear of annihilation from the outside: from bombs and warheads, from poisoned water reservoirs, communist armies, and invaders from outer space. The threat to society was perceived as external. Horror movies—the thermometers of anxiety in popular culture—featured alien invasions, parasitic occupations of the brain, and body snatching: *It Came from Outer Space* or *The Man from Planet X*.

But by the early 1970s, the locus of anxiety—the "object of horror," as Salecl describes it—had dramatically shifted from the outside to the inside. The rot, the horror—the biological decay and its concomitant spiritual decay—was now relocated *within* the corpus of society and, by extension, within the body of man. American society was still threatened, but this time, the threat came from inside. The names of horror films reflected the switch: *The Exorcist*; *They Came from Within*.

Cancer epitomized this internal horror. It was the ultimate emergence of the enemy from within—a marauding cell that crawled out of one's own body and occupied it from the inside, an internal alien. The "Big Bomb," a columnist wrote, was replaced by "the Big C":

"When I was growing up in the 1950s, it was The Bomb. This thing, The Bomb, belonged to a generation of war babies. . . . But we are fickle even about fear. We seem to have dropped our bombphobia now without, in any way, reducing the reasons for it. Cancer now leads this macabre hit parade. The middle-sized children I know seem to think that death comes, not with a bang but with a tumor. . . . Cancer is the obsession of people who sense that disaster may not be a purposeful instrument of public policy but a matter of accidental, random carelessness."

These metaphorical shifts were more powerful, more pervasive, and more influential than the Laskerites could even have imagined. The *Times* ad represented a strategic realignment of power. By addressing their letter to the president on behalf of "millions of Americans," the Laskerites performed a tactically brilliant about-face. In the past, they had pleaded *to* the nation for funds for cancer. Now, as they pleaded *for* the nation for a more coordinated attack on cancer, they found themselves colossally empowered in the public imagination. The cure for cancer became incorporated into the very fabric of the American dream. "To oppose big spending against cancer," one observer told the historian James Patterson, was to "oppose Mom, apple pie, and the flag." In America, this was a triumvirate too powerful for even the president to ignore.

Impatient, aggressive, and goal-driven, the president, Richard Milhous Nixon, was inherently partial to impatient, aggressive, and goal-driven projects. The notion of science as an open-ended search for obscure truths bothered and befuddled him. Nixon often groused that scientists didn't "know a goddamn thing" about the management of science. Nor was he particularly sympathetic to open-ended scientific funding. Corn-fed and fattened on increasingly generous federal grants, scientists (often called "nuts" or "bastards" by members of his administration) were thought to have become arrogant and insular. Nixon wanted them "to shape up."

For Nixon, this "shaping up" meant wresting the control of science out of the hands of academic "nutcases" and handing it over to a new cadre of scientific bureaucrats—science managers who would bring discipline and accountability to science. The replacement of Nixon's science adviser, Lee DuBridge, a scholarly, old-school atomic physicist from Caltech, with Ed David, an impulsive, fast-paced engineer-turned-manager from the Bell research labs, was meant as a signal to the scientific community to get into shape. David was the first presidential science adviser to emerge out of an industrial lab and to have no direct connection with a university. His mandate was to get an effective science operation that would redirect its energies toward achieving defined national goals. What scientists needed—what the public demanded—was not an "endless frontier" (à la Vannevar Bush) but a discipline with pragmatic frontiers and well-defined ends.

Lasker's job, then, was to convert the already converted. In 1969, deploying her typical strategic genius, Mary Lasker proposed that a "neutral" committee of experts, called a Commission on the Conquest of Cancer, be created to advise the president on the most efficient strategy to mount a systematic response to cancer. The commission, she wrote, should "include space scientists, industrialists, administrators, planners, and cancer research specialists . . . entrusted to outline the possibilities for the conquest of cancer for the Congress of the United States at whatever cost."

Of course, Lasker ensured that there was nothing neutral about the commission (eventually called the Panel of Consultants). Its members, chosen with exquisite deliberateness, were all Lasker's friends, associates, and sympathizers—men and women already sold on the War on Cancer. Sidney Farber was selected as the cochairman, along with Senator Ralph Yarborough from Texas (Yarborough, like Lister Hill, was one of the Laskers' oldest allies in Congress). Solomon Garb was appointed on account of his book. Joseph Burchenal was brought in from Memorial Hospital, James Holland from Roswell Park, Henry Kaplan from Stanford. Benno Schmidt, a partner in a prominent New York investment firm and a major donor to Memorial Hospital, joined the group. (An energetic organizer, Schmidt was eventually asked to replace Farber and Yarborough to head the panel; that Schmidt was a Republican and a close confidant of President Nixon's was a marked plus.) Politics, science, medicine, and finance were thus melded together to craft a national response. To reinforce the facade of neutrality, Yarborough wrote to Mary Lasker in the summer of 1970, "asking" her to join (although he scribbled at the bottom, "Your letter should have been the first mailed. It was your genius, energy and will to help.")

The panel's final report, entitled the *National Program for the Conquest of Cancer*, was issued in the winter of 1970, and its conclusions were predictable: "In the past, when the Federal Government has desired to give top priority to a major scientific project of the magnitude of that involved in the conquest of cancer, it has, on occasion, with considerable success, given the responsibility for the project to an independent agency." While tiptoeing around the idea, the panel was proposing the creation of an independent cancer agency—a NASA for cancer.

The agency would start with a budget of $400 million, then its allocations would increase by $100 million to $150 million per year, until, by the mid-1970s, it would stand at $1 billion. When Schmidt was asked if he thought that the country could "afford such a program," he was unhesitant in his reply: "Not only can we afford the effort, we cannot afford *not* to do it."

ॐ

On March 9, 1971, acting on the panel's recommendations, Ted Kennedy and Jacob Javits floated a Senate Bill—S 1828, the Conquest of Cancer Act—to create a National Cancer Authority, an independent, self-governing agency for cancer research. The director of the authority would be appointed by the president and confirmed by the Senate—again underscoring an extraordinary level of autonomy. (Usually, disease-specific institutes, such as the National Heart Institute, were overseen by the NIH.) An advisory board of eighteen members would report back to Congress about progress on cancer. That panel would comprise scientists, administrators, politicians, physicians—and, most controversially, "lay individuals," such as Lasker, Foote, and Bobst, whose sole task would be to keep the public eye trained sharply on the war. The level of funding, public scrutiny, and autonomy would be unprecedented in the history of the NIH—and arguably in the history of American science.

Mary Lasker was busy maneuvering behind the scenes to whip up support for the Kennedy/Javits bill. In January 1971, she fired off a cavalcade of letters to her various friends seeking support for the independent cancer agency. In February, she hit upon another tactical gem: she persuaded her close friend Ann Landers (her real name was Eppie Lederer), the widely read advice columnist from Chicago, to publish a column about cancer and the Kennedy bill, positioning it exactly at the time that the vote was fermenting in the Senate.

Landers's column appeared on April 20, 1971. It began solemnly, "Dear Readers: If you are looking for a laugh today, you'd better skip Ann Landers. If you want to be part of an effort that might save millions of lives—maybe your own—please stay with me. . . . How many of us have asked the question, 'If this great country of ours can put a man on the moon why can't we find a cure for cancer?'"

Landers's answer to that question—echoing the Laskerites—was that cancer was missing not merely a medical cure but a political cure. "If enough citizens let their senators know they want Bill S-34 passed, it will pass. . . . Vote for S-34," she pleaded. "And sign your name please."

Even Landers and Lasker were shocked by the ensuing "blizzard" of mail. "I saw trucks arriving at the Senate," the journalist Barbara Walters recalled. Letters poured in by the bagful—about a million in all—pushing the Senate mailroom to its breaking point. One senator wrote that he received sixty thousand letters. An exasperated secretary charged with sorting the mail hung up the sign IMPEACH ANN LANDERS on her desk. Stuart Symington, the senator from Missouri, wrote to Landers begging her to post another column advising people to stop writing. "Please Eppie," he begged, "I got the message."

The Senate was also getting the message. In June 1971, a modified version of the Kennedy/Javits bill appeared on the floor. On Wednesday afternoon, July 7, after dozens of testimonies by scientists and physicians, the motion was finally put to a vote. At five thirty that evening, the votes were counted: 79 in favor and 1 against.

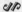

The swift and decisive victory in the Senate was precisely as the Laskerites had planned it. The cancer bill was now destined for the House, but its passage there promised to be a much tougher hurdle. The Laskerites had few allies and little influence in the lower chamber. The House wanted more testimony—and not just testimony from the Laskerites' carefully curated panel. It solicited opinions from physicians, scientists, administrators and policymakers—and those opinions, it found, diverged sharply from the ones presented to the Senate. Philip Lee, the former assistant secretary of health complained, "Cancer is not simply an island waiting in isolation for a crash program to wipe it out. It is in no way comparable to a moon shot—to a Gemini or an Apollo program—which requires mainly the mobilization of money, men, and facilities to put together in one imposing package the scientific knowledge we already possess." The Apollo mission and the Manhattan Project, the two models driving this War on Cancer were both *technological* achievements that stood on the shoulders of long and deep scientific discoveries (atomic physics, fluid mechanics, and thermodynamics). In contrast, even a cursory understanding of the process that made cells become malignant was missing. Seizing on the Laskerites' favorite metaphor, Sol Spiegelman, the Columbia University cancer scientist, argued, "An all-out effort at this time would be like trying to land a man on the moon without knowing Newton's laws of gravity." James Watson, who had discovered the structure of DNA, unloosed a verbal rampage against the Senate bill. "Doing 'relevant' research is not necessarily doing 'good' research," Watson would later write. "In particular we must reject the notion that we will be lucky. . . . Instead we will be witnessing a massive expansion of well-intentioned mediocrity."

Others argued that the notion of a targeted war on a particular disease inevitably distracted from natural synergies with other arenas of research, forcing cancer researchers to think "inside the box." An NIH administrator complained, "In a nutshell, [the act] states that all NIH institutes are equal, but one [the NCI] is more equal than the others." Yet others argued that the metaphor of war would inevitably become a distraction. It would whip up a froth of hype and hope, and the letdown would be catastrophic. "I suspect there is trouble ahead for research in cancer," Irvine Page, the editor of a prominent scientific journal wrote. "People have become impatient with what they take to be lack of progress. Having seen what can be achieved by systems analysis, directed research, and great coordinated achievements such as the moon walk, they transfer the same thinking to the conquest of cancer all too readily." This bubble would inevitably burst if the cancer project stalled or failed.

*

Nixon, meanwhile, had reached the edge of his patience. Elections were fast approaching in 1972. Earlier that year, commentators such as Bob Wiedrich from the *Chicago Tribune* had laid down the stakes: "If Richard Milhous Nixon . . . can achieve these two giant goals—an end to the war in Vietnam and defeat of the ravages of cancer—then he will have carved for himself in the history of this nation a niche of Lincolnesque proportions, for he will have done more than put a man on the moon."

An end to the war in Vietnam was nowhere in sight, but a campaign against cancer seemed vastly more tractable, and Nixon was willing to force a cancer bill—*any* cancer bill—through Congress. When the ever-resourceful Schmidt went to visit him in the Oval Office that fall of 1971 (in part, to propose a compromise), Nixon reassured Schmidt that he would finagle—or strong-arm—a solution: "Don't worry about it. I'll take care of that."

In November 1971, Paul Rogers, a Democrat in the House from Florida, crafted a compromise cancer bill. In keeping with the Laskerites' vision, Rogers's bill proposed a vast increase in the budget for cancer research. But in contrast to the Kennedy/Javits bill, it proposed to sharply restrict the autonomy of the National Cancer Institute. There would be no "NASA for cancer." But given the vast increase in money, the focused federal directive, and the staggering rise in hope and energy, the rhetoric of a "war" on cancer would still be fully justified. The Laskerites, their critics, and Nixon would all go home happy.

In December 1971, the House finally put a modified version of Rogers's bill to a vote. The verdict was nearly unanimous: 350 votes for and 5 against. A week later, a House-Senate meeting resolved minor differences in their bills, and the final legislation was sent to the president to sign.

On December 23, 1971, on a cold, windswept afternoon in Washington, Nixon signed the National Cancer Act at a small ceremony in the White House. The doors to the State Dining Room were thrown open, and the president seated himself at a small wooden desk. Photographers parried for positions on the floor around the desk. Nixon leaned over and signed the act with a quick flourish. He handed the pen as a gift to Benno Schmidt, the chair of the Panel of Consultants. Mary Lasker beamed forcefully from her chair. Farber chose not to attend.

For the Laskerites, the date marked a bittersweet vindication. The flood of money authorized for cancer research and control—$400 million for 1972; $500 million for 1973; and $600 million for 1974 (a total of $1.5 billion over the next three years)—was a monumental achievement. If money was "frozen energy," as Mary Lasker often described it, then this, at last, was a pot of energy to be brought to full boil.

But the passage of the bill had also been a reality check. The overwhelming opinion among scientists (outside those on the Panel of Consultants) was that this was a premature attack on cancer. Mary Lasker was bitingly critical of the final outcome. The new bill, she told a reporter, "contained nothing that was useful that gave any guts to the Senate bill."

Humiliated by the defeat, Lasker and Sidney Farber withdrew soon after the House vote from the political world of cancer. Farber went back to Boston and nursed his wounds privately. Lasker retired to her museum-like apartment on Beekman Place in New York—a white box filled with white furniture—and switched the focus of her efforts from cancer to urban beautification projects. She would continue to actively campaign in Washington for health-related legislation and award the Lasker Prize, an annual award given to researchers for breakthroughs in medicine and biological sciences. But the insistent, urgent vigor that she had summoned during the two-decade campaign for a War on Cancer, the near-molten energy capable of flowing into any federal agency and annihilating resistance in its course, dissipated slowly. In April 1974, a young journalist went to Lasker to ask her about one of her many tulip-planting proposals for New York. At the end of the interview, the reporter asked Lasker about her perception of her own power: was she not one of the most powerful women in the country? Lasker cut the journalist short: "Powerful? I don't know. No. If I were really powerful, I'd have gotten more done."

Scientists, too, withdrew from the war—in part, because they had little to contribute to it. The rhetoric of this war implied that its tools, its weapons, its army, its target, and its strategy had already been assembled. Science, the discovery of the unknown, was pushed to the peripheries of this battle. Massive, intensively funded clinical trials with combinations of cell-killing drugs would be heavily prioritized. The quest for universal causes and universal solutions—cancer viruses among them—would be highly funded. "We will in a relatively short period of time make vast inroads on the cancer problem," Farber had announced to Congress in 1970. His army was now "on the march," even if he and Mary Lasker had personally extricated themselves from its front lines.

The act, then, was an anomaly, designed explicitly to please all of its clients, but unable to satisfy any of them. The NIH, the Laskerites, scientists, lobbyists, administrators, and politicians—each for his or her own reasons—felt that what had been crafted was either precisely too little or precisely too much. Its most ominous assessment came from the editorial pages of the *Chicago Tribune*: "A crash program can produce only one result: a crash."

❦

On March 30, 1973, in the late afternoon, a code call, a signal denoting the highest medical emergency, rang through the floors of the Jimmy Fund Building. It sounded urgently through the open doors of the children's clinic, past the corridors with the cartoon portraits on the walls and the ward beds lined with white sheets and children with intravenous lines, all the way to the Brigham and Women's Hospital, where Farber had trained as an intern—in a sense retracing the trajectory of his life.

A group of doctors and nurses in scrubs swung out toward the stairs. The journey took a little longer than usual because their destination was on the far end of the hospital, up on the eighth floor. In the room with tall, airy windows, they found Farber with his face resting on his desk. He had died of a cardiac arrest. His last hours had been spent discussing the future of the Jimmy Fund and the direction of the War on Cancer. His papers were neatly arranged in the shelves all around him, from his first book on the postmortem examination to the most recent article on advances in leukemia therapy, which had arrived that very week.

Obituaries poured out from every corner of the world. Mary Lasker's was possibly the most succinct and heartfelt, for she had lost not just her friend but a part of herself. "Surely," she wrote, "the world will never be the same."

*

From the fellows' office at the Dana-Farber Cancer Institute, just a few hundred feet across the street from where Farber had collapsed in his office, I called Carla Reed. It was August 2005, a warm, muggy morning in Boston. A child's voice answered the phone, then I was put on hold. In the background I could hear the white noise of a household in full tilt: crockery, doorbells, alarms, the radio blaring morning news. Carla came on the phone, her voice suddenly tightening as she recognized mine.

"I have news," I said quickly, "good news."

Her bone marrow results had just returned. A few nodules of normal blood cells were growing back interspersed between cobblestones of bone and fat cells—signs of a regenerating marrow reclaiming its space. But there was no trace of leukemia anywhere. Under the microscope, what had once been lost to cancer was slowly returning to normalcy. This was the first of many milestones that we would cross together, a moment of celebration.

"Congratulations, Carla," I said. "You are in a full remission."

PART THREE

"WILL YOU TURN ME OUT IF I CAN'T GET BETTER?"

Oft expectation fails, and most oft there
Where most it promises; and oft it hits
Where hope is coldest, and despair most sits
  —William Shakespeare,
    All's Well That Ends Well

I have seen the moment of my greatness flicker
And I have seen the eternal Footman hold my coat, and
    snicker,
And in short, I was afraid.

                              —T. S. Eliot

You are absolutely correct, of course, when you say that
we can't go on asking for more money from the President
unless we demonstrate progress.
                  —Frank Rauscher, director of
                    the National Cancer Program,
                    to Mary Lasker, 1974

"In God we trust.
All others [must] have data"

In science, ideology tends to corrupt; absolute ideology,
[corrupts] absolutely.

　　　　　　　　　　　　　　　—Robert Nisbet

Orthodoxy in surgery is like orthodoxy in other depart-
ments of the mind—it . . . begins to almost challenge a
comparison with religion.

　　　　　　　　　　　　　　　—Geoffrey Keynes

You mean I had a mastectomy for nothing?
　　　　　　　　　　—Rose Kushner

Farber was fortunate to have lived in the right time, but he was perhaps even more fortunate to have died at the right time. The year of his death, 1973, marked the beginning of a deeply fractured and contentious period in the history of cancer. Theories were shattered; drug discoveries stagnated; trials languished; and academic meetings degenerated into all-out brawls. Radiotherapists, chemotherapists, and surgeons fought viciously for power and information. The War on Cancer seemed, at times, to have devolved into a war *within* cancer.

The unraveling began at the very center of oncology. Radical surgery, Halsted's cherished legacy, had undergone an astonishing boom in the 1950s and '60s. At surgical conferences around the world, Halsted's descendants—powerful and outspoken surgeons such as Cushman Haagensen and Jerome Urban—had stood up to announce that they had outdone the master himself in their radicalism. "In my own surgical attack on carcinoma of the breast," Haagensen wrote in 1956, "I have followed the fundamental principle that the disease, even in its early stage, is such a formidable enemy that it is my duty to carry out as radical an operation as the . . . anatomy permits."

The radical mastectomy had thus edged into the "superradical" and then into the "ultraradical," an extraordinarily morbid, disfiguring procedure in which surgeons removed the breast, the pectoral muscles, the axillary nodes, the chest wall, and occasionally the ribs, parts of the sternum, the clavicle, and the lymph nodes inside the chest.

Halsted, meanwhile, had become the patron saint of cancer surgery, a deity presiding over his comprehensive "theory" of cancer. He had called it, with his Shakespearean ear for phrasemaking, the "centrifugal theory"—the idea that cancer, like a malevolent pinwheel, tended to spread in ever-growing arcs from a single central focus in the body. Breast cancer, he claimed, spun out from the breast into the lymph nodes under the arm (poetically again, he called these nodes "sentinels"), then cartwheeled mirthlessly through the blood into the liver, lungs, and bones. A surgeon's job was to arrest that centrifugal spread by cutting every piece of it out of the body, as if to catch and break the wheel in midspin. This meant treating early breast cancer aggressively and definitively. The more a surgeon cut, the more he cured.

Even for patients, that manic diligence had become a form of therapy. Women wrote to their surgeons in admiration and awe, begging them not to spare their surgical extirpations, as if surgery were an anagogical ritual that would simultaneously rid them of cancer and uplift them into health. Haagensen transformed from surgeon to shaman: "To some extent," he wrote about his patients, "no doubt, they transfer the burden [of their disease] to me." Another surgeon wrote—chillingly—that he sometimes "operated on cancer of the breast solely for its effect on morale." He also privately noted, "I do not despair of carcinoma being cured somewhere in the future, but this blessed achievement will, I believe, never be wrought by the knife of the surgeon."

*

Halsted may have converted an entire generation of physicians in America to believe in the "blessed achievement" of his surgical knife. But the farther one got from Baltimore, the less, it seemed, was the force of his centrifugal theory; at St. Bartholomew's Hospital in London, a young doctor named Geoffrey Keynes was not so convinced.

In August 1924, Keynes examined a patient with breast cancer, a thin, emaciated woman of forty-seven with an ulcerated malignant lump in her breast. In Baltimore or in New York, such a patient would immediately have been whisked off for radical surgery. But Keynes was concerned about his patient's constitutional frailty. Rather than reaching indiscriminately for a radical procedure (which would likely have killed her at the operating table), he opted for a much more conservative strategy. Noting that radiation therapists, such as Emil Grubbe, had demonstrated the efficacy of X-rays in treating breast cancer, Keynes buried fifty milligrams of radium in her breast to irradiate her tumor and monitored her to observe the effect, hoping, at best, to palliate her symptoms. Surprisingly, he found a marked improvement. "The ulcer rapidly heal[ed]," he wrote, "and the whole mass [became] smaller, softer and less fixed." Her mass reduced so rapidly, Keynes thought he might be able to perform a rather minimal, nonradical surgery on her to completely remove it.

Emboldened by his success, between 1924 and 1928, Keynes attempted other variations on the same strategy. The most successful of these permutations, he found, involved a careful mixture of surgery and radiation, both at relatively small doses. He removed the malignant lumps locally with a minor operation (i.e., without resorting to radical or ultraradical surgery). He followed the surgery with radiation to the breast. There was no stripping of nodes, no cracking or excavation of clavicles, no extirpations that stretched into six or eight hours. Nothing was radical, yet, in case after case, Keynes and his colleagues found that their cancer recurrence rate was at least comparable to those obtained in New York or Baltimore—achieved without grinding patients through the terrifying crucible of radical surgery.

In 1927, in a rather technical report to his department, Keynes reviewed his experience combining local surgery with radiation. For some cases of breast cancer, he wrote, with characteristic understatement, the "extension of [the] operation beyond a local removal might sometimes be unnecessary." Everything about Keynes's sentence was carefully, strategically, almost surgically constructed. Its implication was enormous. If local surgery resulted in the same outcome as radical surgery, then the centrifugal theory had to be reconsidered. Keynes had slyly declared war on radical surgery, even if he had done so by pricking it with a pin-size lancet.

But Halsted's followers in America laughed away Keynes's efforts. They retaliated, by giving his operation a nickname: the lumpectomy. The name was like a low-minded joke, a cartoon surgery in which a white-coated doctor pulls out a body part and calls it a "lump." Keynes's theory and operation were largely ignored by American surgeons. He gained fame briefly in Europe as a pioneer of blood transfusions during the First World War, but his challenge to radical surgery was quietly buried.

Keynes would have remained conveniently forgotten by American surgeons except for a fateful series of events. In 1953, a colleague of Keynes's, on sabbatical from St. Bart's at the Cleveland Clinic in Ohio, gave a lecture on the history of breast cancer, focusing on Keynes's observations on minimal surgery for the breast. In the audience that evening was a young surgeon named George Barney Crile. Crile and Keynes had never met, but they shared old intellectual debts. Crile's father, George Crile Sr., had pioneered the use of blood transfusions in America and written a widely read textbook on the subject. During the First World War, Keynes had learned to transfuse blood in sterilized, cone-shaped glass vessels—an apparatus devised, in part, by the elder Dr. Crile.

Political revolutions, the writer Amitav Ghosh writes, often occur in the courtyards of palaces, in spaces on the cusp of power, located neither outside nor inside. Scientific revolutions, in contrast, typically occur in basements, in buried-away places removed from mainstream corridors of thought. But a surgical revolution must emanate from *within* surgery's inner sanctum—for surgery is a profession intrinsically sealed to outsiders. To even enter the operating theater, one must be soused in soap and water, and surgical tradition. To change surgery, one must *be* a surgeon.

The Criles, father and son, were quintessential surgical insiders. The elder Crile, an early proponent of radical surgery, was a contemporary of Halsted's. The younger had learned the radical mastectomy from students of Halsted himself. The Criles were steeped in Halstedian tradition, upholding the very pole staffs of radical surgery for generations. But like Keynes in London, Crile Jr. was beginning to have his own doubts about the radical mastectomy. Animal studies performed in mice (by Skipper in Alabama, among others) had revealed that tumors implanted in animals did not behave as Halsted might have imagined. When a large tumor was grown in one site, microscopic metastatic deposits from it often skipped over the local nodes and appeared in faraway places such as the liver and the spleen. Cancer didn't move centrifugally by whirling through larger and larger ordered spirals; its spread was more erratic and unpredictable. As Crile pored through Keynes's data, the old patterns suddenly began to make sense: Hadn't Halsted also observed that patients had died four or five years after radical surgery from "occult" metastasis? Could breast cancer in these patients also have metastasized to faraway organs even *before* radical surgery?

The flaw in the logic began to crystallize. If the tumor was locally confined to start with, Crile argued, then it would be adequately removed by local surgery and radiation, and manically stripping away extra nodes and muscles could add no possible benefit. In contrast, if breast cancer had already spread outside the breast, then surgery would be useless anyway, and more aggressive surgery would simply be more aggressively useless. Breast cancer, Crile realized, was either an inherently localized disease—thus curable by a smaller mastectomy—or an inherently systemic disease—thus incurable even by the most exhaustive surgery.

Crile soon gave up on the radical mastectomy altogether and, instead, began to operate in a manner similar to Keynes's, using a limited surgical approach (Crile called it the "simple mastectomy"). Over about six years, he found that his "simple" operation was remarkably similar to Keynes's lumpectomy+radiation combination in its impact: the survival rate of patients treated with either form of local surgery tended to be no different from that of those treated historically with the radical mastectomy. Separated by an ocean and forty years of clinical practice, both Keynes and Crile had seemingly stumbled on the same clinical truth.

But was it a truth? Keynes had had no means to prove it. Until the 1930s, clinical trials had typically been designed to prove *positive* results: treatment A was better than treatment B, or drug X superior to drug Y. But to prove a *negative* result—that radical surgery was no better than conventional surgery—one needed a new set of statistical measures.

The invention of that measure would have a profound influence on the history of oncology, a branch of medicine particularly suffused with hope (and thus particularly prone to unsubstantiated claims of success). In 1928, four years after Keynes had begun his lumpectomies in London, two statisticians, Jerzy Neyman and Egon Pearson, provided a systematic method to evaluate a negative statistical claim. To measure the confidence in a negative claim, Neyman and Pearson invoked a statistical concept called power. "Power" in simplistic terms, is a measure of the ability of a test or trial to reject a hypothesis. Intuitively, Neyman and Pearson reasoned that a scientist's capacity to reject a hypothesis depends most critically on how intensively he has tested the hypothesis—and thus, on the *number* of samples that have independently been tested. If one compares five radical mastectomies against five conventional mastectomies and finds no difference in outcome, it is hard to make a significant conclusion about the result. But if a thousand cases of each produce precisely identical outcomes, then one can make a strong claim about a lack of benefit.

Right there, buried inside that dependence, lies one of the strangest pitfalls of medicine. For any trial to be adequately "powered," it needs to recruit an adequate number of patients. But to recruit patients, a trialist has to convince doctors to participate in the trial—and yet these doctors are often precisely those who have the least interest in having a theory rejected or disproved. For breast cancer, a discipline immersed in the legacy of the radical surgery, these conflicts were particularly charged. No breast cancer trial, for instance, could have proceeded without the explicit blessing and participation of larger-than-life surgeons such as Haagensen and Urban. Yet these surgeons, all enraptured intellectual descendants of Halsted, were the *least* likely to sponsor a trial that might dispute the theory that they had so passionately advocated for decades. When critics wondered whether Haagensen had been biased in his evaluation by selecting only his best cases, he challenged surgeons to replicate his astounding success using their own alternative methods: "Go thou and do likewise."

Thus even Crile—a full forty years after Keynes's discovery—couldn't run a trial to dispute Halsted's mastectomy. The hierarchical practice of medicine, its internal culture, its rituals of practice ("The Gospel[s] of the Surgical Profession," as Crile mockingly called it), were ideally arranged to resist change and to perpetuate orthodoxy. Crile found himself pitted against his own department, against friends and colleagues. The very doctors that he would need to recruit to run such a trial were fervently, often viciously, opposed to it. "Power," in the colloquial sense of the word, thus collided with "power" in the statistical sense. The surgeons who had so painstakingly created the world of radical surgery had absolutely no incentive to revolutionize it.

☙

It took a Pennsylvania surgeon named Bernard Fisher to cut through that knot of surgical tradition. Fisher was brackish, ambitious, dogged, and feisty—a man built after Halsted's image. He had trained at the University of Pittsburgh, a place just as steeped in the glorious Halstedian tradition of radical surgery as the hospitals of New York and Baltimore. But he came from a younger generation of surgeons—a generation with enough critical distance from Halsted to be able to challenge the discipline without undermining its own sense of credibility. Like Crile and Keynes, he, too, had lost faith in the centrifugal theory of cancer. The more he revisited Keynes's and Crile's data, the more Fisher was convinced that radical mastectomy had no basis in biological reality. The truth, he suspected, was quite the opposite. "It has become apparent that the tangled web of threads on the wrong side of the tapestry really represented a beautiful design when examined properly, a meaningful pattern, a hypothesis . . . diametrically opposite to those considered to be 'halstedian,'" Fisher wrote.

The only way to turn the upside-down tapestry of Halstedian theory around was to run a controlled clinical trial to test the radical mastectomy against the simple mastectomy and lumpectomy+radiation. But Fisher also knew that resistance would be fierce to any such trial. Holed away in their operating rooms, their slip-covered feet dug into the very roots of radical surgery, most academic surgeons were least likely to cooperate.

But another person in that operating room was stirring awake: the long-silent, etherized body lying at the far end of the scalpel—the cancer *patient*. By the late 1960s, the relationship between doctors and patients had begun to shift dramatically. Medicine, once considered virtually infallible in its judgment, was turning out to have deep fallibilities—flaws that appeared to cluster pointedly around issues of women's health. Thalidomide, prescribed widely to control pregnancy-associated nausea and "anxiety," was hastily withdrawn from the market in 1961 because of its propensity to cause severe fetal malformations. In Texas, Jane Roe (a pseudonym) sued the state for blocking her ability to abort her fetus at a medical clinic—launching the *Roe v. Wade* case on abortion and highlighting the complex nexus between the state, medical authority, and women's bodies. Political feminism, in short, was birthing medical feminism—and the fact that one of the most common and most disfiguring operations performed on women's bodies had never been formally tested in a trial stood out as even more starkly disturbing to a new generation of women. "Refuse to submit to a radical mastectomy," Crile exhorted his patients in 1973.

And refuse they did. Rachel Carson, the author of *Silent Spring* and a close friend of Crile's, refused a radical mastectomy (in retrospect, she was right: her cancer had already spread to her bones and radical surgery would have been pointless). Betty Rollin and Rose Kushner also refused and soon joined Carson in challenging radical surgeons. Rollin and Kushner—both marvelous writers: provocative, down-to-earth, no-nonsense, witty—were particularly adept at challenging the bloated orthodoxy of surgery. They flooded newspapers and magazines with editorials and letters and appeared (often uninvited) at medical and surgical conferences, where they fearlessly heckled surgeons about their data and the fact that the radical mastectomy had never been put to a test. "Happily for women," Kushner wrote, ". . . surgical custom is changing." It was as if the young woman in Halsted's famous etching—the patient that he had been so "loathe to disfigure"—had woken up from her gurney and begun to ask why, despite his "loathing," the cancer surgeon was so keen to disfigure her.

In 1967, bolstered by the activism of patients and the public attention swirling around breast cancer, Fisher became the new chair of the National Surgical Adjuvant Breast and Bowel Project (NSABP), a consortium of academic hospitals modeled self-consciously after Zubrod's leukemia group that would run large-scale trials in breast cancer. Four years later, the NSABP proposed to test the operation using a systematic, randomized trial. It was, coincidentally, the eightieth "anniversary" of Halsted's original description of the radical mastectomy. The implicit, nearly devotional faith in a theory of cancer was finally to be put to a test. "The clinician, no matter how venerable, must accept the fact that experience, voluminous as it might be, cannot be employed as a sensitive indicator of scientific validity," Fisher wrote in an article. He was willing to have faith in divine wisdom, but not in Halsted *as* divine wisdom. "In God we trust," he brusquely told a journalist. "All others [must] have data."

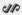

It took Fisher a full ten years to actually gather that data. Recruiting patients for his study was an uphill task. "To get a woman to participate in a clinical trial where she was going to have her breast off or have her breast not taken off, that was a pretty difficult thing to do. Not like testing Drug A versus Drug B," he recalled.

If patients were reluctant, surgeons were almost impossibly so. Immersed in the traditions of radical surgery, many American surgeons put up such formidable barriers to patient recruitment that Canadian surgeons and their patients were added to complete the study. The trial recruited 1,765 patients in thirty-four centers in the United States and Canada. Patients were randomized into three groups: one treated with the radical mastectomy, the second with simple mastectomy, and the third with surgery followed by radiation. Even with all forces in gear, it still took years to recruit adequate numbers. Crippled by forces within surgery itself, the NSABP-04 trial barely hobbled to its end.

In 1981, the results of the trial were finally made public. The rates of breast cancer recurrence, relapse, death, and distant cancer metastasis were statistically identical among all three groups. The group treated with the radical mastectomy had paid heavily in morbidity, but accrued no benefits in survival, recurrence, or mortality.

Between 1891 and 1981, in the nearly one hundred years of the radical mastectomy, an estimated five hundred thousand women underwent the procedure to "extirpate" cancer. Many chose the procedure. Many were forced into it. Many others did not even realize that it *was* a choice. Many were permanently disfigured; many perceived the surgery as a benediction; many suffered its punishing penalties bravely, hoping that they had treated their cancer as aggressively and as definitively as possible. Halsted's "cancer storehouse" grew far beyond its original walls at Hopkins. His ideas entered oncology, then permeated its vocabulary, then its psychology, its ethos, and its self-image. When radical surgery fell, an entire culture of surgery thus collapsed with it. The radical mastectomy is rarely, if ever, performed by surgeons today.

"The smiling oncologist"

> Few doctors in this country seem to be involved with the non-life-threatening side effects of cancer therapy. . . . In the United States, baldness, nausea and vomiting, diarrhea, clogged veins, financial problems, broken marriages, disturbed children, loss of libido, loss of self-esteem, and body image are nurses' turf.
>
> —Rose Kushner

> And it is solely by risking life that freedom is obtained.
>
> —Hegel

The ominous toppling of radical surgery off its pedestal may have given cancer chemotherapists some pause for reckoning. But they had their own fantasy of radicalism to fulfill, their own radical arsenal to launch against cancer. Surgery, the traditional battle-ax against cancer, was considered too primitive, too indiscriminate, and too weary. A "large-scale chemotherapeutic attack," as one doctor put it, was needed to obliterate cancer.

Every battle needs its iconic battleground, and if one physical place epitomized the cancer wars of the late 1970s, it was the chemotherapy ward. It was "our trench and our bunker," a chemotherapist recalls, a space marked indelibly in the history of cancer. To enter the ward was to acquire automatic citizenship—as Susan Sontag might have put it—into the kingdom of the ill.

The journalist Stewart Alsop was confined to one such ward at the NIH in 1973 for the treatment of a rare and unidentifiable blood condition. Crossing its threshold, he encountered a sanitized vision of hell. "Wandering about the NIH clinical center, in the corridors or in the elevator, one comes occasionally on a human monster, on a living nightmare, on a face or body hideously deformed," he wrote. Patients, even disguised in "civilian" clothes, could still be identified by the orange tinge that chemotherapy left on their skin, underneath which lurked the unique pallor of cancer-related anemia. The space was limbolike, with no simple means of egress—no exit. In the glass-paneled sanatorium where patients walked for leisure, Alsop recalled, the windows were covered in heavy wire mesh to prevent the men and women confined in the wards from jumping off the banisters and committing suicide.

A collective amnesia prevailed in these wards. If remembering was an essential requisite for survival, then so was forgetting. "Although this was a cancer ward," an anthropologist wrote, "the word 'cancer' was actively avoided by staff and patients." Patients lived by the regulations—"accepted roles, a predetermined routine, constant stimuli." The artifice of manufactured cheer (a requirement for soldiers in battle) made the wards even more poignantly desolate: in one wing, where a woman lay dying from breast cancer, there were "yellow and orange walls in the corridors; beige and white stripes in the patients' rooms." At the NIH, in an attempt to inject optimism into the wards, the nurses wore uniforms with plastic yellow buttons with the cartoonish outline of a smiling face.

These wards created not just a psychological isolation chamber but also a physical microenvironment, a sterile bubble where the core theory of cancer chemotherapy—eradicating cancer with a death-defying bombardment of drugs—could be adequately tested. It was, undeniably, an experiment. At the NIH, Alsop wrote pointedly, "Saving the individual patient is not the essential mission. Enormous efforts are made to do so, or at least to prolong the patient's life to the last possible moment. But the basic purpose is not to save that patient's particular life but to find means of saving the lives of others."

*

In some cases, the experiment worked. In 1976, the year that the NSABP-04 trial struggled to its midpoint, a novel drug, cisplatin, appeared in the cancer wards. Cisplatin—short for *cis-platinum*—was a new drug forged out of an old one. Its molecular structure, a central planar platinum atom with four "arms" extending outward, had been described back in the 1890s. But chemists had never found an application for cisplatin: the beautiful, satisfyingly symmetric chemical structure had no obvious human use. It had been shelved away in the laboratory in relative obscurity. No one had bothered to test its biological effects.

In 1965, at Michigan State University, a biophysicist, Barnett Rosenberg, began to investigate whether electrical currents might stimulate bacterial cell division. Rosenberg devised a bacterial flask through which an electrical current could be run using two platinum electrodes. When Rosenberg turned the electricity on, he found, astonishingly, that the bacterial cells stopped dividing entirely. Rosenberg initially proposed that the electrical current was the active agent in inhibiting cell division. But the electricity, he soon determined, was merely a bystander. The platinum electrode had reacted with the salt in the bacterial solution to generate a new growth-arresting molecule that had diffused throughout the liquid. That chemical was cisplatin. Like all cells, bacteria need to replicate DNA in order to divide. Cisplatin had chemically attacked DNA with its reactive molecular arms, cross-linking and damaging the molecule irreparably, forcing cells to arrest their division.

For patients such as John Cleland, cisplatin came to epitomize the new breed of aggressive chemotherapeutics of the 1970s. In 1973, Cleland was a twenty-two-year-old veterinary student in Indiana. In August that year, two months after his marriage, he discovered a rapidly expanding lump in his right testis. He saw a urologist on a Tuesday afternoon in November. On Thursday, he was whisked off to the operating room for surgery. He returned with a scar that extended from his abdomen to his breastbone. The diagnosis was metastatic testicular cancer—cancer of the testes that had migrated diffusely into his lymph nodes and lungs.

In 1973, the survival rate from metastatic testes cancer was less than 5 percent. Cleland entered the cancer ward at Indiana University and began treatment with a young oncologist named Larry Einhorn. The regimen, a weather-beaten and toxic three-drug cocktail called ABO that had been derived from the NCI's studies in the 1960s—was only marginally effective. Cleland lived in and out of the hospital. His weight shrank from 158 to 106 pounds. One day in 1974, while he was still receiving chemo, his wife suggested that they sit outside to enjoy the afternoon. Cleland realized, to his utter shame, that he was too weak to stand up. He was carried to his bed like a baby, weeping with embarrassment.

In the fall of 1974, the ABO regimen was stopped. He was switched to another equally ineffective drug. Einhorn suggested a last-ditch effort: a new chemical called cisplatin. Other researchers had seen some responses in patients with testicular cancer treated with single-agent cisplatin, although not durable ones. Einhorn wanted to combine cisplatin with two other drugs to see if he could increase the response rate.

There was the uncertainty of a new combination and the certainty of death. On October 7, 1974, Cleland took the gamble: he enrolled as "patient zero" for BVP, the acronym for a new regimen containing bleomycin, vinblastine, and cisplatin (abbreviated *P* for "platinum"). Ten days later, when he returned for his routine scans, the tumors in his lungs had vanished. Ecstatic and mystified, he called his wife from a hospital phone. "I cannot remember what I said, but I told her."

Cleland's experience was typical. By 1975, Einhorn had treated twenty additional patients with the regimen and found dramatic and sustained responses virtually unheard of in the history of this disease. Einhorn presented his data at the annual meeting of oncologists held in Toronto in the winter of 1975. "Walking up to that podium was like my own walk on the moon," he recalled. By the late winter of 1976, it was becoming progressively clearer that some of these patients would not relapse at all. Einhorn had cured a solid cancer by chemotherapy. "It was unforgettable. In my own naive mind I thought this was the formula that we had been missing all the while."

❦

Cisplatin was unforgettable in more than one sense. The drug provoked an unremitting nausea, a queasiness of such penetrating force and quality that had rarely been encountered in the history of medicine: on *average,* patients treated with the drug vomited twelve times a day. (In the 1970s, there were few effective antinausea drugs. Most patients had to be given intravenous fluids to tide them through the nausea; some survived by smuggling marijuana, a mild antiemetic, into the chemotherapy wards.) In Margaret Edson's play *Wit,* a scathing depiction of a woman's battle with ovarian cancer, an English professor undergoing chemotherapy clutches a nausea basin on the floor of her hospital ward, dry-heaving in guttural agony (prompting her unforgettable aside, "You may think my vocabulary has taken a turn for the Anglo-Saxon"). The pharmacological culprit lurking unmentioned behind that scene is cisplatin. Even today, nurses on oncology floors who tended to patients in the early 1980s (before the advent of newer antiemetics that would somewhat ease the effect of the drug) can vividly recollect the violent jolts of nausea that suddenly descended on patients and brought them dry-heaving to the ground. In nursing slang, the drug came to be known as "cisflatten."

These side effects, however revolting, were considered minor dues to pay for an otherwise miraculous drug. Cisplatin was touted as the epic chemotherapeutic product of the late 1970s, the quintessential example of how curing cancer involved pushing patients nearly to the brink of death. By 1978, cisplatin-based chemotherapy was the new vogue in cancer pharmacology; every conceivable combination was being tested on thousands of patients across America. The lemon-yellow chemical dripping through intravenous lines was as ubiquitous in the cancer wards as the patients clutching their nausea basins afterward.

The NCI meanwhile was turning into a factory of toxins. The influx of money from the National Cancer Act had potently stimulated the institute's drug-discovery program, which had grown into an even more gargantuan effort and was testing hundreds of thousands of chemicals each year to discover new cytotoxic drugs. The strategy of discovery was empirical—throwing chemicals at cancer cells in test tubes to identify cancer killers—but, by now, unabashedly and defiantly so. The biology of cancer was still poorly understood. But the notion that even relatively indiscriminate cytotoxic agents discovered largely by accident would cure cancer had captivated oncology. "We want and need and seek better guidance and are gaining it," Howard Skipper (Frei and Freireich's collaborator on the early leukemia studies) admitted in 1971, "but we cannot afford to sit and wait for the promise of tomorrow so long as stepwise progress can be made with tools at hand today." Ehrlich's seductive phrase—"magic bullet"—had seemingly been foreshortened. What this war needed was simply "bullets," whether magical or not, to annihilate cancer.

Chemicals thus came pouring out of the NCI's cauldrons, each one with a unique personality. There was Taxol, one gram purified from the bark of a hundred Pacific yew trees, whose molecular structure resembled a winged insect. Adriamycin, discovered in 1969, was bloodred (it was the chemical responsible for the orange-red tinge that Alsop had seen at the NCI's cancer ward); even at therapeutic doses, it could irreversibly damage the heart. Etoposide came from the fruit of the poisonous mayapple. Bleomycin, which could scar lungs without warning, was an antibiotic derived from a mold.

"Did we believe we were going to cure cancer with these chemicals?" George Canellos recalled. "Absolutely, we did. The NCI was a charged place. The chief [Zubrod] wanted the boys to move into solid tumors. I proposed ovarian cancer. Others proposed breast cancer. We wanted to get started on the larger clinical problems. We spoke of curing cancer as if it was almost a given."

In the mid-1970s, high-dose combination chemotherapy scored another sentinel victory. Burkitt's lymphoma, the tumor originally discovered in eastern Africa (and rarely found in children and adolescents in America and Europe), was cured with a cocktail of seven drugs, including a molecular cousin of nitrogen mustard—a regimen concocted at the NCI by Ian Magrath and John Ziegler.* The felling of yet another aggressive tumor by combination chemotherapy even more potently boosted the institute's confidence—once again underscoring the likelihood that the "generic solution" to cancer had been found.

Events outside the world of medicine also impinged on oncology, injecting new blood and verve into the institute. In the early 1970s, young doctors who opposed the Vietnam War flooded to the NCI. (Due to an obscure legal clause, enrollment in a federal research program, such as the NIH, exempted someone from the draft.) The undrafted soldiers of one battle were thus channeled into another. "Our applications skyrocketed. They were brilliant and energetic, these new fellows at the institute," Canellos said. "They wanted to run new trials, to test new permutations of drugs. We were a charged place." At the NCI and in its academic outposts around the world, the names of regimens evolved into a language of their own: ABVD, BEP, C-MOPP, ChlaVIP, CHOP, ACT.

"There is no cancer that is not potentially curable," an ovarian cancer chemotherapist self-assuredly told the media at a conference in 1979. "The chances in some cases are infinitesimal, but the potential is still there. This is about all that patients need to know and it is about all that patients want to know."

The greatly expanded coffers of the NCI also stimulated enormous, expensive, multi-institutional trials, allowing academic centers to trot out ever more powerful permutations of cytotoxic drugs. Cancer hospitals, also boosted by the NCI's grants, organized themselves into efficient

---

* Many of these NCI-sponsored trials were carried out in Uganda, where Burkitt's lymphoma is endemic in children.

and thrumming trial-running machines. By 1979, the NCI had recognized twenty so-called Comprehensive Cancer Centers spread across the nation—hospitals with large wards dedicated exclusively to cancer—run by specialized teams of surgeons and chemotherapists and supported by psychiatrists, pathologists, radiologists, social workers, and ancillary staff. Hospital review boards that approved and coordinated human experimentation were revamped to allow researchers to bulldoze their way through institutional delays.

It was trial and error on a giant human scale—with the emphasis, it seemed at times, distinctly on error. One NCI-sponsored trial tried to outdo Einhorn by doubling the dose of cisplatin in testicular cancer. Toxicity doubled, although there was no additional therapeutic effect. In another particularly tenacious trial, known as the eight-in-one study, children with brain tumors were given eight drugs in a single day. Predictably, horrific complications ensued. Fifteen percent of the patients needed blood transfusions. Six percent were hospitalized with life-threatening infections. Fourteen percent of the children suffered kidney damage; three lost their hearing. One patient died of septic shock. Yet, despite the punishing escalation of drugs and doses, the efficacy of the drug regimen remained minimal. Most of the children in the eight-in-one trial died soon afterward, having only marginally responded to chemotherapy.

This pattern was repeated with tiresome regularity for many forms of cancer. In metastatic lung cancer, for instance, combination chemotherapy was found to increase survival by three or four months; in colon cancer, by less than six months; in breast, by about twelve. (I do not mean to belittle the impact of twelve or thirteen months of survival. One extra year can carry a lifetime of meaning for a man or woman condemned to death from cancer. But it took a particularly fanatical form of zeal to refuse to recognize that this was far from a "cure.") Between 1984 and 1985, at the midpoint of the most aggressive expansion of chemotherapy, nearly six thousand articles were published on the subject in medical journals. Not a single article reported a new strategy for the definitive cure of an advanced solid tumor by means of combination chemotherapy alone.

Like lunatic cartographers, chemotherapists frantically drew and redrew their strategies to annihilate cancer. MOPP, the combination that had proved successful in Hodgkin's disease, went through every conceivable permutation for breast, lung, and ovarian cancer. More combinations entered clinical trials—each more aggressive than its precursor and each tagged by its own cryptic, nearly indecipherable name. Rose Kushner (by then, a member of the National Cancer Advisory Board) warned against the growing disconnect between doctors and their patients. "When doctors say that the side effects are tolerable or acceptable, they are talking about life-threatening things," she wrote. "But if you just vomit so hard that you break the blood vessels in your eyes . . . they don't consider that even mentionable. And they certainly don't care if you're bald." She wrote sarcastically, "The smiling oncologist does not know whether his patients vomit or not."

The language of suffering had parted, with the "smiling oncologist" on one side and his patients on the other. In Edson's *Wit*—a work not kind to the medical profession—a young oncologist, drunk with the arrogance of power, personifies the divide as he spouts out lists of nonsensical drugs and combinations while his patient, the English professor, watches with mute terror and fury: "Hexamethophosphacil with Vinplatin to potentiate. Hex at three hundred mg per meter squared. Vin at one hundred. Today is cycle two, day three. Both cycles at the *full dose*."

Knowing the Enemy

It is said that if you know your enemies and know
yourself, you will not be imperiled in a hundred battles;
if you do not know your enemies but do know yourself,
you will win one and lose one; if you do not know your
enemies nor yourself, you will be imperiled in every single
battle.

—Sun Tzu

As the armada of cytotoxic therapy readied itself for even more aggressive battles against cancer, a few dissenting voices began to be heard along its peripheries. These voices were connected by two common themes.

First, the dissidents argued that indiscriminate chemotherapy, the unloading of barrel after barrel of poisonous drugs, could not be the only strategy by which to attack cancer. Contrary to prevailing dogma, cancer cells possessed unique and specific vulnerabilities that rendered them particularly sensitive to certain chemicals that had little impact on normal cells.

Second, such chemicals could only be discovered by uncovering the deep biology of every cancer cell. Cancer-specific therapies existed, but they could only be known from the bottom up, i.e., from solving the basic biological riddles of each form of cancer, rather than from the top down, by maximizing cytotoxic chemotherapy or by discovering cellular poisons empirically. To attack a cancer cell specifically, one needed to begin by identifying its biological behavior, its genetic makeup, and its unique vulnerabilities. The search for magic bullets needed to begin with an understanding of cancer's magical *targets*.

The most powerful such voice arose from the most unlikely of sources, a urological surgeon, Charles Huggins, who was neither a cell biologist nor even a cancer biologist, but rather a physiologist interested in glandular secretions. Born in Nova Scotia in 1901, Huggins attended Harvard Medical School in the early 1920s (where he intersected briefly with Farber) and trained as a general surgeon in Michigan. In 1927, at age twenty-six, he was appointed to the faculty of the University of Chicago as a urological surgeon, a specialist in diseases of the bladder, kidney, genitals, and prostate.

Huggins's appointment epitomized the confidence (and hubris) of surgery: he possessed no formal training in urology, nor had he trained as a cancer surgeon. It was an era when surgical specialization was still a fluid concept; if a man could remove an appendix or a lymph node, the philosophy ran, he could certainly learn to remove a kidney. Huggins thus learned urology on the fly by cramming a textbook in about six weeks. He arrived optimistically in Chicago, expecting to find a busy, flourishing practice. But his new clinic, housed inside a stony neo-Gothic tower, remained empty all winter. (The fluidity of surgical specialization was, perhaps, not as reassuring to patients.) Tired of memorizing books and journals in an empty, drafty waiting room, Huggins changed tracks and set up a laboratory to study urological diseases while waiting for patients to come to his clinic.

To choose a medical specialty is also to choose its cardinal bodily liquid. Hematologists have blood. Hepatologists have bile. Huggins had prostatic fluid: a runny, straw-colored mixture of salt and sugar meant to lubricate and nourish sperm. Its source, the prostate, is a small gland buried deep in the perineum, wrapped around the outlet of the urinary tract in men. (Vesalius was the first to identify it and draw it into human anatomy.) Walnut-shaped and only walnut-sized, it is yet ferociously the site of cancer. Prostate cancer represents a full third of all cancer incidence in men—sixfold that of leukemia and lymphoma. In autopsies of men over sixty years old, nearly one in every three specimens will bear some evidence of prostatic malignancy.

But although an astoundingly common form of cancer, prostate cancer is also highly variable in its clinical course. Most cases are indolent—elderly men usually die *with* prostate cancer than die *of* prostate cancer—but in other patients the disease can be aggressive and invasive, capable of exploding into painful lesions in the bones and lymph nodes in its advanced, metastatic form.

Huggins, though, was far less interested in cancer than in the physiology of prostatic fluid. Female hormones, such as estrogen, were known to control the growth of breast tissue. Did male hormones, by analogy, control the growth of the normal prostate—and thus regulate the secretion of its principal product, prostatic fluid? By the late 1920s, Huggins had devised an apparatus to collect precious drops of prostatic fluid from dogs. (He diverted urine away by inserting a catheter into the bladder and stitched a collection tube to the exit of the prostate gland.) It was the only surgical innovation that he would devise in his lifetime.

Huggins now had a tool to measure prostatic function; he could quantify the amount of fluid produced by the gland. He found that if he surgically removed the testicles of his dogs—and thereby depleted the dogs of the hormone testosterone—the prostate gland involuted and shriveled and the fluid secretion dried up precipitously. If he injected the castrated dogs with purified testosterone, the exogenous hormone saved the prostate from shriveling. Prostate cells were thus acutely dependent on the hormone testosterone for their growth and function. Female sexual hormones kept breast cells alive; male hormones had a similar effect on prostate cells.

Huggins wanted to delve further into the metabolism of testosterone and the prostate cell, but his experiments were hampered by a peculiar problem. Dogs, humans, and lions are the only animals known to develop prostate cancer, and dogs with sizable prostate tumors kept appearing in his lab during his studies. "It was vexatious to encounter a dog with a prostatic tumor during a metabolic study," he wrote. His first impulse was to cull the cancer-afflicted dogs from his study and continue single-mindedly with his fluid collection, but then a question formed in his mind. If testosterone deprivation could shrink normal prostate cells, what might testosterone deprivation do to *cancer* cells?

The answer, as any self-respecting cancer biologist might have informed him, was almost certain: very little. Cancer cells, after all, were deranged, uninhibited, and altered—responsive only to the most poisonous combinations of drugs. The signals and hormones that regulated normal cells had long been flung aside; what remained was a cell driven to divide with such pathological and autonomous fecundity that it had erased all memory of normalcy.

But Huggins knew that certain forms of cancer did not obey this principle. Variants of thyroid cancer, for instance, continued to make thyroid hormone, the growth-stimulating molecule secreted by the normal thyroid gland; even though cancerous, these cells remembered their former selves. Huggins found that prostate cancer cells also retained a physiological "memory" of their origin. When he removed the testicles of prostate cancer-bearing dogs, thus acutely depriving the cancer cells of testosterone, the tumors also involuted within days. In fact, if normal prostate cells were dependent on testosterone for survival, then malignant prostate cells were nearly addicted to the hormone—so much so that the acute withdrawal acted like the most powerful therapeutic drug conceivable. "Cancer is not necessarily autonomous and intrinsically self-perpetuating," Huggins wrote. "Its growth can be sustained and propagated by hormonal function in the host." The link between the growth-sustenance of normal cells and of cancer cells was much closer than previously imagined: cancer could be fed and nurtured by our own bodies.

ಱಳ

Surgical castration, fortunately, was not the only means to starve prostate cancer cells. If male hormones were driving the growth of these cancer cells, Huggins reasoned, then rather than eliminate the male hormones, what if one tricked the cancer into thinking that the body was "female" by suppressing the effect of testosterone?

In 1929, Edward Doisy, a biochemist, had tried to identify the hormonal factors in the estrous cycle of females. Doisy had collected hundreds of gallons of urine from pregnant women in enormous copper vats, then extracted a few milligrams of a hormone called estrogen. Doisy's extraction had sparked a race to produce estrogen or its analogue in large quantities. By the mid-1940s, several laboratories and pharmaceutical companies, jostling to capture the market for the "essence of femininity," raced to synthesize analogues of estrogen or find novel means to purify it efficiently. The two most widely used versions of the drug were diethylstilbestrol (or DES), an artificial estrogen chemically synthesized by biochemists in London, or Premarin, natural estrogen purified from horse's urine in Montreal. (The synthetic analogue, DES, will return in a more sinister form in subsequent pages.)

Both Premarin (its name derived from *pre*gnant *ma*re ur*ine*) and DES were initially marketed as elixirs to cure menopause. But for Huggins, the existence of synthetic estrogens suggested a markedly different use: he could inject them to "feminize" the male body and stop the production of testosterone in patients with prostate cancer. He called the method "chemical castration." And once again, he found striking responses. As with surgical castration, patients with aggressive prostate cancer chemically castrated with feminizing hormones responded briskly to the therapy, often with minimal side effects. (The most prominent complaint among men was the occurrence of menopause-like hot flashes.) Prostate cancer was not cured with these steroids; patients inevitably relapsed with cancer that had become resistant to hormone therapy. But the remissions, which often stretched into several months, proved that hormonal manipulations could choke the growth of a hormone-dependent cancer. To produce a cancer remission, one did not need a toxic, indiscriminate cellular poison (such as cisplatin or nitrogen mustard).

જી

If prostate cancer could be starved to near-death by choking off testosterone, then could hormonal deprivation be applied to starve another hormone-dependent cancer? There was at least one obvious candidate—breast cancer. In the late 1890s, an adventurous Scottish surgeon named George Beatson, trying to devise new surgical methods to treat breast cancer, had learned from shepherds in the Scottish highlands that the removal of the ovaries from cows altered their capacity to lactate and changed the quality of their udders. Beatson did not understand the basis for this phenomenon (estrogen, the ovarian hormone, had not yet been discovered by Doisy), but intrigued by the inexplicable link between ovaries and breasts, Beatson had surgically removed the ovaries of three women with breast cancer.

In an age before the hormonal circuits between the ovary and the breast were even remotely established, this was unorthodox beyond description—like removing the lung to cure a brain lesion. But to Beatson's astonishment, his three cases revealed marked responses to the ovarian removal—the breast tumors shrank dramatically. When surgeons in London tried to repeat Beatson's findings on a larger group of women, though, the operation led to a more nuanced outcome: only about two-thirds of all women with breast cancer responded.

The hit-and-miss quality of the benefit mystified nineteenth-century physiologists. "It is impossible to tell beforehand whether any benefit will result from the operation or not, its effects being quite uncertain," a surgeon wrote in 1902. How might the surgical removal of a faraway organ affect the growth of cancer? And why, tantalizingly, had only a fraction of cases responded? The phenomenon almost brought back memories of a mysterious humoral factor circulating in the body—of Galen's black bile. But why was this humoral factor only active in certain women with breast cancer?

Nearly three decades later, Doisy's discovery of estrogen provided a partial answer to the first question. Estrogen is the principal hormone secreted by the ovaries. As with testosterone for the normal prostate, estrogen was soon demonstrated to be a vital hormone for the maintenance and growth of normal breast tissue. Was breast cancer also fueled by estrogen from the ovaries? If so, what of Beatson's puzzle: why did some breast cancers shrink with ovarian removal while others remained totally unresponsive?

In the mid-1960s, working closely with Huggins, a young chemist in Chicago, Elwood Jensen, came close to solving Beatson's riddle. Jensen began his studies not with cancer cells but with the normal physiology of estrogen. Hormones, Jensen knew, typically work by binding to a receptor in a target cell, but the receptor for the steroid hormone estrogen had remained elusive. Using a radioactively labeled version of the hormone as bait, in 1968 Jensen found the estrogen receptor—the molecule responsible for binding estrogen and relaying its signal to the cell.

Jensen now asked whether breast *cancer* cells also uniformly possessed this receptor. Unexpectedly, some did and some did not. Indeed, breast cancer cases could be neatly divided into two types—ones with cancer cells that expressed high levels of this receptor and those that expressed low levels, "ER-positive" and "ER-negative" tumors.

Jensen's observations suggested a possible solution to Beatson's riddle. Perhaps the marked variation of breast cancer cells in response to ovarian removal depended on whether the cancer cells expressed the estrogen receptor or not. ER-positive tumors, possessing the receptor, retained their "hunger" for estrogen. ER-negative tumors had rid themselves of both the receptor and the hormone dependence. ER-positive tumors thus responded to Beatson's surgery, Jensen proposed, while ER-negative tumors were unresponsive.

The simplest way to prove this theory was to launch an experiment—to perform Beatson's surgery on women with ER-positive and ER-negative tumors and determine whether the receptor status of the cancer cells was predictive of the response. But the surgical procedure had fallen out of fashion. (Ovarian removal produced many other severe side effects, such as osteoporosis.) An alternative was to use a *pharmacological* means to inhibit estrogen function, a female version of chemical castration à la Huggins.

But Jensen had no such drug. Testosterone did not work, and no synthetic "antiestrogen" was in development. In their dogged pursuit of cures for menopause and for new contraceptive agents (using synthetic estrogens), pharmaceutical companies had long abandoned the development of an antiestrogen, and there was no interest in developing an antiestrogen for cancer. In an era gripped by the hypnotic promise of cytotoxic chemotherapy, as Jensen put it, "there was little enthusiasm about developing endocrine [hormonal] therapies to treat cancer. Combination chemotherapy was [thought to be] more likely to be successful in curing not only breast cancer but other solid tumors." Developing an antiestrogen, an antagonist to the fabled elixir of female youth, was widely considered a waste of effort, money, and time.

Scarcely anyone paid notice, then, on September 13, 1962, when a team of talented British chemists from Imperial Chemical Industries (ICI) filed a patent for the chemical named ICI 46474, or tamoxifen. Originally invented as a birth control pill, tamoxifen had been synthesized by a team led by the hormone biologist Arthur Walpole and a synthetic chemist, Dora Richardson, both members of the "fertility control program" at the ICI. But even though structurally designed to be a potent stimulator of estrogen—its winged, birdlike skeleton designed to perch perfectly into the open arms of the estrogen receptor—tamoxifen had turned out to have exactly the opposite effect: rather than turning on the estrogen signal, a requirement for a contraceptive drug, it had, surprisingly, shut it off in many tissues. It was an estrogen *antagonist*—thus considered a virtually useless drug.

Yet the connection between fertility drugs and cancer preoccupied Walpole. He knew of Huggins's experiments with surgical castration for prostate cancer. He knew of Beatson's riddle—almost solved by Jensen. The antiestrogenic properties of his new drug raised an intriguing possibility. ICI 46474 may be a useless contraceptive, but perhaps, he reasoned, it might be useful against estrogen-sensitive breast cancer.

To test that idea, Walpole and Richardson sought a clinical collaborator. The natural site for such a trial was immediately apparent, the sprawling Christie Hospital in Manchester, a world-renowned cancer center just a short ride through the undulating hills of Cheshire from ICI's research campus at Alderley Park. And there was a natural collaborator: Mary Cole, a Manchester oncologist and radiotherapist with a particular interest in breast cancer. Known affectionately as Moya by her patients and colleagues, Cole had a reputation as a feisty and meticulous physician intensely dedicated to her patients. She had a ward full of women with advanced, metastatic breast cancer, many of them hurtling inexorably toward their death. Moya Cole was willing to try anything—even an abandoned contraceptive—to save the lives of these women.

Cole's trial was launched at Christie in the late summer of 1969. Forty-six women with breast cancer were treated with tablets of ICI 46474. Cole expected little from the drug—at best, a partial response. But in ten patients, the response was almost immediately obvious. Tumors shriveled visibly in the breast. Lung metastases shrank. Bone pain flickered away and lymph nodes softened.

Like Huggins's prostate cancer patients, many of the women who responded to the drug eventually relapsed. But the success of the trial was incontrovertible—and the proof of principle historic. A drug designed to target a specific pathway in a cancer cell—not a cellular poison discovered empirically by trial and error—had successfully driven metastatic tumors into remission.

Tamoxifen's journey came full circle in a little-known pharmaceutical laboratory in Shrewsbury, Massachusetts. In 1973, V. Craig Jordan, a biochemist working at the lab of the Worcester Foundation (a research institute involved in the development of new contraceptives), investigated the pattern behind cancers that did or did not respond to tamoxifen therapy. Jordan used a simple molecular technique to stain breast cancer cells for the estrogen receptor that Elwood Jensen had discovered in Chicago, and the answer to Beatson's riddle finally leapt out of the experiment. Cancer cells that expressed the estrogen receptor were highly responsive to tamoxifen, while cells that lacked the estrogen receptor did not respond. The reason behind the slippery, hit-and-miss responses in women with breast cancer observed in England nearly a century earlier was now clear. Cells that expressed the estrogen receptor could bind tamoxifen, and the drug, an estrogen antagonist, shut off estrogen responsiveness, thus choking the cells' growth. But ER-negative cells lacked the receptor for the drug and thus were insensitive to it. The schema had a satisfying simplicity. For the first time in the history of cancer, a drug, its target, and a cancer cell had been conjoined by a core molecular logic.

Halsted's Ashes

I would rather be ashes than dust.
—Jack London

Will you turn me out if I can't get better?
—A cancer patient to
her physician, 1960s

Moya Cole's tamoxifen trial was initially designed to treat women with advanced, metastatic breast cancer. But as the trial progressed, Cole began to wonder about an alternative strategy. Typically, clinical trials of new cancer drugs tend to escalate inexorably toward sicker and sicker patients (as news of a novel drug spreads, more and more desperate patients lurch toward last-ditch efforts to save their lives). But Cole was inclined to journey in the opposite direction. What if women with *earlier-stage* tumors were treated with tamoxifen? If a drug could halt the progression of diffusely metastatic and aggressive stage IV cancers, might it work even better on more localized, stage II breast cancers, cancers that had spread only to the regional lymph nodes?

Unwittingly, Cole had come full circle toward Halsted's logic. Halsted had invented the radical mastectomy based on the premise that early breast cancer needed to be attacked exhaustively and definitively—by surgically "cleansing" every conceivable reservoir of the disease, even when no visible cancer was present. The result had been the grotesque and disfiguring mastectomy, foisted indiscriminately on women with even small, locally restricted tumors to stave off relapses and metastasis into distant organs. But Cole now wondered whether Halsted had tried to cleanse the Augean stables of cancer with all the right intentions, but with the wrong tools. Surgery could not eliminate invisible reservoirs of cancer. But per-

218

haps what was needed was a potent chemical—a systemic therapy, Willy Meyer's dreamed-about "after-treatment" from 1932.

A variant of this idea had already gripped a band of renegade researchers at the NCI even before tamoxifen had appeared on the horizon. In 1963, nearly a decade before Moya Cole completed her experiments in Manchester, a thirty-three-year-old oncologist at the NCI, Paul Carbone, had launched a trial to see if chemotherapy might be effective when administered to women after an early-stage primary tumor had been completely removed surgically—i.e., women with no visible tumor remaining in the body. Carbone had been inspired by the patron saint of renegades at the NCI: Min Chiu Li, the researcher who had been expelled from the institute for treating women with placental tumors with methotrexate long after their tumors had visibly disappeared.

Li had been packed off in ignominy, but the strategy that had undone him—using chemotherapy to "cleanse" the body of residual tumor—had gained increasing respectability at the institute. In his small trial, Carbone found that adding chemotherapy after surgery decreased the rate of relapse from breast cancer. To describe this form of treatment, Carbone and his team used the word *adjuvant*, from the Latin phrase "to help." Adjuvant chemotherapy, Carbone conjectured, could be the surgeon's little helper. It would eradicate microscopic deposits of cancer left behind after surgery, thus extirpating any remnant reservoirs of malignancy in the body in early breast cancer—in essence, completing the Herculean cancer-cleansing task that Halsted had set for himself.

But surgeons had no interest in getting help from anyone—least of all chemotherapists. By the mid-1960s, as radical surgery became increasingly embattled, most breast surgeons had begun to view chemotherapists as estranged rivals that could not be trusted with anything, least of all improving surgical outcomes. And since surgeons largely dominated the field of breast cancer (and saw all the patients upon diagnosis), Carbone could not ramp up his trial because he could barely recruit any patients. "Except for an occasional woman who underwent a mastectomy at the NCI . . . the study never got off the ground," Carbone recalled.

But Carbone found an alternative. Shunned by surgeons, he now turned to the surgeon who had shunned his own compatriots—Bernie Fisher, the man caught in the controversial swirl of testing radical breast surgery. Fisher was instantly interested in Carbone's idea. Indeed, Fisher had been trying to run a trial along similar lines—combining chemotherapy with surgical mastectomy. But even Fisher could pick only one fight at a time. With his own trial, the NSABP-04 (the trial to test radical surgery versus nonradical surgery) barely limping along, he could hardly convince surgeons to join a trial to combine chemo and surgery in breast cancer.

An Italian team came to the rescue. In 1972, as the NCI was scouring the nation for a site where "adjuvant chemotherapy" after surgery could be tested, the oncologist Gianni Bonadonna came to Bethesda to visit the institute. Suave, personable, and sophisticated, impeccably dressed in custom-cut Milanese suits, Bonadonna made an instant impression at the NCI. He learned from DeVita, Canellos, and Carbone that they had been testing combinations of drugs to treat advanced breast cancer and had found a concoction that would likely work: Cytoxan (a cousin of nitrogen mustard), methotrexate (a variant of Farber's aminopterin), and fluorouracil (an inhibitor of DNA synthesis). The regimen, called CMF, could be tolerated with relatively minimal side effects, yet was active enough in combination to thwart microscopic tumors—an ideal combination to be used as an adjuvant in breast cancer.

Bonadonna worked at a large cancer center in Milan called the Istituto Tumori, where he had a close friendship with the chief breast surgeon, Umberto Veronesi. Convinced by Carbone (who was still struggling to get a similar trial launched in America), Bonadonna and Veronesi, the only surgeon-chemotherapist pair seemingly on talking terms with each other, proposed a large randomized trial to study chemotherapy after breast surgery for early-stage breast cancer. They were immediately awarded the contract for the NCI trial.

The irony of that award could hardly have escaped the researchers at the institute. In America, the landscape of cancer medicine had become so deeply gashed by internal rifts that the most important NCI-sponsored trial of cytotoxic chemotherapy to be launched after the announcement of the War on Cancer had to be relocated to a foreign country.

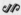

Bonadonna began his trial in the summer of 1973. By the early winter that year, he had randomized nearly four hundred women to the trial—half to no treatment and half to treatment with CMF. Veronesi was a crucial supporter, but there was still little interest from other breast surgeons. "The surgeons were not just skeptical," Bonadonna recalled. "They were hostile. [They] did not want to know. At the time there were very few chemotherapists, and they were not rated highly, and the attitude among surgeons was 'chemotherapists deliver drugs in advanced disease [while] surgeons operate and we have complete remission for the entire life of the patient. . . . Surgeons rarely saw their patients again, and I think they didn't want to hear about how many patients were being failed by surgery alone. It was a matter of prestige.' "

On an overcast morning in the winter of 1975, Bonadonna flew to Brussels to present his results at a conference of European oncologists. The trial had just finished its second year. But the two groups, Bonadonna reported, had clearly parted ways. Nearly half the women treated with no therapy had relapsed. In contrast, only a third of the women treated with the adjuvant regimen had relapsed. Adjuvant chemotherapy had prevented breast cancer relapses in about one in every six treated women.

The news was so unexpected that it was greeted by a stunned silence in the auditorium. Bonadonna's presentation had shaken the terra firma of cancer chemotherapy. It was only on the flight back to Milan, ten thousand feet above the earth, that Bonadonna was finally inundated with questions about his trial by other researchers on his flight.

✒

Gianni Bonadonna's remarkable Milanese trial left a question almost begging to be answered. If adjuvant CMF chemotherapy could decrease relapses in women with early-stage breast cancer, then might adjuvant tamoxifen—the other active breast cancer drug established by Cole's group—also decrease relapses in women with localized ER-positive breast cancer after surgery? Had Moya Cole been right about her instinct in treating early-stage breast cancer with antiestrogen therapy?

This was a question that Bernie Fisher, although embroiled in several other trials, could not resist trying to answer. In January 1977, five years after Cole had published her results on tamoxifen in metastatic cancer, Fisher recruited 1,891 women with estrogen receptor–positive (ER-positive) breast cancer that had spread only to the axillary nodes. He treated half with adjuvant tamoxifen and the other half with no tamoxifen. By 1981, the two groups had deviated sharply. Treatment with tamoxifen after surgery reduced cancer relapse rates by nearly 50 percent. The effect was particularly pronounced among women above fifty years old—a group most resistant to standard chemotherapy regimens and most likely to relapse with aggressive, metastatic breast cancer.

Three years later, in '85, when Fisher reanalyzed the deviating curves of relapse and survival, the effect of tamoxifen treatment was even more dramatic. Among the five-hundred-odd women older than fifty assigned to each group, tamoxifen had prevented fifty-five relapses and deaths. Fisher had altered the biology of breast cancer after surgery using a targeted hormonal drug that had barely any significant side effects.

By the early 1980s, brave new paradigms of treatment had thus arisen out of the ashes of old paradigms. Halsted's fantasy of attacking early-stage cancers was reborn as adjuvant therapy. Ehrlich's "magic bullet" for cancer was reincarnated as antihormone therapy for breast and prostate cancer.

Neither method of treatment professed to be a complete cure. Adjuvant therapy and hormonal therapy typically did not obliterate cancer. Hormonal therapy produced prolonged remissions that could stretch into years or even decades. Adjuvant therapy was mainly a cleansing method to purge the body of residual cancer cells; it lengthened survival, but many patients eventually relapsed. In the end, often after decades of remission, chemotherapy-resistant and hormone-resistant cancers grew despite the prior interventions, flinging aside the equilibrium established during the treatment.

But although these alternatives did not offer definitive cures, several important principles of cancer biology and cancer therapy were firmly cemented in these powerful trials. First, as Kaplan had found with Hodgkin's disease, these trials again clearly etched the message that cancer was enormously heterogeneous. Breast or prostate cancers came in an array of forms, each with unique biological behaviors. The heterogeneity was genetic: in breast cancer, for instance, some variants responded to hormonal treatment, while others were hormone-unresponsive. And the heterogeneity was anatomic: some cancers were localized to the breast when detected, while others had a propensity to spread to distant organs.

Second, understanding that heterogeneity was of deep consequence. "Know thine enemy" runs the adage, and Fisher's and Bonadonna's trials had shown that it was essential to "know" the cancer as intimately as possible before rushing to treat it. The meticulous separation of breast cancer into distinct stages, for instance, was a crucial prerequisite to the success of Bonadonna's study: early-stage breast cancer could not be treated like late-stage breast cancer. The meticulous separation of ER-positive and

ER-negative cancers was crucial to Fisher's study: if tamoxifen had indiscriminately been tested on ER-negative breast cancer, the drug would have been discarded as having no benefit.

This nuanced understanding of cancer underscored by these trials had a sobering effect on cancer medicine. As Frank Rauscher, the director of the NCI, put it in 1985, "We were all more naive a decade ago. We hoped that a single application of drugs would result in a dramatic benefit. We now understand it's much more complicated than that. People are optimistic but we're not expecting home runs. Right now, people would be happy with a series of singles or doubles."

Yet the metaphorical potency of battling and obliterating cancer relatively indiscriminately ("one cause, one cure") still gripped oncology. Adjuvant chemotherapy and hormonal therapy were like truces declared in the battle—signs, merely, that a more aggressive attack was necessary. The allure of deploying a full armamentarium of cytotoxic drugs—of driving the body to the edge of death to rid it of its malignant innards—was still irresistible. So cancer medicine charged on, even if it meant relinquishing sanctity, sanity, or safety. Pumped up with self-confidence, bristling with conceit, and hypnotized by the potency of medicine, oncologists pushed their patients—and their discipline—to the brink of disaster. "We shall so poison the atmosphere of the first act," the biologist James Watson warned about the future of cancer in 1977, "that no one of decency shall want to see the play through to the end."

For many cancer patients caught in the first act, there was little choice but to see the poisonous play to its end.

ↂ

More is more, a patient's daughter told me curtly. (I had suggested to her delicately that for some patients with cancer, "Less might be more.") The patient was an elderly Italian woman with liver cancer that had metastasized widely throughout her abdomen. She had come to the Massachusetts General Hospital seeking chemotherapy, surgery, or radiation—if possible, all three. She spoke halting, heavily accented English, often pausing between her words to catch her breath. Her skin had a yellow-gray tinge—a tinge, I was worried, that would bloom into a bright jaundice if the tumor obstructed her bile duct fully and her blood began to fill up with bile pigments. Exhausted, she drifted in and out of sleep even while I was examining her. I asked her to hold the palms of her hands straight upward, as if halting traffic, looking for signs of a subtle flapping motion that often predates liver failure. Thankfully, there was no tremor, but the abdomen had a dull, full sound of fluid building up inside it, likely full of malignant cells.

The daughter was a physician, and she watched me with intense, hawk-like eyes while I finished the exam. She was devoted to her mother, with the reversed—and twice as fierce—maternal instinct that marks the poignant moment of midlife when the roles of mother and daughter begin to switch. The daughter wanted the best possible care for her mother—the best doctors, the best room with the best view of Beacon Hill, and the best, strongest, and toughest medicine that privilege and money could buy.

The elderly woman, meanwhile, would hardly tolerate even the mildest drug. Her liver had not failed yet but was on the verge of doing so, and subtle signs suggested her kidneys were barely functioning. I suggested that we try a palliative drug, perhaps a single chemotherapeutic agent that might just ameliorate her symptoms rather than pushing for a tougher regimen to try to cure an incurable disease.

The daughter looked at me as if I were mad. "I came here to get treatment, not consolations about hospice," she finally said, glowering with fury.

I promised to reconsider by asking more experienced doctors to weigh in. Perhaps I had been too hasty in my caution. But in a few weeks, I learned that she and her daughter had found another doctor, presumably someone who had acquiesced more readily to their demands. I do not know whether the elderly woman died from cancer or its cure.

જી

Yet a third voice of dissent arose in oncology in the 1980s, although this voice had skirted the peripheries of cancer for several centuries. As trial after trial of chemotherapy and surgery failed to chisel down the mortality rate for advanced cancers, a generation of surgeons and chemotherapists, unable to cure patients, began to learn (or relearn) the art of *caring* for patients.

It was a fitful and uncomfortable lesson. Palliative care, the branch of medicine that focuses on symptom relief and comfort, had been perceived as the antimatter of cancer therapy, the negative to its positive, an admission of failure to its rhetoric of success. The word *palliate* comes from the Latin *palliare*, "to cloak"—and providing pain relief was perceived as cloaking the essence of the illness, smothering symptoms rather than attacking disease. Writing about pain relief, a Boston surgeon thus reasoned in the 1950s: "If there is persistent pain which cannot be relieved by direct surgical attack on the pathological lesion itself . . . , relief can be obtained only by surgical interruption of sensory pathways." The only alternative to surgery was more surgery—fire to fight fire. Pain-relieving opiate drugs such as morphine or fentanyl were deliberately denied. "If surgery is withheld," the writer continued, "the sufferer is doomed to opiate addiction, physical deterioration or even suicide"—an ironic consideration, since Halsted himself, while devising his theory of radical surgery, had swiveled between his twin addictions to cocaine and morphine.

The movement to restore sanity and sanctity to the end-of-life care of cancer patients emerged, predictably, not from cure-obsessed America but from Europe. Its founder was Cecily Saunders, a former nurse who had retrained as a physician in England. In the late 1940s, Saunders had tended to a Jewish refugee from Warsaw dying of cancer in London. The man had left Saunders his life savings—£500—with a desire to be "a window in [her] home." As Saunders entered and explored the forsaken cancer wards of London's East End in the fifties, she began to decipher that cryptic request in a more visceral sense: she encountered terminally ill patients denied dignity, pain relief, and often even basic medical care—their lives confined, sometimes literally, to rooms without windows. These "hopeless" cases, Saunders found, had become the pariahs of oncology, unable to find any place in its rhetoric of battle and victory, and thus pushed, like useless, wounded soldiers, out of sight and mind.

Saunders responded to this by inventing, or rather resurrecting, a counterdiscipline—palliative medicine. (She avoided the phrase *palliative care* because *care*, she wrote, "is a soft word" that would never win respectability in the medical world.) If oncologists could not bring themselves to provide care for their terminally ill patients, she would leverage other specialists—psychiatrists, anesthesiologists, geriatricians, physical therapists, and neurologists—to help patients die painlessly and gracefully. And she would physically remove the dying from the oncology wards: in 1967, she created a hospice in London to care specifically for the terminally ill and dying, evocatively naming it St. Christopher's—not after the patron saint of death, but after the patron saint of travelers.

It would take a full decade for Saunders's movement to travel to America and penetrate its optimism-fortified oncology wards. "The resistance to providing palliative care to patients," a ward nurse recalls, "was so deep that doctors would not even look us in the eye when we recommended that they stop their efforts to save lives and start saving dignity instead . . . doctors were allergic to the smell of death. Death meant failure, defeat—*their* death, the death of medicine, the death of oncology."

Providing end-of-life care required a colossal act of reimagination and reinvention. Trials on pain and pain relief—trials executed with no less rigor or precision than those launched to test novel drugs and surgical protocols—toppled several dogmas about pain and revealed new and unexpected foundational principles. Opiates, used liberally and compassionately on cancer patients, did not cause addiction, deterioration, and suicide; instead, they relieved the punishing cycle of anxiety, pain, and despair. New antinausea drugs were deployed that vastly improved the lives of patients on chemotherapy. The first hospice in the United States was launched at Yale–New Haven Hospital in 1974. By the early 1980s, hospices for cancer patients built on Saunders's model had sprouted up worldwide—most prominently in Britain, where nearly two hundred hospice centers were operating by the end of that decade.

Saunders refused to recognize this enterprise as pitted "against" cancer. "The provision of . . . terminal care," she wrote, "should not be thought of as a separate and essentially negative part of the attack on cancer. This is not merely the phase of defeat, hard to contemplate and unrewarding to carry out. In many ways its principles are fundamentally the same as those which underlie all other stages of care and treatment, although its rewards are different."

This, too, then, was knowing the enemy.

Counting Cancer

> *We must learn to count the living with that same particular attention with which we number the dead.*
> —Audre Lorde

> *Counting is the religion of this generation. It is its hope and its salvation.*
> —Gertrude Stein

In November 1985, with oncology caught at a pivotal crossroads between the sobering realities of the present and the hype of past promises, a Harvard biologist named John Cairns resurrected the task of measuring progress in the War on Cancer.

The word *resurrection* implies a burial, and since the *Fortune* article of 1937, composite assessments of the War on Cancer had virtually been buried—oddly, in an overwhelming excess of information. Every minor footfall and every infinitesimal step had been so obsessively reported in the media that it had become nearly impossible to discern the trajectory of the field as a whole. In part, Cairns was reacting to the *overgranularity* of the view from the prior decade. He wanted to pull away from the details and offer a bird's-eye view. Were patients with cancer surviving longer in general? Had the enormous investments in the War on Cancer since 1971 translated into tangible clinical achievements?

To quantify "progress," an admittedly hazy metric, Cairns began by revitalizing a fusty old record that had existed since World War II, the cancer registry, a state-by-state statistical record of cancer-related deaths subclassified by the type of cancer involved. "These registries," Cairns wrote in an article in *Scientific American,* "yield a rather precise picture of the natural history of cancer, and that is a necessary starting point for any discussion of treatment." By poring through that record, he hoped to draw a portrait of cancer over time—not over days or weeks, but over decades.

Cairns began by using the cancer registry to estimate the number of lives saved by the therapeutic advances in oncology since the 1950s. (Since surgery and radiation therapy preceded the 1950s, these were excluded; Cairns was more interested in advances that had emerged from the brisk expansion in biomedical research since the fifties.) He divided these therapeutic advances into various categories, then made numerical conjectures about their relative effects on cancer mortality.

The first of these categories was "curative" chemotherapy—the approach championed by Frei and Freireich at the NCI and by Einhorn and his colleagues at Indiana. Assuming relatively generous cure rates of about 80 or 90 percent for the subtypes of cancer curable by chemotherapy, Cairns estimated that between 2,000 and 3,000 lives were being saved overall every year—700 children with acute lymphoblastic leukemia, about 1,000 men and women with Hodgkin's disease, 300 men with advanced testicular cancer, and 20 to 30 women with choriocarcinoma. (Variants of non-Hodgkin's lymphomas, which were curable with polychemotherapy by 1986, would have added another 2,000 lives, bringing the total up to about 5,000, but Cairns did not include these cures in his initial metric.)

"Adjuvant" chemotherapy—chemotherapy given after surgery, as in the Bonadonna and Fisher breast cancer trials—contributed to another 10,000 to 20,000 lives saved annually. Finally, Cairns factored in screening strategies such as Pap smears and mammograms that detected cancer in its early stages. These, he estimated loosely, saved an additional 10,000 to 15,000 cancer-related deaths per year. The grand tally, generously speaking, amounted to about 35,000 to 40,000 lives per year.

That number was to be contrasted with the annual incidence of cancer in 1985—448 new cancer cases diagnosed for every 100,000 Americans, or about 1 million every year—and the mortality from cancer in 1985—211 deaths for every 100,000, or 500,000 deaths every year. In short, even with relatively liberal estimates about lives saved, less than one in twenty patients diagnosed with cancer in America, and less than one in ten of the total number of patients who would die of cancer, had benefited from the advances in therapy and screening.

Cairns wasn't surprised by the modesty of that number; in fact, he claimed, no self-respecting epidemiologist should be. In the history of medicine, no significant disease had ever been eradicated by a treatment-related program alone. If one plotted the decline in deaths from tuberculosis, for instance, the decline predated the arrival of new antibiotics by several decades. Far more potently than any miracle medicine, relatively uncelebrated shifts in civic arrangements—better nutrition, housing, and sanitation, improved sewage systems and ventilation—had driven TB mortality down in Europe and America. Polio and smallpox had also dwindled as a result of vaccinations. Cairns wrote, "The death rates from malaria, cholera, typhus, tuberculosis, scurvy, pellagra and other scourges of the past have dwindled in the US because humankind has learned how to *prevent* these diseases. . . . To put most of the effort into treatment is to deny all precedent."

ↄ⅃ℭ

Cairns's article was widely influential in policy circles, but it still lacked a statistical punch line. What it needed was some measure of the *comparative* trends in cancer mortality over the years—whether more or less people were dying of cancer in 1985 as compared to 1975. In May 1986, less than a year after Cairns's article, two of his colleagues from Harvard, John Bailar and Elaine Smith, provided precisely such an analysis in the *New England Journal of Medicine*.

To understand the Bailar-Smith analysis, we need to begin by understanding what it was not. Right from the outset, Bailar rejected the metric most familiar to patients: changes in survival rates over time. A five-year survival rate is a measure of the fraction of patients diagnosed with a particular kind of cancer who are alive at five years after diagnosis. But a crucial pitfall of survival-rate analysis is that it can be sensitive to biases.

To understand these biases, imagine two neighboring villages that have identical populations and identical death rates from cancer. On average, cancer is diagnosed at age seventy in both villages. Patients survive for ten years after diagnosis and die at age eighty.

Imagine now that in one of those villages, a new, highly specific test for cancer is introduced—say the level of a protein Preventin in the blood as a marker for cancer. Suppose Preventin is a perfect detection test. Preventin "positive" men and women are thus immediately counted among those who have cancer.

Preventin, let us further suppose, is an exquisitely sensitive test and reveals very early cancer. Soon after its introduction, the average age of cancer *diagnosis* in village 1 thus shifts from seventy years to sixty years, because earlier and earlier cancer is being caught by this incredible new test. However, since no therapeutic intervention is available even after the introduction of Preventin tests, the average age of death remains identical in both villages.

To a naive observer, the scenario might produce a strange effect. In village 1, where Preventin screening is active, cancer is now detected at age sixty and patients die at age eighty—i.e., there is a twenty-year survival. In village 2, without Preventin screening, cancer is detected at age seventy and patients die at age eighty—i.e., a ten-year survival. Yet the "increased" survival cannot be real. How can Preventin, by its mere existence, have increased survival without any therapeutic intervention?

The answer is immediately obvious: the increase in survival is, of course, an artifact. Survival rates seem to increase, although what has really increased is the *time from diagnosis to death* because of a screening test.

A simple way to avoid this bias is to not measure survival rates, but overall mortality. (In the example above, mortality remains unchanged, even after the introduction of the test for earlier diagnosis.)

But here, too, there are profound methodological glitches. "Cancer-related death" is a raw number in a cancer registry, a statistic that arises from the diagnosis entered by a physician when pronouncing a patient dead. The problem with comparing that raw number over long stretches of time is that the American population (like any) is gradually aging overall, and the rate of cancer-related mortality naturally increases with it. Old age inevitably drags cancer with it, like flotsam on a tide. A nation with a larger fraction of older citizens will seem more cancer-ridden than a nation with younger citizens, even if actual cancer mortality has not changed.

To compare samples over time, some means is needed to *normalize* two populations to the same standard—in effect, by statistically "shrinking" one into another. This brings us to the crux of the innovation in Bailar's analysis: to achieve this scaling, he used a particularly effective form of normalization called age-adjustment.

To understand age-adjustment, imagine two very different populations. One population is markedly skewed toward young men and women. The second population is skewed toward older men and women. If one measures the "raw" cancer deaths, the older-skewed population obviously has more cancer deaths.

Now imagine normalizing the second population such that this age skew is eliminated. The first population is kept as a reference. The second population is adjusted: the age-skew is eliminated and the death rate shrunk proportionally as well. Both populations now contain identical age-adjusted populations of older and younger men, and the death rate, adjusted accordingly, yields identical cancer-specific death rates. Bailar performed this exercise repeatedly over dozens of years: he divided the population for every year into age cohorts—20–29 years, 30–39 years, 40–49, and so forth—then used the population distribution from 1980 (chosen arbitrarily as a standard) to convert the population distributions for all other years into the same distribution. Cancer rates were adjusted accordingly. Once all the distributions were fitted into the same standard demographic, the populations could be studied and compared over time.

❧

Bailar and Smith published their article in May 1986—and it shook the world of oncology by its roots. Even the moderately pessimistic Cairns had expected at least a small decrease in cancer-related mortality over time. Bailar and Smith found that even Cairns had been overgenerous: between 1962 and 1985, cancer-related deaths had *increased* by 8.7 percent. That increase reflected many factors—most potently, an increase in smoking rates in the 1950s that had resulted in an increase in lung cancer.

One thing was frightfully obvious: cancer mortality was not declining in the United States. There is "no evidence," Bailar and Smith wrote darkly, "that some thirty-five years of intense and growing efforts to improve the treatment of cancer have had much overall effect on the most fundamental measure of clinical outcome—death." They continued, "We are losing the war against cancer notwithstanding progress against several uncommon forms of the disease [such as childhood leukemia and Hodgkin's disease], improvements in palliation and extension of productive years of life. . . . Some thirty-five years of intense effort focused largely on improving treatment must be judged a qualified failure."

That phrase, "qualified failure," with its mincing academic ring, was deliberately chosen. In using it, Bailar was declaring his own war—against the cancer establishment, against the NCI, against a billion-dollar cancer-treatment industry. One reporter described him as "a thorn in the side of the National Cancer Institute." Doctors railed against Bailar's analysis, describing him as a naysayer, a hector, a nihilist, a defeatist, a crank.

Predictably, a torrent of responses appeared in medical journals. One camp of critics contended that the Bailar-Smith analysis appeared dismal not because cancer treatment was ineffective, but because it was not being implemented aggressively enough. Delivering chemotherapy, these critics argued, was a vastly more complex process than Bailar and Smith had surmised—so complex that even most oncologists often blanched at the prospect of full-dose therapy. As evidence, they pointed to a survey from 1985 that had estimated that only one-third of cancer doctors were using the most effective combination regimen for breast cancer. "I estimate that 10,000 lives could be saved by the early aggressive use of polychemotherapy in breast cancer, as compared with the negligible number of lives, perhaps several thousand, now being saved," one prominent critic wrote.

In principle, this might have been correct. As the '85 survey suggested, many doctors were indeed underdosing chemotherapy—at least by the standards advocated by most oncologists, or even by the NCI. But the obverse idea—that *maximizing* chemotherapy would maximize gains in survival—was also untested. For some forms of cancer (some subtypes of breast cancer, for instance) increasing the intensity of dosage would eventually result in increasing efficacy. But for a vast majority of cancers, more intensive regimens of standard chemotherapeutic drugs did not necessarily mean more survival. "Hit hard and hit early," a dogma borrowed from the NCI's experience with childhood leukemia, was not going to be a general solution to all forms of cancer.

A more nuanced critique of Bailar and Smith came, unsurprisingly, from Lester Breslow, the UCLA epidemiologist. Breslow reasoned that while age-adjusted mortality was one method of appraising the War on Cancer, it was by no means the only measure of progress or failure. In fact, by highlighting only one measure, Bailar and Smith had created a fallacy of their own: they had oversimplified the measure of progress. "The problem with reliance on a single measure of progress," Breslow wrote, "is that the impression conveyed can vary dramatically when the measure is changed."

To illustrate his point, Breslow proposed an alternative metric. If chemotherapy cured a five-year-old child of ALL, he argued, then it saved a full sixty-five years of potential life (given an overall life expectancy of about seventy). In contrast, the chemotherapeutic cure in a sixty-five-year-old man contributed only five additional years given a life expectancy of seventy. But Bailar and Smith's chosen metric—age-adjusted mortality—

could not detect any difference in the two cases. A young woman cured of lymphoma, with fifty additional years of life, was judged by the same metric as an elderly woman cured of breast cancer, who might succumb to some other cause of death in the next year. If "years of life saved" was used as a measure of progress on cancer, then the numbers turned far more palatable. Now, instead of losing the War on Cancer, it appeared that we were winning it.

Breslow, pointedly, wasn't recommending one form of calculus over another; his point was to show that measurement itself was subjective. "Our purpose in making these calculations," he wrote, "is to indicate how sensitive one's conclusions are to the choice of measure. In 1980, cancer was responsible for 1.824 million lost years of potential life in the United States to age 65. If, however, the cancer mortality rates of 1950 had prevailed, 2.093 million years of potential life would have been lost."

The measurement of illness, Breslow was arguing, is an inherently subjective activity: it inevitably ends up being a measure of ourselves. Objective decisions come to rest on normative ones. Cairns or Bailar could tell us how many absolute lives were being saved or lost by cancer therapeutics. But to decide whether the investment in cancer research was "worth it," one needed to start by questioning the notion of "worth" itself: was the life extension of a five-year-old "worth" more than the life extension of a sixty-year-old? Even Bailar and Smith's "most fundamental measure of clinical outcome"—death—was far from fundamental. Death (or at least the social meaning of death) could be counted and recounted with other gauges, often resulting in vastly different conclusions. The appraisal of diseases depends, Breslow argued, on our *self*-appraisal. Society and illness often encounter each other in parallel mirrors, each holding up a Rorschach test for the other.

∂ℓ℘

Bailar might have been willing to concede these philosophical points, but he had a more pragmatic agenda. He was using the numbers to prove a principle. As Cairns had already pointed out, the only intervention ever known to reduce the aggregate mortality for a disease—*any* disease—at a population level was prevention. Even if other measures were chosen to evaluate our progress against cancer, Bailar argued that it was indubitably true that prevention, as a strategy, had been neglected by the NCI in its ever-manic pursuit of cures.

A vast majority of the institute's grants, 80 percent, were directed toward treatment strategies for cancer; prevention research received about 20 percent. (By 1992, this number had increased to 30 percent; of the NCI's $2 billion research budget, $600 million was being spent on prevention research.) In 1974, describing to Mary Lasker the comprehensive activities of the NCI, the director, Frank Rauscher, wrote effusively about its three-pronged approach to cancer: "Treatment, Rehabilitation and Continuing Care." That there was no mention of either prevention or early detection was symptomatic: the institute did not even consider cancer prevention a core strength.

A similarly lopsided bias existed in private research institutions. At Memorial Sloan-Kettering in New York, for instance, only one laboratory out of nearly a hundred identified itself as having a prevention research program in the 1970s. When one researcher surveyed a large cohort of doctors in the early 1960s, he was surprised to learn that "not one" was able to suggest an "idea, lead or theory on cancer prevention." Prevention, he noted drily, was being carried out "on a part-time basis."*

This skew of priorities, Bailar argued, was the calculated by-product of 1950s-era science; of books, such as Garb's *Cure for Cancer*, that had forecast impossibly lofty goals; of the Laskerites' near-hypnotic conviction that cancer could be cured within the decade; of the steely, insistent enthusiasm of researchers such as Farber. The vision could be traced back to Ehrlich, ensconced in the semiotic sorcery of his favorite phrase: "magic bullet." Progressive, optimistic, and rationalistic, this vision—of magic bullets and miracle cures—had admittedly swept aside the pessimism around cancer and radically transformed the history of oncology. But the notion of the "cure" as the singular solution to cancer had degenerated into a sclerotic dogma. Bailar and Smith noted, "A shift in research emphasis, from research on treatment to research on prevention, seems necessary if substantial progress against cancer is to be forthcoming. . . . Past disappointments must be dealt with in an objective, straightforward and comprehensive manner before we go much further in pursuit of a cure that always seems just out of reach."

---

* Although this line of questioning may be intrinsically flawed since it does not recognize the interrelatedness of preventive and therapeutic research.

PART FOUR

PREVENTION IS
THE CURE

*It should first be noted, however, that the 1960s and 1970s
did not witness so much a difficult* birth *of approaches
to prevention that focused on environmental and lifestyle
causes of cancer, as a difficult* reinvention *of an older
tradition of interest in these possible causes.*

—David Cantor

*The idea of preventive medicine is faintly un-American.
It means, first, recognizing that the enemy is us.*

—Chicago Tribune, *1975*

*The same correlation could be drawn to the intake of
milk. . . . No kind of interviewing [can] get satisfactory
results from patients. . . . Since nothing had been proved
there exists no reason why experimental work should be
conducted along this line.*

—U.S. surgeon general
Leonard Scheele on the link
between smoking and cancer

"Coffins of black"

When my mother died I was very young,
And my father sold me while yet my tongue,
Could scarcely cry weep weep weep weep,
So your chimneys I sweep & in soot I sleep . . .

And so he was quiet, & that very night.
As Tom was a sleeping he had such a sight
That thousands of sweepers Dick, Joe, Ned, & Jack
Were all of them lock'd up in coffins of black
　　　　　　　　　　　　　　　　　—William Blake

In 1775, more than a century before Ehrlich fantasized about chemotherapy or Virchow espoused his theory of cancer cells, a surgeon at St. Bartholomew's Hospital named Percivall Pott noticed a marked rise in cases of scrotal cancer in his clinic. Pott was a methodical, compulsive, reclusive man, and his first impulse, predictably, had been to try to devise an elegant operation to excise the tumors. But as cases streamed into his London clinic, he noticed a larger trend. His patients were almost invariably chimney sweeps or "climbing-boys"—poor, indentured orphans apprenticed to sweeps and sent up into chimneys to clean the flues of ash, often nearly naked and swathed in oil. The correlation startled Pott. It is a disease, he wrote, "peculiar to a certain set of people . . . ; I mean the chimney-sweepers' cancer. It is a disease which always makes its first attack on . . . the inferior part of the scrotum; where it produces a superficial, painful, ragged, ill-looking sore, with hard and rising edges. . . . I never saw it under the age of puberty, which is, I suppose, one reason why it is generally taken, both by patient and surgeon, for venereal; and being treated with mercurials, is thereby soon and much exasperated."

Pott might easily have accepted this throwaway explanation. In

Georgian England, sweeps and climbing-boys were regarded as general cesspools of disease—dirty, consumptive, syphilitic, pox-ridden—and a "ragged, ill-looking sore," easily attributed to some sexually transmitted illness, was usually treated with a toxic mercury-based chemical and otherwise shrugged off. ("Syphilis," as the saying ran, "was one night with Venus, followed by a thousand nights with mercury.") But Pott was searching for a deeper, more systematic explanation. If the illness was venereal, he asked, why, of all things, the predilection for only one trade? If a sexual "sore," then why would it get "exasperated" by standard emollient drugs?

Frustrated, Pott transformed into a reluctant epidemiologist. Rather than devise new methods to operate on these scrotal tumors, he began to hunt for the cause of this unusual disease. He noted that sweeps spent hours in bodily contact with grime and ash. He recorded that minute, invisible particles of soot could be found lodged under their skin for days, and that scrotal cancer typically burst out of a superficial skin wound that tradesmen called a soot wart. Sifting through these observations, Pott eventually pinned his suspicion on chimney soot lodged chronically in the skin as the most likely cause of scrotal cancer.

Pott's observation extended the work of the Paduan physician Bernardino Ramazzini. In 1713, Ramazzini had published a monumental work—*De Morbis Artificum Diatriba*—that had documented dozens of diseases that clustered around particular occupations. Ramazzini called these diseases *morbis artificum*—man-made diseases. Soot cancer, Pott claimed, was one such *morbis artificum*—only in this case, a man-made disease for which the inciting agent could be identified. Although Pott lacked the vocabulary to describe it as such, he had discovered a carcinogen.*

The implication of Pott's work was far-reaching. If soot, and not some mystical, numinous humor (à la Galen), caused scrotal cancer, then two facts had to be true. First, external agents, rather than imbalances of internal fluids, had to lie at the root of carcinogenesis—a theory so radical for its time that even Pott hesitated to believe it. "All this makes it (at first) a very different case from a cancer which appears in an elderly man, whose fluids are become acrimonious from time," he wrote (paying sly homage to Galen, while undermining Galenic theory).

Second, if a foreign substance was truly the cause, then cancer was

---

* Soot is a mixture of chemicals that would eventually be found to contain several carcinogens.

potentially preventable. There was no need to purge the body of fluids. Since the illness was man-made, its solution could also be man-made. Remove the carcinogen—and cancer would stop appearing.

But the simplest means of removing the carcinogen was perhaps the most difficult to achieve. Eighteenth-century England was a land of factories, coal, and chimneys—and by extension, of child labor and chimney sweeps servicing these factories and chimneys. Chimney sweeping, though still a relatively rare occupation for children—by 1851, Britain had about eleven hundred sweeps under the age of fifteen—was emblematic of an economy deeply dependent on children's labor. Orphans, often as young as four and five years old, were "apprenticed" to master sweeps for a small price. ("I wants a 'prentis, and I am ready to take him," says Mr. Gamfield, the dark, malevolent chimney sweep in Dickens's *Oliver Twist*. By an odd stroke of luck, Oliver is spared from being sold to Gamfield, who has already sent two previous apprentices to their deaths by asphyxiation in chimneys.)

But political winds changed. By the late eighteenth century, the embarrassing plight of London's climbing-boys was publicly exposed, and social reformers in England sought to create laws to regulate the occupation. In 1788, the Chimney Sweepers Act was passed in Parliament, preventing master sweeps from employing children under eight (children over eight were allowed to be apprenticed). In 1834, the age was raised to fourteen, and in 1840 to sixteen years. By 1875, the use of young climbing-boys was fully forbidden and the profession vigorously policed to prevent infractions. Pott did not live to see the changes—he contracted pneumonia and died in 1788—but the man-made epidemic of scrotal cancer among sweeps vanished over several decades.

ℐℛ

If soot could cause cancer, then were such preventable causes—and their cancer *"artificia"*—strewn about in the world?

In 1761, more than a decade before Pott had published his study on soot cancer, an amateur scientist and apothecary in London, John Hill, claimed that he had found one such carcinogen concealed in another innocuous-seeming substance. In a pamphlet entitled *Cautions against the Immoderate Use of Snuff*, Hill argued that snuff—oral tobacco—could also cause lip, mouth, and throat cancer.

Hill's evidence was no weaker or stronger than Pott's. He, too, had drawn a conjectural line between a habit (snuff use), an exposure (tobacco), and a particular form of cancer. His culprit substance, often smoked as well as chewed, even *resembled* soot. But Hill—a self-professed "Bottanist, apothecary, poet, stage player, or whatever you please to call him"—was considered the court jester of British medicine, a self-promoting amateur dabbler, part scholar and part buffoon. While Pott's august monograph on soot cancer circulated through the medical annals of England drawing admiration and praise, Hill's earlier pamphlet, written in colorful, collo-quial language and published without the backing of any medical author-ity, was considered a farce.

In England, meanwhile, tobacco was rapidly escalating into a national addiction. In pubs, smoking parlors, and coffeehouses—in "close, clouded, hot, narcotic rooms"—men in periwigs, stockings, and lace ruffs gath-ered through the day and night to pull smoke from pipes and cigars or sniff snuff from decorated boxes. The commercial potential of this habit was not lost on the Crown or its colonies. Across the Atlantic, where the tobacco had originally been discovered and the conditions for cultivat-ing the plant were almost providentially optimal, production increased exponentially decade by decade. By the mid-1700s, the state of Virginia was producing thousands of tons of tobacco every year. In England, the import of tobacco escalated dramatically between 1700 and 1770, nearly tripling from 38 million pounds to more than 100 million per year.

It was a relatively minor innovation—the addition of a piece of trans-lucent, combustible paper to a plug of tobacco—that further escalated tobacco consumption. In 1855, legend runs, a Turkish soldier in the Crimean War, having run out of his supply of clay pipes, rolled up tobacco in a sheet of newspaper to smoke it. The story is likely apocryphal, and the idea of packing tobacco in paper was certainly not new. (The papirossi, or papelito, had traveled to Turkey through Italy, Spain, and Brazil.) But the context was pivotal: the war had squeezed soldiers from three continents into a narrow, blasted peninsula, and habits and mannerisms were des-tined to spread quickly through its trenches like viruses. By 1855, English, Russian, and French soldiers were all puffing their tobacco rations rolled up in paper. When these soldiers returned from the war, they brought their habits, like viruses again, to their respective homelands with them.

The metaphor of infection is particularly apposite, since cigarette smok-ing soon spread like a fierce contagion through all those nations and then leapt across the Atlantic to America. In 1870, the per capita consumption in America was less than one cigarette per year. A mere thirty years later, Americans were consuming 3.5 billion cigarettes and 6 billion cigars every year. By 1953, the average annual consumption of cigarettes had reached thirty-five hundred per person. On average, an adult American smoked ten cigarettes every day, an average Englishman twelve, and a Scotsman nearly twenty.

Like a virus, too, the cigarette mutated, adapting itself to diverse contexts. In the Soviet gulags, it became an informal currency; among English suffragettes, a symbol of rebellion; among American suburbanites, of rugged machismo, among disaffected youth, of generational rift. In the turbulent century between 1850 and 1950, the world offered conflict, atomization, and disorientation. The cigarette offered its equal and opposite salve: camaraderie, a sense of belonging, and the familiarity of habits. If cancer is the quintessential product of modernity, then so, too, is its principal preventable cause: tobacco.

༄ᐧ

It was precisely this rapid, viral ascendancy of tobacco that made its medical hazards virtually invisible. Our intuitive acuity about statistical correlations, like the acuity of the human eye, performs best at the margins. When rare events are superposed against rare events, the association between them can be striking. Pott, for instance, had discovered the link between scrotal cancer and chimney sweeping because chimney sweeping (the profession) and scrotal cancer (the disease) were both uncommon enough that the juxtaposition of the two stood out starkly like a lunar eclipse—two unusual occurrences in precise overlap.

But as cigarette consumption escalated into a national addiction, it became harder and harder to discern an association with cancer. By the early twentieth century, four out of five—and, in some parts of the world, nearly nine of ten—men were smoking cigarettes (women would soon follow). And when a risk factor for a disease becomes so highly prevalent in a population, it paradoxically begins to disappear into the white noise of the background. As the Oxford epidemiologist Richard Peto put it: "By the early 1940s, asking about a connection between tobacco and cancer was like asking about an association between sitting and cancer." If nearly all men smoked, and only some of them developed cancer, then how might one tease apart the statistical link between one and the other?

Even surgeons, who encountered lung cancer most frequently, could no longer perceive any link. In the 1920s, when Evarts Graham, the renowned surgeon in St. Louis who had pioneered the pneumonectomy (the resection of the lung to remove tumors), was asked whether tobacco smoking had caused the increased incidence of lung cancer, he countered dismissively, "So has the use of nylon stockings."

Tobacco, like the nylon stockings of cancer epidemiology, thus vanished from the view of preventive medicine. And with its medical hazards largely hidden, cigarette usage grew even more briskly, rising at a dizzying rate throughout the western hemisphere. By the time the cigarette returned to visibility as arguably the world's most lethal carrier of carcinogens, it would be far too late. The lung cancer epidemic would be in full spate, and the world would be deeply, inextricably ensconced, as the historian Allan Brandt once characterized it, in "the cigarette century."

The Emperor's Nylon Stockings

Whether epidemiology alone can, in strict logic, ever prove
causality, even in this modern sense, may be questioned,
but the same must also be said of laboratory experiments
on animals.

—Richard Doll

In the early winter of 1947, government statisticians in Britain alerted the Ministry of Health that an unexpected "epidemic" was slowly emerging in the United Kingdom: lung cancer morbidity had risen nearly fifteen-fold in the prior two decades. It is a "matter that ought to be studied," the deputy registrar wrote. The sentence, although couched in characteristic English understatement, was strong enough to provoke a response. In February 1947, in the midst of a bitterly cold winter, the ministry asked the Medical Research Council to organize a conference of experts on the outskirts of London to study this inexplicable rise of lung cancer rates and to hunt for a cause.

The conference was a lunatic comedy. One expert, having noted parenthetically that large urban towns (where cigarette consumption was the highest) had much higher rates of lung cancer than villages (where consumption was the lowest), concluded that "the only adequate explanation" was the "smokiness or pollution of the atmosphere." Others blamed influenza, the fog, lack of sunshine, X-rays, road tar, the common cold, coal fires, industrial pollution, gasworks, automobile exhaust—in short, every breathable form of toxin except cigarette smoke.

Befuddled by this variance in opinions, the council charged Austin Bradford Hill, the eminent biostatistician who had devised the randomized trial in the 1940s, to devise a more systematic study to identify the risk factor for lung cancer. Yet the resources committed for the study were almost comically minimal: on January 1, 1948, the council authorized a part-time salary of £600 for a student, £350 each for two social workers, and £300 for incidental expenses and supplies. Hill recruited a thirty-six-year-old medical researcher, Richard Doll, who had never performed a study of comparable scale or significance.

Across the Atlantic, too, the link between smoking and cancer was seemingly visible only to neophytes—young interns and residents "uneducated" in surgery and medicine who seemed to make an intuitive connection between the two. In the summer of 1948, Ernst Wynder, a medical student on a surgical rotation in New York, encountered an unforgettable case of a forty-two-year-old man who had died of bronchogenic carcinoma—cancer of the airways of the lung. The man had been a smoker, and as in most autopsies of smokers, his body had been scarred with the stigmata of chronic smoking: tar-stained bronchi and soot-blackened lungs. The surgeon who was operating on the case made no point of it. (As with most surgeons, the association had likely become invisible to him.) But for Wynder, who had never encountered such a case before, the image of cancer growing out of that soot-stained lung was indelible; the link was virtually staring him in the face.

Wynder returned to St. Louis, where he was in medical school, and applied for money to study the association between smoking and lung cancer. He was brusquely told that the effort would be "futile." He wrote to the U.S. surgeon general quoting prior studies that had hypothesized such an association, but was told that he would be unable to prove anything. "The same correlation could be drawn to the intake of milk. . . . No kind of interviewing [can] get satisfactory results from patients. . . . Since nothing had been proved there exists no reason why experimental work should be conducted along this line."

Thwarted in his attempts to convince the surgeon general's office, Wynder recruited an unlikely but powerful mentor in St. Louis: Evarts Graham, of "nylon stockings" fame. Graham didn't believe the connection between smoking and cancer either. The great pulmonary surgeon, who operated on dozens of lung cancer cases every week, was rarely seen without a cigarette himself. But he agreed to help Wynder with the study in part to conclusively *disprove* the link and lay the issue to rest. Graham also reasoned the trial would teach Wynder about the complexities and nuances of study design and allow him to design a trial to capture the real risk factor for lung cancer in the future.

Wynder and Graham's trial followed a simple methodology. Lung cancer patients and a group of control patients without cancer were asked about their history of smoking. The ratio of smokers to nonsmokers within the two groups was measured to estimate whether smokers were overrepresented in lung cancer patients compared to other patients. This setup (called a case-control study) was considered methodologically novel, but the trial itself was thought to be largely unimportant. When Wynder presented his preliminary ideas at a conference on lung biology in Memphis, not a single question or comment came from the members of the audience, most of whom had apparently slept through the talk or cared too little about the topic to be roused. In contrast, the presentation that followed Wynder's, on an obscure disease called pulmonary adenomatosis in sheep, generated a lively, half-hour debate.

♇

Like Wynder and Graham in St. Louis, Doll and Hill could also barely arouse any interest in their study in London. Hill's department, called the Statistical Unit, was housed in a narrow brick house in London's Bloomsbury district. Hefty Brunsviga calculators, the precursors of modern computers, clacked and chimed in the rooms, ringing like clocks each time a long division was performed. Epidemiologists from Europe, America, and Australia thronged the statistical seminars. Just a few steps away, on the gilded railings of the London School of Tropical Medicine, the seminal epidemiological discoveries of the nineteenth century—the mosquito as the carrier for malaria, or the sand fly for black fever—were celebrated with plaques and inscriptions.

But many epidemiologists argued that such cause-effect relationships could only be established for infectious diseases, where there was a known pathogen and a known carrier (called a vector) for a disease—the mosquito for malaria or the tsetse fly for sleeping sickness. Chronic, noninfectious diseases such as cancer and diabetes were too complex and too variable to be associated with single vectors or causes, let alone "preventable" causes. The notion that a chronic disease such as lung cancer might have a "carrier" of its own sort, to be gilded and hung like an epidemiological trophy on one of those balconies, was dismissed as nonsense.

In this charged, brooding atmosphere, Hill and Doll threw themselves

245

into work. They were an odd couple, the younger Doll formal, dispassionate, and cool, the older Hill lively, quirky, and humorous, a pukka Englishman and his puckish counterpart. The postwar economy was brittle, and the treasury on the verge of a crisis. When the price of cigarettes was increased by a shilling to collect additional tax revenues, "tobacco tokens" were issued to those who declared themselves "habitual users." During breaks in the long hours and busy days, Doll, a "habitual user" himself, stepped out of the building to catch a quick smoke.

Doll and Hill's study was initially devised as mainly a methodological exercise. Patients with lung cancer ("cases") versus patients admitted for other illnesses ("controls") were culled from twenty hospitals in and around London and interviewed by a social worker in a hospital. And since even Doll believed that tobacco was unlikely to be the true culprit, the net of associations was spread widely. The survey included questions about the proximity of gasworks to patients' homes, how often they ate fried fish, and whether they preferred fried bacon, sausage, or ham for dinner. Somewhere in that haystack of questions, Doll buried a throwaway inquiry about smoking habits.

By May 1, 1948, 156 interviews had come in. And as Doll and Hill sifted through the preliminary batch of responses, only one solid and indisputable statistical association with lung cancer leapt out: cigarette smoking. As more interviews poured in week after week, the statistical association strengthened. Even Doll, who had personally favored road-tar exposure as the cause of lung cancer, could no longer argue with his own data. In the middle of the survey, sufficiently alarmed, he gave up smoking.

In St. Louis, meanwhile, the Wynder-Graham team had arrived at similar results. (The two studies, performed on two populations across two continents, had converged on almost precisely the same magnitude of risk—a testament to the strength of the association.) Doll and Hill scrambled to get their paper to a journal. In September of that year, their seminal study, "Smoking and Carcinoma of the Lung," was published in the *British Medical Journal*. Wynder and Graham had already published their study a few months earlier in the *Journal of the American Medical Association*.

☙

It is tempting to suggest that Doll, Hill, Wynder, and Graham had rather effortlessly proved the link between lung cancer and smoking. But they had, in fact, proved something rather different. To understand that difference—and it is crucial—let us return to the methodology of the case-control study.

In a case-control study, risk is estimated post hoc—in Doll's and Wynder's case by asking patients with lung cancer whether they had smoked. In an often-quoted statistical analogy, this is akin to asking car accident victims whether they had been driving under the influence of alcohol—but interviewing them *after* their accident. The numbers one derives from such an experiment certainly inform us about a potential link between accidents and alcohol. But it does not tell a drinker his or her actual chances of being involved in an accident. It is risk viewed as if from a rearview mirror, risk assessed backward. And as with any distortion, subtle biases can creep into such estimations. What if drivers tend to overestimate (or underestimate) their intoxication at the time of an accident? Or what if (to return to Doll and Hill's case) the interviewers had unconsciously probed lung cancer victims more aggressively about their smoking habits while neglecting similar habits in the control group?

Hill knew the simplest method to counteract such biases: he had invented it. If a cohort of people could be *randomly* assigned to two groups, and one group forced to smoke cigarettes and the other forced not to smoke, then one could follow the two groups over time and determine whether lung cancer developed at an increased rate in the smoking group. That would prove causality, but such a ghoulish human experiment could not even be conceived, let alone performed on living people, without violating fundamental principles of medical ethics.

But what if, recognizing the impossibility of that experiment, one could settle for the next-best option—for a half-perfect experiment? Random assignment aside, the problem with the Doll and Hill study thus far was that it had estimated risk retrospectively. But what if they could set the clocks back and launch their study *before* any of the subjects developed cancer? Could an epidemiologist watch a disease such as lung cancer develop from its moment of inception, much as an embryologist might observe the hatching of an egg?

ɔſɒ

In the early 1940s, a similar notion had gripped the eccentric Oxford geneticist Edmund Ford. A firm believer in Darwinian evolution, Ford nonetheless knew that Darwin's theory suffered from an important limitation: thus far, the evolutionary progression had been inferred indirectly from the fossil record, but never demonstrated directly on a population of organisms. The trouble with fossils, of course, is that they are fossilized—static and immobile in time. The existence of three fossils A, B, and C, representing three distinct and progressive stages of evolution, might suggest that fossil A *generated* B and fossil B *generated* C. But this proof is retrospective and indirect; that three evolutionary stages exist suggests, but cannot prove, that one fossil had *caused* the genesis of the next.

The only formal method to prove the fact that populations undergo defined genetic changes over time involves capturing that change in the real world in real time—*prospectively*. Ford became particularly obsessed with devising such a prospective experiment to watch Darwin's cogwheels in motion. To this end, he persuaded several students to tramp through the damp marshes near Oxford collecting moths. Each time a moth was captured, it was marked with a cellulose pen and released back into the wild. Year after year, Ford's students had returned with galoshes and moth nets, recapturing and studying the moths that they had marked in the prior years and their unmarked descendants—in effect, creating a "census" of wild moths in the field. Minute changes in that cohort of moths, such as shifts in wing markings or variations in size, shape, and color, were recorded each year with great care. By charting those changes over nearly a decade, Ford had begun to watch evolution in action. He had documented gradual changes in the color of moth coats (and thus changes in genes), grand fluctuations in populations and signs of natural selection by moth predators—a macrocosm caught in a marsh.*

Both Doll and Hill had followed this work with deep interest. And the notion of using a similar cohort of humans occurred to Hill in the winter of 1951—purportedly, like most great scientific notions, while in his bath. Suppose a large group of men could be marked, à la Ford, with some fantastical cellulose pen, and followed, decade after decade after decade. The group would contain some natural mix of smokers and nonsmokers. If smoking truly predisposed subjects to lung cancer (much like brightwinged moths might be predisposed to being hunted by predators), then the smokers would begin to succumb to cancer at an increased rate. By following that cohort over time—by peering into that natural marsh of

* It was Ford's student Henry B. D. Kettlewell who used this moth-labeling technique to show that dark-colored moths—better camouflaged on pollution-darkened trees—tended to be spared by predatory birds, thus demonstrating "natural selection" in action.

human pathology—an epidemiologist could calculate the precise relative risk of lung cancer among smokers versus nonsmokers.

But how might one find a large enough cohort? Again, coincidences surfaced. In Britain, efforts to nationalize health care had resulted in a centralized registry of all doctors, containing more than sixty thousand names. Every time a doctor in the registry died, the registrar was notified, often with a relatively detailed description of the cause of death. The result, as Doll's collaborator and student Richard Peto described it, was the creation of a "fortuitous laboratory" for a cohort study. On October 31, 1951, Doll and Hill mailed out letters to about 59,600 doctors containing their survey. The questions were kept intentionally brief: respondents were asked about their smoking habits, an estimation of the amount smoked, and little else. Most doctors could respond in less than five minutes.

An astonishing number—41,024 of them—wrote back. Back in London, Doll and Hill created a master list of the doctors' cohort, dividing it into smokers and nonsmokers. Each time a death in the cohort was reported, they contacted the registrar's office to determine the precise cause of death. Deaths from lung cancer were tabulated for smokers versus nonsmokers. Doll and Hill could now sit back and watch cancer unfold in real time.

In the twenty-nine months between October 1951 and March 1954, 789 deaths were reported in Doll and Hill's original cohort. Thirty-six of these were attributed to lung cancer. When these lung cancer deaths were counted in smokers versus nonsmokers, the correlation virtually sprang out: all thirty-six of the deaths had occurred in smokers. The difference between the two groups was so significant that Doll and Hill did not even need to apply complex statistical metrics to discern it. The trial designed to bring the most rigorous statistical analysis to the cause of lung cancer barely required elementary mathematics to prove its point.

"A thief in the night"

> *By the way, [my cancer] is a squamous cell cancer apparently like all the other smokers' lung cancers. I don't think anyone can bring up a very forcible argument against the idea of a causal connection with smoking because after all I had smoked for about 50 years before stopping.*
>
> —Evarts Graham to Ernst Wynder, 1957

> *We believe the products that we make are not injurious to health. We always have and always will cooperate closely with those whose task it is to safeguard public health.*
>
> —"A Frank Statement to Cigarette Smokers,"
> a full-page advertisement produced
> by the tobacco industry in 1954

Richard Doll and Bradford Hill published their prospective study on lung cancer in 1956—the very year that the fraction of smokers in the adult American population reached its all-time peak at 45 percent. It had been an epochal decade for cancer epidemiology, but equally, an epochal decade for tobacco. Wars generally stimulate two industries, ammunition and cigarettes, and indeed both the World Wars had potently stimulated the already bloated tobacco industry. Cigarette sales had climbed to stratospheric heights in the mid-1940s and continued to climb in the '50s. In a gargantuan replay of 1864, as tobacco-addicted soldiers returned to civilian life, they brought even more public visibility to their addiction.

To stoke its explosive growth in the postwar period, the cigarette industry poured tens, then hundreds, of millions of dollars into advertising. And if advertising had transformed the tobacco industry in the past, the tobacco industry now transformed advertising. The most striking innovation of this era was the targeting of cigarette advertising to highly stratified consumers, as if to achieve exquisite specificity. In the past, cigarettes had been advertised quite generally to all consumers. By the early 1950s, though, cigarette ads, and cigarette brands, were being "designed" for segmented groups: urban workers, housewives, women, immigrants, African-Americans—and, to preemptively bell the medical cat—doctors themselves. "More doctors smoke Camels," one advertisement reminded consumers, thus reassuring patients of the safety of *their* smoking. Medical journals routinely carried cigarette advertisements. At the annual conferences of the American Medical Association in the early 1950s, cigarettes were distributed free of charge to doctors, who lined up outside the tobacco booths. In 1955, when Philip Morris introduced the Marlboro Man, its most successful smoking icon to date, sales of the brand shot up by a dazzling 5,000 percent over eight months. Marlboro promised a nearly erotic celebration of tobacco and machismo rolled into a single, seductive pack: "Man-sized taste of honest tobacco comes full through. Smooth-drawing filter feels right in your mouth. Works fine but doesn't get in the way." By the early 1960s, the gross annual sale of cigarettes in America peaked at nearly $5 billion, a number unparalleled in the history of tobacco. On average, Americans were consuming nearly four thousand cigarettes per year or about eleven cigarettes per day—nearly one for every waking hour.

♉

Public health organizations in America in the mid-1950s were largely unperturbed by the link between tobacco and cancer delineated by the Doll and Hill studies. Initially, few, if any, organizations highlighted the study as an integral part of an anticancer campaign (although this would soon change). But the tobacco industry was far from complacent. Concerned that the ever-tightening link between tar, tobacco, and cancer would eventually begin to frighten consumers away, cigarette makers began to proactively tout the benefits of filters added to the tips of their cigarettes as a "safety" measure. (The iconic Marlboro Man, with his hypermasculine getup of lassos and tattoos, was an elaborate decoy set up to prove that there was nothing effeminate or sissy about smoking filter-tipped cigarettes.)

On December 28, 1953, three years before Doll's prospective study had been released to the public, the heads of several tobacco companies met preemptively at the Plaza Hotel in New York. Bad publicity was clearly looming on the horizon. To counteract the scientific attack, an equal and opposite counterattack was needed.

The centerpiece of that counterattack was an advertisement titled "A Frank Statement," which saturated the news media in 1954, appearing simultaneously in more than four hundred newspapers over a few weeks. Written as an open letter from tobacco makers to the public, the statement's purpose was to address the fears and rumors about the possible link between lung cancer and tobacco. In about six hundred words, it would nearly rewrite the research on tobacco and cancer.

"A Frank Statement" was anything but frank. The speciousness began right from its opening lines: "Recent reports on experiments with mice have given wide publicity to a theory that cigarette smoking is in some way linked with lung cancer in human beings." Nothing, in fact, could have been further from the truth. The most damaging of the "recent experiments" (and certainly the ones that had received the "widest publicity") were the Doll/Hill and Wynder/Graham retrospective studies—both of which had been performed not on mice, but on humans. By making the science seem obscure and arcane, those sentences sought to render its results equally arcane. Evolutionary distance would force emotional distance: after all, who could possibly care about lung cancer in mice? (The epic perversity of all this was only to be revealed a decade later when, confronted with a growing number of superlative *human* studies, the tobacco lobby would counter that smoking had never been effectively shown to cause lung cancer in, of all things, mice.)

Obfuscation of facts, though, was only the first line of defense. The more ingenious form of manipulation was to gnaw at science's own self-doubt: "The statistics purporting to link cigarette smoking with the disease could apply with equal force to any one of many other aspects of modern life. Indeed the validity of the statistics themselves is questioned by numerous scientists." By half revealing and half concealing the actual disagreements among scientists, the advertisement performed a complex dance of veils. What, precisely, was being "questioned by numerous scientists" (or what link was being claimed between lung cancer and other features of "modern life") was left entirely to the reader's imagination.

Obfuscation of facts and the reflection of self-doubt—the proverbial combination of smoke and mirrors—might have sufficed for any ordinary public relations campaign. But the final ploy was unrivaled in its genius. Rather than discourage further research into the link between tobacco and cancer, tobacco companies proposed letting scientists have more of it: "We are pledging aid and assistance to the research effort into all phases of tobacco use and health . . . in addition to what is already being contributed by individual companies." The implication was that if more research was needed, then the issue was still mired in doubt—and thus unresolved. Let the public have its addiction, and let the researchers have theirs.

To bring this three-pronged strategy to fruition, the tobacco lobby had already formed a "research committee," which it called the Tobacco Industry Research Committee, or the TIRC. Ostensibly, the TIRC would act as an intermediary between an increasingly hostile academy, an increasingly embattled tobacco industry, and an increasingly confused public. In January 1954, after a protracted search, the TIRC announced that it had finally chosen a director, who had—as the institute never failed to remind the public—been ushered in from the deepest realms of science. Their choice, as if to close the circle of ironies, was Clarence Cook Little, the ambitious contrarian that the Laskerites had once deposed as president of the American Society for the Control of Cancer (ASCC).

* handle*

If Clarence Little had not been discovered by the tobacco lobbyists in 1954, then they might have needed to invent him: he came preformed to their precise specifications. Opinionated, forceful, and voluble, Little was a geneticist by training. He had set up a vast animal research laboratory at Bar Harbor in Maine, which served as a repository for purebred strains of mice for medical experiments. Purity and genetics were Little's preoccupations. He was a strong proponent of the theory that all diseases, including cancer, were essentially hereditary, and that these illnesses, in a form of medical ethnic-cleansing, would eventually carry away those with such predispositions, leaving a genetically enriched population resistant to diseases. This notion—call it eugenics lite—was equally applied to lung cancer, which he also considered principally the product of a genetic aberration. Smoking, Little argued, merely unveiled that inherent aberration, causing that bad germ to emerge and unfold in a human body. Blaming cigarettes for lung cancer, then, was like blaming umbrellas for bringing on the rain. The TIRC and the tobacco lobby vociferously embraced that view. Doll and Hill, and Wynder and Graham, had certainly correlated smoking and lung cancer. But correlation, Little insisted, could not be equated with cause. In a guest editorial written for the journal *Cancer Research* in 1956, Little argued that if the tobacco industry was being blamed for scientific dishonesty, then antitobacco activists bore the blame for scientific disingenuousness. How could scientists so easily conflate a mere confluence of two events—smoking and lung cancer—with a causal relationship?

Graham, who knew Little from his days at the ASCC, was livid. In a stinging rebuttal written to the editor, he complained, "A causal relationship between heavy cigarette smoking and cancer of the lung is stronger than for the efficacy of vaccination against smallpox, which is only statistical."

Indeed, like many of his epidemiologist peers, Graham was becoming exasperated with the exaggerated scrutiny of the word *cause*. That word, he believed, had outlived its original utility and turned into a liability. In 1884, the microbiologist Robert Koch had stipulated that for an agent to be defined as the "cause" of a disease, it would need to fulfill at least three criteria. The causal agent had to be present in diseased animals; it had to be isolated from diseased animals; and it had to be capable of transmitting the disease when introduced into a secondary host. But Koch's postulates had arisen, crucially, from the study of infectious diseases and infectious agents; they could not simply be "repurposed" for many noninfectious diseases. In lung cancer, for instance, it would be absurd to imagine a carcinogen being isolated from a cancerous lung after months, or years, of the original exposure. Transmission studies in mice were bound to be equally frustrating. As Bradford Hill argued, "We may subject mice, or other laboratory animals, to such an atmosphere of tobacco smoke that they can—like the old man in the fairy story—neither sleep nor slumber; they can neither breed nor eat. And lung cancers may or may not develop to a significant degree. What then?"

Indeed, what then? With Wynder and other coworkers, Graham *had* tried to expose mice to a toxic "atmosphere of tobacco smoke"—or at least its closest conceivable equivalent. Persuading mice to chain-smoke was obviously unlikely to succeed. So, in an inspired experiment performed in his lab in St. Louis, Graham had invented a "smoking machine," a contraption that would puff the equivalent of hundreds of cigarettes all day (Lucky Strikes were chosen) and deposit the tarry black residue, through a maze of suction chambers, into a distilling flask of acetone. By serially painting the tar on the skins of mice, Graham and Wynder had found that they could create tumors on the backs of mice. But these studies had, if anything, fanned up even more controversy. *Forbes* magazine had famously spoofed the research by asking Graham, "How many men distill their tar from their tobacco and paint it on their backs?" And critics such as Little might well have complained that this experiment was akin to distilling an orange to a millionth of a million parts and then inferring, madly, that the original fruit was too poisonous to eat.

Epidemiology, like the old man in Hill's fairy story, was thus itself huffing against the stifling economy of Koch's postulates. The classical triad—association, isolation, retransmission—would simply not suffice; what preventive medicine needed was its own understanding of "cause."

Once again, Bradford Hill, the éminence grise of epidemiology, proposed a solution to this impasse. For studies on chronic and complex human diseases such as cancer, Hill suggested, the traditional understanding of causality needed to be broadened and revised. If lung cancer would not fit into Koch's straitjacket, then the jacket needed to be loosened. Hill acknowledged epidemiology's infernal methodological struggle with causation—this was not an experimental discipline at its core—but he rose beyond it. At least in the case of lung cancer and smoking, he argued, the association possessed several additional features:

It was strong: the increased risk of cancer was nearly five- or tenfold in smokers.

It was consistent: Doll and Hill's study, and Wynder and Graham's study, performed in vastly different contexts on vastly different populations, had come up with the same link.

It was specific: tobacco was linked to lung cancer—precisely the site where tobacco smoke enters the body.

It was temporal: Doll and Hill had found that the longer one smoked, the greater the increase in risk.

It possessed a "biological gradient": the more one smoked in quantity, the greater the risk for lung cancer.

It was plausible: a mechanistic link between an inhaled carcinogen and a malignant change in the lung was not implausible.

It was coherent; it was backed by experimental evidence: the epidemiological findings and the laboratory findings, such as Graham's tar-painting experiments in mice, were concordant.

It behaved similarly in analogous situations: smoking had been correlated with lung cancer, and also with lip, throat, tongue, and esophageal cancer.

Hill used these criteria to advance a radical proposition. Epidemiologists, he argued, could *infer* causality by using that list of nine criteria. No single item in that list proved a causal relationship. Rather, Hill's list functioned as a sort of à la carte menu, from which scientists could pick and choose criteria to strengthen (or weaken) the notion of a causal relationship. For scientific purists, this seemed rococo—and, like all things rococo, all too easy to mock: imagine a mathematician or physicist choosing from a "menu" of nine criteria to infer causality. Yet Hill's list would charge epidemiological research with pragmatic clarity. Rather than fussing about the metaphysical idea about causality (what, in the purest sense, constitutes "cause"?), Hill changed its emphasis to a functional or operational idea. Cause is what cause *does,* Hill claimed. Often, like the weight of proof in a detective case, the preponderance of small bits of evidence, rather than a single definitive experiment, clinched cause.

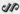

Amid this charged and historic reorganization of epidemiology, in the winter of 1956, Evarts Graham suddenly fell ill with what he thought was the flu. He was at the pinnacle of his career, a surgeon in full. His legacy was far-reaching: he had revolutionized lung cancer surgery by stitching together surgical procedures learned from nineteenth-century TB wards. He had investigated mechanisms by which cancer cells arose, using tobacco as his chosen carcinogen. And with Wynder, he had firmly established the epidemiological link between cigarettes and lung cancer.

In the end, though, it was his prior aversion to the theory that he himself had proved that undid Evarts Graham. In January 1957, when the "flu" refused to remit, Graham underwent a battery of tests at Barnes Hospital. An X-ray revealed the cause of his troubles: a large, coarse rind of a tumor clogging the upper bronchioles and both lungs riddled with hundreds of metastatic deposits of cancer. Keeping the identity of the patient hidden, Graham showed his films to a surgical colleague. The surgeon looked at the X-rays and deemed the tumor inoperable and hopeless. Graham then informed him quietly, "[The tumor] is mine."

On February 14, with his condition deteriorating weekly, Graham wrote to his friend and collaborator the surgeon Alton Ochsner: "Perhaps you have heard that I have recently been a patient at Barnes Hospital because of bilateral bronchogenic carcinoma which sneaked up on me like a thief in the night.... You know I quit smoking more than five years ago, but the trouble is that I smoked for 50 years."

Two weeks later, Graham grew dizzy, nauseated, and confused while shaving. He was brought to Barnes again, to a room a few floors above the operating rooms so beloved by him. He was given intravenous chemotherapy with nitrogen mustard, but to little avail. The "thief" had widely marauded; cancer was growing in his lungs, lymph nodes, adrenal glands, liver, and brain. On February 26, confused, lethargic, and incoherent, he drifted into a coma and died in his room. He was seventy-four years old. By his request, his body was donated to the department of anatomy as an autopsy specimen for other students.

ॐ

In the winter of 1954, three years before his untimely death, Evarts Graham wrote a strikingly prescient essay in a book entitled *Smoking and Cancer*. At the end of the essay, Graham wondered about how the spread of tobacco in human societies might be combated in the future. Medicine, he concluded, was not powerful enough to restrict tobacco's spread. Academic investigators could provide data about risks and argue incessantly about proof and causality, but the solution had to be political. "The obstinacy of [policymakers]," he wrote, "compels one to conclude that it is their own addiction . . . which blinds them. They have eyes to see, but see not because of their inability or unwillingness to give up smoking. All of this leads to the question . . . are the radio and the television to be permitted to continue carrying the advertising material of the cigarette industry? Isn't it time that the official guardian of the people's health, the United States Public Health Service, at least make a statement of warning?"

"A statement of warning"

*Our credulity would indeed be strained by an assumption
that a fatal case of lung cancer could have developed . . .
after the alleged smoking by Cooper of Camel cigarettes
in reliance upon representations by the defendant in the
various forms of advertising.*

—Jury verdict on Cooper case, 1956

*Certainly, living in America in the last half of the 20th
century, one would have to be deaf, dumb and blind not
to be aware of the asserted dangers, real or imagined, of
cigarette smoking. Yet the personal choice to smoke is . . .
the same kind of choice as the driver who downed the beers,
and then the telephone pole.*

—Open letter from the tobacco industry, 1988

In the summer of 1963, seven years after Graham's death, a team of three
men traveled to East Orange, New Jersey, to visit the laboratory of Oscar
Auerbach. A careful man of few words, Auerbach was a widely respected
lung pathologist who had recently completed a monumental study comparing lung specimens from 1,522 autopsies of smokers and nonsmokers.

Auerbach's paper describing the lesions he had found was a landmark
in the understanding of carcinogenesis. Rather than initiating his studies
with cancer in its full-blown form, Auerbach had tried to understand the
genesis of cancer. He had begun not with cancer but with its past incarnation, its precursor lesion—*precancer*. Long before lung cancer grew overtly
and symptomatically out of a smoker's lung, Auerbach found, the lung contained layer upon layer of precancerous lesions in various states of evolution—like a prehistoric shale of carcinogenesis. The changes began in the

bronchial airways. As smoke traveled through the lung, the outermost layers, exposed to the highest concentrations of tar, began to thicken and swell. Within these thickened layers, Auerbach found the next stage of malignant evolution: atypical cells with ruffled or dark nuclei in irregular patches. In a yet smaller fraction of patients, these atypical cells began to show the characteristic cytological changes of cancer, with bloated, abnormal nuclei often caught dividing furiously. In the final stage, these cell clusters broke through the thin lining of the basement membranes and transformed into frankly invasive carcinoma. Cancer, Auerbach argued, was a disease unfolded slowly in time. It did not run, but rather slouched to its birth.

Auerbach's three visitors that morning were on a field trip to understand that slouch of carcinogenesis as comprehensively as possible. William Cochran was an exacting statistician from Harvard; Peter Hamill, a pulmonary physician from the Public Health Service; Emmanuel Farber,* a pathologist. Their voyage to Auerbach's laboratory marked the beginning of a long scientific odyssey. Cochran, Hamill, and Farber were three members of a ten-member advisory committee appointed by the U.S. surgeon general. (Hamill was the committee's medical coordinator.) The committee's mandate was to review the evidence connecting smoking to lung cancer so that the surgeon general could issue an official report on smoking and lung cancer—the long-due "statement of warning" that Graham had urged the nation to produce.

❦

In 1961, the American Cancer Society, the American Heart Association, and the National Tuberculosis Association sent a joint letter to President Kennedy asking him to appoint a national commission to investigate the link between smoking and health. The commission, the letter recommended, should seek "a solution to this health problem that would interfere least with the freedom of industry or the happiness of individuals." The "solution," inconceivably, was meant to be both aggressive and conciliatory—clearly publicizing the link between cancer, lung disease, heart disease, and smoking, yet posing no obvious threat to the freedom of the tobacco industry. Suspecting an insolvable task, Kennedy (whose own political base in the tobacco-rich South was thin) quickly assigned it to his surgeon general, Luther Terry.

* No relation of Sidney Farber's.

Soft-spoken, conciliatory, and rarely combative, Luther Terry was an Alabaman who had picked tobacco as a child. Enthralled from early childhood by the prospect of studying medicine, he had graduated from Tulane University in 1935, then interned in St. Louis, where he had encountered the formidable Evarts Graham in his surgical prime. Terry had moved to the Public Health Service after graduation, then to the NIH in 1953, where, at the Clinical Center, his laboratory had neighbored the clinic buildings where Zubrod, Frei, and Freireich had been waging their battle against leukemia. Terry had thus spent his childhood in the penumbra of tobacco and his academic life in the penumbra of cancer.

Kennedy's assignment left Terry with three choices. He could quietly skirt the issue—thus invoking the wrath of the nation's three major medical organizations. He could issue a unilateral statement from the surgeon general's office about the health risks of tobacco—knowing that powerful political forces would quickly converge to neutralize that report. (In the early sixties, the surgeon general's office was a little-known and powerless institution; tobacco-growing states and tobacco-selling companies, in contrast, wielded enormous power, money, and influence.) Or he could somehow leverage the heft of science to reignite the link between tobacco and cancer in the public eye.

Hesitantly at first, but with growing confidence—"a reluctant dragon," as Kenneth Endicott, the NCI director, would characterize him—Terry chose the third path. Crafting a strategy that seemed almost reactionary at first glance, he announced that he would appoint an advisory committee to summarize the evidence on the links between smoking and lung cancer. The committee's report, he knew, would be scientifically redundant: nearly fifteen years had passed since the Doll and Wynder studies, and scores of studies had validated, confirmed, and reconfirmed their results. In medical circles, the link between tobacco and cancer was such stale news that most investigators had begun to focus on *secondhand* smoke as a risk factor for cancer. But by "revisiting" the evidence, Terry's commission would vivify it. It would intentionally create a show trial out of real trials, thus bringing the tragedy of tobacco back into the public eye.

Terry appointed ten members to his committee. Charles LeMaistre, from the University of Texas, was selected as an authority on lung physiology. Stanhope Bayne-Jones, the senior-most member of the committee, was a bearded, white-haired bacteriologist who had moderated several prior committees for the NIH. Louis Fieser, an organic chemist from Harvard, was an expert on chemical carcinogenesis. Jacob Furth from Columbia, a pathologist, was an authority on cancer genetics; John Hickam was a clinical specialist with a particular interest in heart and lung physiology; Walter Burdette, a Utah surgeon; Leonard Schuman, a widely respected epidemiologist; Maurice Seevers, a pharmacologist; William Cochran, a Harvard statistician; Emmanuel Farber, a pathologist who specialized in cell proliferation.

For nine sessions spanning thirteen months, the team met in a sparsely furnished, neon-lit room of the National Library of Medicine, a modern concrete building on the campus of the NIH. Ashtrays filled with cigarette butts littered the tables. (The committee was split exactly five to five among nonsmokers and smokers—men whose addiction was so deep that it could not be shaken even when deliberating the carcinogenesis of smoke.) The committee visited dozens of labs. Data, interviews, opinions, and testimonies were drawn from some 6,000 articles, 1,200 journals, and 155 biologists, chemists, physicians, mathematicians, and epidemiologists. In total, the trials used for the report encompassed studies on about 1,123,000 men and women—one of the largest cohorts ever analyzed in an epidemiological report.

Each member of the committee brought insight to a unique dimension of the puzzle. The precise and meticulous Cochran devised a new mathematical insight to judge the trials. Rather than privilege any particular study, he reasoned, perhaps one could use a method to estimate the relative risk as a composite number through *all* trials in the aggregate. (This method, termed meta-analysis, would deeply influence academic epidemiology in the future.) The organic chemist in Fieser was similarly roused: his discussion of chemicals in smoke remains one of the most authoritative texts on the subject. Evidence was culled from animal experiments, from autopsy series, from thirty-six clinical studies, and, crucially, from seven independent prospective trials.

Piece by piece, a highly incontrovertible and consistent picture emerged. The relationship between smoking and lung cancer, the committee found, was one of the strongest in the history of cancer epidemiology—remarkably significant, remarkably conserved between diverse populations, remarkably durable over time, and remarkably reproducible in trial after trial. Animal experiments demonstrating a causal link between smoking and lung cancer were inconclusive at best. But an experiment was not needed— at least not a laboratory experiment in the traditional sense of that word.

"The word 'cause,'" the report read, leaning heavily on Hill's prior work, "is capable of conveying the notion of a significant, effectual relationship between an agent and an associated disorder or disease in the host. . . . Granted that these complexities were recognized, it is to be noted clearly that the Committee's considered decision [was] to use the words 'a cause,' or 'a major cause,' . . . in certain conclusions about smoking and health."

In that single, unequivocal sentence, the report laid three centuries of doubt and debate to rest.

ↁ

Luther Terry's report, a leatherbound, 387-page "bombshell" (as he called it), was released on January 11, 1964, to a room packed with journalists. It was a cool Saturday morning in Washington, deliberately chosen so that the stock market would be closed (and thus bolstered against the financial pandemonium expected to accompany the report). To contain the bomb, the doors to the State Department auditorium were locked once the reporters filed in. Terry took the podium. The members of the advisory committee sat behind him in dark suits with name tags. As Terry spoke, in cautious, measured sentences, the only sound in the room was the dull scratch of journalists furiously scribbling notes. By the next morning, as Terry recalled, the report "was front-page news and a lead story on every radio and television station in the United States and many abroad."

In a nation obsessed with cancer, the attribution of a vast preponderance of a major cancer to a single, preventable cause might have been expected to provoke a powerful and immediate response. But front-page coverage notwithstanding, the reaction in Washington was extraordinarily anergic. "While the propaganda blast was tremendous," George Weissman, a public relations executive, wrote smugly to Joseph Cullman, the president of Philip Morris, ". . . I have a feeling that the public *reaction* was not as severe nor did it have the emotional depth I might have feared. Certainly, it is not of a nature that caused prohibitionists to go out with axes and smash saloons."

Even if the report had temporarily sharpened the scientific debate, the prohibitionists' legislative "axes" had long been dulled. Ever since the spectacularly flawed attempts to regulate alcohol during Prohibition, Congress had conspicuously disabled the capacity of any federal agency to regulate an industry. Few agencies wielded direct control over any industry. (The Food and Drug Administration was the most significant exception to this rule. Drugs were strictly regulated by the FDA, but the cigarette had narrowly escaped being defined as a "drug.") Thus, even if the surgeon general's report provided a perfect rationale to control the tobacco industry, there was little that Washington would do—or, importantly, *could* do—to achieve that goal.

It fell upon an altogether odd backwater agency of Washington to cobble together the challenge to cigarettes. The Federal Trade Commission (FTC) was originally conceived to regulate advertisements and claims made by various products: whether Carter's liver pills truly contained liver, or whether a product advertised for balding truly grew new hair. For the large part, the FTC was considered a moribund, torpid entity, thinning in authority and long in the tooth. In 1950, for instance, the year that the Doll/Hill and Wynder/Graham reports had sent shock waves through academic medicine, the commission's shining piece of lawmaking involved policing the proper use of the various words to describe health tonics, or (perhaps more urgently) the appropriate use of the terms "slip-proof" and "slip-resistant" versus "slip-retardant" to describe floor wax.

The FTC's destiny changed in the summer of 1957. By the mid-1950s, the link between smoking and cancer had sufficiently alarmed cigarette makers that many had begun to advertise new filter tips on cigarettes—to supposedly filter away carcinogens and make cigarettes "safe." In 1957, John Blatnik, a Minnesota chemistry teacher turned congressman, hauled up the FTC for neglecting to investigate the veracity of this claim. Federal agencies could not directly regulate tobacco, Blatnik acknowledged. But since the FTC's role was to regulate tobacco *advertisements,* it could certainly investigate whether "filtered" cigarettes were truly as safe as advertised. It was a brave, innovative attempt to bell the cat, but as with so much of tobacco regulation, the actual hearings that ensued were like a semiotic circus. Clarence Little was asked to testify, and with typically luminous audacity, he argued that the question of testing the efficacy of filters was immaterial because, after all, there was nothing harmful to be filtered anyway.

The Blatnik hearings thus produced few immediate results in the late 1950s. But, having been incubated over six years, they produced a powerful effect. The publication of the surgeon general's report in 1964 revived Blatnik's argument. The FTC had been revamped into a younger, streamlined agency, and within days of the report's release, a team of youthful lawmakers began to assemble in Washington to revisit the notion of regulating tobacco advertising. A week later, in January 1964, the FTC announced that it would pursue the lead. Given the link between cigarettes and cancer—a causal link, as recently acknowledged by the surgeon general's report—cigarette makers would need to acknowledge this risk directly in advertising for their products. The most effective method to alert consumers about this risk, the commission felt, was to imprint the message onto the product itself. Cigarette packages were thus to be labeled with *Caution: Cigarette Smoking Is Dangerous to Health. It May Cause Death from Cancer and Other Diseases.* The same warning label was to be attached to all advertisements in the print media.

As news of the proposed FTC action moved through Washington, panic spread through the tobacco industry. Lobbying and canvassing by cigarette manufacturers to prevent any such warning label reached a febrile pitch. Desperate to halt the FTC's juggernaut, the tobacco industry leaned on Abe Fortas, President Johnson's friend and legal adviser (and soon to be Supreme Court justice), and Earle Clements, the former governor of Kentucky who had become Little's replacement at the TIRC in 1959. Led by Clements and Fortas, tobacco makers crafted a strategy that, at first glance, seemed counterintuitive: rather than being regulated by the FTC, they voluntarily requested regulation by Congress.

The gambit had a deeply calculated logic. Congress, it was well-known, would inherently be more sympathetic to the interests of tobacco makers. Tobacco was the economic lifeblood of Southern states, and the industry had bribed politicians and funded campaigns so extensively over the years that negative political action was inconceivable. Conversely, the FTC's unilateral activism on tobacco had turned out to be such a vexing embarrassment to politicians that Congress was expected to at least symbolically rap the wrist of the vigilante commission—in part, by lightening its blow to tobacco. The effect would be a double boon. By voluntarily pushing for congressional control, the tobacco industry would perform a feat of political acrobatics—a leap from the commission's hostile fire to the much milder frying pan of Congress.

So it proved to be. In Congress, the FTC's recommendation was diluted and reduluted as it changed hands from hearing to hearing and committee to subcommittee, leading to a denervated and attenuated shadow of the bill's former self. Entitled the Federal Cigarette Labeling and Advertising Act (FCLAA) of 1965, it changed the FTC's warning label to *Caution: Cigarette smoking may be hazardous to your health.* The dire, potent language of the original label—most notably the words *cancer, cause,* and *death*—was expunged. To ensure uniformity, state laws were also enfolded into the FCLAA—in effect, ensuring that no stronger warning label could exist in any state in America. The result, as the journalist Elizabeth Drew noted in the *Atlantic Monthly,* was "an unabashed act to protect private industry from government regulation." Politicians were far more protective of the narrow interests of tobacco than of the broad interest of public health. Tobacco makers need not have bothered inventing protective filters, Drew wrote drily: Congress had turned out to be "the best filter yet."

∽

The FCLAA bill was a disappointment, but it galvanized antitobacco forces. The twisting of an unknown piece of trade law into a regulatory noose for tobacco was both symbolic and strategic: an unregulatable industry had been brought to heel—even if partially so. In 1966, a young attorney barely out of law school, John Banzhaf, pushed that strategy even further. Brash, self-confident, and iconoclastic, Banzhaf was lounging at home during the Thanksgiving holiday of 1966 (watching the omnipresent cigarette ads) when his mind raced to an obscure legal clause. In 1949, Congress had issued the "fairness doctrine," which held that public broadcast media had to allow "fair" airtime to opposing viewpoints on controversial issues. (Congress had reasoned that since the broadcast media used a public resource—airwaves—they should reciprocate by performing a public function, by providing balanced information on controversial issues.) The doctrine was little known and little used. But Banzhaf began to wonder whether it could be applied to cigarette advertising. The FTC had attacked the disingenuousness of the tobacco industry's advertising efforts. Could a parallel strategy be used to attack the disproportionality of its media presence?

In the early summer of 1967, Banzhaf dashed off a letter to the Federal Communications Commission (the agency responsible for enforcing the fairness doctrine) complaining that a New York TV station was dedicating disproportional airtime to tobacco commercials with no opposing antitobacco commercials. The complaint was so unusual that Banzhaf, then on a four-week cruise, expected no substantial response. But Banzhaf's letter had landed, surprisingly, on sympathetic ears. The FCC's general counsel, Henry Geller, an ambitious reformer with a long-standing interest in public-interest broadcasting, had privately been investigating the possibility of attacking tobacco advertising. When Banzhaf returned from the Bahamas, he found a letter from Geller:

"The advertisements in question clearly promote the use of a particular cigarette as attractive and enjoyable. Indeed, they understandably have no other purpose. We believe that a station which presents such advertisements has the duty of informing its audience of the other side of this controversial issue of public importance—that, however enjoyable, such smoking may be a hazard to the smoker's health."

With Geller's consent, Banzhaf filed his case against the TV station in court. Predictably, tobacco companies protested vociferously, arguing that legal action of this sort would have a chilling effect on free speech and vowing to fight the case to its bitter end. Faced with the prospect of a prolonged court battle, Banzhaf approached the American Cancer Society, the American Lung Association, and several other public health organizations for support. In all cases, he was rebuffed.

Banzhaf chose to go to trial anyway. Dragged into court in 1968, he squared off against "a squadron of the best-paid lawyers in the country, row after row of them in pinstripe suits and cuff links"—and, to the utter shock of the tobacco industry, won his case. The court held that "proportional airtime" had to be given to protobacco and antitobacco advertising. The FCC and Geller leapt back into the arena. In February 1969, the commission issued a public announcement that it would rigorously police the "proportional airtime" clause and, given the public-health hazard of tobacco, seek to ban cigarette commercials from television altogether. Tobacco makers appealed and reappealed the Banzhaf decision, but the Supreme Court refused to hear the case, letting the decision stand.

The industry tried to mount an aggressive countercampaign. An unpublicized internal report drawn up in 1969 to respond to the looming threat of the FCC advertising ban concluded, "Doubt is our product, since it is the best means of competing with the 'body of fact.'" But antismoking advocates had also learned the tricks of the trade; if tobacco sellers had "doubt" to sow into public minds, then tobacco opponents had something just as visceral: fear—in particular, fear of the ultimate illness. A barrage of antismoking commercials appeared on television. In 1968, a worn and skeletal-looking William Talman, a veteran actor and former smoker, announced in a prime-time advertisement that he was dying from lung cancer. Narcotized on painkilling medicines, his words slurring, Talman nonetheless had a clear message for the public: "If you do smoke—quit. Don't be a loser."

In late 1970, faced with the daily brunt of negative publicity, tobacco makers voluntarily withdrew cigarette advertising from broadcast media (thus nullifying the need for a proportional representation of antitobacco commercials). The last cigarette commercial was broadcast on television on January 1, 1971. At 11:59 p.m., on the first night of the New Year, the Virginia Slims slogan *You've come a long way, baby* flashed momentarily on TV screens, then vanished forever.

Talman did not live to see that final advertisement. He had already died in 1968 of lung cancer that had metastasized to his liver, bones, and brain.

❦

The mid-1970s thus marked the beginning of the end of an extraordinary era for the tobacco industry. The surgeon general's report, the FCLAA label warning, and the attack on cigarette advertising represented high-impact, sequential assaults on an industry once thought virtually impregnable. It is difficult to quantify the precise impact of any of these individual strategies, but these attacks coincided with a notable change in the trajectory of tobacco consumption: having risen unfailingly for nearly six decades, annual cigarette consumption in America plateaued at about four thousand cigarettes per capita.

The campaign against tobacco now needed one last strategy to consolidate these victories and drive them home to the public. "Statistics," the journalist Paul Brodeur once wrote, "are human beings with the tears wiped off," and thus far the antitobacco campaign had offered plenty of statistics, but with the human victims of tobacco somehow effaced. Litigation and regulation had occurred seemingly in the abstract; the FCLAA warning-label action and the fairness-doctrine case had been fought on *behalf* of cigarette "victims," but faceless and nameless ones. The final rondo of legal assaults against tobacco would, at long last, introduce the American public to the real victims of tobacco, men and women who had quietly been succumbing to lung cancer while Congress had deliberated the pros and cons of attaching a nine-word sentence to a packet of cigarettes.

❦

Rose Cipollone, born Rose DeFrancesco in New York, tasted her first cigarette as a teenager in 1942. She represented the midpoint of a steeply rising curve: between 1940 and 1944, the fraction of female smokers in the United States more than doubled, from 15 to 36 percent. That astonishing rise was the product of arguably the most successful targeted campaign ever launched in the history of American advertising—to persuade women to smoke. In this, tobacco rode on the back of a much deeper social change: in a world increasingly unsteady for women—with women juggling personal identity, child care, homemaking, and work—tobacco was marketed as a normalizing, steadying, even liberating force. Camel's campaign depicted a naval officer firing a torpedo in the high seas, while his wife at home calmed *her* stormy nerves with a cigarette. "[It's] a game only for steady nerves," the copy ran. "But, then, what isn't in these days—with all of us fighting, working, living at the highest tempo in years." Rosie the Riveter, the quintessential symbol of wartime womanhood, was now recast as Rosie the Smoker, depicted in Chesterfield's advertisements with a cigarette in hand. Smoking was a form of national service, and perhaps even Rosie's perpetual composure in the face of intense pressure ("never twittery, nervous or jittery," as the advertising song ran) could also be chalked up to the calming influence of her cigarette.

Like the eponymous Rosie looming larger than life on the twenty-foot billboards above her, Cipollone also chose to calm herself with Chesterfields. She began as a schoolgirl, rebelliously smuggling a few cigarettes here and there after classes. But as the economy soured and dipped in the 1930s, she dropped out of school, taking up jobs as a packer in a scarf factory and then as a billing clerk, and her habit escalated. Within just a few years, she had ramped up her consumption to dozens of cigarettes a day.

If Cipollone *was* ever nervous or jittery, it was in those rare moments when she confronted the health warnings about cigarettes. After her marriage, her husband, Anthony Cipollone, ran a quiet countercampaign, leaving her newspaper clippings that warned against the many hazards of smoking. Rose tried to quit, but relapsed each time with even greater dependency. When she ran out of cigarettes, she scoured the trash to smoke the burnt butts.

What bothered Cipollone was not her addiction, but, oddly, her choice of filters. In 1955, when Liggett introduced a new filter-tip cigarette named L&M, she switched brands expectantly, hoping that the advertised "milder, low tar, low nicotine" would be safer. The quest for the "safe cigarette" turned into a minor obsession for Cipollone. Like a serial monogamist of cigarettes, she bounced and rebounded from brand to brand, hoping to find the one that might protect her. In the mid-1960s, she switched

Humors in tumors

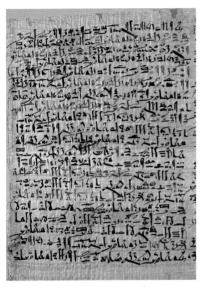

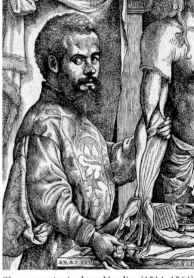

The first medical description of cancer was found in an Egyptian text originally written in 2500 BC: "a bulging tumor in [the] breast . . . like touching a ball of wrappings." Discussing treatment, the ancient scribe noted: "[There] is none."

The anatomist Andreas Vesalius (1514–1564) tried to discover the source for black bile, the fluid thought to be responsible for cancer. Unable to find it, Vesalius launched a new search for cancer's real cause and cure.

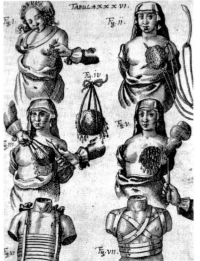

Medieval surgeons attacked cancer using primitive surgical methods. Johannes Scultetus (1595–1645) describes a mastectomy, the surgical removal of breast cancer, using fire, acid and leather bindings.

The rise of radical surgery

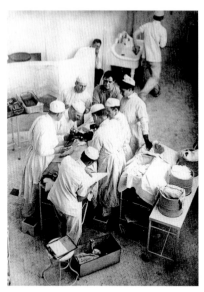

Between 1800 and 1900, surgeons devised increasingly aggressive operations to attack the roots of cancer in the body. In the 1890s, William Stewart Halsted at Johns Hopkins University devised the radical mastectomy—an operation to extirpate the breast, the muscles beneath the breast and the associated lymph nodes.

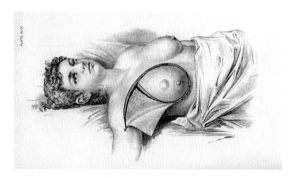

"The patient was a young lady whom I was loath to disfigure," Halsted wrote. In this etching, Halsted presented an idealized patient. Real cancer patients tended to be older women with larger tumors, far less able to withstand this radical attack.

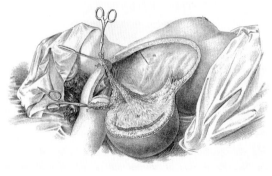

New arms in the battle

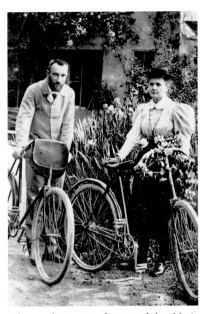

When radium was discovered by Marie and Pierre Curie, oncologists and surgeons began to deliver high doses of radiation to tumors. Yet radiation was itself carcinogenic: Marie Curie died from a leukemia caused by decades of X-ray exposure.

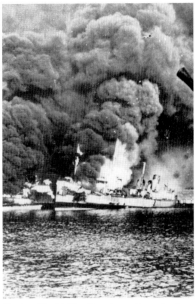

During World War Two, tons of mustard gas were released on the Bari harbor in Italy during an air raid. The gas decimated normal white blood cells in the body, leading pharmacologists to fantasize about using a similar chemical to kill cancers of white blood cells. Chemotherapy—chemical warfare on cancer cells—was inspired, literally, by war.

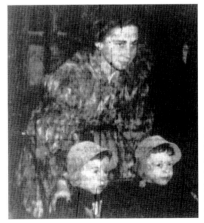

In 1947, Sidney Farber discovered that a folic acid analog called aminopterin killed rapidly dividing cells in the bone marrow. Using aminopterin, Farber obtained brief, tantalizing remissions in acute lymphoblastic leukemia. One of Farber's first patients was two-year-old Robert Sandler.

Building the edifice

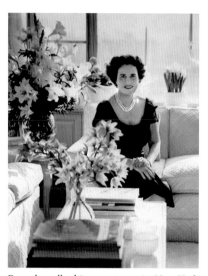

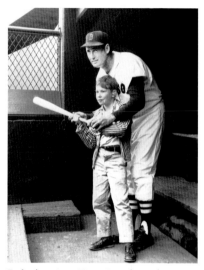

From her all-white apartment in New York City, Mary Lasker, a legendary entrepreneur, socialite, lobbyist and advocate, helped launch a national battle against cancer. Lasker would become the "fairy godmother" of cancer research; she would coax and strong-arm the nation to initiate a War on Cancer.

Farber's patient, Einar Gustafson—known as "Jimmy"—a baseball fan, became the unofficial mascot for children's cancer. The Jimmy Fund, founded in 1948, was one of the most powerful cancer advocacy organizations, with Ted Williams a vocal supporter.

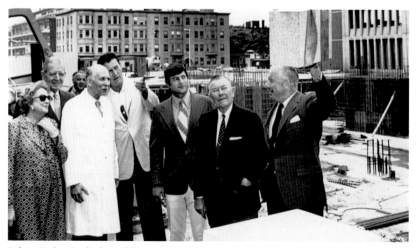

Sidney Farber, Lasker's confidant, mentor and co-conspirator, provided medical legitimacy to the War on Cancer and oversaw the building of a new cancer ward in Boston.

Early victories

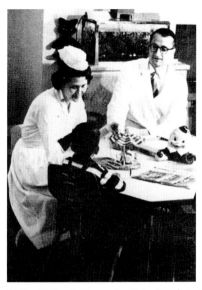

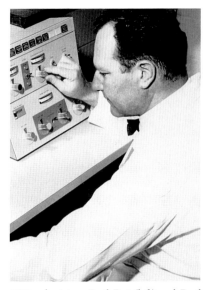

At the National Cancer Institute (NCI) in the 1960s physicians Emil Frei (left) and Emil Freireich (right) forged a strategy to cure acute lymphoblastic leukemia using highly toxic drugs.

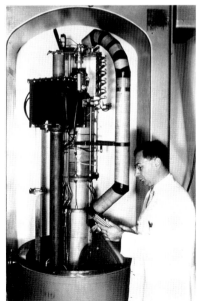

Henry Kaplan, a physician-scientist, used radiation therapy to cure Hodgkin's lymphoma. The cures of lymphoblastic leukemia and Hodgkin's lymphoma invigorated the War on Cancer, raising the possibility of Farber's "universal cure."

The politics of war

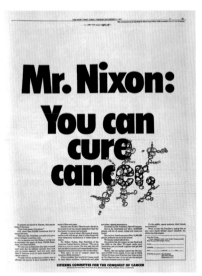

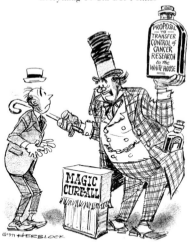

Inspired by the early victories of chemotherapy, cancer advocates, led by Lasker and Farber, urged the nation to launch a War on Cancer. In 1970, the Laskerites published a full-page advertisement in the *New York Times,* coaxing Nixon to support their war.

Many scientists criticized the War on Cancer as premature, arguing that a political cure would not lead to a medical cure.

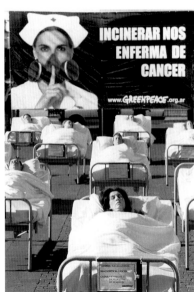

Lasker's use of canny advertising and potent imagery still inspires generations of advocates, including Greenpeace.

Prevention is the cure

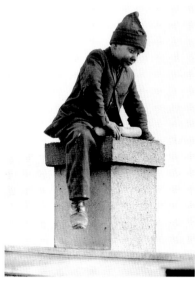

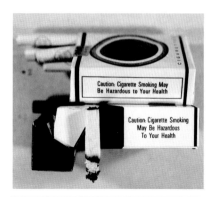

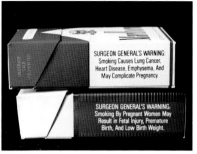

In 1775, the London surgeon Percivall Pott observed that scrotal cancer occurred disproportionately in adolescent chimney sweeps, and proposed a link between soot and scrotal cancer, launching the hunt for preventable carcinogens in the environment.

Innovative studies in the 1950s established the link between cigarette smoking and lung cancer. Yet early warning labels affixed on packages in the 1960s avoided the word "cancer." Explicit warning labels were not required until decades later.

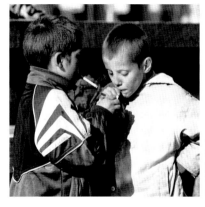

Although smoking rates have fallen in most developed nations, active marketing and bold political lobbying allows the tobacco industry to flourish in others, creating a new generation of smokers (and of future cancer victims).

The fruits of long endeavors

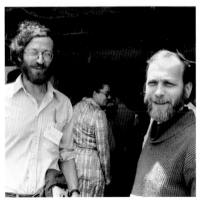

Harold Varmus and J. Michael Bishop discovered that cancer is caused by the activation of endogenous precursor genes that exist in all normal cells. Cancer, Varmus wrote, is a "distorted version" of our normal selves.

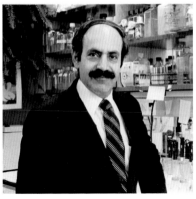

Working with collaborators across the globe, Robert Weinberg, of MIT, discovered distorted genes in mouse and human cancer cells.

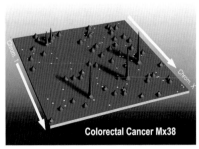

Colorectal Cancer Mx38

Scientists have sequenced the entire genomes of many cancer specimens (all 23,000 genes), making it possible to document every genetic change (relative to normal genes). Dots represent mutations in genes found in colon cancer, with commonly mutated genes becoming "hills" and then "mountains."

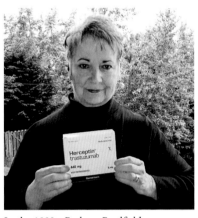

In the 1990s, Barbara Bradfield was among the first women to be treated with a drug, Herceptin, that specifically attacks breast cancer cells. She is the longest survivor of that treatment, with no hint of her cancer remaining.

to Virginia Slims, reasoning perhaps that a cigarette marketed exclusively for women might contain less tar. In 1972, she switched yet again to Parliaments, which promised a longer, recessed filter that might "insulate" a smoker's lips from the smoking tip. Two years later, she switched again, this time to True cigarettes because, as she would later describe in court to an astounded jury, "The doctor recommended them. . . . He said to me, 'You smoke and you might as well smoke these,' and he took out of his coat pocket a package of cigarettes."

In the winter of 1981, Cipollone developed a cough. A routine chest X-ray to evaluate the cough revealed a mass in the upper lobe of her right lung. A surgical biopsy revealed lung cancer. In August 1983, metastatic lung cancer was found all over Cipollone's body—malignant masses in her lungs, bones, and liver. She started chemotherapy, but had a poor response. As the cancer advanced into her marrow and burrowed into her brain and spinal cord, she was confined to bed, with shots of morphine to relieve her pain. Cipollone died on the morning of October 21, 1984. She was fifty-eight years old.

⁂

Marc Edell, a New Jersey attorney, heard of Cipollone's diagnosis eleven months before her death. Ambitious, canny, and restless, Edell possessed a deep knowledge of tort litigation (he had defended asbestos manufacturers against product-liability suits in the 1970s) and was looking for an iconic "victim" of cigarette smoke to launch a legal attack on tobacco. In the summer of 1983, Edell thus traveled to the sleepy suburban town of Little Ferry to visit Rose Cipollone and her family. Realizing that she was dying, he urged the Cipollones to file their suit against the three cigarette manufacturers whose products Rose had extensively used—Liggett, Lorillard, and Philip Morris.

Edell's case, filed in 1983, was ingeniously crafted. Previous cases against tobacco companies had followed a rather stereotypical pattern: plaintiffs had argued that they had personally been unaware of the risks of smoking. Cigarette makers had countered that the victims would have had to be "deaf, dumb and blind" not to have known about them, and juries had universally sided with cigarette makers, acknowledging that the packaging labels provided adequate warnings for consumers. For the plaintiffs, the record was truly dismal. In the three decades between 1954 and 1984, more than three hundred product-liability cases had been launched against tobacco companies. Sixteen of these cases had gone to trial. Not a single case had resulted in a judgment against a tobacco company, and not one had been settled out of court. The tobacco industry had all but declared absolute victory: "Plaintiff attorneys can read the writing on the wall," one report crowed, "they have no case."

Edell, however, refused to read any writing on any walls. He acknowledged openly that Rose Cipollone was aware of the risks of smoking. Yes, she had read the warning labels on cigarettes and the numerous magazine articles cut out so painstakingly by Tony Cipollone. Yet, unable to harness her habit, she had remained addicted. Cipollone was far from innocent, Edell conceded. But what mattered was not how much Rose Cipollone knew about tobacco risks; what mattered was what *cigarette makers* knew, and how much of the cancer risk they had revealed to consumers such as Rose.

The argument took the tobacco companies by surprise. Edell's insistence that he needed to know what cigarette makers knew about smoking risks allowed him to ask the courts for unprecedented access to the internal files of Philip Morris, Liggett, and Lorillard. Armed with powerful legal injunctions to investigate these private files, Edell unearthed a saga of epic perversity. Many of the cigarette makers had not only known about the cancer risks of tobacco and the potent addictive properties of nicotine, but had also actively tried to quash internal research that proved it. Document after document revealed frantic struggles within the industry to conceal risks, often leaving even its own employees feeling morally queasy.

In one letter, Fred Panzer, a public relations manager at the Tobacco Research Institute, wrote to Horace Kornegay, its president, to explain the industry's three-pronged marketing strategy—"creating doubt about the health charge without actually denying it, advocating the public's right to smoke without actually urging them to take up the practice [and] encouraging objective scientific research as the only way to resolve the question of health hazard." In another internal memorandum (marked "confidential"), the assertions were nearly laughably perverse: "In a sense, the tobacco industry may be thought of as a specialized, highly ritualized and stylized segment of the pharmaceutical industry. Tobacco products, uniquely, contain and deliver nicotine, a potent drug with a variety of physiological effects."

Pharmacological research on nicotine left no doubt about why women such as Rose Cipollone found it so difficult to quit tobacco—not because they were weak-willed, but because nicotine subverted will itself. "Think of the cigarette pack as a storage container for a day's supply of nicotine," a researcher at Philip Morris wrote. "Think of the cigarette as a dispenser for a dose unit of nicotine. . . . Think of a puff of smoke as the vehicle of nicotine."

In a particularly memorable exchange, Edell quizzed Liggett's president about why the company had spent nearly $5 million to show that tobacco could cause tumors to sprout on the backs of mice, and then systematically chose to ignore any implications for carcinogenesis in humans:

Edell: What was the purpose of this [experiment]?
Dey: To try to reduce tumors on the backs of mice.
Edell: It had nothing to do with the health and welfare of human beings? Is that correct?
Dey: That's correct. . . .
Edell: And this was to save rats, right? Or mice? You spent all this money to save mice the problem of developing tumors?

Exchanges such as this epitomized the troubles of the tobacco industry. As the cigarette industry mavens muddled their way through Edell's cross-examination, the depth of deception made even the industry's own attorneys cringe in horror. Cover-ups were covered up with nonsensical statistics; lies concealed within other lies. Edell's permission to exhume the internal files of tobacco makers created a historic legal precedent, allowing others to potentially raid that same cabinet of horrors to pull out their own sooty exhibits for future tort cases.

After four long years of legal wrangling, the Cipollone cancer trial appeared before the court in 1987. Despite the hopes and predictions of many observers, the verdict was a terrible disappointment for Edell and Cipollone's family. The jury found Rose Cipollone 80 percent responsible for her cancer. Liggett, the maker of the brand that she had smoked before 1966 (i.e., before the warning labels had been mandated), was assigned the rest of the responsibility—20 percent. Philip Morris and Lorillard got off scot-free. The jury awarded Anthony Cipollone $400,000 in damages— barely enough to cover even the clerical costs of four years of obsessive litigation. If this was counted as a win, then, as the tobacco industry pointed out gleefully, it was the very definition of a Pyrrhic victory.

Yet the real legacy of the Cipollone case had little to do with legal victories or losses. Lampooned in court as a weak-willed, ill-informed, and dim-witted addict unaware of the "obvious" dangers of tobacco, Rose Cipollone nonetheless turned into a heroic icon of a cancer victim battling her disease—even from her grave.

A flurry of cases followed the Cipollone case. The tobacco industry defended itself vigorously against these cases, reflexively waving the warning labels on cigarette packets as proof that their liability was negligible. But the precedents set by these cases fueled even more tort suits. Demonized, demoralized, and devastated by the negative publicity, cigarette makers found themselves increasingly beleaguered and increasingly the butt of blame and liability.

By 1994, the per capita consumption of cigarettes in America had dropped for twenty straight years (from 4,141 in 1974 to 2,500 in 1994), representing the most dramatic downturn in smoking rates in history. It had been a long and slow battle of attrition. No intervention had single-handedly decimated tobacco, but the cumulative force of scientific evidence, political pressure, and legal inventiveness had worn the industry down over a decade.

Yet, old sins have long shadows, and carcinogenic sins especially so. The lag time between tobacco exposure and lung cancer is nearly three decades, and the lung cancer epidemic in America will have an afterlife long after smoking incidence has dropped. Among men, the age-adjusted incidence of lung adenocarcinoma, having peaked at 102 per 100,000 in 1984, dropped to 77 in 2002. Among women, though, the epidemic still runs unabated. The stratospheric rise of smoking among women in Rose Cipollone's generation is still playing itself out in the killing fields of lung cancer.

✺

Twenty-seven years have passed since Marc Edell filed his unusual case in the New Jersey courtroom, and tort lawsuits against tobacco companies have now grown into a deluge. In 1994, in yet another landmark case in the history of tobacco litigation, the state of Mississippi filed suit against several tobacco companies seeking to recover over a billion dollars of health-care costs incurred by the state from smoking-related illnesses—including, most prominently, lung cancer. (Michael Moore, the attorney general, summarized the argument for tobacco companies: "You caused the health crisis; you pay for it.") Several other states then followed, notably Florida, Texas, and Minnesota.

In June 1997, facing a barrage of similar suits, tobacco companies proposed a global agreement. In 1998, forty-six states thus signed the Master Settlement Agreement (MSA) with four of the largest cigarette manufacturers—Philip Morris, R. J. Reynolds, Brown & Williamson, and Lorillard Tobacco Company. (Since 1998, an additional forty-seven cigarette manufacturing companies have joined the agreement.) The agreement includes strong restrictions on cigarette advertising, disbands trade associations and industry lobby groups, allows for free access to internal research documents, and proposes the creation of a national forum to educate the public on the health hazards of tobacco. The MSA represents one of the largest liability settlements ever reached, and, perhaps more profoundly, the most public admission of collusion and guilt in the history of the tobacco industry.

Does the MSA constitute Rose Cipollone's long-awaited legal victory over tobacco? In some respects, quite precisely not. In a perverse recapitulation of the FCLAA "warning labels act" of the 1970s, in fact, the agreement likely creates yet another safe harbor for the tobacco industry. By granting relative protection from future legal action, by restricting cigarette advertising, and by allowing its signatory companies to fix prices, the agreement provides a virtual monopoly to the companies that have signed the MSA. Small independent manufacturers dare not enter or compete in the business, leaving big tobacco to become even bigger tobacco. The influx of annual settlement payments from cigarette makers creates "client-states" that depend on this money to fund escalating medical costs. Indeed, the real cost of the agreement is borne by addicted smokers who now pay more for cigarettes, and then pay with their lives.

Nor has the MSA signaled the death of the industry in a more global sense; beleaguered in America, the Marlboro Man has simply sought out new Marlboro countries. With their markets and profits dwindling and their legal costs mounting, cigarette manufacturers have increasingly targeted developing countries as new markets, and the number of smokers in many of these nations has risen accordingly. Tobacco smoking is now a major preventable cause of death in both India and China. Richard Peto, an epidemiologist at Oxford and a close collaborator of Richard Doll's (until Doll's death in 2005), recently estimated that the number of smoking-related deaths among adults in India would rise to 1 million per year in the 2010s and continue to rise in the next decade. In China, lung cancer is already a leading cause of death attributable to smoking in men.

This steady assault of tobacco on the developing world has been accompanied by bold political maneuvering backstage. In 2004, tobacco companies signed a barely publicized agreement with the Ministry of Health in Mexico that provides generous "contributions" from the tobacco makers to a public health-insurance program in return for sharply reduced regulations on cigarette-packet warnings and advertisements—in effect "robbing Pedro to pay Paolo," as a recent editorial noted. In the early 1990s, a study noted, British American Tobacco signed a similar agreement with the government of Uzbekistan to establish a production monopoly, then lobbied vigorously to overturn recent laws that banned tobacco advertising. Cigarette smoking grew by about 8 percent a year in Uzbekistan after the BAT investment, and cigarette sales increased by 50 percent between 1990 and 1996.

In a recent editorial in the *British Medical Journal,* Stanton Glantz, an epidemiologist at the University of California, San Francisco, described this as yet another catastrophe in the making: "Multinational cigarette companies act as a vector that spreads disease and death throughout the world. This is largely because the tobacco industry uses its wealth to influence politicians to create a favourable environment to promote smoking. The industry does so by minimising restrictions on advertising and promotion and by preventing effective public policies for tobacco control such as high taxes, strong graphic warning labels on packets, smoke-free workplaces and public places, aggressive countermarketing media campaigns, and advertising bans. Unlike mosquitoes, another vector of worldwide disease, the tobacco companies quickly transfer the information and strategies they learn in one part of the world to others."

It is difficult for me to convey the range and depth of devastation that I witnessed in the cancer wards that could be directly attributed to cigarette smoking. An ebullient, immaculately dressed young advertising executive who first started smoking to calm his nerves had to have his jawbone sliced off to remove an invasive tongue cancer. A grandmother who taught her grandchildren to smoke and then shared cigarettes with them was diagnosed with esophageal cancer. A priest with terminal lung cancer swore that smoking was the only vice that he had never been able to overcome. Even as these patients were paying the ultimate price for their habit, the depth of denial in some of them remained astonishing; many of my patients continued to smoke, often furtively, during their treatment for cancer (I could smell the acrid whiff of tobacco on their clothes as they signed the consent forms for chemotherapy). A surgeon who practiced in Britain in the seventies—a time when lung cancer incidence was ascending to its macabre peak—recalled his first nights in the wards when patients awoke from their cancer operations and then walked like zombies through the corridors begging the nurses for cigarettes.

Yet despite the evident seriousness of this addiction and its long-term consequences, tobacco consumption continues relatively unfettered even today. Smoking rates, having plateaued for decades, have begun to rise again in certain demographic pockets, and lackluster antismoking campaigns have lost their grip on public imagination. The disjunction between the threat and the response is widening. It remains an astonishing, disturbing fact that in America—a nation where nearly every new drug is subjected to rigorous scrutiny as a potential carcinogen, and even the bare hint of a substance's link to cancer ignites a firestorm of public hysteria and media anxiety—one of the most potent and common carcinogens known to humans can be freely bought and sold at every corner store for a few dollars.

"Curiouser and curiouser"

You're under a lot of stress, my dear. You haven't really got anything wrong with yourself. We'll give you an antidepressant.
— Barry Marshall on the treatment of women with gastritis, a precancerous lesion, in the 1960s

The classification of tobacco smoke as a potent carcinogen—and the slow avalanche of forces unleashed to regulate cigarettes in the 1980s—is rightfully counted as one of cancer prevention's seminal victories. But it equally highlighted an important lacuna in cancer epidemiology. Statistical methods to identify risk factors for cancer are, by their very nature, descriptive rather than mechanistic: they describe correlations, not causes. And they rely on a certain degree of foreknowledge. To run a classical "case-control" trial to identify an unknown risk factor, paradoxically, an epidemiologist must know the questions to ask. Even Doll and Hill, in devising their classic case-control and prospective studies, had relied on decades of prior knowledge—centuries, if one counts John Hill's pamphlet—about the possible link between tobacco and cancer.

This does not diminish the incredible power of the case-control method. In the early 1970s, for instance, a series of studies definitively identified the risk factor for a rare and fatal form of lung cancer called mesothelioma. When mesothelioma "cases" were compared to "controls," this cancer appeared to cluster densely in certain professions: insulation installers, firefighters, shipyard workers, heating equipment handlers, and chrysolite miners. As with Pott and scrotal cancer, the statistical confluence of a rare profession and a rare tumor swiftly identified the causal agent in this cancer: exposure to asbestos. Tort litigation and federal oversight soon followed, precipitating a reduction in the occupational exposure to asbestos that, in turn, reduced the risk of mesothelioma.

In 1971, yet another such study identified an even more unusual carcinogen, a synthetic hormonal medicine called diethylstilbestrol (DES). DES was widely prescribed to pregnant women in the 1950s to prevent premature deliveries (although it was of only questionable benefit in this regard). A generation later, when women with vaginal and uterine cancer were questioned about their exposures to estrogens, a peculiar pattern emerged: the women had not been exposed to the chemical directly, but their *mothers* had been. The carcinogen had skipped a generation. It had caused cancers not in the DES-treated women, but in their daughters exposed to the drug in utero.

But what if the behavior or exposure responsible for the cancer is completely unknown? What if one did not even know enough about the natural history of mesothelioma, or the link between estrogen and vaginal cancer, to ask those afflicted about their occupational history, or their exposure to asbestos and estrogen? Could carcinogens be discovered a priori—not by the statistical analysis of cancer-afflicted populations, but by virtue of some intrinsic property of all carcinogens?

ↄ

In the late 1960s, a bacteriologist named Bruce Ames at Berkeley, working on an unrelated problem, stumbled on a test for chemical carcinogens. Ames was studying mutations in *Salmonella,* a bacterial genus. *Salmonella,* like any bacteria, possesses genes that allow it to grow under certain conditions—a gene to "digest" galactose, for instance, is essential for a bacterium to survive on a petri dish where the only sugar source is galactose.

Ames observed that mutations in these essential genes could enable or disable the growth of bacteria on a petri dish. A strain of *Salmonella* normally unable to grow on galactose, say, could *acquire* a gene mutation that enabled this growth. Once growth-enabled, a single bacterium would form a minuscule colony on a petri dish. By counting the number of growth-enabled colonies formed, Ames could quantify the mutation rate in any experiment. Bacteria exposed to a certain substance might produce six such colonies, while bacteria exposed to another substance might produce sixty. This second substance, in other words, had a tenfold capacity to initiate changes in genes—or a tenfold rate of mutation.

Ames could now test thousands of chemicals to create a catalog of chemicals that increased the mutation rate—mutagens. And as he populated his catalog, he made a seminal observation: *chemicals that scored as mutagens in his test tended to be carcinogens as well*. Dye derivatives, known to be potent human carcinogens, scored floridly, causing hundreds of colonies of bacteria. So did X-rays, benzene compounds, and nitroso-guanidine derivatives—all known to cause cancers in rats and mice. In the tradition of all good tests, Ames's test transformed the unobservable and immeasurable into the observable and measurable. The invisible X-rays that had killed the Radium girls in the 1920s could now be "seen" as revertant colonies on a petri dish.

Ames's test was far from perfect. Not every known carcinogen scored in the test: neither DES nor asbestos sprinkled on the disabled *Salmonella* caused significant numbers of mutant bacteria. (In contrast, chemical constituents of tobacco smoke did cause mutation in the bacteria, as noted by several cigarette manufacturers who ran the test and, finding it disconcertingly positive, quickly buried the results.) But despite its shortcomings, the Ames test provided an important link between a purely descriptive approach toward cancer prevention and a mechanistic approach. Carcinogens, Ames suggested, had a common, distinctive functional property: they altered genes. Ames could not fathom the deeper reason behind this observation: why was the capacity to cause mutations linked to the ability to induce cancer? But he had demonstrated that carcinogens could be found experimentally—not retrospectively (by investigating cases and controls in human subjects) but by *prospectively* identifying chemicals that could cause mutations in a rather simple and elegant biological assay.

৶৹

Chemicals, it turned out, were not the only carcinogens; nor was Ames's test the only method to find such agents. In the late 1960s, Baruch Blumberg, a biologist working in Philadelphia, discovered that a chronic, smoldering inflammation caused by a human hepatitis virus could also cause cancer.

A biochemistry student at Oxford in the 1950s, Blumberg had become interested in genetic anthropology, the study of genetic variations in human populations. Traditional biological anthropology in the 1950s mainly involved collecting, measuring, and categorizing human anatomical specimens. Blumberg wanted to collect, measure, and categorize human *genes*—and he wanted to link genetic variations in humans to the susceptibility for diseases.

The problem, as Blumberg soon discovered, was the lack of human genes to be measured or categorized. Bacterial genetics was still in its infancy in the 1950s—even the structure of DNA and the nature of the genes was still largely undiscovered—and human genes had not even been seen or analyzed. The only tangible hint of variations in human genetics came from an incidental observation. Proteins in the blood, called blood antigens, varied between individuals and were inherited in families, thus implying a genetic source for this variation. These blood proteins could be measured and compared across populations using relatively simple tests.

Blumberg began to scour far-flung places in the world for blood, drawing tubes of serum from Fulani tribesmen in Africa one month and Basque shepherds the next. In 1964, after a brief tenure at the NIH, he moved to the Institute for Cancer Research in Philadelphia (later renamed the Fox Chase Cancer Center) to systematically organize the variant blood antigens that he had cataloged, hoping to link them to human diseases. It was a curiously inverted approach, like scouring a dictionary for a word and then looking for a crossword puzzle into which that word might fit.

One blood antigen that intrigued him was present in several Australian aboriginal subjects and found frequently in Asian and African populations, but was typically absent in Europeans and Americans. Suspecting that this antigen was the fingerprint of an ancient genetic factor inherited in families, Blumberg called it the Australia antigen or *Au* for short.

In 1966, Blumberg's lab set out to characterize the aboriginal antigen in greater detail. He soon noted an odd correlation: individuals carrying the *Au* antigen often suffered from chronic hepatitis, an inflammation of the liver. These inflamed livers, studied pathologically, showed signs of chronic cycles of injury and repair—death of cells in some pockets and compensatory attempts to repair and regenerate liver cells in others, resulting in scarred, shrunken, and burnt-out livers, a condition termed chronic cirrhosis.

A link between an ancient antigen and cirrhosis suggested a genetic susceptibility for liver disease—a theory that would have sent Blumberg off on a long and largely fruitless tangent. But a chance incident overturned that theory and radically changed the course of Blumberg's studies. The lab had been following a young patient at a mental-disability clinic in New Jersey. Initially, the man had tested negative for the *Au* antigen. But during one of the serial blood draws in the summer of 1966, his serum suddenly converted from "*Au* negative" to "*Au* positive." When his liver function was measured, an acute, fulminant hepatitis was discovered.

But how could an "intrinsic" gene cause sudden seroconversion and hepatitis? Genes, after all, do not typically flicker on and off at will. Blumberg's beautiful theory about genetic variation had been slain by an ugly fact. *Au*, he realized, could not mark an inherent variation in a human gene. In fact, *Au* was soon found to be neither a human protein nor a blood antigen. *Au* was a piece of a viral protein floating in the blood, the sign of an infection. The New Jersey man had been infected by this microbe and thus converted from *Au* negative to positive.

Blumberg now raced to isolate the organism responsible for the infection. By the early 1970s, working with a team of collaborators, his lab had purified particles of a new virus, which he called hepatitis B virus, or HBV. The virus was structurally simple—"roughly circular . . . about forty-two nanometers in diameter, one of the smallest DNA viruses that infect humans"—but the simple structure belied extraordinarily complex behavior. In humans, HBV infection caused a broad spectrum of diseases, ranging from asymptomatic infection to acute hepatitis to chronic cirrhosis in the liver.

The identification of a new human virus set off a storm of activity for epidemiologists. By 1969, Japanese researchers (and subsequently Blumberg's group) had learned that the virus was transmitted from one individual to another through blood transfusions. By screening blood before transfusion—using the now familiar *Au* antigen as one of the early biomarkers in serum—the blood-borne infection could be blocked, thereby reducing the risk of hepatitis B.

But another illness soon stood out as linked to HBV: a fatal, insidious form of liver cancer endemic in parts of Asia and Africa that arose out of scarred, ashen livers often decades after chronic viral infection. When cases of hepatocellular cancer were compared to controls using classical statistical methods, chronic infection with HBV, and the associated cycle of injury and repair in liver cells, stood out as a clear risk factor—at about five- to tenfold the risk for uninfected controls. HBV, then, was a carcinogen—although a live carcinogen, capable of being transmitted from one host to another.[*]

---

[*] In the1970s, Harald zur Hausen discovered yet another virus—HPV—that causes cervical cancer. Vaccination against some HPV strains can drastically decrease cervical cancer risk.

⁂

The discovery of HBV was an embarrassment to the NCI. The institute's highly targeted and heavily funded Special Virus Cancer Program, having inoculated thousands of monkeys with human cancer extracts, had yet to find a single cancer-associated virus. Yet a genetic anthropologist exploring aboriginal antigens had found a highly prevalent virus associated with a highly prevalent human cancer. Blumberg was acutely aware of the NCI's embarrassment, and of the serendipity in his work. His departure from the NIH in 1964, although cordial, had been driven by precisely such conflicts; his interdisciplinary curiosity had chafed against the "discipline-determined rigidity of the constituent institutes," among which the NCI, with its goal-directed cancer virus hunt, was the worst culprit. Worse still for the strongest enthusiasts of the cancer virus theory, it appeared as if Blumberg's virus itself was not the proximal cause of the cancer. The *inflammation* induced by the virus in liver cells, and the associated cycle of death and repair, appeared to be responsible for the cancer—a blow to the notion that viruses directly cause cancer.*

But Blumberg had little time to mull over these conflicts, and he certainly had no theoretical axes to grind about viruses and cancer. A pragmatist, he directed his team toward finding a vaccine for HBV. By 1979, his group had devised one. Like the blood-screening strategy, the vaccine did not, of course, alter the course of the cancer after its genesis, but it sharply reduced the susceptibility to HBV infection in uninfected men and women. Blumberg had thus made a critical link from cause to prevention. He had identified a viral carcinogen, found a method to detect it before transmission, then found a means to thwart transmission.

⁂

The strangest among the newly discovered "preventable" carcinogens, though, was not a virus or a chemical but a cellular organism—a bacterium. In 1979, the year that Blumberg's hepatitis B vaccine was beginning its trial in America, a junior resident in medicine named Barry Marshall and a gastroenterologist, Robin Warren, both at the Royal Perth Hospital in Australia, set out to investigate the cause of stomach inflammation, gas-

---

* HBV can cause cancer in noncirrhotic livers. This virus is now thought to have direct carcinogenic effects as well.

tritis, a condition known to predispose patients to peptic ulcers and to stomach cancer.

For centuries, gastritis had rather vaguely been attributed to stress and neuroses. (In popular use, the term *dyspeptic* still refers to an irritable and fragile psychological state.) By extension, then, cancer of the stomach was cancer unleashed by neurotic stress, in essence a modern variant of the theory of clogged melancholia proposed by Galen.

But Warren had convinced himself that the true cause of gastritis was a yet unknown species of bacteria, an organism that, according to dogma, could not even exist in the inhospitable acidic lumen of the stomach. "Since the early days of medical bacteriology, over one hundred years ago," Warren wrote, "it was taught that bacteria do not grow in the stomach. When I was a student, this was taken as so obvious as to barely rate a mention. It was a 'known fact,' like 'everyone knows that the earth is flat.'"

But the flat-earth theory of stomach inflammation made little sense to Warren. When he examined biopsies of men and women with gastritis or gastric ulcers, he found a hazy, blue layer overlying the craterlike depressions of the ulcers in the stomach. When he looked even harder at that bluish layer, he inevitably saw spiral organisms teeming within it.

Or had he imagined it? Warren was convinced that these organisms represented a new species of bacterium that caused gastritis and peptic ulcers. But he could not isolate the bacteria in any form on a plate, dish, or culture. Others could not see the organism; Warren could not grow it; the whole theory, with its blue haze of alien organisms growing above craters in the stomach, smacked of science fiction.

Barry Marshall, in contrast, had no pet theory to test or disprove. The son of a Kalgoorlie boilermaker and a nurse, he had trained in medicine in Perth and was an unwhetted junior investigator looking for a project. Intrigued by Warren's data (although skeptical of the link with an unknown, phantasmic bacteria), he started to collect brushings from patients with ulcers and spread out the material on petri dishes, hoping to grow a bacterium. But as with Warren, no bacteria grew out. Week after week, Marshall's dishes piled up in the incubator and were discarded in large stacks after a few days of examination.

But then serendipity intervened: over an unexpectedly busy Easter weekend in 1982, with the hospital overflowing with medical admissions, Marshall forgot to examine his plates and left them in the incubator. When he remembered and returned to examine them, he found tiny, translucent pearls of bacterial colonies growing on the agar. The long incubation period had been critical. Under the microscope, the bacterium growing on the plate was a minuscule, slow-growing, fragile organism with a helical tail, a species that had never been described by microbiologists. Warren and Marshall called it *Helicobacter pylori*—*helicobacter* for its appearance, and *pylorus* from the Latin for "gatekeeper," for its location near the outlet valve of the stomach.

But the mere existence of the bacteria, or even its association with ulcers, was not proof enough that it caused gastritis. Koch's third postulate stipulated that to be classified as a bona fide causal element for a disease, an organism needed to re-create the disease when introduced into a naive host. Marshall and Warren inoculated pigs with the bacteria and performed serial endoscopies. But the pigs—seventy pounds of porcine weight that did not take kindly to weekly endoscopies—did not sprout any ulcers. And testing the theory on humans was ethically impossible: how could one justify infecting a human with a new, uncharacterized species of bacteria to prove that it caused gastritis and predisposed to cancer?

In July 1984, with his experiments stalled and his grant applications in jeopardy, Marshall performed the ultimate experiment: "On the morning of the experiment, I omitted my breakfast. . . . Two hours later, Neil Noakes scraped a heavily inoculated 4 day culture plate of *Helicobacter* and dispersed the bacteria in alkaline peptone water (a kind of meat broth used to keep bacteria alive). I fasted until 10 am when Neil handed me a 200 ml beaker about one quarter full of the cloudy brown liquid. I drank it down in one gulp then fasted for the rest of the day. A few stomach gurgles occurred. Was it the bacteria or was I just hungry?"

ঞ৵

Marshall was not "just hungry." Within a few days of swallowing the turbid bacterial culture, he was violently ill, with nausea, vomiting, night sweats, and chills. He persuaded a colleague to perform serial biopsies to document the pathological changes, and he was diagnosed with highly active gastritis, with a dense overlay of bacteria in his stomach and ulcerating craters beneath—precisely what Warren had found in his patients. In late July, with Warren as coauthor, Marshall submitted his own case report to the *Medical Journal of Australia* for publication ("a normal volunteer [has] swallowed a pure culture of the organism," he wrote). The critics had at last been silenced. *Helicobacter pylori* was indisputably the cause of gastric inflammation.

The link between *Helicobacter* and gastritis raised the possibility that bacterial infection and chronic inflammation caused stomach cancer.* Indeed, by the late 1980s, several epidemiological studies had linked *H. pylori*–induced gastritis with stomach cancer. Marshall and Warren had, meanwhile, tested antibiotic regimens (including the once-forsaken alchemical agent bismuth) to create a potent multidrug treatment for the *H. pylori* infection.† Randomized trials run on the western coast of Japan, where stomach and *H. pylori* infection are endemic, showed that antibiotic treatment reduced gastric ulcers and gastritis.

The effect of antibiotic therapy on cancer, though, was more complex. The eradication of *H. pylori* infection in young men and women reduced the incidence of gastric cancer. In older patients, in whom chronic gastritis had smoldered for several decades, eradication of the infection had little effect. In these elderly patients, presumably the chronic inflammation had already progressed to a point that its eradication made no difference. For cancer prevention to work, Auerbach's march—the prodrome of cancer—had to be halted early.

॰ঌৎ

Although unorthodox in the extreme, Barry Marshall's "experiment"— swallowing a carcinogen to create a precancerous state in his own stomach —encapsulated a growing sense of impatience and frustration among cancer epidemiologists. Powerful strategies for cancer prevention arise, clearly, from a deep understanding of causes. The identification of a carcinogen is only the first step toward that understanding. To mount a successful strategy against cancer, one needs to know not only what the carcinogen *is*, but what the carcinogen *does*.

But the set of disparate observations—from Blumberg to Ames to Warren and Marshall—could not simply be stitched together into a coherent theory of carcinogenesis. How could DES, asbestos, radiation, hepatitis virus, and a stomach bacterium all converge on the same pathological state, although in different populations and in different organs? The list of

---

* *H. pylori* infection is linked to several forms of cancer, including gastric adenocarcinoma and mucosa-associated lymphoma.

†Marshall later treated himself with the regimen and eradicated his infection.

cancer-causing agents seemed to get—as another swallower of unknown potions might have put it—"curiouser and curiouser."

There was little precedent in other diseases for such an astonishing diversity of causes. Diabetes, a complex illness with complex manifestations, is still fundamentally a disease of abnormal insulin signaling. Coronary heart disease occurs when a clot, arising from a ruptured and inflamed atherosclerotic plaque, occludes a blood vessel of the heart. But the search for a unifying mechanistic description of cancer seemed to be sorely missing. What, beyond abnormal, dysregulated cell division, was the common pathophysiological mechanism underlying cancer?

To answer this question, cancer biologists would need to return to the birth of cancer, to the very first steps of a cell's journey toward malignant transformation—to carcino*genesis*.

"A spider's web"

The long, slow march of carcinogenesis—the methodical, step-by-step progression of early-stage lesions of cancer into frankly malignant cells—inspired another strategy to prevent cancer. If cancer truly slouched to its birth, as Auerbach suspected, then perhaps one could still intervene on that progression in its earliest stages—by attacking *pre*cancer rather than cancer. Could one thwart the march of carcinogenesis in midstep?

Few scientists had studied this early transition of cancer cells as intensively as George Papanicolaou, a Greek cytologist at Cornell University in New York. Robust, short, formal, and old-worldly, Papanicolaou had trained in medicine and zoology in Athens and in Munich and arrived in New York in 1913. Penniless off the boat, he had sought a job in a medical laboratory but had been relegated to selling carpets at the Gimbels store on Thirty-third Street to survive. After a few months of truly surreal labor (he was, by all accounts, a terrible carpet salesman), Papanicolaou secured a research position at Cornell that may have been just as surreal as carpet selling: he was assigned to study the menstrual cycle of guinea pigs, a species that neither bleeds visibly nor sheds tissue during menses. Using a nasal speculum and Q-tips, Papanicolaou had nonetheless learned to scrape off cervical cells from guinea pigs and spread them on glass slides in thin, watery smears.

The cells, he found, were like minute watch-hands. As hormones rose and ebbed in the animals cyclically, the cells shed by the guinea pig cervix changed their shapes and sizes cyclically as well. Using their morphology as a guide, he could foretell the precise stage of the menstrual cycle often down to the day.

By the late 1920s, Papanicolaou had extended his technique to human patients. (His wife, Maria, in surely one of the more grisly displays of conjugal fortitude, reportedly allowed herself to be tested by cervical smears every day.) As with guinea pigs, he found that cells sloughed off by the human cervix could also foretell the stages of the menstrual cycle in women.

But all of this, it was pointed out to him, amounted to no more than an elaborate and somewhat useless invention. As one gynecologist archly remarked, "in primates, including women," a diagnostic smear was hardly needed to calculate the stage or timing of the menstrual cycle. Women had been timing their periods—without Papanicolaou's cytological help—for centuries.

Disheartened by these criticisms, Papanicolaou returned to his slides. He had spent nearly a decade looking obsessively at normal smears; perhaps, he reasoned, the real value of his test lay not in the normal smear, but in pathological conditions. What if he could diagnose a *pathological* state with his smear? What if the years of staring at cellular normalcy had merely been a prelude to allow him to identify cellular abnormalities?

Papanicolaou thus began to venture into the world of pathological conditions, collecting slides from women with all manners of gynecological diseases—fibroids, cysts, tubercles, inflammations of the uterus and cervix, streptococcal, gonococcal, and staphylococcal infections, tubal pregnancies, abnormal pregnancies, benign and malignant tumors, abscesses and furuncles, hoping to find some pathological mark in the exfoliated cells.

Cancer, he found, was particularly prone to shedding abnormal cells. In nearly every case of cervical cancer, when Papanicolaou brushed cells off the cervix, he found "aberrant and bizarre forms" with abnormal, bloated nuclei, ruffled membranes, and shrunken cytoplasm that looked nothing like normal cells. It "became readily apparent," he wrote, that he had stumbled on a new test for malignant cells.

Thrilled by his results, Papanicolaou published his method in an article entitled "New Cancer Diagnosis" in 1928. But the report, presented initially at an outlandish "race betterment" eugenics conference, generated only further condescension from pathologists. The Pap smear, as he called the technique, was neither accurate nor particularly sensitive. If cervical cancer was to be diagnosed, his colleagues argued, then why not perform a biopsy of the cervix, a meticulous procedure that, even if cumbersome and invasive, was considered far more precise and definitive than a grubby smear? At academic conferences, experts scoffed at the crude alternative. Even Papanicolaou could hardly argue the point. "I think this work will be carried a little further," he wrote self-deprecatingly at the end of his 1928 paper. Then, for nearly two decades, having produced two perfectly useless inventions over twenty years, he virtually disappeared from the scientific limelight.

*

Between 1928 and 1950, Papanicolaou delved back into his smears with nearly monastic ferocity. His world involuted into a series of routines: the daily half-hour commute to his office with Maria at the wheel; the weekends at home in Long Island with a microscope in the study and a microscope on the porch; evenings spent typing reports on specimens with a phonograph playing Schubert in the background and a glass of orange juice congealing on his table. A gynecologic pathologist named Herbert Traut joined him to help interpret his smears. A Japanese fish and bird painter named Hashime Murayama, a colleague from his early years at Cornell, was hired to paint watercolors of his smears using a camera lucida.

For Papanicolaou, too, this brooding, contemplative period was like a personal camera lucida that magnified and reflected old experimental themes onto new ones. A decades-old thought returned to haunt him: if normal cells of the cervix changed morphologically in graded, stepwise fashion over time, might cancer cells also change morphologically in time, in a slow, stepwise dance from normal to malignant? Like Auerbach (whose work was yet to be published), could he identify intermediate stages of cancer—lesions slouching their way toward full transformation?

At a Christmas party in the winter of 1950, challenged by a tipsy young gynecologist in his lab to pinpoint the precise use of the smear, Papanicolaou verbalized a strand of thought that he had been spinning internally for nearly a decade. The thought almost convulsed out of him. The real use of the Pap smear was not to find cancer, but rather to detect its antecedent, its precursor—the portent of cancer.

"It was a revelation," one of his students recalled. "A Pap smear would give a woman a chance to receive preventive care [and] greatly decrease the likelihood of her ever developing cancer." Cervical cancer typically arises in an outer layer of the cervix, then grows in a flaky, superficial whirl before burrowing inward into the surrounding tissues. By sampling asymptomatic women, Papanicolaou speculated that his test, albeit imperfect, might capture the disease at its first stages. He would, in essence, push the diagnostic clock backward—from incurable, invasive cancers to curable, preinvasive malignancies.

◊◊

In 1952, Papanicolaou convinced the National Cancer Institute to launch the largest clinical trial of secondary prevention in the history of cancer using his smearing technique. Nearly every adult female resident of Shelby County, Tennessee—150,000 women spread across eight hundred square miles—was tested with a Pap smear and followed over time. Smears poured in from hundreds of sites: from one-room doctor's offices dotted among the horse farms of Germantown to large urban community clinics scattered throughout the city of Memphis. Temporary "Pap clinics" were set up in factories and office buildings. Once collected, the samples were funneled into a gigantic microscope facility at the University of Tennessee, where framed photographs of exemplary normal and abnormal smears had been hung on the walls. Technicians read slides day and night, looking up from the microscopes at the pictures. At the peak, nearly a thousand smears were read every day.

As expected, the Shelby team found its fair share of advanced cancerous lesions in the population. In the initial cohort of about 150,000, invasive cervical cancer was found in 555 women. But the real proof of Papanicolaou's principle lay in another discovery: astonishingly, 557 women were found to have preinvasive cancers or even precancerous changes—early-stage, localized lesions curable by relatively simple surgical procedures. Nearly all these women were asymptomatic; had they never been tested, they would never have been suspected of harboring preinvasive lesions. Notably, the average age of diagnosis of women with such preinvasive lesions was about twenty years lower than the average age of women with invasive lesions—once again corroborating the long march of carcinogenesis. The Pap smear had, in effect, pushed the clock of cancer detection forward by nearly two decades, and changed the spectrum of cervical cancer from predominantly incurable to predominantly curable.

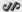

A few miles from Papanicolaou's laboratory in New York, the core logic of the Pap smear was being extended to a very different form of cancer. Epidemiologists think about prevention in two forms. In primary prevention, a disease is prevented by attacking its cause—smoking cessation for lung cancer or a vaccine against hepatitis B for liver cancer. In secondary prevention (also called screening), a disease is prevented by screening for its early, presymptomatic stage. The Pap smear was invented as a means of secondary prevention for cervical cancer. But if a microscope could detect a presymptomatic state in scraped-off cervical tissue, then could another means of "seeing" cancer detect an early lesion in another cancer-afflicted organ?

In 1913, a Berlin surgeon named Albert Salomon had certainly tried. A dogged, relentless champion of the mastectomy, Salomon had whisked away nearly three thousand amputated breasts after mastectomies to an X-ray room where he had photographed them after surgery to detect the shadowy outlines of cancer. Salomon had detected stigmata of cancer in his X-rays—microscopic sprinkles of calcium lodged in cancer tissue ("grains of salt," as later radiologists would call them) or thin crustacean fingerlings of malignant cells reminiscent of the root of the word *cancer*.

The next natural step might have been to image breasts *before* surgery as a screening method, but Salomon's studies were rudely interrupted. Abruptly purged from his university position by the Nazis in the mid-1930s, Salomon escaped the camps to Amsterdam and vanished underground—and so, too, did his shadowy X-rays of breasts. Mammography, as Salomon called his technique, languished in neglect. It was hardly missed:

in a world obsessed with radical surgery, since small or large masses in the breast were treated with precisely the same gargantuan operation, screening for small lesions made little sense.

For nearly two decades, the mammogram thus lurked about in the far peripheries of medicine—in France and England and Uruguay, places where radical surgery held the least influence. But by the mid-1960s, with Halsted's theory teetering uneasily on its pedestal, mammography reentered X-ray clinics in America, championed by pioneering radiographers such as Robert Egan in Houston. Egan, like Papanicolaou, cast himself more as an immaculate craftsman than a scientist—a photographer, really, who was taking photographs of cancer using X-rays, the most penetrating form of light. He tinkered with films, angles, positions, and exposures, until, as one observer put it, "trabeculae as thin as a spider's web" in the breast could be seen in the images.

But could cancer be caught in that "spider's web" of shadows, trapped early enough to prevent its spread? Egan's mammograms could now detect tumors as small as a few millimeters, about the size of a grain of barley. But would screening women to detect such early tumors and extricating the tumors surgically save lives?

♨

Screening trials in cancer are among the most slippery of all clinical trials—notoriously difficult to run, and notoriously susceptible to errors. To understand why, consider the odyssey from the laboratory to the clinic of a screening test for cancer. Suppose a new test has been invented in the laboratory to detect an early, presymptomatic stage of a particular form of cancer, say, the level of a protein secreted by cancer cells into the serum. The first challenge for such a test is technical: its performance in the real world. Epidemiologists think of screening tests as possessing two characteristic performance errors. The first error is overdiagnosis—when an individual tests positive in the test but does not have cancer. Such individuals are called "false positives." Men and women who falsely test positive find themselves trapped in the punitive stigma of cancer, the familiar cycle of anxiety and terror (and the desire to "do something") that precipitates further testing and invasive treatment.

The mirror image of overdiagnosis is *underdiagnosis*—an error in which a patient truly has cancer but does not test positive for it. Underdiagnosis falsely reassures patients of their freedom from disease. These men and women ("false negatives" in the jargon of epidemiology) enter a different punitive cycle—of despair, shock, and betrayal—once their disease, undetected by the screening test, is eventually uncovered when it becomes symptomatic.

The trouble is that overdiagnosis and underdiagnosis are often intrinsically conjoined, locked perpetually on two ends of a seesaw. Screening tests that strive to limit overdiagnosis—by narrowing the criteria by which patients are classified as positive—often pay the price of increasing underdiagnosis because they miss patients that lie in the gray zone between positive and negative. An example helps to illustrate this trade-off. Suppose—to use Egan's vivid metaphor—a spider is trying to invent a perfect web to capture flies out of the air. Increasing the density of that web, she finds, certainly increases the chances of catching real flies (true positives) but it also increases the chances of capturing junk and debris floating through the air (false positives). Making the web less dense, in contrast, decreases the chances of catching real prey, but every time something *is* captured, chances are higher that it is a fly. In cancer, where both overdiagnosis and underdiagnosis come at high costs, finding that exquisite balance is often impossible. We want every cancer test to operate with perfect specificity and sensitivity. But the technologies for screening are not perfect. Screening tests thus routinely fail because they cannot even cross this preliminary hurdle—the rate of over- or underdiagnosis is unacceptably high.

Suppose, however, our new test does survive this crucial bottleneck. The rates of overdiagnosis and underdiagnosis are deemed acceptable, and we unveil the test on a population of eager volunteers. Suppose, moreover, that as the test enters the public domain, doctors immediately begin to detect early, benign-appearing, premalignant lesions—in stark contrast to the aggressive, fast-growing tumors seen before the test. Is the test to be judged a success?

No; merely *detecting* a small tumor is not sufficient. Cancer demonstrates a spectrum of behavior. Some tumors are inherently benign, genetically determined to never reach the fully malignant state; and some tumors are intrinsically aggressive, and intervention at even an early, presymptomatic stage might make no difference to the prognosis of a patient. To address the inherent behavioral heterogeneity of cancer, the screening test must go further. It must increase survival.

Imagine, now, that we have designed a trial to determine whether our screening test increases survival. Two identical twins, call them Hope and Prudence, live in neighboring houses and are offered the trial. Hope chooses to be screened by the test. Prudence, suspicious of overdiagnosis and underdiagnosis, refuses to be screened.

Unbeknownst to Hope and Prudence, identical forms of cancer develop in both twins at the exact same time—in 1990. Hope's tumor is detected by the screening test in 1995, and she undergoes surgical treatment and chemotherapy. She survives five additional years, then relapses and dies ten years after her original diagnosis, in 2000. Prudence, in contrast, detects her tumor only when she feels a growing lump in her breast in 1999. She, too, has treatment, with some marginal benefit, then relapses and dies at the same moment as Hope in 2000.

At the joint funeral, as the mourners stream by the identical caskets, an argument breaks out among Hope's and Prudence's doctors. Hope's physicians insist that she had a five-year survival: her tumor was detected in 1995 and she died in 2000. Prudence's doctors insist that *her* survival was one year: Prudence's tumor was detected in 1999 and she died in 2000. Yet both cannot be right: the twins died from the same tumor at the exact same time. The solution to this seeming paradox—called lead-time bias— is immediately obvious. Using *survival* as an end point for a screening test is flawed because early detection pushes the clock of diagnosis backward. Hope's tumor and Prudence's tumor possess exactly identical biological behavior. But since doctors detected Hope's tumor earlier, it seems, falsely, that she lived longer and that the screening test was beneficial.

So our test must now cross an additional hurdle: it must improve *mortality,* not survival. The only appropriate way to judge whether Hope's test was truly beneficial is to ask whether Hope *lived longer* regardless of the time of her diagnosis. Had Hope lived until 2010 (outliving Prudence by a decade), we could have legitimately ascribed a benefit to the test. Since both women died at the exact same moment, we now discover that screening produced no benefit.

A screening test's path to success is thus surprisingly long and narrow. It must avoid the pitfalls of overdiagnosis and underdiagnosis. It must steer past the narrow temptation to use early detection as an end in itself. Then, it must navigate the treacherous straits of bias and selection. "Survival," seductively simple, cannot be its end point. And adequate randomization at each step is critical. Only a test capable of meeting all these criteria—proving mortality benefit in a genuinely randomized setting with an acceptable over- and underdiagnosis rate—can be judged a success. With the odds stacked so steeply, few tests are powerful enough to withstand this level of scrutiny and truly provide benefit in cancer.

ంౢౢ

In the winter of 1963, three men set out to test whether screening a large cohort of asymptomatic women using mammography would prevent mortality from breast cancer. All three, outcasts from their respective fields, were seeking new ways to study breast cancer. Louis Venet, a surgeon trained in the classical tradition, wanted to capture early cancers as a means to avert the large and disfiguring radical surgeries that had become the norm in the field. Sam Shapiro, a statistician, sought to invent new methods to mount statistical trials. And Philip Strax, a New York internist, had perhaps the most poignant of reasons: he had nursed his wife through the torturous terminal stages of breast cancer in the mid-1950s. Strax's attempt to capture preinvasive lesions using X-rays was a personal crusade to unwind the biological clock that had ultimately taken his wife's life.

Venet, Strax, and Shapiro were sophisticated clinical trialists: right at the onset, they realized that they would need a randomized, prospective trial using mortality as an end point to test mammography. Methodologically speaking, their trial would recapitulate Doll and Hill's famous smoking trial of the 1950s. But how might such a trial be logistically run? The Doll and Hill study had been the fortuitous by-product of the nationalization of health care in Great Britain—its stable cohort produced, in large part, by the National Health Service's "address book" of registered doctors across the United Kingdom. For mammography, in contrast, it was the sweeping wave of privatization in postwar America that provided the opportunity to run the trial. In the summer of 1944, lawmakers in New York unveiled a novel program to provide subscriber-based health insurance to groups of employees in New York. This program, called the Health Insurance Plan (HIP), was the ancestor of the modern HMO.

The HIP filled a great void in insurance. By the mid-1950s, a triad of forces—immigration, World War II, and the Depression—had brought women out of their homes to comprise nearly one-third of the total workforce in New York. These working women sought health insurance, and the HIP, which allowed its enrollees to pool risks and thereby reduce costs, was a natural solution. By the early 1960s, the plan had enrolled more than three hundred thousand subscribers spread across thirty-one medical groups in New York—nearly eighty thousand of them women.

Strax, Shapiro, and Venet were quick to identify the importance of the resource: here was a defined—"captive"—cohort of women spread across New York and its suburbs that could be screened and followed over a prolonged time. The trial was kept deliberately simple: women enrollees in the HIP between the ages of forty and sixty-four were divided into two groups. One group was screened with mammography while the other was left unscreened. The ethical standards for screening trials in the 1960s made the identification of the groups even simpler. The unscreened group—i.e., the one not offered mammography—was not even required to give consent; it could just be enrolled passively in the trial and followed over time.

The trial, launched in December 1963, was instantly a logistic nightmare. Mammography was cumbersome: a machine the size of a full-grown bull; photographic plates like small windowpanes; the slosh and froth of toxic chemicals in a darkroom. The technique was best performed in dedicated X-ray clinics, but unable to convince women to travel to these clinics (many of them located uptown), Strax and Venet eventually outfitted a mobile van with an X-ray machine and parked it in midtown Manhattan, alongside the ice-cream trucks and sandwich vendors, to recruit women into the study during lunch breaks.*

Strax began an obsessive campaign of recruitment. When a subject refused to join the study, he would call, write, and call her again to persuade her to join. The clinics were honed to a machinelike precision to allow thousands of women to be screened in a day:

"Interview . . . 5 stations X 12 women per hour = 60 women. . . . Undress-Dress cubicles: 16 cubicles X 6 women per hour = 96 women per hour. Each cubicle provides one square of floor space for dress-undress and contains four clothes lockers for a total of 64. At the close of the 'circle,' the woman enters the same cubicle to obtain her clothes and dress. . . . To expedite turnover, the amenities of chairs and mirrors are omitted."

Curtains rose and fell. Closets opened and closed. Chairless and mirrorless rooms let women in and out. The merry-go-round ran through the day and late into the evening. In an astonishing span of six years, the trio completed a screening that would ordinarily have taken two decades to complete.

---

* In addition to mammography, women also received a breast exam, typically performed by a surgeon.

If a tumor was detected by mammography, the woman was treated according to the conventional intervention available at the time—surgery, typically a radical mastectomy, to remove the mass (or surgery followed by radiation). Once the cycle of screening and intervention had been completed, Strax, Venet, and Shapiro could watch the experiment unfold over time by measuring breast cancer mortality in the screened versus unscreened groups.

ↀ

In 1971, eight years after the study had been launched, Strax, Venet, and Shapiro revealed the initial findings of the HIP trial. At first glance, it seemed like a resounding vindication of screening. Sixty-two thousand women had been enrolled in the trial; about half had been screened by mammography. There had been thirty-one deaths in the mammography-screened group and fifty-two deaths in the control group. The absolute number of lives saved was admittedly modest, but the fractional reduction in mortality from screening—almost 40 percent—was remarkable. Strax was ecstatic: "The radiologist," he wrote, "has become a potential savior of women—and their breasts."

The positive results of the HIP trial had an explosive effect on mammography. "Within 5 years, mammography has moved from the realm of a discarded procedure to the threshold of widespread application," a radiologist wrote. At the National Cancer Institute, enthusiasm for screening rose swiftly to a crescendo. Arthur Holleb, the American Cancer Society's chief medical officer, was quick to note the parallel to the Pap smear. "The time has come," Holleb announced in 1971, "for the . . . Society to mount a massive program on mammography just as we did with the Pap test. . . . No longer can we ask the people of this country to tolerate a loss of life from breast cancer each year equal to the loss of life in the past ten years in Viet Nam. The time has come for greater national effort. I firmly believe that time is now."

The ACS's massive campaign was called the Breast Cancer Detection and Demonstration Project (BCDDP). Notably, this was not a trial but, as its name suggested, a "demonstration." There was no treatment or control group. The project intended to screen nearly 250,000 women in a single year, nearly eight times the number screened by Strax in three years, in large part to show that it was possible to muscle through mammographic screening at a national level. Mary Lasker backed it strongly, as did virtually every cancer organization in America. Mammography, the "discarded procedure," was about to become enshrined in the mainstream.

◈

But even as the BCDDP forged ahead, doubts were gathering over the HIP study. Shapiro, recall, had chosen to randomize the trial by placing the "test women" and "control" women into two groups and comparing mortality. But, as was common practice in the sixties, the control group had not been informed of its participation in a trial. It had been a virtual group—a cohort drawn out of the HIP's records. When a woman had died of breast cancer in the control group, Strax and Shapiro had dutifully updated their ledgers, but—trees falling in statistical forests—the group had been treated as an abstract entity, unaware even of its own existence.

In principle, comparing a virtual group to a real group would have been perfectly fine. But as the trial enrollment had proceeded in the mid-1960s, Strax and Shapiro had begun to worry whether some women *already* diagnosed with breast cancer might have entered the trial. A screening examination would, of course, be a useless test for such women since they already carried the disease. To correct for this, Shapiro had begun to selectively remove such women from both arms of the trial.

Removing such subjects from the mammography test group was relatively easy: the radiologist could simply ask a woman about her prior history before she underwent mammography. But since the control group was a virtual entity, there could be no virtual asking. It would have to be culled "virtually." Shapiro tried to be dispassionate and rigorous by pulling equal numbers of women from the two arms of the trial. But in the end, he may have chosen selectively. Possibly, he overcorrected: more patients with prior breast cancer were eliminated from the screened group. The difference was small—only 434 patients in a trial of 30,000—but statistically speaking, fatal. Critics now charged that the excess mortality in the unscreened group was an artifact of the culling. The unscreened group had been mistakenly *overloaded* with more patients with prior breast cancer—and the excess death in the untreated group was merely a statistical artifact.

Mammography enthusiasts were devastated. What was needed, they admitted, was a fair reevaluation, a retrial. But where might such a trial be performed? Certainly not in the United States—with two hundred thousand women already enrolled in the BCDDP (and therefore not eligible for another trial), and its bickering academic community shadowboxing over the interpretation of shadows. Scrambling blindly out of controversy, the entire community of mammographers overcompensated as well. Rather than build experiments methodically on other experiments, they launched a volley of parallel trials that came tumbling out over each other. Between 1976 and 1992, enormous parallel trials of mammography were launched in Europe: in Edinburgh, Scotland, and in several sites in Sweden—Malmö, Kopparberg, Östergötland, Stockholm, and Göteborg. In Canada, meanwhile, researchers lurched off on their own randomized trial of mammography, called the National Breast Screening Study (CNBSS). As with so much in the history of breast cancer, mammographic trial-running had turned into an arms race, with each group trying to better the efforts of the others.

∂ℓℓ

Edinburgh was a disaster. Balkanized into hundreds of isolated and disconnected medical practices, it was a terrible trial site to begin with. Doctors assigned blocks of women to the screening or control groups based on seemingly arbitrary criteria. Or, worse still, women assigned themselves. Randomization protocols were disrupted. Women often switched between one group and the other as the trial proceeded, paralyzing and confounding any meaningful interpretation of the study as a whole.

The Canadian trial, meanwhile, epitomized precision and attention to detail. In the summer of 1980, a heavily publicized national campaign involving letters, advertisements, and personal phone calls was launched to recruit thirty-nine thousand women to fifteen accredited centers for screening mammography. When a woman presented herself at any such center, she was asked some preliminary questions by a receptionist, asked to fill out a questionnaire, then examined by a nurse or physician, after which her name was entered into an open ledger. The ledger—a blue-lined notebook was used in most clinics—circulated freely. Randomized assignment was thus achieved by alternating lines in that notebook. One woman was assigned to the screened group, the woman on the next line to the control group, the third line to the screened, the fourth to the control, and so forth.

Note carefully that sequence of events: a woman was typically randomized *after* her medical history and examination. That sequence was neither anticipated nor prescribed in the original protocol (detailed manuals of instruction had been sent to each center). But that minute change completely undid the trial. The allocations that emerged after those nurse interviews were no longer random. Women with abnormal breast or lymph node examinations were disproportionately assigned to the mammography group (seventeen to the mammography group; five to the control arm, at one site). So were women with prior histories of breast cancer. So, too, were women known to be at "high risk" based on their past history or prior insurance claims (eight to mammography; one to control).

The reasons for this skew are still unknown. Did the nurses allocate high-risk women to the mammography group to confirm a suspicious clinical examination—to obtain a second opinion, as it were, by X-ray? Was that subversion even conscious? Was it an unintended act of compassion, an attempt to help high-risk women by forcing them to have mammograms? Did high-risk women skip their turn in the waiting room to purposefully fall into the right line of the allocation book? Were they instructed to do so by the trial coordinators—by their examining doctors, the X-ray technicians, the receptionists?

Teams of epidemiologists, statisticians, radiologists, and at least one group of forensic experts have since pored over those scratchy notebooks to try to answer these questions and decipher what went wrong in the trial. "Suspicion, like beauty, lies in the eye of the beholder," one of the trial's chief investigators countered. But there was plenty to raise suspicion. The notebooks were pockmarked with clerical errors: names changed, identities reversed, lines whited out, names replaced or overwritten. Testimonies by on-site workers reinforced these observations. At one center, a trial coordinator selectively herded her friends to the mammography group (hoping, presumably, to do them a favor and save their lives). At another, a technician reported widespread tampering with randomization with women being "steered" into groups. Accusations and counteraccusations flew through the pages of academic journals. "One lesson is clear," the cancer researcher Norman Boyd wrote dismissively in a summary editorial: "randomization in clinical trials should be managed in a manner that makes subversion impossible."

But such smarting lessons aside, little else was clear. What emerged from that fog of details was a study even more imbalanced than the HIP study. Strax and Shapiro had faltered by selectively depleting the mammography group of high-risk patients. The CNBSS faltered, skeptics now charged, by succumbing to the opposite sin: by selectively *enriching* the mammography group with high-risk women. Unsurprisingly, the result of the CNBSS was markedly negative: if anything, more women died of breast cancer in the mammography group than in the unscreened group.

ℐℐℙ

It was in Sweden, at long last, that this stuttering legacy finally came to an end. In the winter of 2007, I visited Malmö, the site for one of the Swedish mammography trials launched in the late 1970s. Perched almost on the southern tip of the Swedish peninsula, Malmö is a bland, gray-blue industrial town set amid a featureless, gray-blue landscape. The bare, sprawling flatlands of Skåne stretch out to its north, and the waters of the Øresund strait roll to the south. Battered by a steep recession in the mid-1970s, the region had economically and demographically frozen for nearly two decades. Migration into and out of the city had shrunk to an astonishingly low 2 percent for nearly twenty years. Malmö had been in limbo with a captive cohort of men and women. It was the ideal place to run a difficult trial.

In 1976, forty-two thousand women enrolled in the Malmö Mammography Study. Half the cohort (about twenty-one thousand women) was screened yearly at a small clinic outside the Malmö General Hospital, and the other half not screened—and the two groups have been followed closely ever since. The experiment ran like clockwork. "There was only one breast clinic in all of Malmö—unusual for a city of this size," the lead researcher, Ingvar Andersson, recalled. "All the women were screened at the same clinic year after year, resulting in a highly consistent, controlled study—the most stringent study that could be produced."

In 1988, at the end of its twelfth year, the Malmö study reported its results. Overall, 588 women had been diagnosed with breast cancer in the screened group, and 447 in the control group—underscoring, once again, the capacity of mammography to detect early cancers. But notably, at least at first glance, early detection had not translated into overwhelming numbers of lives saved. One hundred and twenty-nine women had died of breast cancer—sixty-three in the screened and sixty-six in the unscreened—with no statistically discernible difference overall.

But there was a pattern behind the deaths. When the groups were analyzed by age, women above fifty-five years had benefited from screening, with a reduction in breast cancer deaths by 20 percent. In younger women, in contrast, screening with mammography showed no detectable benefit.

This pattern—a clearly discernible benefit for older women, and a barely detectable benefit in younger women—would be confirmed in scores of studies that followed Malmö. In 2002, twenty-six years after the launch of the original Malmö experiment, an exhaustive analysis combining all the Swedish studies was published in the *Lancet*. In all, 247,000 women had been enrolled in these trials. The pooled analysis vindicated the Malmö results. In aggregate, over the course of fifteen years, mammography had resulted in 20 to 30 percent reductions in breast cancer mortality for women aged fifty-five to seventy. But for women below fifty-five, the benefit was barely discernible.

Mammography, in short, was not going to be the unequivocal "savior" of all women with breast cancer. Its effects, as the statistician Donald Berry describes it, "are indisputable for a certain segment of women—but also indisputably modest in that segment." Berry wrote, "Screening is a lottery. Any winnings are shared by the minority of women. . . . The overwhelming proportion of women experience no benefit and they pay with the time involved and the risks associated with screening. . . . The risk of not having a mammogram until after age 50 is about the same as riding a bicycle for 15 hours without a helmet." If all women across the nation chose to ride helmetless for fifteen hours straight, there would surely be several more deaths than if they had all worn helmets. But for an individual woman who rides her bicycle helmetless to the corner grocery store once a week, the risk is so minor that some would dismiss it outright.

In Malmö, at least, this nuanced message has yet to sink in. Many women from the original mammographic cohort have died (of various causes), but mammography, as one Malmö resident described it, "is somewhat of a religion here." On the windy winter morning that I stood outside the clinic, scores of women—some over fifty-five and some obviously younger—came in religiously for their annual X-rays. The clinic, I suspect, still ran with the same efficiency and diligence that had allowed it, after disastrous attempts in other cities, to rigorously complete one of the most seminal and difficult trials in the history of cancer prevention. Patients streamed in and out effortlessly, almost as if running an afternoon errand. Many of them rode off on their bicycles—oblivious of Berry's warnings—without helmets.

✑

Why did a simple, reproducible, inexpensive, easily learned technique—an X-ray image to detect the shadow of a small tumor in the breast—

have to struggle for five decades and through nine trials before any benefit could be ascribed to it?

Part of the answer lies in the complexity of running early-detection trials, which are inherently slippery, contentious, and prone to error. Edinburgh was undone by flawed randomization; the BCDDP by nonrandomization. Shapiro's trial was foiled by a faulty desire to be dispassionate; the Canadian trial by a flawed impulse to be compassionate.

Part of the answer lies also in the old conundrum of over- and underdiagnosis—although with an important twist. A mammogram, it turns out, is not a particularly good tool for detecting early breast cancer. Its false-positive and false-negative rates make it far from an ideal screening test. But the fatal flaw in mammography lies in that these rates are not absolute: *they depend on age*. For women above fifty-five, the incidence of breast cancer is high enough that even a relatively poor screening tool can detect an early tumor and provide a survival benefit. For women between forty and fifty years, though, the incidence of breast cancer sinks to a point that a "mass" detected on a mammogram, more often than not, turns out to be a false positive. To use a visual analogy: a magnifying lens designed to make small script legible does perfectly well when the font size is ten or even six points. But then it hits a limit. At a certain size font, chances of reading a letter correctly become about the same as reading a letter incorrectly. In women above fifty-five, where the "font size" of breast cancer incidence is large enough, a mammogram performs adequately. But in women between forty and fifty, the mammogram begins to squint at an uncomfortable threshold—exceeding its inherent capacity to become a discriminating test. No matter how intensively we test mammography in this group of women, it will always be a poor screening tool.

But the last part of the answer lies, surely, in how we imagine cancer and screening. We are a visual species. Seeing is believing, and to see cancer in its early, incipient form, we believe, must be the best way to prevent it. As the writer Malcolm Gladwell once described it, "This is a textbook example of how the battle against cancer is supposed to work. Use a powerful camera. Take a detailed picture. Spot the tumor as early as possible. Treat it immediately and aggressively. . . . The danger posed by a tumor is represented visually. Large is bad; small is better."

But powerful as the camera might be, cancer confounds this simple rule. Since metastasis is what kills patients with breast cancer, it is, of course, generally true that the ability to detect and remove premetastatic tumors saves women's lives. But it is also true that just because a tumor is small does not mean that it is premetastatic. Even relatively small tumors barely detectable by mammography can carry genetic programs that make them vastly more likely to metastasize early. Conversely, large tumors may inherently be genetically benign—unlikely to invade and metastasize. Size matters, in other words—but only to a point. The difference in the behavior of tumors is not just a consequence of quantitative growth, but of qualitative growth.

A static picture cannot capture this qualitative growth. Seeing a "small" tumor and extracting it from the body does not guarantee our freedom from cancer—a fact that we still struggle to believe. In the end, a mammogram or a Pap smear is a portrait of cancer in its infancy. Like any portrait, it is drawn in the hopes that it might capture something essential about the subject—its psyche, its inner being, its future, its *behavior*. "All photographs are accurate," the artist Richard Avedon liked to say, "[but] none of them is the truth."

❦

But if the "truth" of every cancer is imprinted in its behavior, then how might one capture this mysterious quality? How could scientists make that crucial transition between simply visualizing cancer and knowing its malignant potential, its vulnerabilities, its patterns of spread—its future?

By the late 1980s, the entire discipline of cancer prevention appeared to have stalled at this critical juncture. The missing element in the puzzle was a deeper understanding of carcinogenesis—a *mechanistic* understanding that would explain the means by which normal cells become cancer cells. Chronic inflammation with hepatitis B virus and *H. pylori* initiated the march of carcinogenesis, but by what route? The Ames test proved that mutagenicity was linked to carcinogenicity, but mutations in which genes, and by what mechanism?

And if such mutations were known, could they be used to launch more intelligent efforts to prevent cancer? Instead of running larger trials of mammography, for instance, could one run smarter trials of mammography—by risk-stratifying women (identifying those with predisposing mutations for breast cancer) such that high-risk women received higher levels of surveillance? Would that strategy, coupled with better technology, capture the identity of cancer more accurately than a simple, static portrait?

Cancer therapeutics, too, had seemingly arrived at the same bottleneck. Huggins and Walpole had shown that knowing the inner machinery of the cancer cell could reveal unique vulnerabilities. But the discovery had to come from the bottom up—*from* the cancer cell *to* its therapy. "As the decade ended," Bruce Chabner, former director of the NCI's Division of Cancer Treatment, recalled, "it was as if the whole discipline of oncology, both prevention and cure, had bumped up against a fundamental limitation of knowledge. We were trying to combat cancer without understanding the cancer cell, which was like launching rockets without understanding the internal combustion engine."

But others disagreed. With screening tests still faltering, with carcinogens still at large, and with the mechanistic understanding of cancer in its infancy, the impatience to deploy a large-scale therapeutic attack on cancer grew to its bristling tipping point. A chemotherapeutic poison was a poison was a poison, and one did not need to understand a cancer cell to poison it. So, just as a generation of radical surgeons had once shuttered the blinds around itself and pushed the discipline to its terrifying limits, so, too, did a generation of radical chemotherapists. If every dividing cell in the body needed to be obliterated to rid it of cancer, then so be it. It was a conviction that would draw oncology into its darkest hour.

STAMP

*Then did I beat them as small as the dust of the earth, I
did stamp them as the mire of the street, and did spread
them abroad.*

—Samuel 22:43

*Cancer therapy is like beating the dog with a stick to get
rid of his fleas.*
—Anna Deavere Smith, *Let Me Down Easy*

February was my cruelest month. The second month of 2004 arrived with
a salvo of deaths and relapses, each marked with the astonishing, punctu-
ated clarity of a gunshot in winter. Steve Harmon, thirty-six, had esophageal cancer growing at the inlet of his stomach. For six months, he had
soldiered through chemotherapy as if caught in a mythical punishment
cycle devised by the Greeks. He was debilitated by perhaps the severest
forms of nausea that I had ever encountered in a patient, but he had to
keep eating to avoid losing weight. As the tumor whittled him down week
by week, he became fixated, absurdly, on the measurement of his weight
down to a fraction of an ounce, as if gripped by the fear that he might vanish altogether by reaching zero.

Meanwhile, a growing retinue of family members accompanied him
to his clinic visits: three children who came with games and books and
watched, unbearably, as their father shook with chills one morning; a
brother who hovered suspiciously, then accusingly, as we shuffled and
reshuffled medicines to keep Steve from throwing up; a wife who bravely
shepherded the entire retinue through the whole affair as if it were a family trip gone horribly wrong.

One morning, finding Steve alone on one of the reclining chairs of the infusion room, I asked him whether he would rather have the chemotherapy alone, in a private room. Was it, perhaps, too much for his family—for his children?

He looked away with a flicker of irritation. "I know what the statistics are." His voice was strained, as if tightening against a harness. "Left to myself, I would not even try. I'm doing this *because* of the kids."

✑

"If a man die," William Carlos Williams once wrote, "it is because death / has first possessed his imagination." Death possessed the imagination of my patients that month, and my task was to repossess imagination from death. It is a task almost impossibly difficult to describe, an operation far more delicate and complex than the administration of a medicine or the performance of surgery. It was easy to repossess imagination with false promises; much harder to do so with nuanced truths. It demanded an act of exquisite measuring and remeasuring, filling and unfilling a psychological respirator with oxygen. Too much "repossession" and imagination might bloat into delusion. Too little and it might asphyxiate hope altogether.

In his poignant memoir of his mother's illness, Susan Sontag's son, David Rieff, describes a meeting between Sontag and a prominent doctor in New York. Sontag, having survived uterine and breast cancer, had been diagnosed with myelodysplasia, a precancerous disease that often sours into full-blown leukemia. (Sontag's myelodysplasia was caused by the high-dose chemotherapy that she had received for the other cancers.) The doctor—Rieff calls him Dr. A.—was totally pessimistic. There was no hope, he told her flatly. And not just that; there was nothing to do but wait for cancer to explode out of the bone marrow. All options were closed. His word—the Word—was final, immutable, static. "Like so many doctors," Rieff recalls, "he spoke to us as if we were children but without the care that a sensible adult takes in choosing what words to use with a child."

The sheer inflexibility of that approach and the arrogance of its finality was a nearly fatal blow for Sontag. Hopelessness became breathlessness, especially for a woman who wanted to live twice as energetically, to breathe the world in twice as fast as anyone else—for whom stillness *was* mortality. It took months before Sontag found another doctor whose attitude was vastly more measured and who was willing to negotiate with her psyche. Dr. A. was right, of course, in the formal, statistical sense. A moody, saturnine leukemia eventually volcanoed out of Sontag's marrow, and, yes, there were few medical options. But Sontag's new physician also told her precisely the same information, without ever choking off the possibility of a miraculous remission. He moved her in succession from standard drugs to experimental drugs to palliative drugs. It was all masterfully done, a graded movement toward reconciliation with death, but a movement nonetheless—statistics without stasis.

Of all the clinicians I met during my fellowship, the master of this approach was Thomas Lynch, a lung cancer doctor, whom I often accompanied to clinic. Clinics with Lynch, a youthful-looking man with a startling shock of gray hair, were an exercise in medical nuance. One morning, for instance, a sixty-six-year-old woman, Kate Fitz, came to the clinic having just recovered from surgery for a large lung mass, which had turned out to be cancerous. Sitting alone in the room, awaiting news of her next steps, she looked nearly catatonic with fear.

I was about to enter the room when Lynch caught me by the shoulder and pulled me into the side room. He had looked through her scan and her reports. Everything about the excised tumor suggested a high risk of recurrence. But more important, he had seen Fitz folded over in fear in the waiting room. Right now, he said, she needed something else. "Resuscitation," he called it cryptically as he strode into her room.

I watched him resuscitate. He emphasized process over outcome and transmitted astonishing amounts of information with a touch so slight that you might not even feel it. He told Fitz about the tumor, the good news about the surgery, asked about her family, then spoke about his own. He spoke about his child who was complaining about her long days at school. Did Fitz have a grandchild? he inquired. Did a daughter or a son live close by? And then, as I watched, he began to insert numbers here and there with a light-handedness that was a marvel to observe.

"You might read somewhere that for your particular form of cancer, there is a high chance of local recurrence or metastasis," he said. "Perhaps even fifty or sixty percent."

She nodded, tensing up.

"Well, there are ways that we will tend to it when that happens."

I noted that he had said "when," not "if." The numbers told a statistical truth, but the sentence implied nuance. "We will tend to it," he said, not "we will obliterate it." Care, not cure. The conversation ran for nearly an hour. In his hands, information was something live and molten, ready to freeze into a hard shape at any moment, something crystalline yet nego-tiable; he nudged and shaped it like glass in the hands of a glassblower.

An anxious woman with stage III breast cancer needs her imagina-tion to be repossessed before she will accept chemotherapy that will likely extend her life. A seventy-six-year-old man attempting another round of aggressive experimental chemotherapy for a fatal, drug-resistant leu-kemia needs his imagination to be reconciled to the reality that his dis-ease cannot be treated. Ars longa, vita brevis. The art of medicine is long, Hippocrates tells us, "and life is short; opportunity fleeting; the experi-ment perilous; judgment flawed."

∽

For cancer therapeutics, the mid and late 1980s were extraordinarily cruel years, mixing promise with disappointment, and resilience with despair. As physician-writer Abraham Verghese wrote, "To say this was a time of unreal and unparalleled confidence, bordering on conceit, in the Western medical world is to understate things.... When the outcome of treatment was not good, it was because the host was aged, the protoplasm frail, or the patient had presented too late—never because medical science was impotent.

"There seemed to be little that medicine could not do.... Surgeons, like Tom Starzl . . . were embarking on twelve- to fourteen-hour 'cluster oper-ations' where liver, pancreas, duodenum and jejunum were removed en bloc from a donor and transplanted into a patient whose belly, previously riddled with cancer, had now been eviscerated, scooped clean in prepara-tion for this organ bouquet.

"Starzl was an icon for that period in medicine, the pre-AIDS days, the frontier days of every-other-night call."

Yet even the patients eviscerated and reimplanted with these "organ bouquets" did not make it: they survived the operation, but not the dis-ease.

The chemotherapeutic equivalent of that surgical assault—of eviscerat-ing the body and replacing it with an implant—was a procedure known as autologous bone marrow transplant, or ABMT, which roared into national and international prominence in the mid-1980s. At its core, ABMT was based on an audacious conjecture. Ever since high-dose, multidrug regi-mens had succeeded in curing acute leukemia and Hodgkin's disease in the 1960s, chemotherapists had wondered whether solid tumors, such as breast or lung cancer, had remained recalcitrant to chemotherapeutic obliteration simply because the bludgeon of drugs used was not powerful enough. What if, some had fantasized, one could tip the human body even closer to the brink of death with even higher doses of cytotoxic drugs? Might it be dragged back from that near-lethal brink, leaving cancer behind? What if one could double, or even quadruple, the dosage of drugs?

The dose limit of a drug is set by its toxicity to normal cells. For most chemotherapy drugs, that dose limit rested principally on a single organ— the bone marrow, whose whirring cellular mill, as Farber had found, was so exquisitely sensitive to most drugs that patients administered drugs to kill cancer were left with no normal blood-forming cells. For a while, then, it was the bone marrow's sensitivity to cytotoxic drugs that had defined the outer horizon of chemotherapeutic dosage. The bone marrow represented the frontier of toxicity, an unbreachable barrier that limited the capacity to deliver obliterative chemotherapy—the "red ceiling" as some oncologists called it.

But by the late 1960s, even that ceiling had seemed to lift. In Seattle, one of Farber's early protégés, E. Donnall Thomas, had shown that bone marrow, much like a kidney or liver, could be harvested from one patient and transplanted back—either into the same patient (called autologous transplantation) or into another patient (termed allogeneic transplantation).

Allogeneic transplantation (i.e., transplanting foreign marrow into a patient) was temperamental—tricky, mercurial, often deadly. But in some cancers, particularly leukemias, it was potentially curative. One could, for instance, obliterate a marrow riddled with leukemia using high-dose chemo and replace it with fresh, clean marrow from another patient. Once the new marrow had engrafted, the recipient ran the risk of that foreign marrow turning and attacking his or her own body as well as any residual leukemia left in the marrow, a deadly complication termed graft-versus-host disease or GVHD. But in some patients, that trifecta of assaults— obliterative chemotherapy, marrow replacement, and the attack on the tumor by foreign cells—could be fashioned into an exquisitely potent therapeutic weapon against cancer. The procedure carried severe risks. In Thomas's initial trial at Seattle, only twelve out of a hundred patients had survived. But by the early 1980s, doctors were using the procedure for refractory leukemias, multiple myeloma, and myelodysplastic syndrome—diseases inherently resistant to chemotherapy. Success was limited, but at least some patients were eventually cured.

Autologous bone marrow transplantation was, if conceivable, the lighter fraternal twin of allogeneic transplantation. Here, the patient's *own* marrow was harvested, frozen, and transplanted back into his or her body. No donor was needed. The principal purpose was not to replace diseased marrow (using a foreign marrow) but to maximize chemotherapeutic dosage. A patient's own marrow, containing blood-forming cells, was harvested and frozen. Then blisteringly high levels of drugs were administered to kill cancer. The frozen marrow was thawed and implanted. Since the frozen marrow cells were spared the brunt of chemotherapy, transplantation allowed doctors, theoretically at least, to push doses of chemo to their ultimate end.

For advocates of megadose chemotherapy, ABMT breached a final and crucial roadblock. It was now possible to give five- or even tenfold the typical doses of drugs, in poisonous cocktails and combinations once considered incompatible with survival. Among the first and most fervent proponents of this strategy was Tom Frei—cautious, levelheaded Frei, who had moved from Houston to Boston as the director of Farber's institute. By the early 1980s, Frei had convinced himself that a megadose combination regimen, bolstered by marrow transplantation, was the only conceivable solution in cancer therapy.

To test this theory, Frei hoped to launch one of the most ambitious trials in the history of chemotherapy. With his ear for catchy acronyms, Frei christened the protocol the Solid Tumor Autologous Marrow Program—or STAMP. Crystallized in that name was the storm and rage of cancer medicine; if brute force was needed, then brute force would be summoned. With searing doses of cytotoxic drugs, STAMP would trample its way over cancer. "We have a cure for breast cancer," Frei told one of his colleagues in the summer of 1982. Uncharacteristically, he had already let his optimism fly to the far edge of brinkmanship. The first patient had not even been enrolled on trial.

cy&*p*

VAMP had succeeded, Frei privately believed, not just because of the unique chemotherapeutic synergy among the drugs, but also because of the unique human synergy at the NCI—that cocktail of brilliant young minds and risk-taking bodies that had coalesced in Bethesda between 1955 and 1960. In Boston, two decades later, Frei assiduously set about re-creating that same potent atmosphere, tossing out deadwood faculty and replacing it with fresh new blood. "It was an intensely competitive place," Robert Mayer, the oncologist, recalled, "a pressure cooker for junior and senior faculty." Trial-running was the principal currency of academic advancement, and volley after volley of trials were launched at the institute with a grim, nearly athletic, determination. Metaphors of war permeated the Farber. Cancer was the ultimate enemy, and this was its ultimate crucible, its epic battleground. Laboratory space and clinical space were deliberately intermingled through the floors to create the impression of a highly sophisticated interlocking machine dedicated to a single cause. On blackboards mounted on laboratory walls, complex diagrams with zigzagging arrows and lines depicted the life line of a cancer cell. To walk through the narrow corridors of the institute was to feel immersed in a gigantic, subterranean war room, where technological prowess was on full display and every molecule of air seemed poised for a battle.

In 1982, Frei recruited William Peters, a young doctor from New York, as a fellow at the institute. Peters was an academic all-star. He had graduated from Pennsylvania State University with three majors, in biochemistry, biophysics, and philosophy, then steamrollered his way through the College of Physicians and Surgeons at Columbia, earning both an M.D. and a Ph.D. Affable, determined, enthusiastic, and ambitious, he was considered the most able corporal among the troops of junior faculty at the Farber. The relationship between Frei and Peters was almost instantly magnetic, perhaps even parental. Peters was instinctually drawn to Frei's reputation, creativity, and unorthodox methods; Frei, to Peters's energy and enthusiasm. Each saw in the other an earlier or later incarnation of himself.

❧

On Thursday afternoons, fellows and faculty at the Farber gathered in a conference room on the sixteenth floor. The room was symbolically set on the highest floor of the building, its large windows, overlooking the evergreen fens of Boston, and its wood-paneled walls, blond and reflective, creating a light-immersed casket suspended midair. Lunch was catered. The doors were closed. It was a time dedicated to academic thinking, sealed away from the daily whir of labs and clinics in the floors below.

It was at these afternoon conferences that Frei began to introduce the idea of megadose combination chemotherapy with autologous marrow support to the fellows and junior faculty. In the fall of 1983, he invited

Howard Skipper, the soft-spoken "mouse doctor" who had so deeply influenced Frei's early work, to speak. Skipper was inching toward higher and higher doses of cytotoxic drugs in his mouse models and spoke enthusiastically about the possibility of curative treatment with these megadose regimens. He was soon after followed by Frank Schabel, another scientist who had demonstrated that combining agents, in doses lethal for the marrow, possessed synergistic effects on mouse tumors. Schabel's lecture was particularly galvanizing, a "seminal event," as Peters described it. After the talk, as Frei recalled, the room was abuzz with excitement; Schabel was surrounded by young, eager investigators mesmerized by his ideas. Among the youngest, and by far the most eager, was Bill Peters.

Yet the surer Frei became about megadose chemotherapy, the less sure some others around him seemed to get. George Canellos, for one, was wary, right from the outset. Wiry and tall, with a slight stoop and a commanding basso-profundo voice, Canellos was the closest to Frei's equal at the institute, an original member of the NCI from its heady early days in the mid-1960s. Unlike Frei, though, Canellos had turned from advocate to adversary of megadose chemo regimens, in part because he had been among the first to notice a devastating long-term side effect: as doses escalated, some chemotherapeutic drugs damaged the marrow so severely that, in time, these regimens could precipitate a premalignant syndrome called myelodysplasia, a condition that tended to progress to leukemia. The leukemias that arose from the ashes of chemotherapy-treated marrows carried such grotesque and aberrant mutations that they were virtually resistant to any drugs, as if their initial passage through that fire had tempered them into immortality.

With Canellos arguing one side and Frei the other, the institute split into bitterly opposing camps. But Peters and Frei were unstoppably enthusiastic. By late 1982, with Frei's guidance, Peters had written a detailed protocol for the STAMP regimen. A few weeks later, the Institutional Review Board at the Farber approved STAMP, giving Peters and Frei the green light to begin their trial. "We were going to swing and go for the ring," Peters recalled. "That drove us. You had to believe you were going to pull off something that was going to change history."

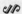

The first patient to "change history" with STAMP was a thirty-year-old commercial driver from Massachusetts with breast cancer. A grim, determined, hefty woman hardened by the gritty culture of truck stops and highways, she had been treated and re-treated with multiple standard and escalating regimens of chemotherapy. Her tumor, a friable, inflamed disk of tissue, was nearly six centimeters wide, hanging visibly off her chest wall. But having "failed" all the conventional treatments, she had become virtually invisible to the institute. Her case was considered so terminal that she had been written off from every other experimental protocol. When she signed on to Peters's protocol, no one objected.

Marrow transplantation begins, of course, by "harvesting" bone marrow. On the morning of the first harvest, Peters went down to the leukemia clinic and gathered his arms full of bone marrow needles. He wheeled his first patient over to the operating room at the neighboring Beth Israel hospital (the Farber had no operating rooms) and began pulling out the marrow, plunging a steel trocar repeatedly into the hip and drawing out the cells, leaving a hip pockmarked with red bruises. Each time he pulled, a few droplets of reddish sludge gathered in the syringe.

Then disaster struck. As Peters pulled out a specimen, the marrow needle broke, leaving a piece of steel buried deeply in his patient's hip. For a few minutes, pandemonium broke out in the operating room. Nurses made frantic phone calls to the floors, asking for surgeons to step in to help. An hour later, using a pair of orthopedic pliers to dig into the hip, Peters recovered the needle.

Later that evening, the full impact of that moment struck Peters. It had been a close shave. "The ultimate trial of chemotherapeutic intensification," Peters said, "almost broke its back on an old needle." For Peters and Frei, it was an all-too-obvious metaphor for the rustiness and obsolescence of the status quo. The War on Cancer was being waged by timorous doctors (unwilling to maximize chemotherapy) with blunt, outmoded weapons.

For a few weeks after that initial tumult, Peters's life fell into a reasonably stable routine. Early mornings, dodging Canellos and other muttering skeptics, he rounded on his patients on the far corner of the twelfth floor, where a few rooms had been set aside for the trial. Evenings were spent at home with *Masterpiece Theatre* playing in the background as he sharpened needles physically and sharpened the trial intellectually. As the trial gathered speed, it also gained visibility. Peters's first few patients had been last-ditch, hopeless cases, women with tumors so deeply recalcitrant to all drugs that they were readily enrolled in experimental trials as a last resort in the hope of obtaining even a minor remission. But as rumors of the trial coursed through networks of patients and friends, cancer patients began to contact Peters and Frei to try the megadose strategy *up front*—not after they had failed more conventional regimens, but before they had even tried anything else. In the late summer of 1983, when a previously untreated woman with metastatic breast cancer enrolled in STAMP, as Peters recalled, the institute stood up to take notice. "Suddenly, everything broke loose and things came apart."

The woman was thirty-six years old—charming, sophisticated, intense, coiled and tightened into a spring by her yearlong battle with illness. She had watched her mother die of an aggressive breast cancer that had been fiercely resistant to conventional therapy. Instinctually, she was convinced that hers would be just as virulent and just as resistant. She wanted to live and wanted the most aggressive therapy up front, without soldiering through trials that would, she was convinced, fail anyway. When Peters offered her STAMP, she grasped at it without hesitation.

Her clinical course was among the most closely watched in the history of the institute. Fortunately for Peters, chemotherapy and transplantation went smoothly. On the seventh day after megadose chemotherapy, when Frei and Peters hurried down to the basement to look at the first chest X-ray after treatment, they found that they had been beaten to it. An entire congregation of curious doctors had gathered in the room like a jury and was huddled around the films. Against the sharp, fluorescent light, her chest X-ray showed a marked response. The metastatic deposits peppered around in her lung had shrunk visibly, and even the swollen lymph nodes around it had visibly recessed. It was, as Peters recalls, "the most beautiful remission you could have imagined."

As the year drew on, Peters treated and transplanted more cases and obtained beautiful remissions. By the summer of 1984, the database of transplanted cases was large enough to begin to discern patterns. The medical complications of the STAMP regimen had, of course, been predictably ghastly: near-lethal infections, severe anemia, pneumonias, and hemorrhages in the heart. But under the clouds of X-rays, blood tests, and CT scans, Peters and Frei saw a silvery inkling. The remissions produced by STAMP, they were convinced, had all been more durable than those produced by conventional chemotherapy. It was only an impression—at best, a guess. To prove that point, Peters needed a randomized trial. In 1985, with Frei's encouragement, he left Boston to set up a STAMP program at Duke University in North Carolina. He wanted to leave the Farber's "pressure cooker" behind for a quiet and stable academic place where he could run a trial in peace.

ঞ্চ

As William Peters dreamed of a quiet and stable environment to test megadose chemotherapy, the world of medicine was overturned by an unexpected and seemingly unrelated event. In March 1981, in the journal *Lancet,* a team of doctors reported eight cases of a highly unusual form of cancer called Kaposi's sarcoma in a cohort of men in New York. The disease was not new: named after a nineteenth-century Hungarian dermatologist, Kaposi's sarcoma had long been recognized as a slow-growing, violet-colored, indolent tumor that crept along the skin of elderly Italian men that, while occasionally serious, was often considered a somewhat glorified form of a mole or carbuncle. But all the *Lancet* cases were virtually unrecognizable forms of the disease, violent and aggressive variants that had exploded into bleeding, metastatic, blue-black macules spread all over the bodies of these young men. All eight of the men were homosexual. The eighth case drew particular alarm and interest: this man, with lesions on his head and back, was also diagnosed with a rare pneumonia called PCP caused by the organism *Pneumocystis carinii.* An outbreak of one obscure illness in a cluster of young men was already outlandish. The confluence of two suggested a deeper and darker aberration—not just a disease, but a syndrome.

Far away from New York, the sudden appearance of *Pneumocystis carinii* was also raising eyebrows at the Centers for Disease Control in Atlanta, Georgia. The CDC is the nation's medical radar screen, an agency that tracks emerging diseases to discern patterns and contain their spread. *Pneumocystis* pneumonia only occurs in humans when the immune system is severely compromised. The principal victims had been cancer patients whose white blood cells had been decimated by chemotherapy. (DeVita had encountered it in Hodgkin's patients treated with four-drug chemo.) The new cases of PCP made little sense: these were young, previously healthy men who had suddenly succumbed to PCP with their immune systems on the verge of collapse.

By the late summer of that year, as the coastal cities sweltered in a heat wave, the CDC began to sense that an epidemiological catastrophe was forming out of thin air. Between June and August 1981, the weather vane of strange illnesses swung frantically around its pivot: additional clusters of PCP, Kaposi's sarcoma, cryptococcal meningitis, and rare lymphomas were reported in young men in cities throughout America. The common pattern behind all these diseases, aside from their disproportionate predilection for gay men, was a massive, near-total collapse of the immune system. A letter in *Lancet* called the disease "gay compromise syndrome." Others called it GRID (gay-related immune deficiency) or, more cruelly, gay cancer. In July 1982, with an understanding of the cause still missing, the disease finally stumbled upon its modern name, acquired immunodeficiency syndrome, or AIDS.

Twinned conspicuously at this birth, the trajectories of AIDS and cancer were destined to crisscross and intersect at many levels. And it was Sontag, again, writing piercingly from her New York apartment (from whose terraced windows she could observe the AIDS epidemic whirling through the streets of Chelsea below), who immediately recognized the symbolic parallels between the two diseases. In a trenchant essay written as a reply to her earlier *Illness as Metaphor,* Sontag argued that AIDS, like cancer, was becoming not just a biological disease but something much larger—a social and political category replete with its own punitive metaphors. Like cancer patients, AIDS patients were also paralyzed and shrouded by those metaphors—stripped bare, like the cancer patient in Solzhenitsyn's *Cancer Ward,* then forced to don the ghoulish uniform of their disease. The stigmas attached to cancer—guilt, secrecy, shame—were recycled and refitted for AIDS, acquiring tenfold force and potency: *sexual* guilt, *sexual* secrecy, *sexual* shame. If cancer, as Sontag had once argued, was perceived as the product of spoiled germ, of biological mutability gone wild, then AIDS was the result of contaminated germ, of social mutability gone wild: men unmoored from the usual conventions of society, metastasizing from coast to coast on airplanes, carrying disease and devastation within them. A patient afflicted with AIDS thus evaporated from individual existence and morphed instantly into an imagined archetype—a young gay man, fresh out of the bathhouses, defiled and ravaged by profligacy, now lying namelessly in the hospital wards of New York or San Francisco.

Sontag concerned herself with metaphorical parallels, but down in those wards, the medical battles also paralleled the battles fought against cancer. In the early days, among the first doctors to encounter and treat AIDS patients were oncologists. One of the "sentinel" diseases of immunodeficiency was Kaposi's sarcoma, an explosive variant of an indolent cancer that had appeared without warning on the bodies of young men. In San Francisco, at the epicenter of the epidemic, the first clinic to be organized for AIDS patients was thus a sarcoma clinic that began to meet weekly beginning in September 1981 led by a dermatologist, Marcus Conant, and an oncologist, Paul Volberding. Volberding personified the crisscrossing fates of the two diseases. Trained as an oncologist at the University of California, San Francisco, he had spent a rather disappointing stint in the laboratory studying mouse retroviruses and, frustrated, switched from the lab to clinical oncology at San Francisco General Hospital.

For Volberding, and for many of his earliest patients, AIDS *was* cancer. To treat his sarcoma patients, Volberding borrowed various chemotherapy regimens from the NCI's protocols.* But more than chemotherapy protocols, Volberding borrowed something more ineffable—an ethos. At San Francisco General, at the end of a long linoleum-floored corridor with chipped paint on the walls and naked lightbulbs dangling from wires, Volberding and his team created the world's first AIDS ward, called Ward 5A, which was explicitly modeled after the cancer wards that he had seen as a fellow. "What we did here," he recalls, was "exactly like an oncology unit, but with a different focus, AIDS. . . . But it really was modeled on oncology units, where you have complex medical diseases with a lot of psychosocial overlay, a lot of use of drugs that are complex and require a sophisticated nursing staff and psychosocial support staff."

Nurses, many of them gay men, gravitated to Ward 5A to tend their friends (or returned poignantly, as the epidemic bloomed, as patients themselves). Doctors reinvented medicine here, pitting their wits against a hostile, mysterious disease that they couldn't quite fathom that was plaguing a community that they didn't quite understand. As the patients boiled up with bizarre, spectral fevers, rules were unshackled and reinvented, creating a ward that came to resemble the unorthodox lives of the men who inhabited it. Fixed visiting hours were eliminated. Friends, companions, lovers, and family members were allowed, even encouraged, to sleep overnight in accompanying cots to help patients through those burning, hallucinatory nights. On Sunday afternoons, a San Francisco dancer catered elaborate brunches featuring tap dancing, feather boas, and marijuana-laced brownies. Farber may not have envisioned these particular

---

* The notion of using a "cocktail" of drugs against HIV was borrowed from oncology—although it would be several years before anti-HIV drugs were available.

innovations, but this, too, in a community drenched with grief, was its own, inimitable interpretation of "total care."

Politically, too, AIDS activists borrowed language and tactics from cancer lobbyists, and then imbued this language with their own urgency and potency. In January 1982, as AIDS cases boomed, a group of six men founded Gay Men's Health Crisis in New York, a volunteer organization dedicated to fighting AIDS through advocacy, lobbying, campaigning, and protest. Early volunteers decamped outside discos, bars, and bathhouses soliciting donations and distributing posters. From its office in a crumbling Chelsea brownstone, GMHC coordinated an extraordinary national effort to bring AIDS awareness to the masses. These were the Laskerites of AIDS, albeit without the gray suits and pearls.

The seminal scientific breakthrough in the AIDS epidemic was, meanwhile, unfolding in a laboratory at the Institut Pasteur in Paris. In January 1983, Luc Montagnier's group found the sign of a virus in a lymph node biopsy from a young gay man with Kaposi's sarcoma and in a Zairean woman who had died of immune deficiency. Montagnier soon deduced that this was an RNA virus that could convert its genes into DNA and lodge into the human genome—a retrovirus. He called his virus IDAV, immunodeficiency associated viruses, arguing that it was likely the cause of AIDS.

At the National Cancer Institute, a group led by Robert Gallo was also circling around the same virus, although under a different name. In the spring of 1984, the two efforts converged dramatically. Gallo also found a retrovirus in AIDS patients—Montagnier's IDAV. A few months later, the identity of the virus was confirmed by yet another group in San Francisco. On April 23, 1984, Margaret Heckler, the Health and Human Services secretary, thus appeared before the press with a bold statement about the future of the epidemic. With a causal agent in hand, a cure seemed just a few steps away. "The arrow of funds, medical personnel, research . . . has hit the target," she said. "We hope to have a vaccine ready for testing in about two years. . . . Today's discovery represents the triumph of science over dread disease."

But AIDS activists, facing the lethal upswirl of the epidemic that was decimating their community, could not afford to wait. In the spring of 1987, a group of volunteers splintered away from GMHC to form a group named the AIDS Coalition to Unleash Power, or ACT UP. Led by a sardonic and hyperarticulate writer named Larry Kramer, ACT UP promised to transform the landscape of AIDS treatment using a kind of militant activism unprecedented in the history of medicine. Kramer blamed many forces for aiding and abetting the epidemic—he called it "genocide by neglect"—but chief among the neglecters was the FDA. "Many of us who live in daily terror of the AIDS epidemic," Kramer wrote in the *Times*, "cannot understand why the Food and Drug Administration has been so intransigent in the face of this monstrous tidal wave of death."

Symptomatic of this intransigence was the process by which the FDA evaluated and approved lifesaving drugs for AIDS, a process that Kramer characterized as terminally lazy and terminally slow. And terminally gaga: the slow, contemplative "academic" mechanism of drug testing, Kramer groused, was becoming life-threatening rather than lifesaving. Randomized, placebo-controlled trials were all well and good in the cool ivory towers of medicine, but patients afflicted by a deadly illness needed drugs *now*. "Drugs into bodies; drugs into bodies," ACT UP chanted. A new model for accelerated clinical trials was needed. "The FDA is fucked-up, the NIH is fucked-up . . . the boys and girls who are running this show have been unable to get whatever system they're operating to work," Kramer told his audience in New York. "Double-blind studies," he argued in an editorial, "were not created with terminal illnesses in mind." He concluded, "AIDS sufferers who have nothing to lose, are more than willing to be guinea pigs."

Even Kramer knew that that statement was extraordinary; Halsted's ghost had, after all, barely been laid to rest. But as ACT UP members paraded through the streets of New York and Washington, frothing with anger and burning paper effigies of FDA administrators, their argument ricocheted potently through the media and the public imagination. And the argument had a natural spillover to other, equally politicized diseases. If AIDS patients demanded direct access to drugs and treatments, should other patients with terminal illnesses not also make similar demands? Patients with AIDS wanted drugs into bodies, so why should bodies with cancer be left without drugs?

In Durham, North Carolina, a city barely touched by the AIDS epidemic in 1987, the sound and fury of these demonstrations may have seemed like a distant thunderclap. Deeply ensconced in his trial of megadose chemotherapy at Duke University, William Peters could not possibly have predicted that this very storm was about to turn south and beat its way to his door.

◈

The STAMP regimen—mega-dose chemotherapy for breast cancer—was gathering momentum day by day. By the winter of 1984, thirty-two women had completed the Phase I "safety" study—a trial designed to document whether STAMP could safely be administered. The data looked promising: although clearly toxic, selected patients could survive the regimen. (Phase I studies are not designed to assess efficacy.) In December that year, at the fifth annual Breast Cancer Symposium in San Antonio, Texas, there was abundant optimism about efficacy as well. "There was so much excitement within the cancer community that some were already convinced," the statistician Donald Berry recalls. Peters was his typically charming self at the conference—boyish, exuberant, cautious, but inveterately positive. He called the meeting a "small victory."

After San Antonio, the early-phase trials gathered speed. Emboldened by the positive response, Peters pushed for evaluating STAMP not just for metastatic breast cancer, but as an adjuvant therapy for high-risk patients with locally advanced cancer (patients with more than ten cancer-afflicted lymph nodes). Following Peters's initial observations, several groups across the nation also hotly pursued megadose chemotherapy with bone marrow transplantation. Two years later, with early-phase trials completed successfully, a randomized, blinded, Phase III trial was needed. Peters approached the Cancer and Leukemia Group B (CALGB), the centralized group that acted as a clearinghouse for clinical trials, to sponsor a definitive multicenter, randomized clinical trial.

On a winter afternoon, Peters flew up from Duke to Boston to detail a STAMP trial to the CALGB for its approval. As expected, vicious arguments broke out in the room. Some clinicians still contended that STAMP was, in fact, no different from cytotoxic chemotherapy taken to its extreme brink—stale wine being sold in a new bottle. Others contended that the chemotherapeutic battle against cancer *needed* to be taken to the brink. The meeting stretched hour upon hour, each side hotly debating its points. In the end, the CALGB agreed to sponsor the trial. Peters left the conference room on the sixth floor of the Massachusetts General Hospital feeling bewildered but relieved. When the hinged saloon door of the room swung closed behind him, it was as if he had just emerged out of a nasty barroom brawl.

The Map and the Parachute

Oedipus: What is the rite of purification? How shall it be done?
Creon: By banishing a man, or expiation of blood by blood.
                                        —Sophocles, *Oedipus the King*

William Peters was trying to convince himself, using a strict randomized trial, that megadose chemotherapy worked. But others were already convinced. Many oncologists had long assumed that the regimen was so obviously effective that no trial could possibly be needed. After all, if the deepest reservoirs of the marrow could be depleted by the searing doses of drugs, how could cancer possibly resist?

By the late 1980s, hospitals and, increasingly, private clinics offering marrow transplantation for breast cancer had sprouted up all around America, Great Britain, and France with waiting lists that stretched into several hundreds of women. Among the most prominent and successful of the megadose transplanters was Werner Bezwoda, an oncologist at the University of Witwatersrand in Johannesburg, South Africa, who was recruiting dozens of women into his trial every month. Transplant was big business: big medicine, big money, big infrastructure, big risks. At large academic centers, such as the Beth Israel hospital in Boston, entire floors were refitted into transplant units, with case volumes that ran into several dozens each week. Minimizing the risks of the procedure using creative phrasing became a cottage industry. As private clinics lined up to perform transplants on women, they christened the procedure a "minitransplant" or "transplant lite" or even "drive-thru transplant." Transplanters, as one oncologist put it, "became gods at hospitals."

This frantic landscape was tipped into further disarray as patients began to file requests for insurance providers to pay for the procedure, priced anywhere between $50,000 to $400,000 per patient. In the summer of 1991, a public-school teacher named Nelene Fox in Temecula,

California, was diagnosed with advanced breast cancer. Fox was thirty-eight years old, the mother of three children. When she relapsed with metastatic breast cancer after exhausting all conventional therapies, her doctors suggested an autologous bone marrow transplant as a last resort. Fox lunged at the suggestion. But when she applied to Health Net, her insurance provider, to pay for the transplant, Health Net refused, stating that the procedure was still "investigational" and thus not covered by the HMO's standard list of clinically proven protocols.

In another decade and with any other disease, Fox's case may have garnered scarcely any public attention. But something fundamental about the relationship between patients and medicine had changed in the aftermath of AIDS. Until the late 1980s, an experimental drug or procedure had been considered precisely that, experimental, and therefore unavailable for general public use. But AIDS activism had transformed that idea. An investigational agent, AIDS activists insisted, was no longer a hothouse flower meant to be cultivated only in the rarefied greenhouses of academic medicine, but rather a public resource merely waiting in the warming antechamber of science while doctors finished clinical trials that would, in the end, prove the efficacy of said drugs or procedures anyway.

Patients, in short, had lost patience. They did not want trials; they wanted drugs and cures. ACT UP, parading on the streets of New York and Washington, had made the FDA out to be a woolly bureaucratic grandfather—exacting but maddeningly slow, whose sole purpose was to delay access to critical medicines. Health Net's denial of Nelene Fox's transplant thus generated a visceral public reaction. Furious and desperate, Fox decided to raise the money privately by writing thousands of letters. By mid-April 1992, an enormous fund-raising effort to pay for Fox's transplant had swung into gear. Temecula, a quiet hamlet of golf courses and antique shops, was gripped by a mission. Money poured in from softball matches and pie sales; from lemonade stands and car washes; from a local Sizzler restaurant; from a yogurt shop that donated a portion of its profits. On June 19, a retinue of Fox's supporters, chanting, "Transplant, transplant," and Fox's name, staged a rally outside Health Net's corporate headquarters. A few days later, Fox's brother, an attorney named Mark Hiepler, filed a lawsuit against Health Net to force the HMO to pay for his sister's transplant. "You marketed this coverage to her when she was well," Hiepler wrote. "Please provide it now that she is ill."

In the late summer of 1992, when Health Net refused yet another request for coverage, once again citing lack of clinical evidence, Fox chose to go ahead on her own. By then, she had raised $220,000 from nearly twenty-five hundred friends, neighbors, relatives, coworkers, and strangers—enough to afford the transplant on her own.

In August 1992, Nelene Fox thus underwent high-dose chemotherapy and a bone marrow transplant for metastatic breast cancer, hoping for a new lease on her life.

☙

In the gleaming new wards of the Norris Center in Los Angeles, where Fox was undergoing her transplant, the story of Werner Bezwoda's remarkable success with megadose chemotherapy was already big news. In Bezwoda's hands, everything about the regimen seemed to work like a perfectly cast spell. A stocky, intense, solitary man capable, Oz-like, of inspiring both charm and suspicion, Bezwoda was the self-styled wizard of autologous transplantation who presided over an ever-growing clinical empire at Witwatersrand in Johannesburg with patients flying in from Europe, Asia, and Africa. As Bezwoda's case series swelled, so, too, did his reputation. By the mid-1990s, he was regularly jetting up from South Africa to discuss his experience with megadose chemotherapy at meetings and conferences organized all around the world. "The dose-limiting barrier," Bezwoda announced audaciously in 1992, had been "overcome"—instantly rocketing himself and his clinic into stratospheric fame.

Oncologists, scientists, and patients who thronged to his packed seminars found themselves mesmerized by his results. Bezwoda lectured slowly and dispassionately, in a bone-dry, deadpan drone, looking occasionally at the screen with his characteristic sideways glance, delivering the most exhilarating observations in the world of clinical oncology as if reading the Soviet evening news. At times the ponderous style seemed almost deliberately mismatched, for even Bezwoda knew that his results were astounding. As the lights flickered on for the poster session at the annual oncology meeting held in San Diego in May 1992, clinicians flocked around him, flooding him with questions and congratulations. In Johannesburg, more than 90 percent of women treated with the megadose regimen had achieved a complete response—a rate that even the powerhouse academic centers in the United States had been unable to achieve. Bezwoda, it seemed, was going to lead oncology out of its decades-long impasse with cancer.

Nelene Fox, though, was not so fortunate. She soldiered through the punishing regimen of high-dose chemotherapy and its multiple complications. But less than one year after her transplant, breast cancer relapsed explosively all over her body, in her lungs, liver, lymph nodes, and, most important, in her brain. On April 22, eleven months after Bezwoda's poster was hung up in nearby San Diego, Fox passed away in her home in a shaded cul-de-sac in Temecula. She was only forty years old. She left behind a husband and three daughters, aged four, nine, and eleven. And a lawsuit against Health Net, now winding its way through the California court system.

∂∫∂

Juxtaposed against Bezwoda's phenomenal results, Fox's agonizing struggle and untimely death seemed an even more egregious outcome. Convinced that the *delayed* transplant—not cancer—had hastened his sister's demise, Hiepler broadened his claims against Health Net and vigorously pushed for a court trial. The crux of Hiepler's case rested on the definition of the word "investigational." High-dose chemotherapy could, he argued, hardly be considered an "investigational" procedure if nearly every major clinical center in the nation was offering it to patients, both on and off trial. In 1993 alone, 1,177 papers in medical journals had been written on the subject. In certain hospitals, entire wards were dedicated to the procedure. The label "experimental" was slapped on, Hiepler contended, by HMOs to save money by denying coverage. "If all you have is a cold or the flu, sure, they will take good care of you. But when you get breast cancer, what happens? Out comes 'investigative.' Out comes 'experimental.'"

On the morning of December 28, 1993, Mark Hiepler spent nearly two hours in the courtroom describing the devastating last year of his sister's life. The balconies and benches overflowed with Fox's friends and supporters and with patients, many of them weeping with anger and empathy. The jury took less than two hours to deliberate. That evening, it returned a verdict awarding Fox's family $89 million in damages—the second-highest amount in the history of litigation in California and one of the highest ever awarded in a medical case in America.

Eighty-nine million dollars was largely symbolic (the case was eventually settled out of court for an undisclosed smaller amount), but it was also the kind of symbolism that any HMO could readily understand. In 1993, patient advocacy groups urged women to battle similar cases around the country. Understandably, most insurers began to relent. In Massachusetts, Charlotte Turner, a forty-seven-year-old nurse diagnosed with metastatic breast cancer, lobbied ferociously for her transplant, rushing on a wheelchair from one legislator's office to another with sheaves of medical articles in her arms. In late 1993, as a result of Turner's efforts, the Massachusetts state legislature enacted the so-called Charlotte's Law, mandating coverage for transplantation for eligible patients within the state. By the mid-1990s, seven states required HMOs to pay for bone marrow transplantation, with similar legislation pending in seven additional states. Between 1988 and 2002, eighty-six cases were filed by patients against HMOs that had denied transplants. In forty-seven instances, the patient won the case.

That this turn of events—aggressive chemotherapy and marrow transplantation *mandated* by law—was truly extraordinary was not lost on many observers. It was, at face value, a liberating moment for many patients and patient advocates. But medical journals ran rife with scorching critiques of the protocol. It is a "complicated, costly and potentially dangerous technology," one article complained pointedly. The litany of complications was grim: infections, hemorrhage, blood clots in the arteries and the liver, heart failure, scarring of lungs, skin, kidneys, and tendons. Infertility was often permanent. Patients were confined to the hospital for weeks, and most ominous perhaps, between 5 and 10 percent of women ran the risk of developing a second cancer or precancerous lesion as a result of the treatment itself—cancers doggedly recalcitrant to any therapy.

But as autologous transplantation for cancer exploded into a major enterprise, the scientific evaluation of the protocol fell further and further behind. Indeed the trials were caught in an old and perverse quagmire. Everyone—patients, doctors, HMOs, advocacy groups—wanted trials in principle. But no one wanted to be *in* trials, in practice. The more health insurance plans opened their floodgates for bone marrow transplantation, the more women fled from clinical trials, fearing that they might be assigned to the nontreatment arm by what amounted to a coin flip.

Between 1991 and 1999, roughly forty thousand women around the world underwent marrow transplantation for breast cancer, at an estimated cost of between $2 billion and $4 billion (at the higher estimate, about twice the yearly budget of the NCI). Meanwhile, patient accrual for the clinical trials, including Peters's trial at Duke, nearly trickled to a halt. The disjunction was poignant. Even as clinics overflowed with women being treated with high-dose chemotherapy and wards filled their beds with transplanted patients, the seminal measure to test the efficacy of that regimen was pushed aside, almost as if it were an afterthought. "Transplants, transplants, everywhere," as Robert Mayer put it, "but not a patient to test."

☙

When Bezwoda returned to the annual cancer meeting in Atlanta in May 1999, he was clearly triumphant. He rose to the podium confidently, feigning irritation that his name had been mispronounced during the introduction, and flashed his opening slides. As Bezwoda presented the data—his monotone voice washing over the vast sea of faces in front of him—a spell of silence fell over the audience. The wizard of Wits had worked magic again. At Witwatersrand hospital, young women with high-risk breast cancer treated with bone marrow transplants had showed staggeringly successful results. At eight and a half years, nearly 60 percent of patients in the megadose/transplant arm were still alive, versus only 20 percent in the control arm. For patients treated with the Bezwoda regimen, the line of survival had plateaued at about seven years with no further deaths, suggesting that many of the remaining patients were not just alive, but likely cured. Applause broke out among transplanters.

But Bezwoda's triumph felt odd, for although the Witwatersrand results were unequivocally spectacular, three other trials presented that afternoon, including Peters's, were either equivocal or negative. At Duke, embarrassingly enough, the trial had not even been finished because of low accrual. And while it was too soon to assess the survival benefits of transplantation, its darker face was readily evident: of the three-hundred-odd patients randomized to the transplant arm, thirty-one women had died of complications—of infections, blood clots, failed organs, and leukemias. The news from Philadelphia was even more grim. The megadose chemotherapy regimen had not produced a hint of benefit, not "even a modest improvement," as the investigators glumly informed the audience. A complex and tangled trial from Sweden, with patients divided into groups and subgroups, was also headed inexorably toward failure with no obvious survival benefit in sight.

How, then, to reconcile these vastly disparate results? The president of the American Society of Clinical Oncology (ASCO) had asked a panel of discussants to try to hammer all the contradictory data into a single cohesive shape, but even the experts threw up their hands. "My goal here," one discussant began, frankly befuddled, "is to critique the data just presented, to maintain some credibility in the field, and to continue to remain friends with both the presenters and the discussants."

But even that would be a tall order. On and off the stage, the presenters and discussants bickered about small points, hurling critiques at each other's trials. Nothing was resolved and certainly no friendships were made. "People who like to transplant will continue to transplant, and people who don't will continue not to," Larry Norton, the powerful breast oncologist and president of the National Alliance of Breast Cancer Organizations (NABCO), told a journalist from the *New York Times*. The conference had been a disaster. As the exhausted audience trickled out of the massive auditorium in Atlanta, it was already dark outside and the warm, muggy blast of air provided no relief.

∽

Bezwoda left the Atlanta meeting in a hurry, leaving behind a field awash with confusion and tumult. He had underestimated the impact of his data, for it was now the sole fulcrum on which an entire theory of cancer therapy, not to mention a $4 billion industry, rested. Oncologists had come to Atlanta for clarity. They left exasperated and confused.

In December 1999, with the benefits of the regimen still uncertain and thousands of women clamoring for treatment, a team of American investigators wrote to Bezwoda at Witwatersrand to ask if they could travel to Johannesburg to examine the data from his trial in person. Bezwoda's transplants were the only ones that had succeeded. Perhaps important lessons could be learned and brought back to America.

Bezwoda readily agreed. On the first day of the visit, when the investigators requested the records and logbooks of the 154 patients in his study, Bezwoda sent them only 58 files—all, oddly, from the treatment arm of the trial. When the team pressed for records from the control arm, Bezwoda claimed that they had been "lost."

Mystified, the team probed further, and the picture began to turn disturbing. The records provided were remarkably shoddy: scratched-out, one-page notes with random scribbles written almost as an afterthought, summarizing six or eight months of supposed care. Criteria for eligibility for the trial were virtually always missing in the records. Bezwoda had claimed to have transplanted equal numbers of black and white women, yet nearly all the records belonged to poor, barely literate black women treated at the Hillbrow Hospital in Johannesburg. When the reviewers asked for consent forms for a procedure known to have deadly consequences, no such forms could be found. The hospital's review boards, meant to safeguard such protocols, certainly had no copies. No one, it seemed, had approved the procedure or possessed even the barest knowledge of the trial. Many of the patients counted as "alive" had long been discharged to terminal-care facilities with advanced, fungating lesions of breast cancer, presumably to die, with no designated follow-up. One woman counted in the treatment arm had never been treated with any drugs. Another patient record, tracked back to its origin, belonged to a man—not a patient with breast cancer.

The whole thing was a fraud, an invention, a sham. In late February 2000, with the trial unraveling and the noose of the investigation tightening around him every day, Werner Bezwoda wrote a terse typewritten letter to his colleagues at Witwatersrand admitting to having falsified parts of the study (he would later claim that he had altered his records to make the trial more "accessible" to American researchers). "I have committed a serious breach of scientific honesty and integrity," he wrote. He then resigned from his university position and promptly stopped giving interviews, referring all questions to his attorney. His phone number was unlisted in Johannesburg. In 2008, when I tried to reach him for an interview, Werner Bezwoda was nowhere to be found.

The epic fall of Werner Bezwoda was a terminal blow to the ambitions of megadose chemotherapy. In the summer of 1999, a final trial was designed to examine whether STAMP might increase survival among women with breast cancer that had spread to multiple lymph nodes. Four years later, the answer was clear. There was no discernible benefit. Of the five hundred patients assigned to the high-dose group, nine died of transplantation-related complications. An additional nine developed highly aggressive, chemotherapy-resistant acute myeloid leukemias as a consequence of their treatments—cancers far worse than the cancers that they had begun with. (Although entirely unsuccessful in breast cancers and many solid tumors, ABMT was subsequently shown to cure some lymphomas—again, highlighting the heterogeneity of cancers.)

"By the late 1990s, the romance was already over," Robert Mayer said.

"The final trials were merely trials meant to hammer the nails into the coffin. We had suspected the result for nearly a decade."

Maggie Keswick Jencks witnessed the end of the transplant era in 1995. Jencks, a landscape artist who lived in Scotland, created fantastical and desolate gardens—futuristic swirls of sticks, lakes, stones, and earth shored up against the disordered forces of nature. Diagnosed with breast cancer in 1988, she was treated with a lumpectomy and then a mastectomy. For several months, she considered herself cured. But five years later, just short of her fifty-second birthday, she relapsed with metastatic breast cancer in her liver, bones, and spine. At the Western General Hospital in Edinburgh, she was treated with high-dose chemotherapy followed with autologous transplant. Jencks did not know that the STAMP trial would eventually fail. "Dr. Bill Peters . . . had already treated several hundred patients with [transplantation]," she wrote, ever hopeful for a cure. "The average length of remission for his patients after treatment was eighteen months. It seemed like a lifetime." But Jencks's remission did not last a lifetime: in 1994, just short of her eighteenth month after transplantation, she relapsed again. She died in July 1995.

In an essay titled *A View from the Front Line,* Jencks described her experience with cancer as like being woken up midflight on a jumbo jet and then thrown out with a parachute into a foreign landscape without a map:

"There you are, the future patient, quietly progressing with other passengers toward a distant destination when, astonishingly (Why me?) a large hole opens in the floor next to you. People in white coats appear, help you into a parachute and—no time to think—*out you go.*

"You descend. You hit the ground. . . . But where is the enemy? *What* is the enemy? What is it up to? . . . No road. No compass. No map. No training. Is there something you should know and don't?

"The white coats are far, far away, strapping others into their parachutes. Occasionally they wave but, even if you ask them, *they don't know the answers.* They are up there in the Jumbo, involved with parachutes, not map-making."

The image captured the desolation and desperation of the era. Obsessed with radical and aggressive therapies, oncologists were devising newer and newer parachutes, but with no systematic maps of the quagmire to guide patients and doctors. The War on Cancer was "lost"—in both senses of the word.

Summer is a season of sequels, but no one, frankly, was looking forward to John Bailar's. Sequestered away at the University of Chicago, Bailar had been smoldering quietly in his office since his first article—"Progress Against Cancer?"—had sent a deep gash through the NCI's brow in May 1986. But eleven years had passed since the publication of that article, and Bailar, the nation's reminder-in-chief on cancer, was expected to explode with an update any day. In May 1997, exactly eleven years after the publication of his first article, Bailar was back in the pages of the *New England Journal of Medicine* with another appraisal of the progress on cancer.

The punch line of Bailar's article (coauthored with an epidemiologist named Heather Gornik) was evident in its title: "Cancer Undefeated." "In 1986," he began pointedly, "when one of us reported on trends in the incidence of cancer in the United States from 1950 through 1982, it was clear that some 40 years of cancer research, centered primarily on treatment, had failed to reverse a long, slow increase in mortality. Here we update that analysis through 1994. Our evaluation begins with 1970, both to provide some overlap with the previous article and because passage of the National Cancer Act of 1971 marked a critical increase in the magnitude and vigor of the nation's efforts in cancer research."

Little had changed in methodology from Bailar's earlier analysis. As before, Bailar and Gornik began by "age-adjusting" the U.S. population, such that every year between 1970 and 1994 contained exactly the same distribution of ages (the method is described in more detail in earlier pages). Cancer mortality for each age bracket was also adjusted proportionally, in effect, creating a frozen, static population so that cancer mortality could be compared directly from one year to the next.

The pattern that emerged from this analysis was sobering. Between 1970 and 1994, cancer mortality had, if anything, *increased* slightly, about 6 percent, from 189 deaths per 100,000 to 201 deaths. Admittedly, the death rate had plateaued somewhat in the last ten years, but even so, this could hardly be construed as a victory. Cancer, Bailar concluded, was still reigning "undefeated." Charted as a graph, the nation's progress on cancer was a flat line; the War on Cancer had, thus far, yielded a stalemate.

But was the flat line of cancer mortality truly inanimate? Physics teaches us to discriminate a static equilibrium from a dynamic equilibrium; the product of two equal and opposite reactions can seem to sit perfectly still until the opposing forces are uncoupled. What if the flat line of cancer mortality represented a dynamic equilibrium of counterbalanced forces pushing and pulling against each other?

As Bailar and Gornik probed their own data further, they began to discern such forces counterpoised against each other with almost exquisite precision. When cancer mortality between 1970 and 1994 was split into two age groups, the counterbalancing of forces was immediately obvious: in men and women above fifty-five, cancer mortality had increased, while in men and women under fifty-five, cancer mortality had decreased by exactly the same proportion. (Part of the reason for this will become clear below.)

A similar dynamic equilibrium was apparent when cancer mortality was reassessed by the *type* of cancer involved. Mortality had decreased for some forms, plateaued for others, and increased for yet others, offsetting nearly every gain with an equal and opposite loss. Death rates from colon cancer, for instance, had fallen by nearly 30 percent, and from cervical and uterine cancer by 20. Both diseases could be detected by screening tests (colonoscopy for colon cancer, and Pap smears for cervical cancer) and at least part of the decrease in mortality was the likely consequence of earlier detection.

Death rates for most forms of children's cancer had also declined since the 1970s, with declines continuing over the decade. So, too, had mortality from Hodgkin's disease and testicular cancer. Although the net number of such cancers still represented a small fraction of the total cancer mortality, treatment had fundamentally altered the physiognomy of these diseases.

The most prominent countervailing ballast against these advances was lung cancer. Lung cancer was still the single biggest killer among cancers, responsible for nearly one-fourth of all cancer deaths. Overall mortality for lung cancer had increased between 1970 and 1994. But the distribution of deaths was markedly skewed. Death rates among men had peaked and dropped off by the mid-1980s. In contrast, lung cancer mortality had dramatically risen in women, particularly in older women, and it was still rising. Between 1970 and 1994, lung cancer deaths among women over the age of fifty-five had increased by 400 percent, more than the rise in the rates of breast and colon cancer *combined*. This exponential upswing in mortality had effaced nearly all gains in survival not just for lung cancer, but for all other types of cancer.

Alterations in the pattern of lung cancer mortality also partially explained the overall age skew of cancer mortality. The incidence of lung cancer was highest in those above fifty-five, and was lower in men and women below fifty-five, a consequence of changes in smoking behavior since the 1950s. The decrease in cancer mortality in younger men and women had been perfectly offset by the increase in cancer mortality in older men and women.

Taken in balance, "Cancer Undefeated" was an article whose title belied its message. The national stalemate on cancer was hardly a stalemate, but rather the product of a frantic game of death in progress. Bailar had set out to prove that the War on Cancer had reached terminal stagnancy. Instead, he had chronicled a dynamic, moving battle in midpitch against a dynamic, moving target.

So even Bailar—*especially* Bailar, the fiercest and most inventive critic of the war—could not deny the fierce inventiveness of this war. Pressed on public television, he begrudgingly conceded the point:

> Interviewer: Why do you think they're going down a little bit, or plateau-ing?
> Bailar: We think they have gone down perhaps one percent. I would like to wait a little bit longer to see this downturn confirmed, but if it isn't here yet, it's coming. . . .
> Interviewer: Dr. Bailar?
> Bailar: I think we might agree that the cup is half-full.

જ્ઞ

No single strategy for prevention or cure had been a runaway success. But undeniably this "half-full cup" was the product of an astonishingly inge-nious array of forces that had been deployed against cancer. The vaunted promises of the 1960s and 1970s and the struggles of the 1980s had given way to a more grounded realism in the 1990s—but this new reality had brought its own promises.

Sharply critiquing the defeatism of Bailar and Gornik's assessment, Richard Klausner, the director of the NCI, pointed out:

"'Cancer' is, in truth, a variety of diseases. Viewing it as a single disease that will yield to a single approach is no more logical than viewing neu-ropsychiatric disease as a single entity that will respond to one strategy. It is unlikely that we will soon see a 'magic bullet' for the treatment of can-cer. But it is just as unlikely that there will be a magic bullet of prevention or early detection that will knock out the full spectrum of cancers. . . . We are making progress. Although we also have a long way to go, it is facile to claim that the pace of favorable trends in mortality reflects poor policies or mistaken priorities."

An era of oncology was coming to a close. Already, the field had turned away from its fiery adolescence, its entrancement with universal solutions and radical cures, and was grappling with fundamental questions about cancer. What were the underlying principles that governed the root behavior of a particular form of cancer? What was common to all cancers, and what made breast cancer different from lung or prostate cancer? Might those common pathways, or differences for that matter, establish new road maps to cure and prevent cancer?

The quest to combat cancer thus turned inward, toward basic biology, toward fundamental mechanisms. To answer these questions, we must turn inward, too. We must, at last, return to the cancer cell.

PART FIVE

"A DISTORTED VERSION OF OUR NORMAL SELVES"

It is in vain to speak of cures, or think of remedies, until such time as we have considered of the causes . . . cures must be imperfect, lame, and to no purpose, wherein the causes have not first been searched.
—Robert Burton,
The Anatomy of Melancholy, 1893

You can't do experiments to see what causes cancer. It's not an accessible problem and it's not the sort of thing scientists can afford to do.
—I. Hermann,
cancer researcher, 1978

What can be the "why" of these happenings?
—Peyton Rous,
1966, on the mystery
of the origin of cancer

"A unitary cause"

It is the spring of 2005—a pivot point in the medical oncology fellowship. Our paths are about to divide. Three of us will continue in the clinic, with a primary focus in clinical research and in the day-to-day care of patients. Four will explore cancer in the laboratory, retaining just a minor presence in the clinic, seeing just a handful of patients every week.

The choice between the two paths is instinctual. Some of us inherently perceive ourselves as clinicians; others primarily as scientists. My own inclinations have changed little since the first day of my internship. Clinical medicine moves me viscerally. But I am a lab rat, a nocturnal, peripatetic creature drawn to the basic biology of cancer. I mull over the type of cancer to study in the laboratory, and I find myself gravitating toward leukemia. I may be choosing the laboratory, but my subject of research is governed by a patient. Carla's disease has left its mark on my life.

Even so, in the fading twilight of my full-time immersion in the hospital, there are disquieting moments that remind me how deeply clinical medicine can surprise and engage me. It is late one evening in the fellows' room, and the hospital around us has fallen silent save for the metallic clink of cutlery being brought up for meals. The air outside is heavy with impending rain. The seven of us, close friends by now, are compiling lists of patients to pass on to the next class of fellows when Lauren begins to read her list aloud, calling out the names of those in her care who have died over our two-year fellowship. Suddenly inspired, she pauses and adds a sentence to each name as a sort of epitaph.

It is an impromptu memorial service, and it stirs something in the room. I join in, calling out names of my patients who have died and appending a sentence or two in memory.

Kenneth Armor, sixty-two, an internist with stomach cancer. In his final days, all he wished for was a vacation with his wife and time to play with his cats.

Oscar Fisher, thirty-eight, had small-cell lung cancer. Cognitively impaired since birth, he was his mother's favorite child. When he died, she was threading rosaries through his fingers.

That night I sit alone with my list, remembering the names and faces late into the evening. How does one memorialize a patient? These men and women have been my friends, my interlocutors, my teachers—a surrogate family. I stand up at my desk, as if at a funeral, my ears hot with emotion, my eyes full of tears. I look around the room at the empty desks and note how swiftly the last two years have reshaped all seven of us. Eric, cocksure, ambitious, and smart, is humbler and more introspective. Edwin, preternaturally cheerful and optimistic in his first month, talks openly about resignation and grief. Rick, an organic chemist by training, has become so infatuated with clinical medicine that he doubts that he will return to the laboratory. Lauren, guarded and mature, enlivens her astute assessments with jokes about oncology. Our encounter with cancer has rounded us off; it has smoothed and polished us like river rocks.

ॐ

A few days later, I meet Carla in the infusion room. She is casually chatting with the nurses, as if catching up with old friends. From a distance, she is barely recognizable. The sheet-white complexion I recall from her first visit to the hospital has warmed up several degrees of red. The bruises in her arm from repeated infusions have vanished. Her children are back in their routine, her husband has returned to work, her mother is home in Florida. Carla's life is nearly normal. She tells me that her daughter occasionally wakes up crying from a nightmare. When I ask her if this reflects some remnant trauma from Carla's yearlong ordeal with illness, she shakes her head assertively: "No. It's just monsters in the dark."

It has been a little more than a year since her original diagnosis. She is still taking pills of 6-mercaptopurine and methotrexate—Burchenal's drug and Farber's drug, a combination intended to block the growth of any remnant cancer cells. When she recalls the lowest points of her illness, she shudders in disgust. But something is normalizing and healing inside her. Her own monsters are vanishing, like old bruises.

When her blood counts return from the lab, they are stone-cold normal. Her remission continues. I am astonished and exalted by the news, but I bring it to her cautiously, as neutrally as I can. Like all patients, Carla smells overenthusiasm with deep suspicion: a doctor who raves disproportionately about small victories is the same doctor who might be preparing his patient for some ultimate defeat. But this time there is no reason to be suspicious. I tell her that her counts look perfect, and that no more tests are required today. In leukemia, she knows, no news is the best kind of news.

Late that evening, having finished my notes, I return to the laboratory. It is a beehive of activity. Postdocs and graduate students hover around the microscopes and centrifuges. Medical words and phrases are occasionally recognizable here, but the dialect of the lab bears little resemblance to the dialect of medicine. It is like traveling to a neighboring country—one that has similar mannerisms but speaks a different language:

"But the PCR on the leukemia cells should pick up the band."

"What conditions did you use to run this gel?"

"Agarose, four percent."

"Was the RNA degraded in the centrifugation step?"

I retrieve a plate of cells from the incubator. The plate has 384 tiny wells, each barely large enough to hold two grains of rice. In each well, I have placed two hundred human leukemia cells, then added a unique chemical from a large collection of untested chemicals. In parallel, I have its "twin" plate—containing two hundred normal human blood-forming stem cells, with the same panel of chemicals added to every well.

Several times each day, an automated microscopic camera will photograph each well in the two plates, and a computerized program will calculate the number of leukemia cells and normal stem cells. The experiment is seeking a chemical that can kill leukemia cells but spare normal stem cells—a specifically targeted therapy against leukemia.

I aspirate a few microliters containing the leukemia cells from one well and look at them under the microscope. The cells look bloated and grotesque, with a dilated nucleus and a thin rim of cytoplasm, the sign of a cell whose very soul has been co-opted to divide and to keep dividing with pathological, monomaniacal purpose. These leukemia cells have come into my laboratory from the National Cancer Institute, where they were grown and studied for nearly three decades. That these cells are still growing with obscene fecundity is a testament to the terrifying power of this disease.

The cells, technically speaking, are immortal. The woman from whose body they were once taken has been dead for thirty years.

As early as 1858, Virchow recognized this power of proliferation. Looking at cancer specimens under the microscope, Virchow understood that cancer was cellular hyperplasia, the disturbed, pathological growth of cells. But although Virchow recognized and described the core abnormality, he could not fathom its cause. He argued that inflammation—the body's reaction to a harmful injury, characterized by redness, swelling, and immune-system activation—caused cells to proliferate, leading to the outgrowth of malignant cells. He was almost right: chronic inflammation, smoldering over decades, does cause cancer (chronic hepatitis virus infection in the liver precipitates liver cancer), but Virchow missed the essence of the cause. Inflammation makes cells divide in response to injury, but this cell division is driven as a reaction to an external agent such as a bacteria or a wound. In cancer, the cell acquires *autonomous* proliferation; it is driven to divide by an internal signal. Virchow attributed cancer to the disturbed physiological milieu around the cell. He failed to fathom that the true disturbance lay within the cancer cell itself.

Two hundred miles south of Virchow's Berlin laboratory, Walther Flemming, a biologist working in Prague, tried to uncover the cause of abnormal cell division, although using salamander eggs rather than human cells as his subject. To understand cell division, Flemming had to visualize the inner anatomy of the cell. In 1879, Flemming thus stained dividing salamander cells with aniline, the all-purpose chemical dye used by Paul Ehrlich. The stain highlighted a blue, threadlike substance located deep within the cell's nucleus that condensed and brightened to a cerulean shade just before cell division. Flemming called his blue-stained structures *chromosomes*—"colored bodies." He realized that cells from every species had a distinct number of chromosomes (humans have forty-six; salamanders have fourteen). Chromosomes were duplicated during cell division and divided equally between the two daughter cells, thus keeping the chromosome number constant from generation to generation of cell division. But Flemming could not assign any further function to these mysterious blue "colored bodies" in the cell.

Had Flemming moved his lens from salamander eggs to Virchow's human specimens, he might have made the next crucial conceptual leap in understanding the root abnormality in cancer cells. It was Virchow's former assistant David Paul von Hansemann, following Flemming's and Virchow's trails, who made a logical leap between the two. Examining cancer cells stained with aniline dyes with a microscope, von Hansemann noticed that Flemming's chromosomes were markedly abnormal in cancer. The cells had split, frayed, disjointed chromosomes, chromosomes broken and rejoined, chromosomes in triplets and quadruplets.

Von Hansemann's observation had a profound corollary. Most scientists continued to hunt for parasites in cancer cells. (Bennett's theory of spontaneous suppuration still held a macabre fascination for some pathologists.) But von Hansemann proposed that the real abnormality lay in the structure of these bodies internal to cancer cells—in chromosomes—and therefore in the cancer cell itself.

But was it cause or effect? Had cancer altered the structure of chromosomes? Or had chromosomal changes precipitated cancer? Von Hansemann had observed a correlation between chromosomal change and cancer. What he needed was an experiment to causally connect the two.

The missing experimental link emerged from the lab of Theodor Boveri, yet another former assistant of Virchow's. Like Flemming, who worked with salamander cells, Boveri chose to study simple cells in simple organisms, eggs from sea urchins, which he collected on the windswept beaches near Naples. Urchin eggs, like most eggs in the animal kingdom, are strictly monogamous; once a single sperm has entered the egg, the egg puts up an instant barrier to prevent others from entering. After fertilization, the egg divides, giving rise to two, then four cells—each time duplicating the chromosomes and splitting them equally between the two daughter cells. To understand this natural chromosomal separation, Boveri devised a highly unnatural experiment. Rather than allowing the urchin egg to be fertilized by just one sperm, he stripped the outer membrane of the egg with chemicals and forcibly fertilized the egg with two sperms.

The multiple fertilization, Boveri found, precipitated chromosomal chaos. Two sperms fertilizing an egg results in three of each chromosome—a number impossible to divide evenly. The urchin egg, unable to divide the number of chromosomes appropriately among its daughter cells, was thrown into frantic internal disarray. The rare cell that got the right combination of all thirty-six sea urchin chromosomes developed normally. Cells that got the wrong combinations of chromosomes failed to develop or aborted development and involuted and died. Chromosomes, Boveri concluded, must carry information vital for the proper development and growth of cells.

This conclusion allowed Boveri to make a bold, if far-fetched, conjecture about the core abnormality in cancer cells. Since cancer cells possessed striking aberrations in chromosomes, Boveri argued that these chromosomal abnormalities might be the cause of the pathological growth characteristic of cancer.

Boveri found himself circling back to Galen—to the age-old notion that all cancers were connected by a common abnormality—the "unitary cause of carcinoma," as Boveri called it. Cancer was not "an unnatural group of different maladies," Boveri wrote. Instead, a common feature lurked behind all cancers, a uniform abnormality that emanated from abnormal chromosomes—and was therefore *internal* to the cancer cell. Boveri could not put his finger on the nature of this deeper internal abnormality. But the "unitary cause" of carcinoma lay in this disarray—not a chaos of black bile, but a chaos of blue chromosomes.

Boveri published his chromosomal theory of cancer in an elegant scientific pamphlet entitled "Concerning the Origin of Malignant Tumors" in 1914. It was a marvel of fact, fantasy, and inspired guesswork that stitched sea urchins and malignancy into the same fabric. But Boveri's theory ran into an unanticipated problem, a hard contradictory fact that it could not explain away. In 1910, four years before Boveri had published his theory, Peyton Rous, working at the Rockefeller Institute, had demonstrated that cancer in chickens could be caused by a virus, soon to be named the Rous sarcoma virus, or RSV.

The central problem was this: as causal agents, Rous's virus and Boveri's chromosomes were incompatible. A virus is a pathogen, an external agent, an invader exogenous to the cell. A chromosome is an internal entity, an endogenous structure buried deep inside the cell. The two opposites could not both claim to be the "unitary cause" of the same disease. How could an internal structure, a chromosome, and an external infectious agent, a virus, both create cancer?

In the absence of concrete proof for either theory, a viral cause for cancer seemed far more attractive and believable. Viruses, initially isolated in 1898 as minuscule infectious microbes that caused plant diseases, were becoming increasingly recognized as causes for a variety of animal and human diseases. In 1909, a year before Rous isolated his cancer-causing virus, Karl Landsteiner implicated a virus as the cause for polio. By the early 1920s, viruses that caused cowpox and human herpes infections had been isolated and grown in laboratories, further cementing the connection between viruses and human and animal diseases.

Undeniably, the belief in cause was admixed with the hope for a cure.

If the causal agent was exogenous and infectious, then a cure for cancer seemed more likely. Vaccination with cowpox, as Jenner had shown, prevented the much more lethal smallpox infection, and Rous's discovery of a cancer-causing virus (albeit in chickens) had immediately provoked the idea of a therapeutic cancer vaccine. In contrast, Boveri's theory that cancer was caused by a mysterious problem lurking in the threadlike chromosomes, stood on thin experimental evidence and offered no prospect for a cure.

ℐℓℴ

While the mechanistic understanding of the cancer cell remained suspended in limbo between viruses and chromosomes, a revolution in the understanding of normal cells was sweeping through biology in the early twentieth century. The seeds of this revolution were planted by a retiring, nearsighted monk in an isolated abbey in Brno, Austria, who bred pea plants as a hobby. In the early 1860s, working alone, Gregor Mendel had identified a few characteristics in his purebred plants that were inherited from one generation to the next—the color of the pea flower, the texture of the pea seed, the height of the pea plant. When Mendel intercrossed short and tall, or blue-flowering and green-flowering, plants using a pair of minute forceps, he stumbled on a startling phenomenon. Short plants bred with tall plants did not produce plants of intermediate height; they produced tall plants. Wrinkle-seeded peas crossed with smooth-seeded peas produced only wrinkled peas.

The implication of Mendel's experiment was far-reaching: inherited traits, Mendel proposed, are transmitted in discrete, indivisible packets. Biological organisms transmit "instructions" from one cell to its progeny by transferring these packets of information.

Mendel could only visualize these traits or properties in a descriptive sense—as colors, texture, or height moving from generation to generation; he could not see or fathom what conveyed this information from one plant to its progeny. His primitive lamplit microscope, with which he could barely peer into the interior of cells, had no power to reveal the mechanism of inheritance. Mendel did not even have the name for this unit of inheritance; decades later, in 1909, botanists would christen it a gene. But the name was still just a name; it offered no further explanation about a gene's structure or function. Mendel's studies left a provocative question hanging over biology for half a century: in what corporal, physical form was a "gene"—the particle of inheritance—carried inside the cell?

In 1910, Thomas Hunt Morgan, an embryologist at Columbia University in New York, discovered the answer. Like Mendel, Morgan was a compulsive breeder, but of fruit flies, which he raised by the thousands on rotting bananas in the Fly Room on the far edge of the Columbia campus. Again, like Mendel, Morgan discovered heritable traits moving indivisibly through his fruit flies generation upon generation—eye colors and wing patterns that were conveyed from parents to offspring without blending.

Morgan made another observation. He noted that an occasional rare trait, such as white eye color, was intrinsically linked to the gender of the fly: white eyes were found only in male flies. But "maleness"—the inheritance of sex—Morgan knew, was linked to chromosomes. So genes had to be carried on chromosomes—the threadlike structures identified by Flemming three decades earlier. Indeed, a number of Flemming's initial observations on the properties of chromosomes began to make sense to Morgan. Chromosomes were duplicated during cell division, and genes were duplicated as well and thus transmitted from one cell to the next, and from one organism to the next. Chromosomal abnormalities precipitated abnormalities in the growth and development of sea urchins, and so abnormal genes must have been responsible for this dysfunction. In 1915, Morgan proposed a crucial advance to Mendel's theory of inheritance: genes were borne on chromosomes. It was the transmission of chromosomes during cell division that allowed genes to move from a cell to its progeny.

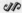

The third vision of the "gene" emerged from the work of Oswald Avery, a bacteriologist at the Rockefeller University in New York. Mendel had found that genes could move from one generation to the next; Morgan had proved that they did so by being carried on chromosomes. In 1926, Avery found that in certain species of bacteria, genes could also be transmitted *laterally* between two organisms—from one bacterium to its neighbor. Even dead, inert bacteria—no more than a conglomeration of chemicals—could transmit genetic information to live bacteria. This implied that an inert chemical was responsible for carrying genes. Avery separated heat-killed bacteria into their chemical components. And by testing each chemical component for its capacity to transmit genes, Avery and his colleagues reported in 1944 that genes were carried by one chemical, deoxyribonucleic acid, or DNA. What scientists had formerly disregarded as a form of cellular stuffing with no real function—a "stupid molecule," as the biologist Max Delbruck once called it dismissively—turned out to be the central conveyor of genetic information between cells, the least stupid of all molecules in the chemical world.

By the mid-1940s, three decades after biologists had coined the word, the molecular nature of the gene had come into focus. Functionally, a gene was a unit of inheritance that carried a biological trait from one cell to another or from one generation to the next. Physically, genes were carried within the cell in the form of chromosomes. Chemically, genes were composed of DNA, deoxyribonucleic acid.

જી૦

But a gene only carries information. The functional, physical, and chemical understanding of the gene begged a mechanistic understanding: How did genetic information become manifest inside the cell? What did a gene "do"—and how?

George Beadle, Thomas Morgan's student, switched from Morgan's fruit flies to an even more primitive organism, the slime mold, to answer these questions. Collaborating with the biochemist Edward Tatum at Stanford University in California, Beadle discovered that genes carried instructions to build proteins—complex, multidimensional macromolecules that were the workhorses of the cell.

Proteins, researchers found in the 1940s, carry out the bulk of cellular functions. They form enzymes, catalysts that speed up biochemical reactions vital to the life of the cell. Proteins are receptors for other proteins or molecules, responsible for transmitting signals from one cell to the next. They can create structural components of the cell, such as the molecular scaffolding that allows a cell to exist in a particular configuration in space. They can regulate other proteins, thus creating minuscule circuits inside the cell responsible for coordinating the life cycle of the cell.

Beadle and Tatum found that a gene "works" by providing the blueprint to build a protein. A protein is a gene realized—the machine built from a gene's instructions. But proteins are not created directly out of genes. In the late 1950s, Jacques Monod and François Jacob, working in Paris, Sydney Brenner and Matthew Meselson at Caltech, and Francis Crick in Cambridge, discovered that the genesis of proteins from genes requires an intermediary step—a molecule called ribonucleic acid, or RNA.

RNA is the working copy of the genetic blueprint. It is through RNA that a gene is translated into a protein. This intermediary RNA copy of a gene is called a gene's "message." Genetic information is transmitted from a cell to its progeny through a series of discrete and coordinated steps. First, genes, located in chromosomes, are duplicated when a cell divides and are transmitted into progeny cells. Next, a gene, in the form of DNA, is converted into its RNA copy. Finally, this RNA message is translated into a protein. The protein, the ultimate product of genetic information, carries out the function encoded by the gene.

An example, borrowed from Mendel and Morgan, helps illustrate the process of cellular information transfer. Red-eyed flies have glowering, ruby-colored eyes because they possess a gene that bears the information to build a red pigment protein. A copy of this gene is created every time a cell divides and it thus moves from a fly to its egg cells, and then into the cells of the offspring fly. In the eye cells of the progeny fly, this gene is "deciphered"—i.e., converted into an intermediate RNA message. The RNA message, in turn, instructs the eye cells to build the red pigment protein, thus giving rise to red-eyed flies of the next generation. Any interruption in this information flow might disrupt the transmission of the red eye trait—producing flies with colorless eyes.

This unidirectional flow of genetic information—DNA → RNA → protein—was found to be universal in living organisms, from bacteria to slime molds to fruit flies to humans. In the mid-1950s, biologists termed this the "central dogma" of molecular biology.

જીૐ

An incandescent century of biological discovery—spanning from Mendel's discovery of genes in 1860 to Monod's identification of the RNA copy of genes in the late 1950s—illuminated the inner workings of a normal cell. But it did little to illuminate the workings of a cancer cell or the cause of cancer—except in two tantalizing instances.

The first came from human studies. Nineteenth-century physicians had noted that some forms of cancer, such as breast and ovarian cancer, tended to run in families. This in itself could not prove a hereditary cause: families share not just genes, but also habits, viruses, foods, exposures to chemicals, and neurotic behaviors—all factors, at some time or another, implicated as causes of cancer. But occasionally, a family history was so striking that a hereditary cause (and, by extension, a *genetic* cause) could not be ignored.

In 1872, Hilário de Gouvêa, a Brazilian ophthalmologist practicing in Rio, treated a young boy with a rare cancer of the eye called a retinoblastoma by removing the eye surgically. The boy had survived, grown up, and married a woman with no family history of cancer. The couple had several children, and two of the daughters developed their father's retinoblastoma in both eyes—and died. De Gouvêa reported this case as a puzzling enigma. He did not possess the language of genetics, but to later observers, the case suggested an inherited factor that "lived" in genes and caused cancer. But such cases were so rare that it was hard to test this hypothesis experimentally, and de Gouvêa's report was largely ignored.

The second time scientists circled around the cause of cancer—almost hitting the nerve spot of carcinogenesis—came several decades after the strange Brazilian case. In the 1910s, Thomas Hunt Morgan, the fruit fly geneticist at Columbia, noticed that mutant flies occasionally appeared within his flock of flies. In biology, mutants are defined as organisms that differ from the normal. Morgan noticed that an enormous flock of flies with normal wings might occasionally give birth to a "monster" with rough or scalloped wings. These mutations, Morgan discovered, were the results of alterations in genes and the mutations could be carried from one generation to the next.

But what caused mutations? In 1928, Hermann Joseph Muller, one of Morgan's students, discovered that X-rays could vastly increase the rate of mutation in fruit flies. At Columbia, Morgan had produced mutant flies spontaneously. (When DNA is copied during cell division, a copying error occasionally generates an accidental change in genes, thus causing mutations.) Muller found that he could accelerate the incidence of these accidents. Using X-rays to bombard flies, he found that he could produce hundreds of mutant flies over a few months—more than Morgan and his colleagues had produced using their vast breeding program over nearly two decades.

The link between X-rays and mutations nearly led Morgan and Muller to the brink of a crucial realization about cancer. Radiation was known to cause cancer. (Recall Marie Curie's leukemia, and the tongue cancers of the radium-watch makers.) Since X-rays also caused mutations in fruit fly genes, could cancer be a disease of *mutations*? And since mutations were changes in genes, could genetic alterations be the "unitary cause" of cancer?

Had Muller and Morgan, student and mentor, pitched their formidable scientific skills together, they might have answered this question and uncovered this essential link between mutations and malignancy. But once close colleagues, they became pitted and embittered rivals. Cantankerous and rigid with old age, Morgan refused to give Muller full recognition for his theory of mutagenesis, which he regarded as a largely derivative observation. Muller, in turn, was sensitive and paranoid; he felt that Morgan had stolen his ideas and taken an undue share of credit. In 1932, having moved his lab to Texas, Muller walked into the nearby woods and swallowed a roll of sleeping pills in an attempted suicide. He survived, but haunted by anxiety and depression, his scientific productivity lapsed in his later years.

Morgan, in turn, remained doggedly pessimistic about the relevance of the fruit fly work in understanding human diseases. In 1933, Morgan received the Nobel Prize in Physiology or Medicine for his far-reaching work on fruit fly genetics. (Muller would receive the Nobel Prize independently in 1946.) But Morgan wrote self-deprecatingly about the medical relevance of his work, "The most important contribution to medicine that genetics has made is, in my opinion, intellectual." At some point far in the future, he imagined a convergence between medicine and genetics. "Possibly," he speculated, "the doctor may then want to call in his geneticist friends for consultation!"

But to oncologists in the 1940s, such a "consultation" seemed far-fetched. The hunt for an internal, genetic cause of cancer had stalled since Boveri. Pathological mitosis was visible in cancerous tissue. But both geneticists and embryologists failed to answer the key question: what caused mitosis to turn so abruptly from such an exquisitely regulated process to chaos?

More deeply, what had failed was a kind of biological imagination. Boveri's mind had so acrobatically leapt from sea urchins to carcinomas, or Morgan's from pea plants to fruit flies, in part because biology itself was leaping from organism to organism, finding systematic cellular blueprints that ran deeply through all the living world. But extending that same blueprint to human *diseases* had turned out to be a much more challenging task. At Columbia, Morgan had assembled a fair collection of fruit fly monsters, but none that even remotely resembled a real human affliction. The notion that the cancer doctor might call in a "genetic friend" to help understand the pathophysiology of cancer seemed laughable.

Cancer researchers would return to the language of genes and mutations again in the 1970s. But the journey back to this language—and to the true "unitary" cause of cancer—would take a bewildering detour through the terrain of new biology, and a further fifty years.

Under the Lamps of Viruses

Unidentified flying objects, abominable snowmen, the
Loch Ness monster and human cancer viruses.
—*Medical World News*, 1974,
on four "mysteries" widely reported
and publicized but never seen

The biochemist Arthur Kornberg once joked that the discipline of modern biology in its early days often operated like the man in the proverbial story who is frantically searching for his keys under a streetlamp. When a passerby asks the man whether he lost his keys at that spot, the man says that he actually lost them at home—but he is looking for the keys under the lamp because "the light there is the brightest."

In the predawn of modern biology, experiments were so difficult to perform on biological organisms, and the results of manipulations so unpredictable, that scientists were severely constrained in their experimental choices. Experiments were conducted on the simplest model organisms—fruit flies, sea urchins, bacteria, slime molds—because the "light" there was the brightest.

In cancer biology, Rous's sarcoma virus represented the only such lamplit spot. Admittedly, it was a rare virus that produced a rare cancer in a species of chicken.* But it was the most reliable way to produce a real cancer in a living organism. Cancer researchers knew that X-rays, soot, cigarette smoke, and asbestos represented vastly more common risk factors for human cancers. They had heard of the odd Brazilian case of a family that seemed to carry retinoblastoma cancer in its genes. But the capacity to *manipulate* cancer in an experimental environment was

---

* Other cancer-causing viruses, such as SV40 and human papillomavirus (HPV), would eventually be discovered in 1960 and 1983, respectively.

unique to the Rous virus, and so it stood center stage, occupying all the limelight.

The appeal of studying Rous virus was further compounded by the formidable force of Peyton Rous's personality. Bulldogish, persuasive, and inflexible, Rous had acquired a near paternal attachment to his virus, and he was unwilling to capitulate to any other theory of cause. He acknowledged that epidemiologists had shown that exogenous carcinogens were *correlated* with cancer (Doll and Hill's study, published in 1950, had clearly shown that smoking was associated with an increase in lung cancer), but this had not offered any mechanistic explanation of cancer causation. Viruses, Rous felt, were the only answer.

By the early 1950s, cancer researchers had thus split into three feuding camps. The virologists, led by Rous, claimed that viruses caused cancer, although no such virus had been found in human studies. Epidemiologists, such as Doll and Hill, argued that exogenous chemicals caused cancer, although they could not offer a mechanistic explanation for their theory or results. The third camp, of Theodor Boveri's successors, stood at the farthest periphery. They possessed weak, circumstantial evidence that genes internal to the cell might cause cancer, but had neither the powerful human data of the epidemiologists nor the exquisite experimental insights of the chicken virologists. Great science emerges out of great contradiction, and here was a gaping rift slicing its way through the center of cancer biology. Was human cancer caused by an infectious agent? Was it caused by an exogenous chemical? Was it caused by an internal gene? How could the three groups of scientists have examined the same elephant and returned with such radically variant opinions about its essential anatomy?

In 1951, a young virologist named Howard Temin, then a postdoctoral researcher, arrived at the California Institute of Technology in Pasadena, California, to study the genetics of fruit flies. Restless and imaginative, Temin soon grew bored with fruit flies. Switching fields, he chose to study Rous sarcoma virus in Renato Dulbecco's laboratory. Dulbecco, a suave, exquisitely mannered Calabrian aristocrat, ran his lab at Caltech with a distant and faintly patrician air. Temin was a perfect fit: if Dulbecco wanted distance, Temin wanted independence. Temin found a house in Pasadena with several other young scientists (including John Cairns, the future author of the *Scientific American* article on the War on Cancer) and spent his time cooking up unusual meals in heavy communal pots and talking volubly about biological riddles late into the night.

In the laboratory, too, Temin was cooking up an unusual experiment that was virtually guaranteed to fail. Until the late fifties, Rous sarcoma virus had been shown to cause tumors only in live chickens. Temin, working closely with Harry Rubin, wanted to study how the virus converted normal cells into cancer cells. To do this, they needed a vastly simplified system—a system free of chickens and tumors, and analogous to bacteria in a petri dish. And so Temin imagined creating *cancer* in a petri dish. In 1958, in his seventh year in Dulbecco's lab, Temin succeeded. He added Rous sarcoma virus to a layer of normal cells in a petri dish. The infection of the cells incited them to grow uncontrollably, forcing them to form tiny distorted heaps containing hundreds of cells that Temin called foci (the plural of *focus*). The foci, Temin reasoned, represented cancer distilled into its essential, elemental form: cells growing uncontrollably, unstoppably—pathological mitosis. It was the sheer, driving power of Temin's imagination that allowed him to look at a tiny heap of cells and reimagine that heap as the essence of the diffuse systemic disease that kills humans. But Temin believed that the cell, and its interaction with the virus, had all the biological components necessary to drive the malignant process. The ghost was out of the organism.

Temin could now use his cancer-in-a-dish to perform experiments that would have been nearly impossible using whole animals. One of his first experiments with this system, performed in 1959, produced an unexpected result. Normally, viruses infect cells, produce more viruses, and infect more cells, but they do not directly affect the genetic makeup, the DNA, of the cell. Influenza virus, for instance, infects lung cells and produces more influenza virus, but it does not leave a permanent fingerprint in our genes; when the virus goes away, our DNA is left untouched. But Rous's virus behaved differently. Rous sarcoma virus, having infected the cells, had *physically* attached itself to the cell's DNA and thereby altered the cell's genetic makeup, its genome. "The virus, in some structural as well as functional sense, becomes part of the genome of the cell," Temin wrote.*

This observation—that a DNA copy of a virus's genes could structurally attach itself to a cell's genes—intrigued Temin and Dulbecco. But it

---

* Temin's statement was speculative, but it bore his unerring biological instinct. Formal proof of the structural attachment of RSV genes into the cellular genome would only come years later.

raised an even more intriguing conceptual problem. In viruses, genes are sometimes carried in their intermediary RNA form. Certain viruses have dispensed with the original DNA copy of genes and keep their genome in the RNA form, which is directly translated into viral proteins once the virus infects a cell.

Temin knew from work performed by other researchers that Rous sarcoma virus is one such RNA virus. But if the virus genes *started* as RNA, then how could a copy of its genes convert into DNA? The central dogma of molecular biology forbade such a transition. Biological information, the dogma proposed, only travels down a one-way street from DNA to RNA to proteins. How on earth, Temin wondered, could RNA turn around acrobatically and make a DNA copy of itself, driving the wrong way down the one-way street of biological information?

Temin made a leap of faith; if the data did not fit the dogma, then the dogma—not the data—needed to be changed. He postulated that Rous sarcoma virus carried a special property, a property unprecedented in any other living organism: it could convert RNA back into DNA. In normal cells, the conversion of DNA into RNA is called transcription. The virus (or the infected cell) therefore had to possess the reverse capacity: *reverse* transcription. "Temin had an inkling, but his proof was so circumstantial—so frail—that he could barely convince anyone," the virologist Michael Bishop recalled twenty-five years later. "The hypothesis had earned him little but ridicule and grief."

৶৶

At first, Temin could barely even convince himself. He had made a bold proposition, but he needed proof. In 1960, determined to find experimental proof, Temin moved his lab to the McArdle laboratory in Wisconsin. Madison, unlike Caltech, was a frozen, faraway place, isolated both physically and intellectually, but this suited Temin. Standing unknowingly at the edge of a molecular revolution, he wanted silence. On his daily walk along Lakeshore path, often blanketed in dense snow, Temin planned experiments to find evidence for this reverse flow of information.

RNA into DNA. Even the thought made him shiver: a molecule that could write history backward, turn back the relentless forward flow of biological information. To prove that such a process existed, Temin would need to isolate in a test tube the viral enzyme that could reverse transcription and prove that it could make a DNA copy out of RNA. In the early 1960s, pursuing the enzyme, he hired a Japanese postdoctoral student named Satoshi Mizutani. Mizutani's task was to purify this reverse transcription enzyme from virus-infected cells.

Mizutani was a catastrophe. Never a cell biologist at heart, as a colleague recalled, he contaminated the cells, infected the cultures, and grew out balls of fungi in the petri dishes. Frustrated, Temin moved Mizutani to a project involving no cells. If Mizutani couldn't manipulate cells, he could try to purify the enzyme out of chemical extracts made from virus-infected cells. The move played to Mizutani's natural skills: he was an incredibly gifted chemist. Overnight, he picked up a weak, flickering enzymatic activity in the cellular extracts of the Rous virus that was capable of converting RNA into DNA. When he added RNA to this cellular extract, he could "see" it creating a DNA copy—reversing transcription. Temin had his proof. Rous sarcoma virus was no ordinary virus. It could write genetic information backward: it was a *retro*virus.*

At MIT, in Boston, another young virologist, David Baltimore, had also picked up the hint of an RNA → DNA conversion activity, although in a different retrovirus. Brilliant, brash, and single-minded, Baltimore had met and befriended Howard Temin in the 1940s at science summer camp in Maine, where Temin had been a teaching assistant and Baltimore a student. They had parted ways for nearly a decade, yet their intellectual paths had kept crisscrossing. As Temin was exploring reverse transcription in Rous sarcoma virus in Madison, Baltimore had begun to amass evidence that his retrovirus also possessed an enzyme that could convert RNA into DNA. He, too, was steps away from isolating the enzyme.

On the afternoon of May 27, 1970, a few weeks after he had found initial evidence for the RNA → DNA converting enzyme in his lab, Temin caught a flight to Houston to present his work at the Tenth International Cancer Congress. The next morning, he walked to the cavernous auditorium at the Houston Civic Center. Temin's talk was entitled "The Role of DNA in the Replication of RNA Viruses," a title left intentionally bland. It was a short, fifteen-minute session. The room was filled mainly with tumor virus specialists, many already dozing off to sleep.

But as Temin began to unfold his findings, the importance of his talk dawned on the audience. On the surface, as one researcher recalled, "It was all very dry biochemistry. . . . Temin spoke in his usual nasal, high-pitched

---

* The term *retrovirus* was coined later by virologists.

monotone, giving no indication of excitement." But the significance of the work crystallized out of the dry biochemical monotone. Temin was not just talking about viruses. He was systematically dismantling one of the fundamental principles of biology. His listeners became restive, unnerved. By the time Temin reached the middle of the talk, there was an awestruck silence. Scientists in the audience were feverishly taking notes, filling page after page with harrowed scribbles. Once outside the conference room, Temin recalled, "You could see people on the telephone. . . . People called people in their laboratories." Temin's announcement that he had identified the long-sought-after enzyme activity in the virus-infected cells left little doubt about the theory. RNA could *generate* DNA. A cancer-causing virus's genome could become a physical part of a cell's genes.

Temin returned to Madison the next morning to find his laboratory inundated with phone messages. The most urgent of these was from David Baltimore, who had heard an inkling of Temin's news from the meeting. Temin called him back.

"You know there is [an enzyme] in the virus particles," Baltimore said.

"I know," said Temin.

Baltimore, who had kept his own work very, very quiet, was stunned. "How do you know?"

"We found it."

Baltimore had also found it. He, too, had identified the RNA → DNA enzymatic activity from the virus particles. Each laboratory, working apart, had converged on the same result. Temin and Baltimore both rushed their observations to publication. Their twin reports appeared back-to-back in *Nature* magazine in the summer of 1970.

In their respective papers, Temin and Baltimore proposed a radical new theory about the life cycle of retroviruses. The genes of retroviruses, they postulated, exist as RNA outside cells. When these RNA viruses infect cells, they make a DNA copy of their genes and attach this copy to the cell's genes. This DNA copy, called a provirus, makes RNA copies, and the virus is regenerated, phoenixlike, to form new viruses. The virus is thus constantly shuttling states, rising from the cellular genome and falling in again—RNA to DNA to RNA; RNA to DNA to RNA—ad infinitum.

It is surely a sign of the prevailing schizophrenia of the time that Temin's work was instantly embraced as a possible mechanistic explanation for cancer by cancer scientists, but largely ignored by clinical oncologists. Temin's presentation in Houston was part of a mammoth meeting on cancer. Both Farber and Frei had flown in from Boston to attend. Yet, the conference epitomized the virtually insurmountable segregation between cancer therapy and cancer science. Chemotherapy and surgery were discussed in one room. Viral carcinogenesis was discussed in another. It was as if a sealed divider had been constructed through the middle of the world of cancer, with "cause" on one side and "cure" on the other. Few scientists or clinical oncologists crossed between the two isolated worlds. Frei and Farber returned to Boston with no significant change in the trajectories of their thoughts about curing cancer.

Yet for some scientists attending the conference, Temin's work, pushed to its logical extreme, suggested a powerful mechanistic explanation for cancer, and thus a well-defined path toward a cure. Sol Spiegelman, a Columbia University virologist known for his incendiary enthusiasm and relentless energy, heard Temin's talk and instantly built a monumental theory out of it—a theory so fiercely logical that Spiegelman could almost conjure it into reality. Temin had suggested that an RNA virus could enter a cell, make a DNA copy of its genes, and attach itself to a cell's genome. Spiegelman was convinced that this process, through a yet unknown mechanism, could activate a viral gene. That activated viral gene must induce the infected cell to proliferate—unleashing pathological mitosis, cancer.

It was a tantalizingly attractive explanation. Rous's viral theory of the origin of cancer would fuse with Boveri's internal genetic theory. The virus, Temin had shown, could *become* an endogenous element attached to a cell's genes, and thus both an internal aberration and an exogenous infection would be responsible for cancer. "Spiegelman's conversion to the new religion [of cancer viruses] took only minutes," Robert Weinberg, the MIT cancer biologist recalled. "The next day [after Temin's conference] he was back in his lab at Columbia University in New York City, setting up a repeat of the work."

Spiegelman raced off to prove that retroviruses caused human cancers. "It became his single-minded preoccupation," Weinberg recalled. The obsession bore fruit quickly. For Spiegelman's schema to work, he would need to prove that human cancers had retrovirus genes hidden inside them. Working fast and hard, Spiegelman found traces of retroviruses in human leukemia, in breast cancer, lymphomas, sarcomas, brain tumors, melanomas—in nearly every human cancer that he examined. The Special

Virus Cancer Program, launched in the 1950s to hunt for human cancer viruses, and moribund for two decades, was swiftly resuscitated: here, at long last, were the thousands of cancer viruses that it had so long waited to discover. Money poured into Spiegelman's lab from the SVCP's coffers. It was a perfect folie à deux—endless funds fueling limitless enthusiasm and vice versa. The more Spiegelman looked for retroviruses in cancer cells, the more he found, and the more funds were sent his way.

In the end, though, Spiegelman's effort turned out to be systematically flawed. In his frenzied hunt for human cancer retroviruses, Spiegelman had pushed the virus-detection test so hard that he saw viruses or traces of viruses that did not exist. When other labs around the nation tried to replicate the work in the mid-1970s, Spiegelman's viruses were nowhere to be found. Only one human cancer, it turned out, was caused by a human retrovirus—a rare leukemia endemic in some parts of the Caribbean. "The hoped-for human virus slipped quietly away into the night," Weinberg wrote. "The hundreds of millions of dollars spent by the SVCP . . . could not make it happen. The rocket never left its launching pad."

Spiegelman's conjecture about human retroviruses was half-right and half-wrong: he was looking for the right kind of virus but in the wrong kind of cell. Retroviruses would turn out to be the cause of a different disease—not cancer. Spiegelman died in 1983 of pancreatic cancer, having heard of a strange illness erupting among gay men and blood-transfusion recipients in New York and San Francisco. One year after Sol Spiegelman's death in New York, the cause of that disease was finally identified. It was a human retrovirus called HIV.

"The hunting of the sarc"

For the Snark was a Boojum, you see.
—Lewis Carroll

Sol Spiegelman had got hopelessly lost hunting for cancer-causing retroviruses in humans. His predicament was symptomatic: cancer biology, the NCI, and the targeted Special Virus Cancer Program had all banked so ardently on the existence of human cancer retroviruses in the early 1970s that when the viruses failed to materialize, it was as if some essential part of their identity or imagination had been amputated. If human cancer retroviruses did not exist, then human cancers must be caused by some other mysterious mechanism. The pendulum, having swung sharply toward an infectious viral cause of cancer, swung just as sharply away.

Temin, too, had dismissed retroviruses as the causal agents for human cancer by the mid-1970s. His discovery of reverse transcription had certainly overturned the dogma of cellular biology, but it had not pushed the understanding of human *carcinogenesis* far. Viral genes could attach themselves to cellular genes, Temin knew, but this could not explain how viruses caused cancer.

Faced with yet another discrepancy between theory and data, Temin proposed another bold conjecture—again, standing on the thinnest foundation of evidence. Spiegelman and the retrovirus hunters, Temin argued, had conflated analogy with fact, confused messenger with message. Rous sarcoma virus could cause cancer by inserting a viral gene into cells. This proved that genetic alterations could cause cancer. But the genetic alteration, Temin proposed, need not originate in a virus. The virus had merely brought a message into a cell. To understand the genesis of cancer, it was that culprit *message*—not the messenger—that needed to be identified. Cancer virus hunters needed to return to their lamplit virus again, but this time with new questions: What was the viral gene that had unleashed pathological mitosis in cells? And how was that gene related to an internal mutation in the cell?

In the 1970s, several laboratories began to home in on that gene. Fortuitously, RSV possesses only four genes in its genome. In California, by then the hotbed of cancer virus research, the virologists Steve Martin, Peter Vogt, and Peter Duesberg made mutants of the Rous virus that replicated normally, but could no longer create tumors—suggesting that the tumor-causing gene had been disrupted. By analyzing the genes altered in these mutant viruses, these groups finally pinpointed RSV's cancer-causing ability to a single gene in the virus. The gene was called *src* (pronounced "sarc"), a diminutive of *sarcoma*.

Src, then, was the answer to Temin's puzzle, the cancer-causing "message" borne by Rous sarcoma virus. Vogt and Duesberg removed or inactivated *src* from the virus and demonstrated that the *src*-less virus could neither induce cell proliferation nor cause transformation. *Src*, they speculated, was some sort of malformed gene acquired by RSV during its evolution and introduced into normal cells. It was termed an oncogene,* a gene capable of causing cancer.

A chance discovery in Ray Erikson's laboratory at the University of Colorado further elucidated *src*'s function. Erikson had been a graduate student in Madison in the early 1960s when Temin had found retroviruses. Erikson had followed the discovery of the *src* gene in California and had been haunted by the function of *src* ever since. In 1977, working with Mark Collett and Joan Brugge, Erikson set out to decipher the function of *src*. *Src*, Erikson discovered, was an unusual gene. It encoded a protein whose most prominent function was to modify other proteins by attaching a small chemical, a phosphate group, to these proteins—in essence, playing an elaborate game of molecular tag.† Indeed, scientists had found a number of similar proteins in normal cells—enzymes that attached phosphate groups to other proteins. These enzymes were called the "kinases," and they were soon found to behave as molecular master switches within a cell. The attachment of the phosphate group to a protein acted like an "on" switch—activating the protein's function. Often, a kinase turned "on" another kinase, which turned "on" another kinase, and so forth. The signal

---

* The term *oncogene* had been coined earlier by two NCI scientists, Robert Huebner and George Todaro, in 1969, although on scant evidence.

† Art Levinson, in Mike Bishop's lab at UCSF, also discovered this phosphorylating activity; we will return to Levinson's discovery in later pages.

was amplified at each step of the chain reaction, until many such molecular switches were thrown into their "on" positions. The confluence of many such activated switches produced a powerful internal signal to a cell to change its "state"—moving, for instance, from a nondividing to a dividing state.

Src was a prototypical kinase—although a kinase on hyperdrive.* The protein made by the viral *src* gene was so potent and hyperactive that it phosphorylated anything and everything around it, including many crucial proteins in the cell. *Src* worked by unleashing an indiscriminate volley of phosphorylation—throwing "on" dozens of molecular switches. In *src*'s case, the activated series of proteins eventually impinged on proteins that controlled cell division. *Src* thus forcibly induced a cell to change its state from nondividing to dividing, ultimately inducing accelerated mitosis, the hallmark of cancer.

By the late 1970s, the combined efforts of biochemists and tumor virologists had produced a relatively simple view of *src*'s ability to transform cells. Rous sarcoma virus caused cancer in chickens by introducing into cells a gene, *src,* that encoded a hyperactive overexuberant kinase. This kinase turned "on" a cascade of cellular signals to divide relentlessly. All of this represented beautiful, careful, meticulously crafted work. But with no human cancer retroviruses in the study, none of this research seemed relevant immediately to human cancers.

∽∾

Yet the indefatigable Temin still felt that viral *src* would solve the mystery of human cancers. In Temin's mind, there was one riddle yet to be solved: the evolutionary origin of the *src* gene. How might a virus have "acquired" a gene with such potent, disturbing qualities? Was *src* a viral kinase gone berserk? Or was it a kinase that the virus had constructed out of bits of other genes like a cobbled-together bomb? Evolution, Temin knew, could build new genes out of old genes. But where had Rous sarcoma virus found the necessary components of a gene to make a chicken cell cancerous?

At the University of California in San Francisco (UCSF), in a building perched high on one of the city's hills, a virologist named J. Michael

---

* Genes encode proteins—but a gene *(src)* and its protein *(src* kinase) are occasionally denoted by the same name. Biologists use context to determine whether one is referring to a gene or its protein.

Bishop became preoccupied with the evolutionary origin of viral *src*. Born in rural Pennsylvania, where his father had been a Lutheran minister, Bishop had studied history at Gettysburg College, then drastically altered his trajectory to attend Harvard Medical School. After a residency at Massachusetts General Hospital, he had trained as a virologist. In the 1960s, Bishop had moved to UCSF to set up a lab to explore viruses.

UCSF was then a little-known, backwater medical school. Bishop's shared office occupied a sliver of space at the edge of the building, a room so cramped and narrow that his office-mate had to stand up to let him through to his desk. In the summer of 1969, when a lanky, self-assured researcher from the NIH, Harold Varmus, then on a hiking trip in California, knocked on Bishop's office door to ask if he might join the lab to study retroviruses, there was hardly any standing room at all.

Varmus had come to California seeking adventure. A former graduate student in literature, he had become enthralled by medicine, obtained his M.D. at Columbia University in New York, then learned virology at the NIH. Like Bishop, he was also an academic itinerant—wandering from medieval literature to medicine to virology. Lewis Carroll's *Hunting of the Snark* tells the story of a motley crew of hunters that launch an agonizing journey to trap a deranged, invisible creature called the Snark. That hunt goes awfully wrong. Unpromisingly, as Varmus and Bishop set off to understand the origins of the *src* gene in the early 1970s, other scientists nicknamed the project "the hunting of the sarc."

Varmus and Bishop launched their hunt using a simple technique—a method invented, in part, by Sol Spiegelman in the 1960s. Their goal was to find cellular genes that were distantly similar to the viral *src* gene—and thus find *src*'s evolutionary precursors. DNA molecules typically exist as paired, complementary strands, like yin and yang, that are "stuck" together by powerful molecular forces. Each strand, if separated, can thus stick to another strand that is complementary in structure. If one molecule of DNA is tagged with radioactivity, it will seek out its complementary molecule in a mixture and stick to it, thereby imparting radioactivity to the second molecule. The sticking ability can be measured by the amount of radioactivity.

In the mid-1970s, Bishop and Varmus began to use the viral *src* gene to hunt for its homologues, using this "sticking" reaction. *Src* was a viral gene, and they expected to find only fragments or pieces of *src* in normal cells—ancestors and distant relatives of the cancer-causing *src* gene. But the hunt soon took a mystifying turn. When Varmus and Bishop looked in normal cells, they did not find a genetic third or fifth cousin of *src*. They found a nearly identical version of viral *src* lodged firmly in the normal cell's genome.

Varmus and Bishop, working with Deborah Spector and Dominique Stehelin, probed more cells, and again the *src* gene appeared in them: in duck cells, quail cells, and geese cells. Closely related homologues of the *src* gene were strewn all over the bird kingdom; each time Varmus's team looked up or down an evolutionary branch, they found some variant of *src* staring back. Soon, the UCSF group was racing through multiple species to look for homologues of *src*. They found *src* in the cells of pheasants, turkeys, mice, rabbits, and fish. Cells from a newborn emu at the Sacramento zoo had *src*. So did sheep and cows. Most important, so did human cells. "*Src*," Varmus wrote in a letter in 1976, ". . . is everywhere."

But the *src* gene that existed in normal cells was not identical to the viral *src*. When Hidesaburo Hanafusa, a Japanese virologist at Rockefeller University in New York, compared the viral *src* gene to the normal cellular *src* gene, he found a crucial difference in the genetic code between the two forms of *src*. Viral *src* carried mutations that dramatically affected its function. Viral *src* protein, as Erikson had found in Colorado, was a disturbed, hyperactive kinase that relentlessly tagged proteins with phosphate groups and thus provided a perpetually blaring "on" signal for cell division. Cellular *src* protein possessed the same kinase activity, but it was far less hyperactive; in contrast to viral *src*, it was tightly regulated—turned "on" and turned "off"—during cell division. The viral *src* protein, in contrast, was a permanently activated switch—"an automaton," as Erikson described it—that had turned the cell into a dividing machine. Viral *src*—the cancer-causing gene—was cellular *src* on overdrive.

A theory began to convulse out of these results, a theory so magnificent and powerful that it would explain decades of disparate observations in a single swoop: *perhaps* src, *the precursor to the cancer-causing gene, was endogenous to the cell.* Perhaps viral *src* had *evolved* out of cellular *src*. Retrovirologists had long believed that the virus had introduced an activated *src* into normal cells to transform them into malignant cells. But the *src* gene had not originated in the virus. It had originated from a precursor gene that existed in a cell—in *all* cells. Cancer biology's decades-long hunt had started with a chicken and ended, metaphorically, in the egg—in a progenitor gene present in all human cells.

Rous's sarcoma virus, then, was the product of an incredible evolutionary accident. Retroviruses, Temin had shown, shuttle constantly out of the cell's genome: RNA to DNA to RNA. During this cycling, they can pick up pieces of the cell's genes and carry them, like barnacles, from one cell to another. Rous's sarcoma virus had likely picked up an activated *src* gene from a cancer cell and carried it in the viral genome, creating more cancer. The virus, in effect, was no more than an accidental courier for a gene that had originated in a cancer cell—a parasite parasitized by cancer. Rous had been wrong—but spectacularly wrong. Viruses did cause cancer, but they did so, typically, by tampering with genes that originate in cells.

✧✧

Science is often described as an iterative and cumulative process, a puzzle solved piece by piece, with each piece contributing a few hazy pixels of a much larger picture. But the arrival of a truly powerful new theory in science often feels far from iterative. Rather than explain one observation or phenomenon in a single, pixelated step, an entire field of observations suddenly seems to crystallize into a perfect whole. The effect is almost like watching a puzzle solve itself.

Varmus and Bishop's experiments had precisely such a crystallizing, zippering effect on cancer genetics. The crucial implication of the Varmus and Bishop experiment was that a precursor of a cancer-causing gene—the "proto-oncogene," as Bishop and Varmus called it—was a normal cellular gene. Mutations induced by chemicals or X-rays caused cancer not by "inserting" foreign genes into cells, but by activating such *endogenous* proto-oncogenes.

"Nature," Rous wrote in 1966, "sometimes seems possessed of a sardonic humor." And the final lesson of Rous sarcoma virus had been its most sardonic by far. For nearly six decades, the Rous virus had seduced biologists—Spiegelman most sadly among them—down a false path. Yet the false path had ultimately circled back to the right destination—from viral *src* toward cellular *src* and to the notion of internal proto-oncogenes sitting omnipresently in the normal cell's genome.

In Lewis Carroll's poem, when the hunters finally capture the deceptive Snark, it reveals itself not to be a foreign beast, but one of the human hunters sent to trap it. And so it had turned out with cancer. Cancer genes came from *within* the human genome. Indeed the Greeks had been peculiarly prescient yet again in their use of the term *oncos*. Cancer was intrinsically "loaded" in our genome, awaiting activation. We were destined to carry this fatal burden in our genes—our own genetic "oncos."

Varmus and Bishop were awarded the Nobel Prize for their discovery of the cellular origin of retroviral oncogenes in 1989. At the banquet in Stockholm, Varmus, recalling his former life as a student of literature, read lines from the epic poem *Beowulf*, recapitulating the slaying of the dragon in that story: "We have not slain our enemy, the cancer cell, or figuratively torn the limbs from his body," Varmus said. "In our adventures, we have only seen our monster more clearly and described his scales and fangs in new ways—ways that reveal a cancer cell to be, like Grendel, a distorted version of our normal selves."

The Wind in the Trees

The fine, fine wind that takes its course through the chaos of the world
Like a fine, an exquisite chisel, a wedge-blade inserted . . .

—D. H. Lawrence

The developments of the summer of 1976 drastically reorganized the universe of cancer biology, returning genes, again, to its center. Harold Varmus and Michael Bishop's proto-oncogene theory provided the first cogent and comprehensive theory of carcinogenesis. The theory explained how radiation, soot, and cigarette smoke, diverse and seemingly unrelated insults, could all initiate cancer—by mutating and thus activating precursor oncogenes within the cell. The theory made sense of Bruce Ames's peculiar correlation between carcinogens and mutagens: chemicals that cause mutations in DNA produce cancers because they alter cellular proto-oncogenes. The theory clarified why the same kind of cancer might arise in smokers and nonsmokers, albeit at different rates: both smokers and nonsmokers have the same proto-oncogenes in their cells, but smokers develop cancer at a higher rate because carcinogens in tobacco increase the mutation rate of these genes.

But what did human cancer genes look like? Tumor virologists had found *src* in viruses and then in cells, but surely other endogenous proto-oncogenes were strewn about in the human cellular genome.

Genetics has two distinct ways to "see" genes. The first is structural: genes can be envisioned as physical structures—pieces of DNA lined up along chromosomes, just as Morgan and Flemming had first envisioned them. The second is functional: genes can be imagined, à la Mendel, as the inheritance of traits that move from one generation to the next. In the decade between 1970 and 1980, cancer genetics would begin to "see" cancer-causing genes in these two lights. Each distinct vision would enhance the mechanistic understanding of carcinogenesis, bringing the field closer and closer to an understanding of the core molecular aberration in human cancers.

Structure—anatomy—came first. In 1973, as Varmus and Bishop were launching their initial studies on *src*, a hematologist in Chicago, Janet Rowley, saw a human cancer gene in a physical form. Rowley's specialty was studying the staining patterns of chromosomes in cells in order to locate chromosomal abnormalities in cancer cells. Chromosome staining, the technique she had perfected, is as much an art as a science. It is also an oddly anachronistic art, like painting with tempera in an age of digital prints. At a time when cancer genetics was zooming off to explore the world of RNA, tumor viruses, and oncogenes, Rowley was intent on dragging the discipline back to its roots—to Boveri's and Flemming's chromosomes dyed in blue. Piling anachronism upon anachronism, the cancer she had chosen to study was chronic myelogenous leukemia (CML)—Bennett's infamous "suppuration of blood."

Rowley's study was built on prior work by a duo of pathologists from Philadelphia who had also studied CML. In the late 1950s, Peter Nowell and David Hungerford had found an unusual chromosomal pattern in this form of leukemia: the cancer cells bore one consistently shortened chromosome. Human cells have forty-six chromosomes—twenty-three matched pairs—one inherited from each parent. In CML cells, Nowell found that one copy of the twenty-second chromosome had its head lopped off. Nowell called the abnormality the Philadelphia chromosome after the place of its discovery. But Nowell and Hungerford could not understand where the decapitated chromosome had come from, or where its missing "head" had gone.

Rowley, following this study, began to trace the headless chromosome in her CML cells. By laying out exquisitely stained photographs of CML chromosomes enlarged thousands of times—she typically spread them on her dining table and then leaned into the pictures, hunting for the missing pieces of the infamous Philadelphia chromosome—Rowley found a pattern. The missing head of chromosome twenty-two had attached itself elsewhere—to the tip of chromosome nine. And a piece of chromosome nine had conversely attached itself to chromosome twenty-two. This genetic event was termed a translocation—the flip-flop transposition of two pieces of chromosomes.

Rowley examined case after case of CML patients. In every single case, she found this same translocation in the cells. Chromosomal abnormalities in cancer cells had been known since the days of von Hansemann and Boveri. But Rowley's results argued a much more profound point. Cancer was not disorganized chromosomal chaos. It was *organized* chromosomal chaos: specific and identical mutations existed in particular forms of cancer.

Chromosomal translocations can create new genes called chimeras by fusing two genes formerly located on two different chromosomes—the "head" of chromosome nine, say, fused with the "tail" of a gene in chromosome thirteen. The CML translocation, Rowley postulated, had created such a chimera. Rowley did not know the identity or function of this new chimeric monster. But she had demonstrated that a novel, unique genetic alteration—later found to be an oncogene—could exist in a human cancer cell, revealing itself purely by virtue of an aberrant chromosome structure.

ॐ

In Houston, Alfred Knudson, a Caltech-trained geneticist, also "saw" a human cancer-causing gene in the early 1970s, although in yet another distinct sense.

Rowley had visualized cancer-causing genes by studying the physical structure of the cancer cell's chromosomes. Knudson concentrated monastically on the function of a gene. Genes are units of inheritance: they shuttle properties—traits—from one generation to the next. If genes cause cancer, Knudson reasoned, then he might capture a pattern in the inheritance of cancer, much as Mendel had captured the idea of a gene by studying the inheritance of flower color or plant height in peas.

In 1969, Knudson moved to the MD Anderson Cancer Center in Texas, where Freireich had set up a booming clinical center for childhood cancers. Knudson needed a "model" cancer, a hereditary malignancy whose underlying pattern of inheritance would reveal how cancer-causing genes worked. The natural choice was retinoblastoma, the odd, rare variant of eye cancer that de Gouvêa had identified in Brazil with its striking tendency to erupt in the same family across generations.

Retinoblastoma is a particularly tragic form of cancer, not just because it assaults children but because it assaults the quintessential organ of childhood: the tumor grows in the eye. Afflicted children are sometimes diagnosed when the world around them begins to blur and fade. But occasionally the cancer is incidentally found in a child's photograph when the eye, lit by a camera flash, glows eerily like a cat's eyes in lamplight, revealing the tumor buried behind the lens. Left untreated, the tumor will crawl backward from the eye socket into the optic nerve, and then climb into the brain. The primary methods of treatment are to sear the tumor with high doses of gamma radiation or to enucleate the eye surgically, leaving behind an empty socket.

Retinoblastoma has two distinct variants, an inherited "familial" form and a sporadic form. De Gouvêa had identified the familial form. Children who suffer from this familial or inherited form may carry strong family histories of the disease—fathers, mothers, cousins, siblings, and kindred affected—and they typically develop tumors in both eyes, as in de Gouvêa's case from Rio. But the tumor also arises in children with no family history of the disease. Children with this sporadic form never carry a history in the family and always have a tumor in only one eye.

This pattern of inheritance intrigued Knudson. He wondered whether he could discern a subtle difference in the development of cancer between the sporadic and the inherited versions using mathematical analyses. He performed the simplest of experiments: he grouped children with the sporadic form into one cohort and children with the familial form in a second. And sifting through old hospital records, Knudson tabulated the ages in which the disease struck the two groups, then plotted them as two curves. Intriguingly, he found that the two cohorts developed the cancers at different "velocities." In inherited retinoblastoma, cancer onset was rapid, with diagnosis typically two to six months after birth. Sporadic retinoblastoma typically appeared two to four years after birth.

But why did the same disease move with different velocities in different children? Knudson used the numbers and simple equations borrowed from physics and probability theory to model the development of the cancer in the two cohorts. He found that the data fit a simple model. In children with the inherited form of retinoblastoma, only one genetic change was required to develop the cancer. Children with the sporadic form required two genetic changes.

This raised another puzzling question: why was only one genetic change needed to unleash cancer in the familial case, while two changes were needed in the sporadic form? Knudson perceived a simple, beautiful explanation. "The number two," he recalled, "is the geneticist's favorite number." Every normal human cell has two copies of each chromosome and thus two copies of every gene. Every normal cell must have two normal copies of the retinoblastoma gene—*Rb*. To develop sporadic retinoblastoma, Knudson postulated, both copies of the gene needed to be inactivated through a mutation in each copy of the *Rb* gene. Hence, sporadic retinoblastoma develops at later ages because two independent mutations have to accumulate in the same cell.

Children with the inherited form of retinoblastoma, in contrast, are born with a defective copy of *Rb*. In their cells, one gene copy is already defective, and only a single additional genetic mutation is needed before the cell senses the change and begins to divide. These children are thus predisposed to the cancer, and they develop cancer faster, producing the "rapid velocity" tumors that Knudson saw in his statistical charts. Knudson called this the two-hit hypothesis of cancer. For certain cancer-causing genes, two mutational "hits" were needed to provoke cell division and thus produce cancer.

Knudson's two-hit theory was a powerful explanation for the inheritance pattern of retinoblastoma, but at first glance it seemed at odds with the initial molecular understanding of cancer. The *src* gene, recall, requires a single activated copy to provoke uncontrolled cell division. Knudson's gene required two. Why was a single mutation in *src* sufficient to provoke cell division, while two were required for *Rb*?

The answer lies in the function of the two genes. *Src activates* a function in cell division. The mutation in *src*, as Ray Erikson and Hidesaburo Hanafusa had discovered, creates a cellular protein that is unable to extinguish its function—an insatiable, hyperactive kinase on overdrive that provokes perpetual cell division. Knudson's gene, *Rb,* performs the opposite function. It *suppresses* cell proliferation, and it is the inactivation of such a gene (by virtue of two hits) that unleashes cell division. *Rb,* then, is a cancer *suppressor* gene—the functional opposite of *src*—an "anti-oncogene," as Knudson called it.

"Two classes of genes are apparently critical in the origin of the cancers of children," he wrote. "One class, that of oncogenes, acts by virtue of abnormal or elevated activity. . . . The other class, that of anti-oncogenes [or tumor suppressors], is recessive in oncogenesis; cancer results when both normal copies have been mutated or deleted. Some persons carry one such mutation in the germline and are highly susceptible to tumor because only one somatic event is necessary. Some children, even though carrying no such mutation in the germline, can acquire tumor as a result of two somatic events."

It was an exquisitely astute hypothesis spun, remarkably, out of statistical reasoning alone. Knudson did not know the molecular identity of his phantasmic anti-oncogenes. He had never looked at a cancer cell to "see" these genes; he had never performed a biological experiment to pin down *Rb*. Like Mendel, Knudson knew his genes only in a statistical sense. He had inferred them, as he put it, "as one might infer the wind from the movement of the trees."

✺

By the late 1970s, Varmus, Bishop, and Knudson could begin to describe the core molecular aberration of the cancer cell, stitching together the coordinated actions of oncogenes and anti-oncogenes. Cancer genes, Knudson proposed, came in two flavors. "Positive" genes, such as *src*, are mutant *activated* versions of normal cellular genes. In normal cells, these genes accelerate cell division, but only when the cell receives an appropriate growth signal. In their mutant form, these genes are driven into perpetual hyperactivity, unleashing cell division beyond control. An activated proto-oncogene, to use Bishop's analogy, is "a jammed accelerator" in a car. A cell with such a jammed accelerator careens down the path of cell division, unable to cease mitosis, dividing and dividing again relentlessly.

"Negative" genes, such as *Rb*, suppress cell division. In normal cells, these anti-oncogenes, or tumor suppressor genes, provide the "brakes" to cellular proliferation, shutting down cell division when the cell receives appropriate signals. In cancer cells, these brakes have been inactivated by mutations. In cells with missing brakes, to use Bishop's analogy again, the "stop" signals for mitosis can no longer be registered. Again, the cell divides and keeps dividing, defying all signals to stop.

Both abnormalities, activated proto-oncogenes and inactivated tumor suppressors ("jammed accelerators" and "missing brakes"), represent the core molecular defects in the cancer cell. Bishop, Knudson, and Varmus did not know how many such defects were ultimately needed to cause human cancers. But a confluence of them, they postulated, causes cancer.

A Risky Prediction

They see only their own shadows or the shadows of one another, which the fire throws on the opposite wall of the cave.

—Plato

The philosopher of science Karl Popper coined the term *risky prediction* to describe the process by which scientists verify untested theories. Good theories, Popper proposed, generate risky predictions. They presage an unanticipated fact or event that runs a real risk of not occurring or being proven incorrect. When this unanticipated fact proves true or the event does occur, the theory gains credibility and robustness. Newton's understanding of gravitation was most spectacularly validated when it accurately presaged the return of Halley's comet in 1758. Einstein's theory of relativity was vindicated in 1919 by the demonstration that light from distant stars is "bent" by the mass of the sun, just as predicted by the theory's equations.

By the late 1970s, the theory of carcinogenesis proposed by Varmus and Bishop had also generated at least one such risky prediction. Varmus and Bishop had demonstrated that precursors of oncogenes—proto-oncogenes—existed in all normal cells. They had found activated versions of the *src* proto-oncogene in Rous sarcoma virus. They had suggested that mutations in such internal genes caused cancer—but a crucial piece of evidence was still missing. If Varmus and Bishop were right, then mutated versions of such proto-oncogenes must exist *inside cancer cells*. But thus far, although other scientists had isolated an assortment of oncogenes from retroviruses, no one had isolated an activated, mutated oncogene out of a cancer cell.

"Isolating such a gene," as the cancer biologist Robert Weinberg put it, "would be like walking out of a cave of shadows. . . . Where scientists had previously only seen oncogenes indirectly, they might see these genes, in flesh and blood, living inside the cancer cell."

Robert Weinberg was particularly concerned with getting out of shadows. Trained as a virologist in an era of great virologists, he had worked in Dulbecco's lab at the Salk Institute in the sixties isolating DNA from monkey viruses to study their genes. In 1970, when Temin and Baltimore had discovered reverse transcriptase, Weinberg was still at the bench, laboriously purifying genes out of monkey viruses. Six years later, when Varmus and Bishop had announced the discovery of cellular *src,* Weinberg was still purifying DNA from viruses. Weinberg felt as if he was stuck in a perpetual penumbra, surrounded by fame but never famous himself. The retrovirus revolution, with all its mysteries and rewards, had quietly passed him by.

In 1972, Weinberg moved to MIT, to a small laboratory a few doors down from Baltimore's lab to study cancer-causing viruses. "The chair of the department," he said, "considered me quite a fool. A good fool. A hardworking fool, but still a fool." Weinberg's lab occupied a sterile, uninspiring space at MIT, in a sixties-style brutalist building served by a single creaking elevator. The Charles River was just far enough to be invisible from the windows, but just near enough to send freezing puffs of wind through the quadrangle in the winter. The building's basement connected to a warren of tunnels with airless rooms where keys were cut and machines repaired for other labs.

Labs, too, can become machines. In science, it is more often a pejorative description than a complimentary one: an efficient, thrumming, technically accomplished laboratory is like a robot orchestra that produces perfectly pitched tunes but no music. By the mid-1970s, Weinberg had acquired a reputation among his colleagues as a careful, technically competent scientist, but one who lacked direction. Weinberg felt his work was stagnating. What he needed was a simple, clear question.

Clarity came to him one morning in the midst of one of Boston's infamously blinding blizzards. On a February day in 1978, walking to work, Weinberg was caught in an epic snowstorm. Public transportation had ground to a halt, and Weinberg, in a rubber hat and galoshes, had chosen to plod across the blustering Longfellow Bridge from his home to his lab, slowly planting his feet through the slush. The snow blotted out the landscape and absorbed all sounds, creating a silent, hypnotic interior. And as Weinberg crossed the frozen river, he thought about retroviruses, cancer, and human cancer genes.

Src had been so easy to isolate and identify as a cancer-causing gene, Weinberg knew, because Rous sarcoma virus possesses a measly four genes. One could scarcely turn around in the retroviral genome without bumping into an oncogene. A cancer cell, in contrast, has about twenty thousand genes. Searching for a cancer-causing gene in that blizzard of genes was virtually hopeless.

But an oncogene, by definition, has a special property: it provokes unbridled cellular proliferation in a normal cell. Temin had used this property in his cancer-in-a-dish experiment to induce cells to form "foci." And as Weinberg thought about oncogenes, he kept returning to this essential property.

Of the twenty thousand genes in a cancer cell, Weinberg reasoned the vast majority were likely normal and only a small minority were mutated proto-oncogenes. Now imagine, for a moment, being able to take all twenty thousand genes in the cancer cell, the good, the bad, the ugly, and transferring them into twenty thousand normal cells, such that each cell receives one of the genes. The normal, unmutated genes will have little effect on the cells. But an occasional cell will receive an oncogene, and, goaded by that signal, it will begin to grow and reproduce insatiably. Reproduced ten times, these cells will form a little clump on a petri dish; at twelve cell divisions, that clump will form a visible "focus"—cancer distilled into its primordial, elemental form.

The snowstorm was Weinberg's catharsis; he had rid himself of retroviruses. If activated oncogenes existed within cancer cells, then transferring these genes into normal cells should induce these normal cells to divide and proliferate. For decades, cancer biologists had relied on Rous sarcoma virus to introduce activated *src* into cells and thereby incite cell division. But Weinberg would bypass Rous's virus; he would determine if cancer-causing genes could be transferred *directly* from cancer cells to normal cells. At the end of the bridge, with snow still swirling around him, he found himself at an empty intersection with lights still flashing. He crossed it, heading to the cancer center.

Weinberg's immediate challenge was technical: how might he transfer DNA from a cancer cell to a population of normal cells? Fortunately, this was one of the technical skills that he had so laboriously perfected in the laboratory during his stagnant decade. His chosen method of DNA transfer began with the purification of DNA from cancer cells, grams of it precipitated out of cell extracts in a dense, flocculent suspension, like curdled milk. This DNA was then sheared into thousands of pieces, each piece carrying one or two genes. To transfer this DNA into cells, he next needed a carrier, a molecule that would slip DNA into the interior of a cell. Here, Weinberg used a trick. DNA binds to the chemical calcium phosphate to form minuscule white particles. These particles are ingested by cells, and as the cells ingest these particles, they also ingest the DNA pieces bound to the calcium phosphate. Sprinkled on top of a layer of normal cells growing in a petri dish, these particles of DNA and calcium phosphate resemble a snowglobe of swirling white flakes, the blizzard of genes that Weinberg had so vividly imagined in his walk in Boston.

Once that DNA blizzard had been sprinkled on the cells and internalized by them, Weinberg envisioned a simple experiment. The cell that had received the oncogene would embark on unbridled growth, forming the proliferating focus of cells. Weinberg would isolate such foci and then purify the DNA fragment that had induced the proliferation. He would thus capture a real human oncogene.

In the summer of 1979, Chiaho Shih, a graduate student in Weinberg's lab, began to barrel his way through fifteen different mouse cancer cells, trying to find a fragment of DNA that would produce foci out of normal cells. Shih was laconic and secretive, with a slippery, quicksilver temper, often paranoid about his experiments. He was also stubborn: when he disagreed with Weinberg, colleagues recalled him thickening his accent and pretending not to understand English, a language he spoke with ease and fluency under normal circumstances. But for all his quirks, Shih was also a born perfectionist. He had learned the DNA transfection technique from his predecessors in the lab, but even more important, he had an instinctive feel for his cells, almost a gardener's instinct to discriminate normal versus abnormal growth.

Shih grew enormous numbers of normal cells in petri dishes and sprinkled them weekly with genes derived from his panel of cancer cells. Plate after plate of transfected cells piled up in the laboratory. As Weinberg had imagined in his walk across the river, Shih soon stumbled upon a crucial early result. He found that transferring DNA from mouse cancer cells invariably produced foci in normal cells, proof that oncogenes could be discovered through such a method.*

Excited and mystified, Weinberg and Shih performed a bolder variant of the experiment. Thus far they had been using mouse cancer cell lines to obtain their DNA. Changing tactics and species, they moved on to human cancer cells. "If we were going to trap a real oncogene so laboriously," Weinberg recalled, "we thought that we might as well find it in real human cancers." Shih walked over to the Dana-Farber Cancer Institute and carried back a cancer cell line derived from a patient, Earl Jensen, a long-term smoker who had died of bladder cancer. DNA from these cells was sheared into fragments and transfected into the normal human cell line. Shih returned to his microscope, scouring plate after plate for foci.

The experiment worked yet again. As with the mouse cancer cell lines, prominent, disinhibited foci appeared in the dishes. Weinberg pushed Shih to find the precise gene that could convert a normal cell to a cancer cell. Weinberg's laboratory was now racing to isolate and identify the first native human oncogene.

He soon realized the race had other contenders. At the Farber, across town, Geoff Cooper, a former student of Temin's, had also shown that DNA from cancer cells could induce transformation in cells. So had Michael Wigler at the Cold Spring Harbor Lab in New York. And Weinberg, Cooper, and Wigler had yet other competitors. At the NCI, a little-known Spanish researcher named Mariano Barbacid had also found a fragment of DNA from yet another cancer cell line that would transform normal cells. In the late winter of 1981, all four laboratories rushed to the finish line. By the early spring, each lab had found its sought-after gene.

In 1982, Weinberg, Barbacid, and Wigler independently published their discoveries and compared their results. It was a powerful, unexpected convergence: all three labs had isolated the same fragment of DNA, containing a gene called *ras,* from their respective cancer cells.† Like *src, ras* was also a gene present in all cells. But like *src* again, the *ras* gene in normal

___

* In fact, the "normal" cells that Weinberg had used were not exactly normal. They were already growth-adapted, such that a single activated oncogene could tip them into transformed growth. Truly "normal" cells, Weinberg would later discover, require several genes to become transformed.

† In fact, *ras,* like *src,* had also been discovered earlier in a cancer-causing virus—again underscoring the striking capacity of these viruses to reveal the mechanisms of endogenous oncogenes.

cells was functionally different from the *ras* present in cancer cells. In normal cells, the *ras* gene encoded a tightly regulated protein that turned "on" and "off" like a carefully modulated switch. In cancer cells, the gene was mutated, just as Varmus and Bishop had predicted. Mutated *ras* encoded a berserk, perpetually hyperactive protein permanently locked "on." This mutant protein produced an unquenchable signal for a cell to divide—and to keep dividing. It was the long-sought "native" human oncogene, captured in flesh and blood out of a cancer cell. "Once we had cloned a cancer gene," Weinberg wrote, "the world would be at our feet." New insights into carcinogenesis, and new therapeutic inroads would instantly follow. "It was," as Weinberg would later write, all "a wonderful pipe dream."

In 1983, a few months after Weinberg had purified mutant *ras* out of cancer cells, Ray Erikson traveled to Washington to receive the prestigious General Motors prize for his research on *src* activity and function. The other awardee that evening was Tom Frei, being honored for his advancement of the cure for leukemia.

It was a resplendent evening. There was an elegant candlelit dinner in a Washington banquet hall, followed by congratulatory speeches and toasts. Scientists, physicians, and policymakers, including many of the former Laskerites,* gathered around linen-covered tables. Talk turned frequently to the discovery of oncogenes and the invention of curative chemotherapy. But the two conversations seemed to be occurring in sealed and separate universes, much as they had at Temin's conference in Houston more than a decade earlier. Frei's award, for curing leukemia, and Erikson's award, for identifying the function of a critical oncogene, might almost have been given to two unconnected pursuits. "I don't remember any enthusiasm among the clinicians to reach out to the cancer biologists to synthesize the two poles of knowledge about cancer," Erikson recalled. The two halves of cancer, cause and cure, having feasted and been feted together, sped off in separate taxis into the night.

---

* The Laskerites had largely been disbanded in the aftermath of the 1971 National Cancer Act. Mary Lasker was still involved in science policy, although with nowhere near the force and visceral energy that she had summoned in the sixties.

The discovery of *ras* brought one challenge to a close for cancer geneticists: they had purified a mutated oncogene from a cancer cell. But it threw open another challenge. Knudson's two-hit hypothesis had also generated a risky prediction: that retinoblastoma cancer cells contained two inactivated copies of the *Rb* gene. Weinberg, Wigler, and Barbacid had proved Varmus and Bishop right. Now someone had to prove Knudson's prediction by isolating his fabled tumor suppressor gene and demonstrating that both its copies were inactivated in retinoblastoma.

This challenge, though, came with an odd conceptual twist. Tumor suppressor genes, by their very nature, are asserted in their *absence*. An oncogene, when mutated, provides an "on" signal for the cells to grow. A tumor suppressor gene when mutated, in contrast, removes an "off" signal for growth. Weinberg and Chiaho Shih's transfection assay had worked because oncogenes can cause the normal cells to divide uncontrollably, thus forming a focus of cells. But an anti-oncogene, transfected into a cell, cannot be expected to create an "anti-focus." "How can one capture genes that behave like ghosts," Weinberg wrote, "influencing cells from behind some dark curtain?"

In the mid-1980s, cancer geneticists had begun to glimpse shadowy outlines behind retinoblastoma's "dark curtain." By analyzing chromosomes from retinoblastoma cancer cells using the technique pioneered by Janet Rowley, geneticists had demonstrated that the *Rb* gene "lived" on chromosome thirteen. But a chromosome contains thousands of genes. Isolating a single gene from that vast set—particularly one whose functional presence was revealed only when inactive—seemed like an impossible task. Large laboratories professionally equipped to hunt for cancer genes—Webster Cavenee's lab in Cincinnati, Brenda Gallie's in Toronto, and Weinberg's in Boston—were frantically hunting for a strategy to isolate *Rb*. But these efforts had reached a standstill. "We knew where *Rb* lived," Weinberg recalled, "but we had no idea what *Rb* was."

Across the Charles River from Weinberg's lab, Thad Dryja, an ophthalmologist-turned-geneticist, had also joined the hunt for *Rb*. Dryja's laboratory was perched on the sixth floor of the Massachusetts Eye and Ear Infirmary—the Eyeball, as it was known colloquially among the medical residents. The ophthalmological infirmary was well-known for its clinical research on eye diseases, but was barely recognized for laboratory-based research. Weinberg's Whitehead Institute boasted the power of the latest technologies, an army of machines that could sequence thousands of DNA samples and powerful fluorescent microscopes that could look down into the very heart of the cell. In contrast, the Eyeball, with its proud display of nineteenth-century eyeglasses and lenses in lacquered wooden vitrines, was almost self-indulgently anachronistic.

Dryja, too, was an unlikely cancer geneticist. In the mid-1980s, having completed his clinical fellowship in ophthalmology at the infirmary in Boston, he had crossed town to the science laboratories at Children's Hospital to study the genetics of eye diseases. As an ophthalmologist interested in cancer, Dryja had an obvious target: retinoblastoma. But even Dryja, an inveterate optimist, was hesitant about taking on the search for *Rb*. "Brenda [Gallie] and Web [Cavenee] had both stalled in their attempts [to clone *Rb*]. It was a slow, frustrating time."

Dryja began his hunt for *Rb* with a few key assumptions. Normal human cells, he knew, have two copies of every chromosome (except the sex chromosomes), one from each parent, twenty-three pairs of chromosomes in all, a total of forty-six. Every normal cell thus has two copies of the *Rb* gene, one in each copy of chromosome thirteen.

Assuming Knudson was right in his two-hit hypothesis, every eye tumor should possess two independent inactivating mutations in the *Rb* gene, one in each chromosome. Mutations, Dryja knew, come in many forms. They can be small changes in DNA that can activate a gene. Or they can be large structural deletions in a gene, stretching over a large piece of the chromosome. Since the *Rb* gene had to be *inactivated* to unleash retinoblastoma, Dryja reasoned that the mutation responsible was likely a deletion of the gene. Deleting a sizable piece of a gene, after all, is perhaps the quickest, crudest way to paralyze and inactivate it.

In most retinoblastoma tumors, Dryja suspected, the two deletions in the two copies of the *Rb* gene would lie in different parts of the gene. Since mutations occur randomly, the chance of both mutations lying in precisely the same region of the gene is a little akin to rolling double sixes in dice that have one hundred faces. Typically, one of the deletions would "hit" the front end of the gene, while the other deletion might hit the back end (in both cases, the functional consequences would be the same—inactivating *Rb*). The two "hits" in most tumors would thus be asymmetric—affecting two different parts of the gene on the two chromosomes.

But even hundred-headed dice, rolled many times, can yield double sixes. Rarely, Dryja knew, one might encounter a tumor in which both hits had deleted exactly the same part of the gene on the two sister chromosomes. In that case, that piece of chromosome would be completely missing from the cell. And if Dryja could find a method to identify a completely missing piece of chromosome thirteen in a retinoblastoma tumor cell, he would instantly land on the *Rb* gene. It was the simplest of strategies: to hunt the gene with absent function, Dryja would look for absence in structure.

To identify such a missing piece, Dryja needed structural mileposts along chromosome thirteen—small pieces of DNA called probes, which were aligned along the length of the chromosome. He could use these DNA probes in a variant of the same "sticking" reaction that Varmus and Bishop had used in the 1970s: if the piece of DNA existed in the tumor cell, it would stick; if the piece did not exist, the probe would not stick, identifying the missing piece in the cell. Dryja had assembled a series of such probes. But more than probes, he needed a resource that he uniquely possessed: an enormous bank of frozen tumors. The chances of finding a shared deletion in the *Rb* gene in both chromosomes were slim, so he would need to test a vast sample set to find one.

This, then, was his crucial advantage over the vast professional labs in Toronto and Houston. Laboratory scientists rarely venture outside the lab to find human samples. Dryja, a clinician, had a freezer full of them. "I stored the tumors obsessively," he said with the childlike delight of a collector. "I put news out among patients and doctors that I was looking for retinoblastoma cases. Every time someone saw a case, they would say, 'Get that guy Dryja.' I would then drive or fly or even walk to pick up the samples and bring them here. I even got to know the patients by name. Since the disease ran in families, I would call them at home to see if there was a brother or sister or cousin with retinoblastoma. Sometimes, I would know [about a tumor] even before doctors knew."

Week after week, Dryja extracted the chromosomes from tumors and ran his probe set against the chromosomes. If the probes bound, they usually made a signal on a gel; if a probe was fully missing, the signal was blank. One morning, having run another dozen tumors, Dryja came to the lab and held up the blot against the window and ran his eyes left to right, lane after lane automatically, like a pianist reading a score. In one tumor, he saw a blank space. One of his probes—H3-8, he had called it—was deleted in both chromosomes in that tumor. He felt the brief hot rush of ecstasy, which then tipped into queasiness. "It was at that moment that I had the feeling that we had a gene in our hands. I had landed on retinoblastoma."

cℐℐ℘

Dryja had found a piece of DNA missing in tumor cells. Now he needed to find the corresponding piece present in normal cells, thus isolating the *Rb* gene. Perilously close to the end, Dryja was like an acrobat at the final stretch of his rope. His one-room lab was taut with tension, stretched to its limit. He had inadequate skills in isolating genes and limited resources. To isolate the gene, he would need help, so he took another lunge. He had heard that researchers in the Weinberg lab were also hunting for the retinoblastoma gene. Dryja's choices were stark: he could either team up with Weinberg, or he could try to isolate the gene alone and lose the race altogether.

The scientist in Weinberg's lab trying to isolate *Rb* was Steve Friend. A jovial, medically trained molecular geneticist with a quick wit and an easy manner, Friend had casually mentioned his interest in *Rb* to Dryja at a meeting. Unlike Dryja, working with his growing stash of tumor samples, Friend had been building a collection of normal cells—cells in which the *Rb* gene was completely intact. Friend's approach had been to find genes that were present in normal retinal cells, then to try to identify ones that were abnormal in retinoblastoma tumors—working backward toward Dryja.

For Dryja, the complementarity of the two approaches was obvious. He had identified a missing piece of DNA in tumors. Could Friend and Weinberg now pull the intact, full-length gene out of normal cells? They outlined a potential collaboration between the two labs. One morning in 1985, Dryja took his probe, H3-8, and virtually ran across the Longfellow Bridge (by now, the central highway of oncogenesis), carrying it by hand to Friend's bench at the Whitehead.

It took Friend a quick experiment to test Dryja's probe. Using the DNA "sticking" reaction again, Friend trapped and isolated the normal cellular gene that stuck to the H3-8 probe. The isolated gene "lived" on chromosome thirteen, as predicted. When Dryja further tested the candidate gene through his bank of tumor samples, he found precisely what Knudson had hypothesized more than a decade earlier: all retinoblastoma cells contained inactivations in both copies of the gene—two hits—while normal cells contained two normal copies of the gene. The candidate gene that Friend had isolated was indisputably *Rb*.

In October 1986, Friend, Weinberg, and Dryja published their findings in *Nature*. The article marked the perfect complement to Weinberg's *ras* paper, the yin to its yang—the isolation of an activated proto-oncogene (*ras*) and the identification of the anti-oncogene (*Rb*). "Fifteen years ago," Weinberg wrote, "Knudson provided a theoretical basis for retinoblastoma tumorigenesis by suggesting that minimally two genetic events are required to trigger tumor development." Weinberg noted, "We have isolated [a human gene] apparently representing one of this class of genes"— a tumor suppressor.

What *Rb* does in normal cells is still an unfolding puzzle. Its name, as it turns out, is quite a misnomer. *Rb*, retinoblastoma, is not just mutated in rare eye tumors in children. When scientists tested the gene isolated by Dryja, Friend, and Weinberg in other cancers in the early nineties, they found it widely mutated in lung, bone, esophageal, breast, and bladder cancers in adults. Like *ras*, it is expressed in nearly every dividing cell. And it is inactivated in a whole host of malignancies. Calling it retinoblastoma thus vastly underestimates the influence, depth, and prowess of this gene.

The retinoblastoma gene encodes a protein, also named Rb, with a deep molecular "pocket." Its chief function is to bind to several other proteins and keep them tightly sealed in that pocket, preventing them from activating cell division. When the cell decides to divide, it tags Rb with a phosphate group, a molecular signal that inactivates the gene and thus forces the protein to release its partners. Rb thus acts as a gatekeeper for cell division, opening a series of key molecular floodgates each time cell division is activated and closing them sharply when the cell division is completed. Mutations in *Rb* inactivate this function. The cancer cell perceives its gates as perpetually open and is unable to stop dividing.

ॐ

The cloning of *ras* and *retinoblastoma*—oncogene and anti-oncogene— was a transformative moment in cancer genetics. In the decade between 1983 and 1993, a horde of other oncogenes and anti-oncogenes (tumor suppressor genes) were swiftly identified in human cancers: *myc, neu, fos, ret, akt* (all oncogenes), and p53, VHL, APC (all tumor suppressors). Retroviruses, the accidental carriers of oncogenes, faded far into the distance. Varmus and Bishop's theory—that oncogenes were activated cellular genes—was recognized to be widely true for many forms of cancer. And the two-hit hypothesis—that tumor suppressors were genes that needed to be inactivated in both chromosomes—was also found to be widely applicable in cancer. A rather general conceptual framework for carcinogenesis was slowly becoming apparent. The cancer cell was a broken, deranged machine. Oncogenes were its jammed accelerators and inactivated tumor suppressors its missing brakes.*

In the late 1980s, yet another line of research, resurrected from the past, yielded a further bounty of cancer-linked genes. Ever since de Gouvêa's report of the Brazilian family with eye tumors in 1872, geneticists had uncovered several other families that appeared to carry cancer in their genes. The stories of these families bore a familiar, tragic trope: cancer haunted them generation upon generation, appearing and reappearing in parents, children, and grandchildren. Two features stood out in these family histories. First, geneticists recognized that the spectrum of cancers in every family was limited and often stereotypical: colon and ovarian cancer threading through one family; breast and ovarian through another; sarcomas, leukemias, and gliomas through a third. And second, similar patterns often reappeared in different families, thereby suggesting a common genetic syndrome. In Lynch syndrome (first described by an astute oncologist, Henry Lynch, in a Nebraskan family), colon, ovarian, stomach, and biliary cancer recurred generation upon generation. In Li-Fraumeni syndrome, there were recurrent bone and visceral sarcomas, leukemias, and brain tumors.

Using powerful molecular genetic techniques, cancer geneticists in the 1980s and 1990s could clone and identify some of these cancer-linked genes. Many of these familial cancer genes, like *Rb,* were tumor suppressors (although occasional oncogenes were also found). Most such syndromes were fleetingly rare. But occasionally geneticists identified cancer-predisposing gene alterations that were quite frequently represented in the population. Perhaps the most striking among these, first suggested by the geneticist Mary Claire-King and then definitively cloned by Mark Skolnick's team at the pharma company Myriad Genetics, was BRCA-1, a gene that strongly predisposes humans to breast and ovarian cancer. BRCA-1 (to which we will return in later pages) can be found in up to 1 percent of women in selected populations, making it one of the most common cancer-linked genes found in humans.

---

* Although cancer is not universally caused by viruses, certain viruses cause particular cancers, such as the human papilloma virus (HPV), which causes cervical cancer. When the mechanism driving this cancer was deciphered in the 1990s, HPV turned out to inactivate *Rb*'s and p53's signal—underscoring the importance of endogenous genes in even virally induced cancers.

By the early 1990s, the discoveries of cancer biology had thus traversed the gap between the chicken tumors of Peyton Rous and real human cancers. But purists still complained. The crusty specter of Robert Koch still haunted the genetic theory of cancer. Koch had postulated that for an agent to be identified as the "cause" of a disease, it must (1) be present in the diseased organism, (2) be capable of being isolated from the diseased organism, and (3) re-create the disease in a secondary host when transferred from the diseased organism. Oncogenes had met the first two criteria. They had been found to be present in cancer cells and they had been isolated from cancer cells. But no one had shown that a cancer gene, in and of itself, could create a bona fide tumor in an animal.

In the mid-1980s, a series of remarkable experiments allowed cancer geneticists to meet Koch's final criteria. In 1984, biologists working on stem cells had invented a new technology that allowed them to introduce exogenous genes into early mouse embryos, then create a living mouse out of those modified embryos. This allowed them to produce "transgenic mice," mice in which one or more genes were artificially and permanently modified. Cancer geneticists seized this opportunity. Among the first such genes to be engineered into a mouse was *c-myc*, an oncogene discovered in lymphoma cells.

Using transgenic mouse technology, Philip Leder's team at Harvard altered the *c-myc* gene in mice, but with a twist: cleverly, they ensured that only breast tissue in the mouse would overexpress the gene. (*Myc* could not be activated in all cells. If *myc* was permanently activated in the embryo, the embryo turned into a ball of overproliferating cells, then involuted and died through unknown mechanisms. The only way to activate *myc* in a living mouse was to restrict the activation to only a subset of cells. Since Leder's lab was studying breast cancer, he chose breast cells.) Colloquially, Leder called his mouse the OncoMouse. In 1988, he successfully applied for a patent on the OncoMouse, making it the first animal patented in history.

Leder expected his transgenic mice to explode with cancer, but to his surprise, the oncomice sprouted rather mousy cancers. Even though an aggressive oncogene had been stitched into their chromosomes, the mice developed small, unilateral breast cancers, and not until late in life. Even more surprisingly, Leder's mice typically developed cancers only after pregnancy, suggesting that environmental influences, such as hormones, were strictly required to achieve full transformation of breast cells. "The active *myc* gene does not appear to be sufficient for the development of these tumors," Leder wrote. "If that were the case, we would have expected the uniform development of tumor masses involving the entire bilateral [breast] glands of all five tumor-bearing animals. Rather, our results suggest at least two additional requirements. One of these is likely to be a further transforming event.... The other seems to be a hormonal environment related to pregnancy that is only suggested by these initial studies."

To test the roles of other oncogenes and environmental stimuli, Leder created a second OncoMouse, in which two activated proto-oncogenes, *ras* and *myc,* were engineered into the chromosome and expressed in breast cells. Multiple tumors sprouted up in the breast glands of these mice in months. The requirement for the hormonal milieu of pregnancy was partially ameliorated. Still, only a few distinct clones of cancer sprouted out of the *ras-myc* mice. Millions of breast cells in each mouse possessed activated *ras* and *myc.* Yet, of those millions of cells, each endowed with the most potent oncogenes, only a few dozen turned into real, living tumors.

Even so, this was a landmark experiment: cancer had artificially been created in an animal. "Cancer genetics," as the geneticist Cliff Tabin recalls, "had crossed a new frontier. It was not dealing with just genes and pathways and artificial lumps in the lab, but a real growing tumor in an animal." Peyton Rous's long squabble with the discipline—that cancer had never been produced in a living organism by altering a defined set of cellular genes—was finally laid to its long-overdue rest.

The Hallmarks of Cancer

*I do not wish to achieve immortality through my works. I
wish to achieve immortality by not dying.*
—Woody Allen

Scurrying about in its cage in the vivarium atop Harvard Medical School,
Philip Leder's OncoMouse bore large implications on small haunches.
The mouse embodied the maturity of cancer genetics: scientists had created real, living tumors (not just abstract, etiolated foci in petri dishes) by
artificially manipulating two genes, *ras* and *myc*, in an animal. Yet Leder's
experiment raised further questions about the genesis of cancer. Cancer
is not merely a lump in the body; it is a disease that migrates, evolves,
invades organs, destroys tissues, and resists drugs. Activating even two
potent proto-oncogenes had not recapitulated the full syndrome of cancer in every cell of the mouse. Cancer genetics had illuminated much
about the genesis of cancer, but much, evidently, remained to be understood.

If two oncogenes were insufficient to create cancers, then how many activated proto-oncogenes and inactivated tumor suppressors *were* required?
What were the genetic steps needed to convert a normal cell into a cancer
cell? For human cancers, these questions could not be answered experimentally. One could not, after all, proactively "create" a human cancer and
follow the activation and inactivation of genes. But the questions could
be answered retrospectively. In 1988, using human specimens, a physician-scientist named Bert Vogelstein at Johns Hopkins Medical School
in Baltimore set out to describe the number of genetic changes required
to initiate cancer. The query, in various incarnations, would preoccupy
Vogelstein for nearly two decades.

Vogelstein was inspired by the observations made by George
Papanicolaou and Oscar Auerbach in the 1950s. Both Papanicolaou and

Auerbach, working on different cancers, had noted that cancer did not arise directly out of a normal cell. Instead, cancer often slouched toward its birth, undergoing discrete, transitional stages between the fully normal and the frankly malignant cell. Decades before cervical cancer evolved into its fiercely invasive incarnation, whorls of noninvasive premalignant cells could be observed in the tissue, beginning their first steps in the grisly march toward cancer. (Identifying and eradicating this premalignant stage before the cancer spreads is the basis for the Pap smear.) Similarly, Auerbach had noted, premalignant cells were seen in smokers' lungs long before lung cancer appeared. Colon cancer in humans also underwent graded and discrete changes in its progression, from a noninvasive premalignant lesion called an adenoma to the highly invasive terminal stage called an invasive carcinoma.

Vogelstein chose to study this progression in colon cancer. He collected samples from patients representing each of the stages of colon cancer. He then assembled a series of four human cancer genes—oncogenes and tumor suppressors—and assessed each stage of cancer in his samples for activations and inactivations of these four genes.*

Knowing the heterogeneity of every cancer, one might naively have presumed that every patient's cancer possessed its own sequence of gene mutations and its unique set of mutated genes. But Vogelstein found a strikingly consistent pattern in his colon cancer samples: across many samples and many patients, the transitions in the stages of cancer were paralleled by the same transitions in genetic changes. Cancer cells did not activate or inactivate genes at random. Instead, the shift from a premalignant state to an invasive cancer could precisely be correlated with the activation and inactivation of genes in a strict and stereotypical sequence.

In 1988, in the *New England Journal of Medicine,* Vogelstein wrote: "The four molecular alterations accumulated in a fashion that paralleled the clinical progression of tumors." He proposed, "Early in the neoplastic process one colonic cell appears to outgrow its companions to form a small, benign neoplasm. During the growth of [these] cells, a mutation in the *ras* gene . . . often occurs. Finally, a loss of tumor suppressor genes . . . may be associated with the progression of adenoma to frank carcinoma."

---

* In 1988, the precise identity of only one gene—*ras*—was known. The other three were suspected human anti-oncogenes, although their identity would only become known later.

Since Vogelstein had preselected his list of four genes, he could not enumerate the total number of genes required for the march of cancer. (The technology available in 1988 would not permit such an analysis; he would need to wait two decades before that technology would become available.) But he had proved an important point, that such a discrete genetic march existed. Papanicolaou and Auerbach had described the pathological transition of cancer as a multistep process, starting with premalignancy and marching inexorably toward invasive cancer. Vogelstein showed that the *genetic* progression of cancer was also a multistep process.

This was a relief. In the decade between 1980 and 1990, proto-oncogenes and tumor suppressor genes had been discovered in such astonishing numbers in the human genome—at last count, about one hundred such genes—that their abundance raised a disturbing question: if the genome was so densely littered with such intemperate genes—genes waiting to push a cell toward cancer as if at the flick of a switch—then why was the human body not exploding with cancer every minute?

Cancer geneticists already knew two answers to this question. First, proto-oncogenes need to be activated through mutations, and mutations are rare events. Second, tumor suppressor genes need to be inactivated, but typically two copies exist of each tumor suppressor gene, and thus two independent mutations are needed to inactivate a tumor suppressor, an even rarer event. Vogelstein provided the third answer. Activating or inactivating any single gene, he postulated, produced only the first steps toward carcinogenesis. Cancer's march was long and slow and proceeded though many mutations in many genes over many iterations. In genetic terms, our cells were not sitting on the edge of the abyss of cancer. They were dragged toward that abyss in graded, discrete steps.

ℐℐ

While Bert Vogelstein was describing the slow march of cancer from one gene mutation to the next, cancer biologists were investigating the functions of these mutations. Cancer gene mutations, they knew, could succinctly be described in two categories: either activations of proto-oncogenes or inactivations of tumor suppressor genes. But although dys-regulated cell division is the pathological hallmark of cancer, cancer cells do not merely divide; they migrate through the body, destroy other tissues, invade organs, and colonize distant sites. To understand the full syndrome of cancer, biologists would need to link gene mutations in cancer cells to the complex and multifaceted abnormal behavior of these cells.

Genes encode proteins, and proteins often work like minuscule molecular switches, activating yet other proteins and inactivating others, turning molecular switches "on" and "off" inside a cell. Thus, a conceptual diagram can be drawn for any such protein: protein A turns B on, which turns C on and D off, which turns E on, and so forth. This molecular cascade is termed the signaling pathway for a protein. Such pathways are constantly active in cells, bringing signals in and signals out, thereby allowing a cell to function in its environment.

Proto-oncogenes and tumor suppressor genes, cancer biologists discovered, sit at the hubs of such signaling pathways. Ras, for instance, activates a protein called Mek. Mek in turn activates Erk, which, through several intermediary steps, ultimately accelerates cell division. This cascade of steps, called the Ras-Mek-Erk pathway—is tightly regulated in normal cells, thereby ensuring tightly regulated cell division. In cancer cells, activated "Ras" chronically and permanently activates Mek, which permanently activates Erk, resulting in uncontrolled cell division—pathological mitosis.

But the activated *ras* pathway (Ras→ Mek → Erk) does not merely cause accelerated cell division; the pathway also intersects with other pathways to enable several other "behaviors" of cancer cells. At Children's Hospital in Boston in the 1990s, the surgeon-scientist Judah Folkman demonstrated that certain activated signaling pathways within cancer cells, *ras* among them, could also induce neighboring blood vessels to grow. A tumor could thus "acquire" its own blood supply by insidiously inciting a network of blood vessels around itself and then growing, in grapelike clusters, around those vessels, a phenomenon that Folkman called tumor angiogenesis.

Folkman's Harvard colleague Stan Korsmeyer found other activated pathways in cancer cells, originating in mutated genes, that also blocked cell death, thus imbuing cancer cells with the capacity to resist death signals. Other pathways allowed cancer cells to acquire motility, the capacity to move from one tissue to another—initiating metastasis. Yet other gene cascades increased cell survival in hostile environments, such that cancer cells traveling through the bloodstream could invade other organs and not be rejected or destroyed in environments not designed for their survival.

Cancer, in short, was not merely genetic in its origin; it was genetic in its entirety. Abnormal genes governed all aspects of cancer's behavior. Cascades of aberrant signals, originating in mutant genes, fanned out within the cancer cell, promoting survival, accelerating growth, enabling mobility, recruiting blood vessels, enhancing nourishment, drawing oxygen—sustaining cancer's life.

These gene cascades, notably, were perversions of signaling pathways used by the body under normal circumstances. The "motility genes" activated by cancer cells, for instance, are the very genes that normal cells use when they require movement through the body, such as when immunological cells need to move toward sites of infection. Tumor angiogenesis exploits the same pathways that are used when blood vessels are created to heal wounds. Nothing is invented; nothing is extraneous. Cancer's life is a recapitulation of the body's life, its existence a pathological mirror of our own. Susan Sontag warned against overburdening an illness with metaphors. But this is not a metaphor. Down to their innate molecular core, cancer cells are hyperactive, survival-endowed, scrappy, fecund, inventive copies of ourselves.

By the early 1990s, cancer biologists could begin to model the genesis of cancer in terms of molecular changes in genes. To understand that model, let us begin with a normal cell, say a lung cell that resides in the left lung of a forty-year-old fire-safety-equipment installer. One morning in 1968, a minute sliver of asbestos from his equipment wafts through the air and lodges in the vicinity of that cell. His body reacts to the sliver with an inflammation. The cells around the sliver begin to divide furiously, like a minuscule wound trying to heal, and a small clump of cells derived from the original cell arises at the site.

In one cell in that clump an accidental mutation occurs in the *ras* gene. The mutation creates an activated version of *ras*. The cell containing the mutant gene is driven to grow more swiftly than its neighbors and creates a clump within the original clump of cells. It is not yet a cancer cell, but a cell in which uncontrolled cell division has partly been unleashed—cancer's primordial ancestor.

A decade passes. The small collection of *ras*-mutant cells continues to proliferate, unnoticed, in the far periphery of the lung. The man smokes cigarettes, and a carcinogenic chemical in tar reaches the periphery of the lung and collides with the clump of *ras*-mutated cells. A cell in this clump acquires a second mutation in its genes, activating a second oncogene.

Another decade passes. Yet another cell in that secondary mass of cells is caught in the path of an errant X-ray and acquires yet another mutation, this time inactivating a tumor suppressor gene. This mutation has little effect since the cell possesses a second copy of that gene. But in the next year, another mutation inactivates the second copy of the tumor suppressor gene, creating a cell that possesses two activated oncogenes and an inactive tumor suppressor gene.

Now a fatal march is on; an unraveling begins. The cells, now with four mutations, begin to outgrow their brethren. As the cells grow, they acquire additional mutations and they activate pathways, resulting in cells even further adapted for growth and survival. One mutation in the tumor allows it to incite blood vessels to grow; another mutation within this blood-nourished tumor allows the tumor to survive even in areas of the body with low oxygen.

Mutant cells beget cells beget cells. A gene that increases the mobility of the cells is activated in a cell. This cell, having acquired motility, can migrate through the lung tissue and enter the bloodstream. A descendant of this mobile cancer cell acquires the capacity to survive in the bone. This cell, having migrated through the blood, reaches the outer edge of the pelvis, where it begins yet another cycle of survival, selection, and colonization. It represents the first metastasis of a tumor that originated in the lung.

The man is occasionally short of breath. He feels a tingle of pain in the periphery of his lung. Occasionally, he senses something moving under his rib cage when he walks. Another year passes, and the sensations accelerate. The man visits a physician and a CT scan is performed, revealing a rindlike mass wrapped around a bronchus in the lung. A biopsy reveals lung cancer. A surgeon examines the man and the CT scan of the chest and deems the cancer inoperable. Three weeks after that visit, the man returns to the medical clinic complaining of pain in his ribs and his hips. A bone scan reveals metastasis to the pelvis and the ribs.

Intravenous chemotherapy is initiated. The cells in the lung tumor respond. The man soldiers through a punishing regimen of multiple cell-killing drugs. But during the treatment, one cell in the tumor acquires yet another mutation that makes it resistant to the drug used to treat the cancer. Seven months after his initial diagnosis, the tumor relapses all over the body—in the lungs, the bones, the liver. On the morning of October, 17, 2004, deeply narcotized on opiates in a hospital bed in Boston and surrounded by his wife and his children, the man dies of metastatic lung cancer, a sliver of asbestos still lodged in the periphery of his lung. He is seventy-six years old.

I began this as a hypothetical story of cancer. The genes, carcinogens, and the sequence of mutations in this story are all certainly hypothetical. But the body at its center is real. This man was the first patient to die in my care during my fellowship in cancer medicine at Massachusetts General Hospital.

Medicine, I said, begins with storytelling. Patients tell stories to describe illness; doctors tell stories to understand it. Science tells its own story to explain diseases. This story of one cancer's genesis—of carcinogens causing mutations in internal genes, unleashing cascading pathways in cells that then cycle through mutation, selection, and survival—represents the most cogent outline we have of cancer's birth.

∂∫

In the fall of 1999, Robert Weinberg attended a conference on cancer biology in Hawaii. Late one afternoon, he and Douglas Hanahan, another cancer biologist, trekked through the lava beds of the low, black mountains until they found themselves at the mouth of a volcano, staring in. Their conversation was tinged with frustration. For too long, it seemed, cancer had been talked about as if it were a bewildering hodgepodge of chaos. The biological characteristics of tumors were described as so multifarious as to defy any credible organization. There seemed to be no organizing rules.

Yet, Weinberg and Hanahan knew, the discoveries of the prior two decades had suggested deep rules and principles. Biologists looking directly into cancer's maw now recognized that roiling beneath the incredible heterogeneity of cancer were behaviors, genes, and pathways. In January 2000, a few months after their walk to the volcano's mouth, Weinberg and Hanahan published an article titled "The Hallmarks of Cancer" to summarize these rules. It was an ambitious and iconic work that marked a return, after nearly a century's detour, to Boveri's original notion of a "unitary cause of carcinoma":

"We discuss . . . rules that govern the transformation of normal human cells into malignant cancers. We suggest that research over the past decades has revealed a small number of molecular, biochemical, and cellular traits—acquired capabilities—shared by most and perhaps all types of human cancer."

How many "rules," then, could Weinberg and Hanahan evoke to explain the core behavior of more than a hundred distinct types and subtypes of tumors? The question was audacious in its expansiveness; the answer even more audacious in its economy: six. "We suggest that the vast catalog of cancer cell genotypes is a manifestation of six essential alterations in cell physiology that collectively dictate malignant growth."

1. *Self-sufficiency in growth signals:* cancer cells acquire an autonomous drive to proliferate—pathological mitosis—by virtue of the activation of oncogenes such as *ras* or *myc.*
2. *Insensitivity to growth-inhibitory (antigrowth) signals:* cancer cells inactivate tumor suppressor genes, such as retinoblastoma (*Rb*), that normally inhibit growth
3. *Evasion of programmed cell death (apoptosis):* cancer cells suppress and inactivate genes and pathways that normally enable cells to die.
4. *Limitless replicative potential:* cancer cells activate specific gene pathways that render them immortal even after generations of growth.
5. *Sustained angiogenesis:* cancer cells acquire the capacity to draw out their own supply of blood and blood vessels—tumor angiogenesis.
6. *Tissue invasion and metastasis:* cancer cells acquire the capacity to migrate to other organs, invade other tissues, and colonize these organs, resulting in their spread throughout the body.

Notably, Weinberg and Hanahan wrote, these six rules were not abstract descriptions of cancer's behavior. Many of the genes and pathways that enabled each of these six behaviors had concretely been identified—*ras, myc, Rb,* to name just a few. The task now was to *connect* this causal understanding of cancer's deep biology to the quest for its cure:

"Some would argue that the search for the origin and treatment of this disease will continue over the next quarter century in much the same manner as it has in the recent past, by adding further layers of complexity to a scientific literature that is already complex almost beyond measure. But we anticipate otherwise: those researching the cancer problem will be practicing a dramatically different type of science than we have experienced over the past 25 years."

The mechanistic maturity of cancer science would create a new kind of cancer medicine, Weinberg and Hanahan posited: "With holistic clarity of mechanism, cancer prognosis and treatment will become a rational science, unrecognizable by current practitioners." Having wandered in the darkness for decades, scientists had finally reached a clearing in their understanding of cancer. Medicine's task was to continue that journey toward a new therapeutic attack.

PART SIX

———

THE FRUITS OF
LONG ENDEAVORS

We are really reaping the fruits of our long endeavors.
—Michael Gorman
to Mary Lasker, 1985

The National Cancer Institute, which has overseen
American efforts on researching and combating cancers
since 1971, should take on an ambitious new goal for
the next decade: the development of new drugs that will
provide lifelong cures for many, if not all, major cancers.
Beating cancer now is a realistic ambition because, at
long last, we largely know its true genetic and chemical
characteristics.

—James Watson, 2009

The more perfect a power is, the more difficult it is to quell.
—Saint Aquinas, attributed

"No one had labored in vain"

Have you met Jimmy? . . . Jimmy is any one of thousands
of children with leukemia or any other form of cancer,
from the nation or from around the world.
　　　　　　　　　　—Pamphlet for the Jimmy Fund, 1963

In the summer of 1997, a woman named Phyllis Clauson, from Billerica, Massachusetts, posted a letter to the Dana-Farber Cancer Institute. She was writing on behalf of "Jimmy," Farber's mascot. It had been nearly fifty years since Jimmy had arrived at Farber's clinic in Boston from upstate Maine with a diagnosis of lymphoma of the intestines. Like all his wardmates from the 1950s, Jimmy was presumed long dead.

Not true, Clauson wrote; he was alive and well. Jimmy—Einar Gustafson—was her brother, a truck driver in Maine with three children. For five decades, his family had guarded the knowledge of Jimmy's identity and his survival. Only Sidney Farber had known; Christmas cards from Farber had arrived each winter, until Farber himself had died in 1973. Every year, for decades, Clauson and her siblings had sent in modest donations to the Jimmy Fund, divulging to no one that the silhouetted face on the solicitation card for contributions was their brother's. But with the passage of fifty years, Clauson felt she could no longer keep the secret in good conscience. "Jimmy's story," she recalled, "had become a story that I could not hold. I knew I had to write the letter while Einar was still alive."

Clauson's letter was nearly thrown into the trash. Jimmy "sightings," like Elvis sightings, were reported often, but rarely taken seriously; all had turned out to be hoaxes. Doctors had informed the Jimmy Fund's publicity department that the odds of Jimmy's having survived were nil, and that all claims were to be treated with great skepticism. But Clauson's letter contained details that could not be waved away. She wrote of listening to the radio in New Sweden, Maine, in the summer of 1948 to tune in to the Ralph Edwards broadcast. She recalled her brother's midwinter trips to Boston that often took two days, with Jimmy in his baseball uniform lying patiently in the back of a truck.

When Clauson told her brother about the letter that she had sent, she found him more relieved than annoyed. "It was like an unburdening for him, too," she recalled. "Einar was a modest man. He had kept to himself because he did not want to brag." ("I would read in the papers that they had found me someplace," he said, "and I would smile.")

Clauson's letter was spotted by Karen Cummings, an associate in the Jimmy Fund's development office, who immediately understood its potential significance. She contacted Clauson, and then reached Gustafson.

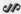

A few weeks later, in January 1998, Cummings arranged to meet Jimmy at a truck stop outside a shopping center in a suburb of Boston. It was six in the morning on a bone-chilling winter day, and Gustafson and his wife piled into Cummings's warm car. Cummings had brought a tape of Jimmy from 1948 singing his favorite song. She played it:

> Take me out to the ball game,
> Take me out with the crowd.
> Buy me some peanuts and Cracker Jack,
> I don't care if I never get back.

Gustafson listened to his own voice with tears in his eyes. Cummings and Jimmy's wife sat in the car, their eyes also welling with silent tears.

Later that month, Cummings drove up to New Sweden, a brutally beautiful town in northern Maine with austere angular houses set against an even more austere landscape. Old-timers in the town also recalled Gustafson's trips to Boston for chemotherapy. He had hitchhiked to and from Boston in cars and trucks and delivery vans anytime someone from the town had driven up or down the coast; it had taken a village to save a child. As Cummings sat in Gustafson's kitchen, he crept upstairs and returned with a cardboard box. Wrapped inside was the battered baseball uniform that the Boston Braves had given Jimmy on the night of the Edwards broadcast. Cummings needed no further proof.

And so it was in May 1998, almost exactly fifty years after he had journeyed from small-town Maine to the Children's Hospital to meet the odd, formal doctor in a three-piece suit, that Jimmy returned with full fanfare to the Jimmy Fund. His wardmates from the hospital—the Sandler twin with his recalcitrant leukemia engorging his spleen, the blond girl in plaits by the television, little Jenny with leukemia—had long ago been buried in small graves in and around Boston. Gustafson walked into the Jimmy Fund Building,* up the low, long steps to the room where the clockwork train had run through the mountain tunnel. Patients, survivors, nurses, and doctors milled around him. Like a latter-day Rip van Winkle, he found the present unfathomable and unrecognizable. "Everything has changed," Clauson recalled him saying. "The rooms, the patients, the drugs." But more than anything, survivorship had changed. "Einar remembered the cancer ward as a place with many curtains," she continued. "When the children were well, the curtains would be spread open. But they would soon close the curtains, and there would be no child when they were opened again."

Here Gustafson was, fifty years later, back in those long hallways with the faded cartoon paintings on the walls, his curtains thrown apart. It is impossible to know whether Jimmy had survived because of surgery, or chemotherapy, or because his cancer had been inherently benign in its behavior. But the facts of his medical history are irrelevant; his return was symbolic. Jimmy had unwittingly been picked to become the icon of the child with cancer. But Einar Gustafson, now sixty-three years old, had returned as the icon of a man beyond cancer.

✌

The Italian memoirist Primo Levi, who survived a concentration camp and then navigated his way through a blasted Germany to his native Turin, often remarked that among the most fatal qualities of the camp was its ability to erase the idea of a life outside and beyond itself. A person's past and his present were annihilated as a matter of course—to be in the camps was to abnegate history, identity, and personality—but it was the erasure of the future that was the most chilling. With that annihilation, Levi wrote, came a moral and spiritual death that perpetuated the status quo of imprisonment. If no life existed beyond the camp, then the distorted logic by which the camp operated became life as usual.

---

* Jimmy began chemo in the Children's Hospital in 1948, but was later followed and treated in the Jimmy Fund Building in 1952.

Cancer is not a concentration camp, but it shares the quality of annihilation: it negates the possibility of life outside and beyond itself; it subsumes all living. The daily life of a patient becomes so intensely preoccupied with his or her illness that the world fades away. Every last morsel of energy is spent tending the disease. "How to overcome him became my obsession," the journalist Max Lerner wrote of the lymphoma in his spleen. "If it was to be a combat then I had to engage it with everything I had—knowledge and guile, ways covert as well as overt."

For Carla, in the midst of the worst phase of her chemotherapy, the day-to-day rituals of survival utterly blotted out any thought of survivorship in the long run. When I asked a woman with a rare form of muscle sarcoma about her life outside the hospital, she told me that she spent her days and nights scouring the Internet for news about the disease. "I am in the hospital," she said, "even when I am outside the hospital." The poet Jason Shinder wrote, "Cancer is a tremendous opportunity to have your face pressed right up against the glass of your mortality." But what patients see through the glass is not a world outside cancer, but a world taken over by it—cancer reflected endlessly around them like a hall of mirrors.

I was not immune to this compulsive preoccupation either. In the summer of 2005, as my fellowship hurtled to its end, I experienced perhaps the singularly transformative event of my life: the birth of my daughter. Glowing, beautiful, and cherubic, Leela was born on a warm night at Massachusetts General Hospital, then swaddled in blankets and brought to the newborn unit on the fourteenth floor. The unit is directly across from the cancer ward. (The apposition of the two is hardly a coincidence. As a medical procedure, childbirth is least likely to involve infectious complications and is thus the safest neighbor to a chemotherapy ward, where any infection can turn into a lethal rampage. As in so much in medicine, the juxtaposition between the two wards is purely functional and yet just as purely profound.)

I would like to see myself at my wife's side awaiting the miraculous moment of my daughter's birth as most fathers do. But in truth I was gowned and gloved like a surgeon, with a blue, sterile sheet spread out in front of me, and a long syringe in my hands, poised to harvest the maroon gush of blood cells from the umbilical cord. When I cut that cord, part of me was the father, but the other part an oncologist. Umbilical blood contains one of the richest known sources of blood-forming stem cells—cells that can be stored away in cryobanks and used for a bone marrow transplant to treat leukemia in the future, an intensely precious resource often flushed down a sink in hospitals after childbirth.

The midwives rolled their eyes; the obstetrician, an old friend, asked jokingly if I ever stopped thinking about work. But I was too far steeped in the study of blood to ignore my instincts. In the bone-marrow-transplant rooms across that very hallway were patients for whom I had scoured tissue banks across the nation for one or two pints of these stem cells that might save their lives. Even in this most life-affirming of moments, the shadows of malignancy—and death—were forever lurking on my psyche.

∂ℓ∂

But not everything was involuting into death. Something transformative was also happening in the fellows' clinics in the summer of 2005: many of my patients, whose faces had so fixedly been pressed up against the glass of their mortality, began to glimpse an afterlife beyond cancer. February, as I said before, had marked the midpoint of an abysmal descent. Cancer had reached its full, lethal bloom that month. Nearly every week had brought news of a mounting toll, culminating chillingly with Steve Harmon's arrival in the emergency room and his devastating spiral into death thereafter. Some days I dreaded walking by the fax machines outside my office, where a pile of death certificates would be waiting for my signature.

But then, like a poisonous tide receding, the bad news ebbed. The nightly phone calls from the hospitals or from ERs and hospice units around Boston bringing news of yet another death ("I'm calling to let you know that your patient arrived here this evening with dizziness and difficulty breathing") suddenly ceased. It was as if the veil of death had lifted—and survivors had emerged from underneath.

Ben Orman had been definitively cured of Hodgkin's lymphoma. It had not been an effortless voyage. His blood counts had dropped calamitously during the midcycle of chemotherapy. For a few weeks it had appeared that the lymphoma had ceased responding—a poor prognostic sign portending a therapy-resistant, fatal variant of the disease. But in the end the mass in his neck, and the larger archipelago of masses in his chest, had all melted away, leaving just minor remnants of scar tissue. The formality of his demeanor had visibly relaxed. When I last saw him in the summer of 2005, he spoke about moving away from Boston to Los Angeles to join a law firm. He assured me that he would visit to follow up, but I wasn't convinced. Orman epitomized the afterlife of cancer—eager to forget the clinic and its bleak rituals, like a bad trip to a foreign country.

Katherine Fitz could also see a life beyond cancer. For Fitz, with the lung tumor wrapped ominously around her bronchus, the biggest hurdle had been the local control of her cancer. The mass had been excised in an incredibly meticulous surgery; she had then finished adjuvant chemotherapy and radiation. Nearly twelve months after the surgery, there was no sign of a local relapse. Nor was there any sign of the woman who had come to the clinic several months earlier, nearly folded over in fear. Tumor out, chemotherapy done, radiation behind her, Fitz's effervescence poured out of every spigot of her soul. At times, watching her personality emerge as if through a nozzle, it seemed abundantly clear why the Greeks had thought of disease as pathological blockades of humors.

Carla returned to see me in July 2005, bringing pictures of her three growing children. She refused to let another doctor perform her bone marrow biopsy, so I walked over from the lab on a warm morning to perform the procedure. She looked relieved when she saw me, greeting me with her anxious half-smile. We had developed a ritualistic relationship; who was I to desecrate a lucky ritual? The biopsy revealed no leukemia in the bone marrow. Her remission, for now, was still intact.

I have chosen these cases not because they were "miraculous" but because of precisely the opposite reason. They represent a routine spectrum of survivors—Hodgkin's disease cured with multidrug chemotherapy; locally advanced lung cancer controlled with surgery, chemotherapy, and radiation; lymphoblastic leukemia in a prolonged remission after intensive chemotherapy. To me, these were miracles enough. It is an old complaint about the practice of medicine that it inures you to the idea of death. But when medicine inures you to the idea of life, to survival, then it has failed utterly. The novelist Thomas Wolfe, recalling a lifelong struggle with illness, wrote in his last letter, "I've made a long voyage and been to a strange country, and I've seen the dark man very close." I had not made the journey myself, and I had only seen the darkness reflected in the eyes of others. But surely, it was the most sublime moment of my clinical life to have watched that voyage in reverse, to encounter men and women *returning* from the strange country—to see them so very close, clambering back.

Incremental advances can add up to transformative changes. In 2005, an avalanche of papers cascading through the scientific literature converged on a remarkably consistent message—the national physiognomy of cancer had subtly but fundamentally changed. The mortality for nearly every major form of cancer—lung, breast, colon, and prostate—had continuously dropped for fifteen straight years. There had been no single, drastic turn but rather a steady and powerful attrition: mortality had declined by about 1 percent every year. The rate might sound modest, but its cumulative effect was remarkable: between 1990 and 2005, the cancer-specific death rate had dropped nearly 15 percent, a decline unprecedented in the history of the disease. The empire of cancer was still indubitably vast—more than half a million American men and women died of cancer in 2005—but it was losing power, fraying at its borders.

What precipitated this steady decline? There was no single answer but rather a multitude. For lung cancer, the driver of decline was primarily prevention—a slow attrition in smoking sparked off by the Doll-Hill and Wynder-Graham studies, fueled by the surgeon general's report, and brought to its full boil by a combination of political activism (the FTC action on warning labels), inventive litigation (the Banzhaf and Cipollone cases), medical advocacy, and countermarketing (the antitobacco advertisements).

For colon and cervical cancer, the declines were almost certainly due to the successes of secondary prevention—cancer screening. Colon cancers were detected at earlier and earlier stages in their evolution, often in the premalignant state, and treated with relatively minor surgeries. Cervical cancer screening using Papanicolaou's smearing technique was being offered at primary-care centers throughout the nation, and as with colon cancer, premalignant lesions were excised using relatively minor surgeries.*

For leukemia, lymphoma, and testicular cancer, in contrast, the declining numbers reflected the successes of chemotherapeutic treatment. In childhood ALL, cure rates of 80 percent were routinely being achieved. Hodgkin's disease was similarly curable, and so, too, were some large-cell aggressive lymphomas. Indeed, for Hodgkin's disease, testicular cancer, and childhood leukemias, the burning question was not how *much* chemotherapy was curative, but how *little*: trials were addressing whether

* Vaccination against human papillomavirus (HPV) has further driven the incidence down.

milder and less toxic doses of drugs, scaled back from the original protocols, could achieve equivalent cure rates.

Perhaps most symbolically, the decline in breast cancer mortality epitomized the cumulative and collaborative nature of these victories—and the importance of attacking cancer using multiple independent prongs. Between 1990 and 2005, breast cancer mortality had dwindled an unprecedented 24 percent. Three interventions had potentially driven down the breast cancer death rate—mammography (screening to catch early breast cancer and thereby prevent invasive breast cancer), surgery, and adjuvant chemotherapy (chemotherapy after surgery to remove remnant cancer cells). Donald Berry, a statistician in Houston, Texas, set out to answer a controversial question: How much had mammography and chemotherapy *independently* contributed to survival? Whose victory was this—a victory of prevention or of therapeutic intervention?*

Berry's answer was a long-due emollient to a field beset by squabbles between the advocates of prevention and the proponents of chemotherapy. When Berry assessed the effect of each intervention independently using statistical models, it was a satisfying tie: both cancer prevention and chemotherapy had diminished breast cancer mortality equally—12 percent for mammography and 12 percent for chemotherapy, adding up to the observed 24 percent reduction in mortality. "No one," as Berry said, paraphrasing the Bible, "had labored in vain."

These were all deep, audacious, and meaningful victories borne on the backs of deep and meaningful labors. But, in truth, they were the victories of another generation—the results of discoveries made in the fifties and sixties. The core conceptual advances from which these treatment strategies arose predated nearly all the significant work on the cell biology of cancer. In a bewildering spurt over just two decades, scientists had unveiled a fantastical new world—of errant oncogenes and tumor suppressor genes that accelerated and decelerated growth to unleash cancer; of chromosomes that could be decapitated and translocated to create new genetic chimeras, of cellular pathways corrupted to subvert the death of cancer. But the *therapeutic* advances that had led to the slow attrition of

---

* Surgery's contribution could not be judged since surgery predated 1990, and nearly all women are treated surgically.

cancer mortality made no use of this novel biology of cancer. There was new science on one hand and old medicine on the other. Mary Lasker had once searched for an epochal shift in cancer. But the shift that had occurred seemed to belong to another epoch.

Mary Lasker died of heart failure in 1994 in her carefully curated home in Connecticut—having removed herself physically from the bristling epicenters of cancer research and policymaking in Washington, New York, and Boston. She was ninety-three years old. Her life had nearly spanned the most transformative and turbulent century of biomedical science. Her potent ebullience had dimmed in her last decade. She spoke rarely about the achievements (or disappointments) of the War on Cancer. But she had expected cancer medicine to have achieved more during her lifetime—to have taken a more assertive step toward Farber's "universal cure" for cancer and marked a more definitive victory in the war. The complexity, the tenacity—the sheer magisterial force of cancer—had made even its most committed and resolute opponent seem circumspect and humbled.

In 1994, a few months after Lasker's death, the cancer geneticist Ed Harlow captured both the agony and the ecstasy of the era. At the end of a weeklong conference at the Cold Spring Harbor Laboratory in New York pervaded by a giddy sense of anticipation about the spectacular achievements of cancer biology, Harlow delivered a sobering assessment: "Our knowledge of . . . molecular defects in cancer has come from a dedicated twenty years of the best molecular biology research. Yet this information does not translate to any effective treatments nor to any understanding of why many of the current treatments succeed or why others fail. It is a frustrating time."

More than a decade later, I could sense the same frustration in the clinic at Mass General. One afternoon, I watched Tom Lynch, the lung cancer clinician, masterfully encapsulate carcinogenesis, cancer genetics, and chemotherapy for a new patient, a middle-aged woman with bronchoalveolar cell cancer. She was a professor of history with a grave manner and a sharp, darting mind. He sat across from her, scribbling a picture as he spoke. The cells in her bronchus, he began, had acquired mutations in their genes that had allowed them to grow autonomously and uncontrollably. They had formed a local tumor. Their propensity was to acquire further mutations that might allow them to migrate, to invade tissues, to metastasize. Chemotherapy with Carboplatin and Taxol (two standard chemotherapy drugs), augmented with radiation, would kill the cells and perhaps prevent them from migrating to other organs to seed metastases. In the best-case scenario, the cells carrying the mutated genes would die, and her cancer would be cured.

She watched Lynch put his pen down with her quick, sharp eyes. The explanation sounded logical and organized, but she had caught the glint of a broken piece in the chain of logic. What was the connection between this explanation and the therapy being proposed? How, she wanted to know, would Carboplatin "fix" her mutated genes? How would Taxol know which cells carried the mutations in order to kill them? How would the mechanistic explanation of her illness connect with the medical interventions?

She had captured a disjunction all too familiar to oncologists. For nearly a decade, practicing cancer medicine had become like living inside a pressurized can—pushed, on one hand, by the increasing force of biological clarity about cancer, but then pressed against the wall of medical stagnation that seemed to have produced no real medicines out of this biological clarity. In the winter of 1945, Vannevar Bush had written to President Roosevelt, "The striking advances in medicine during the war have been possible only because we had a large backlog of scientific data accumulated through basic research in many scientific fields in the years before the war."

For cancer, the "backlog of scientific data" had reached a critical point. The boil of science, as Bush liked to imagine it, inevitably produced a kind of steam—an urgent, rhapsodic pressure that could only find release in technology. Cancer science was begging to find release in a new kind of cancer medicine.

New Drugs for Old Cancers

> *In the story of Patroclus*
> *No one survives, not even Achilles*
> *Who was nearly a god.*
> *Patroclus resembled him; they wore*
> *The same armor*
> —Louise Glück

> *The perfect therapy has not been developed. Most of us*
> *believe that it will not involve toxic cytotoxic therapy,*
> *which is why we support the kinds of basic investigations*
> *that are directed towards more fundamental under-*
> *standing of tumor biology. But . . . we must do the best*
> *with what we now have.*
> —Bruce Chabner to Rose Kushner

In the legend, Achilles was quickly dipped into the river Styx, held up only by the tendon of his heel. Touched by the dark sheath of water, every part of his body was instantly rendered impervious to even the most lethal weapon—except the undipped tendon. A simple arrow targeted to that vulnerable heel would eventually kill Achilles in the battlefields of Troy.

Before the 1980s, the armamentarium of cancer therapy was largely built around two fundamental vulnerabilities of cancer cells. The first is that most cancers originate as local diseases before they spread systemically. Surgery and radiation therapy exploit this vulnerability. By physically excising locally restricted tumors before cancer cells can spread—or by searing cancer cells with localized bursts of powerful energy using X-rays—surgery and radiation attempt to eliminate cancer en bloc from the body.

The second vulnerability is the rapid growth rate of some cancer cells.* Most chemotherapy drugs discovered before the 1980s target this second vulnerability. Antifolates, such as Farber's aminopterin, interrupt the metabolism of folic acid and starve all cells of a crucial nutrient required for cell division. Nitrogen mustard and cisplatin chemically react with DNA, and DNA-damaged cells cannot duplicate their genes and thus cannot divide. Vincristine, the periwinkle poison, thwarts the ability of a cell to construct the molecular "scaffold" required for all cells to divide.

But these two traditional Achilles' heels of cancer—local growth and rapid cell division—can only be targeted to a point. Surgery and radiation are intrinsically localized strategies, and they fail when cancer cells have spread beyond the limits of what can be surgically removed or irradiated. More surgery thus does not lead to more cures, as the radical surgeons discovered to their despair in the 1950s.

Targeting cellular growth also hits a biological ceiling because normal cells must grow as well. Growth may be the hallmark of cancer, but it is equally the hallmark of life. A poison directed at cellular growth, such as vincristine or cisplatin, eventually attacks normal growth, and cells that grow most rapidly in the body begin to bear the collateral cost of chemotherapy. Hair falls out. Blood involutes. The lining of the skin and gut sloughs off. More drugs produce more toxicity without producing cures, as the radical chemotherapists discovered to their despair in the 1980s.

To target cancer cells with novel therapies, scientists and physicians needed new vulnerabilities that were unique to cancer. The discoveries of cancer biology in the 1980s offered a vastly more nuanced view of these vulnerabilities. Three new principles emerged, representing three new Achilles' heels of cancer.

First, cancer cells are driven to grow because of the accumulation of mutations in their DNA. These mutations activate internal proto-oncogenes and inactivate tumor suppressor genes, thus unleashing the "accelerators" and "brakes" that operate during normal cell division. Targeting these hyperactive genes, while sparing their modulated normal precursors, might be a novel means to attack cancer cells more discriminately.

Second, proto-oncogenes and tumor suppressor genes typically lie at the hubs of cellular signaling pathways. Cancer cells divide and grow

* Not all cancers grow rapidly. Slow-growing cancers are often harder to kill with drugs that target growth.

because they are driven by hyperactive or inactive signals in these critical pathways. These pathways exist in normal cells but are tightly regulated. The potential dependence of a cancer cell on such permanently activated pathways is a second potential vulnerability of a cancer cell.

Third, the relentless cycle of mutation, selection, and survival creates a cancer cell that has acquired several additional properties besides uncontrolled growth. These include the capacity to resist death signals, to metastasize throughout the body, and to incite the growth of blood vessels. These "hallmarks of cancer" are not invented by the cancer cell; they are typically derived from the corruption of similar processes that occur in the normal physiology of the body. The acquired dependence of a cancer cell on these processes is a third potential vulnerability of cancer.

The central therapeutic challenge of the newest cancer medicine, then, was to find, among the vast numbers of similarities in normal cells and cancer cells, subtle differences in genes, pathways, and acquired capabilities—and to drive a poisoned stake into that new heel.

❧

It was one thing to identify an Achilles' heel—and quite another to discover a weapon that would strike it. Until the late 1980s, no drug had reversed an oncogene's activation or a tumor suppressor's inactivation. Even tamoxifen, the most specific cancer-targeted drug discovered to that date, works by attacking the dependence of certain breast cancer cells on estrogen, and not by directly inactivating an oncogene or oncogene-activated pathway. In 1986, the discovery of the first oncogene-targeted drug would thus instantly galvanize cancer medicine. Although found largely serendipitously, the mere existence of such a molecule would set the stage for the vast drug-hunting efforts of the next decade.

The disease that stood at the pivotal crossroads of oncology was yet another rare variant of leukemia called acute promyelocytic leukemia— APL. First identified as a distinct form of adult leukemia in the 1950s, the disease has a distinct characteristic: the cells in this form of cancer do not merely divide rapidly, they are also strikingly frozen in immature development. Normal white blood cells developing in the bone marrow undergo a series of maturational steps to develop into fully functional adult cells. One such intermediate cell is termed a promyelocyte, an adolescent cell on the verge of becoming functionally mature. APL is characterized by the malignant proliferation of these immature promyelocytes. Normal promyelocytes are loaded with toxic enzymes and granules that are usually released by adult white blood cells to kill viruses, bacteria, and parasites. In promyelocytic leukemia, the blood fills up with these toxin-loaded promyelocytes. Moody, mercurial, and jumpy, the cells of APL can release their poisonous granules on a whim—precipitating massive bleeding or simulating a septic reaction in the body. In APL, the pathological proliferation of cancer thus comes with a fiery twist. Most cancers contain cells that refuse to stop growing. In APL, the cancer cells also refuse to grow up.

Since the early 1970s, this maturation arrest of APL cells had prompted scientists to hunt for a chemical that might force these cells to mature. Scores of drugs had been tested on APL cells in test tubes, and only one had stood out—retinoic acid, an oxidized form of vitamin A. But retinoic acid, researchers had found, was a vexingly unreliable reagent. One batch of the acid might mature APL cells, while another batch of the same chemical might fail. Frustrated by these flickering, unfathomable responses, biologists and chemists had turned away after their initial enthusiasm for the maturation chemical.

In the summer of 1985, a team of leukemia researchers from China traveled to France to meet Laurent Degos, a hematologist at Saint Louis Hospital in Paris with a long-standing interest in APL. The Chinese team, led by Zhen Yi Wang, was also treating APL patients, at Ruijin Hospital, a busy, urban clinical center in Shanghai, China. Both Degos and Wang had tried standard chemotherapy agents—drugs that target rapidly growing cells—to promote remissions in APL patients, but the results had been dismal. Wang and Degos spoke of the need for a new strategy to attack this whimsical, lethal disease, and they kept circling back to the peculiar immaturity of APL cells and to the lapsed search for a maturation agent for the disease.

Retinoic acid, Wang and Degos knew, comes in two closely related molecular forms, called cis-retinoic acid and trans-retinoic acid. The two forms are compositionally identical, but possess a slight difference in their molecular structure, and they behave very differently in molecular reactions. (Cis-retinoic acid and trans-retinoic acid have the same atoms, but the atoms are arranged differently in the two chemicals.) Of the two forms, cis-retinoic acid had been the most intensively tested, and it had produced the flickering, transient responses. But Wang and Degos wondered if trans-retinoic acid was the true maturation agent. Had the unreliable responses in the old experiments been due to a low and variable amount of the trans-retinoic form present in every batch of retinoic acid?

Wang, who had studied at a French Jesuit school in Shanghai, spoke a lilting, heavily accented French. Linguistic and geographic barriers breached, the two hematologists outlined an international collaboration. Wang knew of a pharmaceutical factory outside Shanghai that could produce pure trans-retinoic acid—without the admixture of cis-retinoic acid. He would test the drug on APL patients at the Ruijin Hospital. Degos's team in Paris would follow after the initial round of testing in China and further validate the strategy on French APL patients.

Wang launched his trial in 1986 with twenty-four patients. Twenty-three experienced a dazzling response. Leukemic promyelocytes in the blood underwent a brisk maturation into white blood cells. "The nucleus became larger," Wang wrote, "and fewer primary granules were observed in the cytoplasm. On the fourth day of culture, these cells gave rise to myelocytes containing specific, or secondary, granules . . . [indicating the development of] fully mature granulocytes."

Then something even more unexpected occurred: having fully matured, the cancer cells began to die out. In some patients, the differentiation and death erupted so volcanically that the bone marrow swelled up with differentiated promyelocytes and then emptied slowly over weeks as the cancer cells matured and underwent an accelerated cycle of death. The sudden maturation of cancer cells produced a short-lived metabolic disarray, which was controlled with medicines, but the only other side effects of trans-retinoic acid were dryness of lips and mouth and an occasional rash. The remissions produced by trans-retinoic acid lasted weeks and often months.

Acute promyelocytic leukemia still relapsed, typically about three to four months after treatment with trans-retinoic acid. The Paris and Shanghai teams next combined standard chemotherapy drugs with trans-retinoic acid—a cocktail of old and new drugs—and remissions were prolonged by several additional months. In about three-fourths of the patients, the leukemia remission began to stretch into a full year, then into five years. By 1993, Wang and Degos concluded that 75 percent of their patients treated with the combination of trans-retinoic acid and standard chemotherapy would never relapse—a percentage unheard of in the history of APL.

Cancer biologists would need another decade to explain the startling Ruijin responses at a molecular level. The key to the explanation lay in the elegant studies performed by Janet Rowley, the Chicago cytologist. In 1984, Rowley had identified a unique translocation in the chromosomes of APL cells—a fragment of a gene from chromosome fifteen fused with a fragment of a gene from chromosome seventeen. This created an activated "chimeric" oncogene that drove the proliferation of promyelocytes and blocked their maturation, thus creating the peculiar syndrome of APL.

In 1990, a full four years after Wang's clinical trial in Shanghai, this culprit oncogene was isolated by independent teams of scientists from France, Italy, and America. The APL oncogene, scientists found, encodes a protein that is tightly bound by trans-retinoic acid. This binding immediately extinguishes the oncogene's signal in APL cells, thereby explaining the rapid, powerful remissions observed in Shanghai.

The Ruijin discovery was remarkable: trans-retinoic acid represented the long-sought fantasy of molecular oncology—an oncogene-targeted cancer drug. But the discovery was a fantasy lived backward. Wang and Degos had first stumbled on trans-retinoic acid through inspired guesswork—and only later discovered that the molecule could directly target an oncogene.

But was it possible to make the converse journey—starting *from* oncogene and going *to* drug? Indeed, Robert Weinberg's lab in Boston had already begun that converse journey, although Weinberg himself was largely oblivious of it.

By the early 1980s, Weinberg's lab had perfected a technique to isolate cancer-causing genes directly out of cancer cells. Using Weinberg's technique, researchers had isolated dozens of new oncogenes from cancer cells. In 1982, a postdoctoral scientist from Bombay working in Weinberg's lab, Lakshmi Charon Padhy, reported the isolation of yet another such oncogene from a rat tumor called a neuroblastoma. Weinberg christened the gene *neu*, naming it after the type of cancer that harbored this gene.

Neu was added to the growing list of oncogenes, but it was an anomaly. Cells are bounded by a thin membrane of lipids and proteins that acts as an oily barrier against the entry of many drugs. Most oncogenes discovered thus far, such as *ras* and *myc*, are sequestered inside the cell (*ras* is bound to the cell membrane but faces into the cell), making them inaccessible to drugs that cannot penetrate the cell membrane. The product of the *neu* gene, in contrast, was a novel protein, not hidden deep inside the cell, but tethered to the cell membrane with a large fragment that hung outside, freely accessible to any drug.

Lakshmi Charon Padhy even had a "drug" to test. In 1981, while iso-lating his gene, he had created an antibody against the new *neu* protein. Antibodies are molecules designed to bind to other molecules, and the binding can occasionally block and inactivate the bound protein. But anti-bodies are unable to cross the cell membrane and need an exposed pro-tein outside the cell to bind. *Neu*, then, was a perfect target, with a large portion, a long molecular "foot," projected tantalizingly outside the cell membrane. It would have taken Padhy no more than an afternoon's exper-iment to add the *neu* antibody to the neuroblastoma cells to determine the binding's effect. "It would have been an overnight test," Weinberg would later recall. "I can flagellate myself. If I had been more studious and more focused and not as monomaniacal about the ideas I had at that time, I would have made that connection."

Despite the trail of seductive leads, Padhy and Weinberg never got around to doing their experiment. Afternoon upon afternoon passed. Introspective and bookish, Padhy shuffled through the lab in a thread-bare coat in the winter, running his experiments privately and saying little about them to others. And although Padhy's discovery was published in a high-profile scientific journal, few scientists noticed that he might have stumbled on a potential anticancer drug (the *neu*-binding antibody was buried in an obscure figure in the article). Even Weinberg, caught in the giddy upswirl of new oncogenes and obsessed with the basic biology of the cancer cell, simply forgot about the *neu* experiment.*

Weinberg had an oncogene and possibly an oncogene-blocking drug, but the twain had never met (in human cells or bodies). In the neuroblas-toma cells dividing in his incubators, *neu* rampaged on monomaniacally, single-mindedly, seemingly invincible. Yet its molecular foot still waved just outside the surface of the plasma membrane, exposed and vulnerable, like Achilles' famous heel.

---

*In 1986, Jeffrey Drebin and Mark Greene showed that treatment with an anti-*neu* antibody arrested the growth of cancer cells. But the prospect of developing this antibody into a human anticancer drug eluded all groups.

A City of Strings

In Ersilia, to establish the relationships that sustain the city's life, inhabitants stretch strings from the corners of the houses, white or black or gray or black-and-white according to whether they mark a relationship of blood, of trade, authority, agency. When the strings become so numerous that you can no longer pass among them, the inhabitants leave: the houses are dismantled.

—Italo Calvino

Weinberg may briefly have forgotten about the therapeutic implication of *neu,* but oncogenes, by their very nature, could not easily be forgotten. In his book *Invisible Cities,* Italo Calvino describes a fictional metropolis in which every relationship between one household and the next is denoted by a piece of colored string stretched between the two houses. As the metropolis grows, the mesh of strings thickens and the individual houses blur away. In the end, Calvino's city becomes no more than an interwoven network of colored strings.

If someone were to draw a similar map of relationships among genes in a normal human cell, then proto-oncogenes and tumor suppressors such as *ras, myc, neu,* and *Rb* would sit at the hub of this cellular city, radiating webs of colored strings in every direction. Proto-oncogenes and tumor suppressors are the molecular pivots of the cell. They are the gatekeepers of cell division, and the division of cells is so central to our physiology that genes and pathways that coordinate this process intersect with nearly every other aspect of our biology. In the laboratory, we call this the six-degrees-of-separation-from-cancer rule: you can ask any biological question, no matter how seemingly distant—what makes the heart fail, or why worms age, or even how birds learn songs—and you will end up, in fewer than six genetic steps, connecting with a proto-oncogene or tumor suppressor.

It should hardly come as a surprise, then, that *neu* was barely forgotten in Weinberg's laboratory when it was resurrected in another. In the summer of 1984, a team of researchers, collaborating with Weinberg, discovered the human homolog of the *neu* gene. Noting its resemblance to another growth-modulating gene discovered previously—the Human EGF Receptor (HER)—the researchers called the gene *Her-2*.

A gene by any other name may still be the same gene, but something crucial had shifted in the story of *neu*. Weinberg's gene had been discovered in an academic laboratory. Much of Weinberg's attention had been focused on dissecting the molecular mechanism of the *neu* oncogene. *Her-2*, in contrast, was discovered on the sprawling campus of the pharmaceutical company Genentech. The difference in venue, and the resulting difference in goals, would radically alter the fate of this gene. For Weinberg, *neu* had represented a route to understanding the fundamental biology of neuroblastoma. For Genentech, *Her-2* represented a route to developing a new drug.

禺

Located on the southern edge of San Francisco, sandwiched among the powerhouse labs of Stanford, UCSF, and Berkeley and the burgeoning start-ups of Silicon Valley, Genentech—short for *Gen*etic *En*gineering *Tech*nology—was born out of an idea imbued with deep alchemic symbolism. In the late 1970s, researchers at Stanford and UCSF had invented a technology termed "recombinant DNA." This technology allowed genes to be manipulated—engineered—in a hitherto unimaginable manner. Genes could be shuttled from one organism to another: a cow gene could be transferred into bacteria, or a human protein synthesized in dog cells. Genes could also be spliced together to create new genes, creating proteins never found in nature. Genentech imagined leveraging this technology of genes to develop a pharmacopoeia of novel drugs. Founded in 1976, the company licensed recombinant DNA technology from UCSF, raised a paltry $200,000 in venture funds, and launched its hunt for these novel drugs.

A "drug," in bare conceptual terms, is any substance that can produce an effect on the physiology of an animal. Drugs can be simple molecules; water and salt, under appropriate circumstances, can function as potent pharmacological agents. Or drugs can be complex, multifaceted chemicals—molecules derived from nature, such as penicillin, or chemicals synthesized artificially, such as aminopterin. Among the most complex drugs in medicine are proteins, molecules synthesized by cells that can exert diverse effects on human physiology. Insulin, made by pancreas cells, is a protein that regulates blood sugar and can be used to control diabetes. Growth hormone, made by the pituitary cells, augments growth by increasing the metabolism of muscle and bone cells.

Before Genentech, protein drugs, although recognizably potent, had been notoriously difficult to produce. Insulin, for instance, was produced by grinding up cow and pig innards into a soup and then extracting the protein from the mix—one pound of insulin from every eight thousand pounds of pancreas. Growth hormone, used to treat a form of dwarfism, was extracted from pituitary glands dissected out of thousands of human cadavers. Clotting drugs to treat bleeding disorders came from liters of human blood.

Recombinant DNA technology allowed Genentech to synthesize human proteins de novo: rather than extracting proteins from animal and human organs, Genentech could "engineer" a human gene into a bacterium, say, and use the bacterial cell as a bioreactor to produce vast quantities of that protein. The technology was transformative. In 1982, Genentech unveiled the first "recombinant" human insulin; in 1984, it produced a clotting factor used to control bleeding in patients with hemophilia; in 1985, it created a recombinant version of human growth hormone—all created by engineering the production of human proteins in bacterial or animal cells.

By the late 1980s, though, after an astonishing growth spurt, Genentech ran out of existing drugs to mass-produce using recombinant technology. Its early victories, after all, had been the result of a *process* and not a product: the company had found a radical new way to produce old medicines. Now, as Genentech set out to invent new drugs from scratch, it was forced to change its winning strategy: it needed to find targets for drugs—proteins in cells that might play a critical role in the physiology of a disease that might, in turn, be turned on or off by other proteins produced using recombinant DNA.

It was under the aegis of this "target discovery" program that Axel Ullrich, a German scientist working at Genentech, rediscovered Weinberg's gene— *Her-2/neu,* the oncogene tethered to the cell membrane.* But having dis-

---

* Ullrich actually found the human homolog of the mouse *neu* gene. Two other groups independently discovered the same gene.

covered the gene, Genentech did not know what to do with it. The drugs that Genentech had successfully synthesized thus far were designed to treat human diseases in which a protein or a signal was absent or low—insulin for diabetics, clotting factors for hemophiliacs, growth hormone for dwarfs. An oncogene was the opposite—not a missing signal, but a signal in overabundance. Genentech could fabricate a missing protein in bacterial cells, but it had yet to learn how to inactivate a hyperactive protein in a human cell.

∂∫∂

In the summer of 1986, while Genentech was still puzzling over a method to inactivate oncogenes, Ullrich presented a seminar at the University of California in Los Angeles. Flamboyant and exuberant, dressed in a dark, formal suit, Ullrich was a riveting speaker. He floored his audience with the incredible story of the isolation of *Her-2,* and the serendipitous convergence of that discovery with Weinberg's prior work. But he left his listeners searching for a punch line. Genentech was a drug company. Where was the drug?

Dennis Slamon, a UCLA oncologist, attended Ullrich's talk that afternoon in 1986. The son of an Appalachian coal miner, Slamon had come to UCLA as a fellow in oncology after medical school at the University of Chicago. He was a peculiar amalgam of smoothness and tenacity, a "velvet jackhammer," as one reporter described him. Early in his academic life he had acquired what he called "a murderous resolve" to cure cancer, but thus far, it was all resolve and no result. In Chicago, Slamon had performed a series of exquisite studies on a human leukemia virus called HTLV-1, the lone retrovirus shown to cause a human cancer. But HTLV-1 was a fleetingly rare cause of cancer. Murdering viruses, Slamon knew, would not cure cancer. He needed a method to kill an oncogene.

Slamon, hearing Ullrich's story of *Her-2,* made a quick, intuitive connection. Ullrich had an oncogene; Genentech wanted a drug—but an intermediate was missing. A drug without a disease is a useless tool; to make a worthwhile cancer drug, both needed a cancer in which the *Her-2* gene was hyperactive. Slamon had a panel of cancers that he could test for *Her-2* hyperactivity. A compulsive pack rat, like Thad Dryja in Boston, Slamon had been collecting and storing samples of cancer tissues from patients who had undergone surgery at UCLA, all saved in a vast freezer. Slamon proposed a simple collaboration. If Ullrich sent him the DNA probes for *Her-2* from Genentech, Slamon could test his collection of cancer cells for samples with hyperactive *Her-2*—thus bridging the gap between the oncogene and a human cancer.

Ullrich agreed. In 1986, he sent Slamon the *Her-2* probe to test on cancer samples. In a few months, Slamon reported back to Ullrich that he had found a distinct pattern, although he did not fully understand it. Cancer cells that become habitually dependent on the activity of a gene for their growth can amplify that gene by making multiple copies of the gene in the chromosome. This phenomenon—like an addict feeding an addiction by ramping up the use of a drug—is called oncogene amplification. *Her-2*, Slamon found, was highly amplified in breast cancer samples, but not in all breast cancers. Based on the pattern of staining, breast cancers could neatly be divided into *Her-2* amplified and *Her-2* unamplified samples— *Her-2* positive and *Her-2* negative.

Puzzled by the "on-off" pattern, Slamon sent an assistant to determine whether *Her-2* positive tumors behaved differently from *Her-2* negative tumors. The search yielded yet another extraordinary pattern: breast tumors that amplified Ullrich's gene tended to be more aggressive, more metastatic, and more likely to kill. *Her-2* amplification marked the tumors with the worst prognosis.

Slamon's data set off a chain reaction in Ullrich's lab at Genentech. The association of *Her-2* with a subtype of cancer—aggressive breast cancer— prompted an important experiment. What would happen, Ullrich wondered, if *Her-2* activity could somehow be shut off? Was the cancer truly "addicted" to amplified *Her-2*? And if so, might squelching the addiction signal using an anti-*Her-2* drug block the growth of the cancer cells? Ullrich was tiptoeing around the afternoon experiment that Weinberg and Padhy had forgotten to perform.

Ullrich knew where he might look for a drug to shut off *Her-2* function. By the mid-1980s, Genentech had organized itself into an astonishing simulacrum of a university. The South San Francisco campus had departments, conferences, lectures, subgroups, even researchers in cutoff jeans playing Frisbee on the lawns. One afternoon, Ullrich walked to the Immunology Division at Genentech. The division specialized in the creation of immunological molecules. Ullrich wondered whether someone in immunology might be able to design a drug to bind *Her-2* and possibly erase its signaling.

Ullrich had a particular kind of protein in mind—an antibody. Antibodies are immunological proteins that bind their targets with exquisite affinity and specificity. The immune system synthesizes antibodies to bind and kill specific targets on bacteria and viruses; antibodies are nature's magic bullets. In the mid-1970s, two immunologists at Cambridge University, Cesar Milstein and George Kohler, had devised a method to produce vast quantities of a single antibody using a hybrid immune cell that had been physically fused to a cancer cell. (The immune cell secreted the antibody while the cancer cell, a specialist in uncontrolled growth, turned it into a factory.) The discovery had instantly been hailed as a potential route to a cancer cure. But to exploit antibodies therapeutically, scientists needed to identify targets unique to cancer cells, and such cancer-specific targets had proved notoriously difficult to identify. Ullrich believed that he had found one such target. *Her-2*, amplified in some breast tumors but barely visible in normal cells, was perhaps Kohler's missing bull's-eye.

At UCLA, meanwhile, Slamon had performed another crucial experiment with *Her-2* expressing cancers. He had implanted these cancers into mice, where they had exploded into friable, metastatic tumors, recapitulating the aggressive human disease. In 1988, Genentech's immunologists successfully produced a mouse antibody that bound and inactivated *Her-2*. Ullrich sent Slamon the first vials of the antibody, and Slamon launched a series of pivotal experiments. When he treated *Her-2* overexpressing breast cancer cells in a dish with the antibody, the cells stopped growing, then involuted and died. More impressively, when he injected his living, tumor-bearing mice with the *Her-2* antibody, the tumors also disappeared. It was as perfect a result as he or Ullrich could have hoped for. *Her-2* inhibition worked in an animal model.

Slamon and Ullrich now had all three essential ingredients for a targeted therapy for cancer: an oncogene, a form of cancer that specifically activated that oncogene, and a drug that specifically targeted it. Both expected Genentech to leap at the opportunity to produce a new protein drug to erase an oncogene's hyperactive signal. But Ullrich, holed away in his lab with *Her-2*, had lost touch with the trajectory of the company outside the lab. Genentech, he now discovered, was abandoning its interest in cancer. Through the 1980s, as Ullrich and Slamon had been hunting for a target specific to cancer cells, several other pharmaceutical companies had tried to develop anticancer drugs using the limited knowledge of the mechanisms driving the growth of cancer cells. Predictably, the drugs that had emerged were largely indiscriminate—toxic to both cancer cells and normal cells—and predictably, all had failed miserably in clinical trials.

Ullrich and Slamon's approach—an oncogene and an oncogene-targeted antibody—was vastly more sophisticated and specific, but Genentech was worried that pouring money into the development of another drug that failed would cripple the company's finances. Chastened by the experience of others—"allergic to cancer," as one Genentech researcher described it—Genentech pulled funding away from most of its cancer projects.

The decision created a deep rift in the company. A small cadre of scientists ardently supported the cancer program, but Genentech's executives wanted to focus on simpler and more profitable drugs. *Her-2* was caught in the cross fire. Drained and dejected, Ullrich left Genentech. He would eventually join an academic laboratory in Germany, where he could work on cancer genetics without the fickle pressures of a pharmaceutical company constraining his science.

Slamon, now working alone at UCLA, tried furiously to keep the *Her-2* effort alive at Genentech, even though he wasn't on the company's payroll. "Nobody gave a shit except him," John Curd, Genentech's medical director, recalled. Slamon became a pariah at Genentech, a pushy, obsessed gadfly who would often jet up from Los Angeles and lurk in the corridors seeking to interest anyone he could in his mouse antibody. Most scientists had lost interest. But Slamon retained the faith of a small group of Genentech scientists, scientists nostalgic for the pioneering, early days of Genentech when problems had been taken on precisely *because* they were intractable. An MIT-educated geneticist, David Botstein, and a molecular biologist, Art Levinson, both at Genentech, had been strong proponents of the *Her-2* project. (Levinson had come to Genentech from Michael Bishop's lab at UCSF, where he had worked on the phosphorylating function of *src*; oncogenes were stitched into his psyche.) Pulling strings, resources, and connections, Slamon and Levinson convinced a tiny entrepreneurial team to push ahead with the *Her-2* project.

Marginally funded, the work edged along, almost invisible to Genentech's executives. In 1989, Mike Shepard, an immunologist at Genentech, improved the production and purification of the *Her-2* antibody. But the purified mouse antibody, Slamon knew, was far from a human drug. Mouse antibodies, being "foreign" proteins, provoke a potent immune response in humans and make terrible human drugs. To circumvent that response, Genentech's antibody needed to be converted into a protein that more closely resembled a human antibody. This process, evocatively called "humanizing" an antibody, is a delicate art, somewhat akin to translating a novel;

what matters is not just the content, but the ineffable essence of the antibody—its form. Genentech's resident "humanizer" was Paul Carter, a quiet, twenty-nine-year-old Englishman who had learned the craft at Cambridge from Cesar Milstein, the scientist who had first produced these antibodies using fused immune and cancer cells. Under Slamon's and Shepard's guidance, Carter set about humanizing the mouse antibody. In the summer of 1990, Carter proudly produced a fully humanized *Her-2* antibody ready to be used in clinical trials. The antibody, now a potential drug, would soon be renamed Herceptin, fusing the words *Her-2, intercept,* and *inhibitor.**

Such was the halting, traumatic birth of the new drug that it was easy to forget the enormity of what had been achieved. Slamon had identified *Her-2* amplification in breast cancer tissue in 1987; Carter and Shepard had produced a humanized antibody against it by 1990. They had moved from cancer to target to drug in an astonishing three years, a pace unprecedented in the history of cancer.

♨

In the summer of 1990, Barbara Bradfield, a forty-eight-year-old woman from Burbank, California, discovered a mass in her breast and a lump under her arm. A biopsy confirmed what she already suspected: she had breast cancer that had spread to her lymph nodes. She was treated with a bilateral mastectomy followed by nearly seven months of chemotherapy. "When I was finished with all that," she recalled, "I felt as if I had crossed a river of tragedy."

But there was more river to ford: Bradfield's life was hit by yet another incommensurate tragedy. In the winter of 1991, driving on a highway not far from their house, her daughter, twenty-three years old and pregnant, was killed in a fiery accident. A few months later, sitting numbly in a Bible-study class one morning, Bradfield let her fingers wander up to the edge of her neck. A new grape-size mass had appeared just above her collarbone. Her breast cancer had relapsed and metastasized—almost certainly a harbinger of death.

Bradfield's oncologist in Burbank offered her more chemotherapy, but she declined it. She enrolled in an alternative herbal-therapy program and bought a vegetable juicer and planned a trip to Mexico. When her oncolo-

---

* The drug is also known by its pharmacological name Trastuzumab; the "ab" suffix is used to denote the fact that this is an *anti*bod*y*.

gist asked if he could send samples of her breast cancer to Slamon's lab at UCLA for a second opinion, she agreed reluctantly. A faraway doctor performing unfamiliar tests on her tumor sample, she knew, could not possibly affect her.

One afternoon in the summer of 1991, Bradfield received a phone call from Slamon. He introduced himself as a researcher who had been analyzing her slides. Slamon told Bradfield about *Her-2*. "His tone changed," she recalled. Her tumor, he said, had one of the highest levels of amplified *Her-2* that he had ever seen. Slamon told her that he was launching a trial of an antibody that bound *Her-2* and that she would be the ideal candidate for the new drug. Bradfield refused. "I was at the end of my road," she said, "and I had accepted what seemed inevitable." Slamon tried to reason with her for a while, but found her unbending. He thanked her for her consideration and rang off.

Early the next morning, though, Slamon was back on the telephone. He apologized for the intrusion, but her decision had troubled him all night. Of all the variants of *Her-2* amplification that he had encountered, hers had been truly extraordinary; Bradfield's tumor was chock-full of *Her-2,* almost hypnotically drunk on the oncogene. He begged her once again to join his trial.

"Survivors look back and see omens, messages they missed," Joan Didion wrote. For Bradfield, Slamon's second phone call was an omen that was not missed; something in that conversation pierced through a shield that she had drawn around herself. On a warm August morning in 1992, Bradfield visited Slamon in his clinic at UCLA. He met her in the hallway and led her to a room in the back. Under the microscope, he showed her the breast cancer that had been excised from her body, with its dark ringlets of *Her-2* labeled cells. On a whiteboard, he drew a step-by-step picture of an epic scientific journey. He began with the discovery of *neu,* its rediscovery in Ullrich's lab, the struggles to produce a drug, culminating in the antibody stitched together so carefully by Shepard and Carter. Bradfield considered the line that stretched from oncogene to drug. She agreed to join Slamon's trial.

It was an extraordinarily fortunate decision. In the four months between Slamon's phone call and the first infusion of Herceptin, Bradfield's tumor had erupted, spraying sixteen new masses into her lung.

❦

Fifteen women, including Bradfield, enrolled in Slamon's trial at UCLA in 1992. (The number would later be expanded to thirty-seven.) The drug was given for nine weeks, in combination with cisplatin, a standard chemotherapy agent used to kill breast cancer cells, both delivered intravenously. As a matter of convenience, Slamon planned to treat all the women on the same day and in the same room. The effect was theatrical; this was a stage occupied by a beleaguered set of actors. Some women had begged and finagled their way into Slamon's trial through friends and relatives; others, such as Bradfield, had been begged to join it. "All of us knew that we were living on borrowed time," Bradfield said, "and so we felt twice as alive and lived twice as fiercely." A Chinese woman in her fifties brought stash after stash of traditional herbs and salves that she swore had kept her alive thus far; she would take oncology's newest drug, Herceptin, only if she could also take its most ancient drugs with it. A frail, thin woman in her thirties, recently relapsed with breast cancer after a bone marrow transplant, glowered silently and intensely in a corner. Some treated their illness reverentially. Some were bewildered, some too embittered to care. A mother from Boston in her midfifties cracked raunchy jokes about her cancer. The daylong drill of infusions and blood tests was exhausting. In the late evening, after all the tests, the women went their own ways. Bradfield went home and prayed. Another woman soused herself with martinis.

The lump on Bradfield's neck—the only tumor in the group that could be physically touched, measured, and watched—became the compass for the trial. On the morning of the first intravenous infusion of the *Her-2* antibody, all the women came up to feel the lump, one by one, running their hands across Bradfield's collarbone. It was a peculiarly intimate ritual that would be repeated every week. Two weeks after the first dose of the antibody, when the group filed past Bradfield, touching the node again, the change was incontrovertible. Bradfield's tumor had softened and visibly shrunk. "We began to believe that something was happening here," Bradfield recalled. "Suddenly, the weight of our good fortune hit us."

Not everyone was as fortunate as Bradfield. Exhausted and nauseous one evening, the young woman with relapsed metastatic cancer was unable to keep down the fluids needed to hydrate her body. She vomited through the night and then, too tired to keep drinking and too sick to understand the consequences, fell back into sleep. She died of kidney failure the next week.

Bradfield's extraordinary response continued. When the CT scans were repeated two months into the trial, the tumor in her neck had virtually disappeared, and the lung metastases had also diminished both in number and size. The responses in many of the thirteen other women were more ambiguous. At the three-month midpoint of the trial, when Slamon reviewed the data with Genentech and the external trial monitors, tough decisions clearly needed to be made. Tumors had remained unchanged in size in some women—not shrunk, but static: was this to be counted as a positive response? Some women with bone metastasis reported diminished bone pain, but pain could not objectively be judged. After a prolonged and bitter debate, the trial coordinators suggested dropping seven women from the study because their responses could not be quantified. One woman discontinued the drug herself. Only five of the original cohort, including Bradfield, continued the trial to its six-month end point. Embittered and disappointed, the others returned to their local oncologists, their hopes for a miracle drug again dashed.

Barbara Bradfield finished eighteen weeks of therapy in 1993. She survives today. A gray-haired woman with crystalline gray-blue eyes, she lives in the small town of Puyallup near Seattle, hikes in the nearby woods, and leads discussion groups for her church. She vividly remembers her days at the Los Angeles clinic—the half-lit room in the back where the nurses dosed the drugs, the strangely intimate touch of the other women feeling the node in her neck. And Slamon, of course. "Dennis is my hero," she said. "I refused his first phone call, but I have never, ever, refused him anything since that time." The animation and energy in her voice crackled across the phone line like an electrical current. She quizzed me about my research. I thanked her for her time, but she, in turn, apologized for the distraction. "Get back to work," she said, laughing. "There are people waiting for discoveries."

Drugs, Bodies, and Proof

Dying people don't have time or energy. We can't keep doing this one woman, one drug, one company at a time.
—Gracia Buffleben

It seemed as if we had entered a brave new world of precisely targeted, less toxic, more effective combined therapies.
—*Breast Cancer Action Newsletter*, 2004

By the summer of 1993, news of Slamon's early-phase trial had spread like wildfire through the community of breast cancer patients, fanning out through official and unofficial channels. In waiting rooms, infusion centers, and oncologists' offices, patients spoke to other patients describing the occasional but unprecedented responses and remissions. Newsletters printed by breast cancer support groups whipped up a frenzy of hype and hope about Herceptin. Inevitably, a tinderbox of expectations was set to explode.

The issue was "compassionate use." *Her-2* positive breast cancer is one of the most fatal and rapidly progressive variants of the disease, and patients were willing to try any therapy that could produce a clinical benefit. Breast cancer activists pounded on Genentech's doors to urge the release of the drug to women with *Her-2* positive cancer who had failed other therapies. These patients, the activists argued, could not wait for the drug to undergo interminable testing; they wanted a potentially lifesaving medicine *now.* "True success happens," as one writer put it in 1995, "only when these new drugs actually enter bodies."

For Genentech, though, "true success" was defined by vastly different imperatives. Herceptin had not been approved by the FDA; it was a molecule in its infancy. Genentech wanted carefully executed early-phase tri-als—not just new drugs entering bodies, but carefully monitored drugs entering carefully monitored bodies in carefully monitored trials. For the next phase of Herceptin trials launched in 1993, Genentech wanted to stay small and focused. The number of women enrolled in these trials had been kept to an absolute minimum: twenty-seven patients at Sloan-Kettering, sixteen at UCSF, and thirty-nine at UCLA, a tiny cohort that the company intended to follow deeply and meticulously over time. "We do not provide . . . compassionate use programs," Curd curtly told a journalist. Most doc-tors involved in the early-phase trials agreed. "If you start making excep-tions and deviating from your protocol," Debu Tripathy, one of the leaders of the UCSF trial, said, "then you get a lot of patients whose results are not going to help you understand whether a drug works or not. All you're doing is delaying . . . being able to get it out into the public."

Outside the cloistered laboratories of Genentech, the controversy ignited a firestorm. San Francisco, of course, was no stranger to this issue of compassionate use versus focused research. In the late 1980s, as AIDS had erupted in the city, filling up Paul Volberding's haunted Ward 5B with scores of patients, gay men had coalesced into groups such as ACT UP to demand speedier access to drugs, in part through compassionate use pro-grams. Breast cancer activists saw a grim reflection of their own struggle in these early battles. As one newsletter put it, "Why do women dying of breast cancer have such trouble getting experimental drugs that could extend their lives? For years, AIDS activists have been negotiating with drug companies and the FDA to obtain new HIV drugs while the thera-pies were still in clinical trials. Surely women with metastatic breast can-cer for whom standard treatments have failed should know about, and have access to, compassionate use programs for experimental drugs."

Or, as another writer put it, "Scientific uncertainty is no excuse for inaction. . . . We cannot wait for 'proof.'"

❧

Marti Nelson, for one, certainly could not afford to wait for proof. An outgoing, dark-haired gynecologist in California, Nelson had discovered a malignant mass in her breast in 1987, when she was just thirty-three. She had had a mastectomy and multiple cycles of chemo, then returned to practicing medicine in a San Francisco clinic. The tumor had disappeared. The scars had healed. Nelson thought that she might have been cured.

In 1993, six years after her initial surgery, Nelson noticed that the scar in her breast had begun to harden. She waved it away. But the hardened line of tissue outlining her breast was relapsed breast cancer, worming its way insidiously along the scar lines and coalescing into small, matted masses in her chest. Nelson, who compulsively followed the clinical literature on breast cancer, had heard of *Her-2*. Reasoning presciently that her tumor might be *Her-2* positive, she tried to have her own specimen tested for the gene.

But Nelson soon found herself inhabiting a Kafkaesque nightmare. Her HMO insisted that because Herceptin was in investigational trials, testing the tumor for *Her-2* was useless. Genentech insisted that without *Her-2* status confirmed, giving her access to Herceptin was untenable.

In the summer of 1993, with Nelson's cancer advancing daily and spewing out metastases into her lungs and bone marrow, the struggle took an urgent, political turn. Nelson contacted the Breast Cancer Action project, a local San Francisco organization connected with ACT UP, to help her get someone to test her tumor and obtain Herceptin for compassionate use. BCA, working through its activist networks, asked several laboratories in and around San Francisco to test Nelson's tumor. In October 1994, the tumor was finally tested for *Her-2* expression at UCSF. It was strikingly *Her-2* positive. She was an ideal candidate for the drug. But the news came too late. Nine days later, still awaiting Herceptin approval from Genentech, Marti Nelson drifted into a coma and died. She was forty-one years old.

◈

For BCA activists, Nelson's death was a watershed event. Livid and desperate, a group of women from the BCA stormed through the Genentech campus on December 5, 1994, to hold a fifteen-car "funeral procession" for Nelson with placards showing Nelson in her chemo turban before her death. The women shouted and honked their horns and drove their cars through the manicured lawns. Gracia Buffleben, a nurse with breast cancer and one of the most outspoken leaders of the BCA, parked her car outside one of the main buildings and handcuffed herself to the steering wheel. A furious researcher stumbled out of one of the lab buildings and shouted, "I'm a scientist working on the AIDS cure. Why are you here? You are making too much noise." It was a statement that epitomized the vast and growing rift between scientists and patients.

Marti Nelson's "funeral" woke Genentech up to a new reality. Outrage, rising to a crescendo, threatened to spiral into a public relations disaster. Genentech had a narrow choice: unable to silence the activists, it was forced to join them. Even Curd admitted, if somewhat begrudgingly, that the BCA was "a tough group [and] their activism is not misguided."

In 1995, a small delegation of Genentech scientists and executives thus flew to Washington to meet Frances Visco, the chair of the National Breast Cancer Coalition (NBCC), a powerful national coalition of cancer activists, hoping to use the NBCC as a neutral intermediary between the company and the local breast cancer activists in San Francisco. Pragmatic, charismatic, and savvy, Visco, a former attorney, had spent nearly a decade immersed in the turbulent politics of breast cancer. Visco had a proposal for Genentech, but her terms were inflexible: Genentech had to provide an expanded access program for Herceptin. This program would allow oncologists to treat patients outside clinical trials. In return, the National Breast Cancer Coalition would act as a go-between for Genentech and its embittered and alienated community of cancer patients. Visco offered to join the planning committee of the phase III trials of Herceptin, and to help recruit patients for the trial using the NBCC's extensive network. For Genentech, this was a long-overdue education. Rather than running trials *on* breast cancer patients, the company learned to run trials *with* breast cancer patients. (Genentech would eventually outsource the compassionate-access program to a lottery system run by an independent agency. Women applied to the lottery and "won" the right to be treated, thus removing the company from any ethically difficult decision-making.)

It was an uneasy triangle of forces—academic researchers, the pharmaceutical industry, and patient advocates—united by a deadly disease. Genentech's next phase of trials involved large-scale, randomized studies on thousands of women with metastatic *Her-2* positive cancer, comparing Herceptin treatment against placebo treatment. Visco sent out newsletters from the NBCC to patients using the coalition's enormous Listservs. Kay Dickersin, a coalition member and an epidemiologist, joined the Data Safety and Monitoring board of the trial, underscoring the new partnership between Genentech and the NBCC, between academic medicine and activism. And an all-star team of breast oncologists was assembled to run the trial: Larry Norton from Sloan-Kettering, Karen Antman from Columbia, Daniel Hayes from Harvard, and, of course, Slamon from UCLA.

In 1995, empowered by the very forces that it had resisted for so long, Genentech launched three independent phase III trials to test Herceptin. The most pivotal of the three was a trial labeled 648, randomizing women newly diagnosed with metastatic breast cancer to standard chemotherapy alone versus chemotherapy with Herceptin added. Trial 648 was launched in 150 breast cancer clinics around the world. The trial would enroll 469 women and cost Genentech $15 million to run.

ᴶᴵᴾ

In May 1998, eighteen thousand cancer specialists flocked to Los Angeles to attend the thirty-fourth meeting of the American Society of Clinical Oncology, where Genentech would unveil the data from the Herceptin trials, including trial 648. On Sunday, May 17, the third day of the meeting, an expectant audience of thousands piled into the stuffy central amphitheater at the convention center to attend a special session dedicated to *Her-2/neu* in breast cancer. Slamon was slated to be the last speaker. A coil of nervous energy, with the characteristic twitch in his mustache, he stood up at the podium.

Clinical presentations at ASCO are typically sanitized and polished, with blue-and-white PowerPoint slides depicting the bottom-line message using survival curves and statistical analyses. But Slamon began—relishing this pivotal moment—not with numbers and statistics, but with forty-nine smudgy bands on a gel run by one of his undergraduate students in 1987. Oncologists slowed down their scribbling. Reporters squinted their eyes to see the bands on the gel.

That gel, he reminded his audience, had identified a gene with no pedigree—no history, no function, no mechanism. It was nothing more than an isolated, amplified signal in a fraction of breast cancer cases. Slamon had gambled the most important years of his scientific life on those bands. Others had joined the gamble: Ullrich, Shepard, Carter, Botstein and Levinson, Visco and the activists, pharma executives and clinicians and Genentech. The trial results to be announced that afternoon represented the result of that gamble. But Slamon wouldn't—he couldn't—rush to the end point of the journey without reminding everyone in the room of the fitful, unsanitized history of the drug.

Slamon paused for a theatrical moment before revealing the results of the trial. In the pivotal 648 study, 469 women had received standard cytotoxic chemotherapy (either Adriamycin and Cytoxan in combination, or Taxol) and were randomized to receive either Herceptin or a placebo. In every conceivable index of response, women treated with the addition of Herceptin had shown a clear and measurable benefit. Response rates to standard chemotherapy had moved up 150 percent. Tumors had shrunk in half the women treated with Herceptin compared to a third of women in the control arm. The progression of breast cancer had been delayed from four to seven and a half months. In patients with tumors heavily resistant to the standard Adriamycin and Cytoxan regimen, the benefit had been the most marked: the combination of Herceptin and Taxol had increased response rates to nearly 50 percent—a rate unheard of in recent clinical experience. The survival rate would also follow this trend. Women treated with Herceptin lived four or five months longer than women in the control group.

At face value, some of these gains might have seemed small in absolute terms—life extended by only four months. But the women enrolled in these initial trials were patients with late-stage, metastatic cancers, often heavily pretreated with standard chemotherapies and refractory to all drugs—women carrying the worst and most aggressive variants of breast cancer. (This pattern is typical: in cancer medicine, trials often begin with the most advanced and refractory cases, where even small benefits of a drug might outweigh risks.) The true measure of Herceptin's efficacy would lie in the treatment of treatment-naive patients—women diagnosed with early-stage breast cancer who had never received any prior treatment.

In 2003, two enormous multinational studies were launched to test Herceptin in early-stage breast cancer in treatment-naive patients. In one of the studies, Herceptin treatment increased breast cancer survival at four years by a striking 18 percent over the placebo group. The second study, although stopped earlier, showed a similar magnitude of benefit. When the trials were statistically combined, overall survival in women treated with Herceptin was increased by 33 percent—a magnitude unprecedented in the history of chemotherapy for *Her-2* positive cancer. "The results," one oncologist wrote, were "simply stunning . . . not evolutionary, but revolutionary. The rational development of molecularly targeted therapies points the direction toward continued improvement in breast cancer therapy. Other targets and other agents will follow."

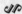

On the evening of May 17, 1998, after Slamon had announced the results of the 648 study to a stunned audience at the ASCO meeting, Genentech threw an enormous cocktail party at the Hollywood Terrace, an open-air restaurant nestled in the hills of Los Angeles. Wine flowed freely, and the conversation was light and breezy. Just a few days earlier, the FDA had reviewed the data from the three Herceptin trials, including Slamon's study, and was on the verge of "fast-tracking" the approval of Herceptin. It was a poignant posthumous victory for Marti Nelson: the drug that would likely have saved her life would become accessible to all breast cancer patients—no longer reserved for clinical trials or compassionate use alone.

"The company," Robert Bazell, the journalist, wrote, "invited all the investigators, as well as most of Genentech's *Her-2* team. The activists came too: Marilyn McGregor and Bob Erwin [Marti Nelson's husband] from San Francisco and Fran Visco from the National Breast Cancer Coalition."

The evening was balmy, clear, and spectacular. "The warm orange glow of the setting sun over the San Fernando Valley set the tone of the festivities. Everyone at the party would celebrate an enormous success. Women's lives would be saved and a huge fortune would be made."

Only one person was conspicuously missing from the party—Dennis Slamon. Having spent the afternoon planning the next phase of Herceptin trials with breast oncologists at ASCO, Slamon had jumped into his run-down Nissan and driven home.

A Four-Minute Mile

*The nontoxic curative compound remains undiscovered
but not undreamt.*

—James F. Holland

*Why, it is asked, does the supply of new miracle drugs
lag so far behind, while biology continues to move from
strength to strength . . . ? There is still the conspicuous
asymmetry between molecular biology and, say, the
therapy of lung cancer.*

—Lewis Thomas,
The Lives of a Cell, 1978

In the summer of 1990, as Herceptin entered its earliest trials, another
oncogene-targeted drug began its long journey toward the clinic. More
than any other medicine in the history of cancer, more even than
Herceptin, the development of this drug—from cancer to oncogene to a
targeted therapy and to successive human trials—would signal the arrival
of a new era in cancer medicine. Yet to arrive at this new era, cancer biologists would again need to circle back to old observations—to the peculiar illness that John Bennett had called a "suppuration of blood," that
Virchow had reclassified as *weisses Blut* in 1847, and that later researchers
had again reclassified as chronic myeloid leukemia or CML.

For more than a century, Virchow's *weisses Blut* had lived on the
peripheries of oncology. In 1973, CML was suddenly thrust center stage.
Examining CML cells, Janet Rowley identified a unique chromosomal
aberration that existed in all the leukemia cells. This abnormality, the so-
called Philadelphia chromosome, was the result of a translocation in which
the "head" of chromosome twenty-two and the "tail" of chromosome nine

had been fused to create a novel gene. Rowley's work suggested that CML cells possess a distinct and unique genetic abnormality—possibly the first human oncogene.

๙๐

Rowley's observation launched a prolonged hunt for the mysterious chimeric gene produced by the 9:22 fusion. The identity of the gene emerged piece by piece over a decade. In 1982, a team of Dutch researchers in Amsterdam isolated the gene on chromosome nine. They called it *abl*.* In 1984, working with American collaborators in Maryland, the same team isolated *abl*'s partner on chromosome twenty-two—a gene called *Bcr*. The oncogene created by the fusion of these two genes in CML cells was named *Bcr-abl*. In 1987, David Baltimore's laboratory in Boston "engineered" a mouse containing the activated *Bcr-abl* oncogene in its blood cells. The mouse developed the fatal spleen-choking leukemia that Bennett had seen in the Scottish slate-layer and Virchow in the German cook more than a century earlier—proving that *Bcr-abl* drove the pathological proliferation of CML cells.

As with the study of any oncogene, the field now turned from structure to function: what did *Bcr-abl* do to cause leukemia? When Baltimore's lab and Owen Witte's lab investigated the function of the aberrant *Bcr-abl* oncogene, they found that, like *src*, it was yet another kinase—a protein that tagged other proteins with a phosphate group and thus unleashed a cascade of signals in a cell. In normal cells, the *Bcr* and *abl* genes existed separately; both were tightly regulated during cell division. In CML cells, the translocation created a new chimera—*Bcr-abl*, a hyperactive, overexuberant kinase that activated a pathway that forced cells to divide incessantly.

๙๐

In the mid-1980s, with little knowledge about the emerging molecular genetics of CML, a team of chemists at Ciba-Geigy, a pharmaceutical company in Basel, Switzerland, was trying to develop drugs that might inhibit kinases. The human genome has about five hundred kinases (of which, about ninety belong to the subclass that contains *src* and *Bcr-abl*).

---

* *Abl*, too, was first discovered in a virus, and later found to be present in human cells— again recapitulating the story of *ras* and *src*. Once more, a retrovirus had "pirated" a human cancer gene and turned into a cancer-causing virus.

Every kinase attaches phosphate tags to a unique set of proteins in the cell. Kinases thus act as molecular master-switches in cells—turning "on" some pathways and turning "off" others—thus providing the cell a coordinated set of internal signals to grow, shrink, move, stop, or die. Recognizing the pivotal role of kinases in cellular physiology, the Ciba-Geigy team hoped to discover drugs that could activate or inhibit kinases selectively in cells, thus manipulating the cell's master-switches. The team was led by a tall, reserved, acerbic Swiss physician-biochemist, Alex Matter. In 1986, Matter was joined in his hunt for selective kinase inhibitors by Nick Lydon, a biochemist from Leeds, England.

Pharmaceutical chemists often think of molecules in terms of faces and surfaces. Their world is topological; they imagine touching molecules with the tactile hypersensitivity of the blind. If the surface of a protein is bland and featureless, then that protein is typically "undruggable"; flat, poker-faced topologies make for poor targets for drugs. But if a protein's surface is marked with deep crevices and pockets, then that protein tends to make an attractive target for other molecules to bind—and is thereby a possible "druggable" target.

Kinases, fortuitously, possess at least one such deep druggable pocket. In 1976, a team of Japanese researchers looking for poisons in sea bacteria had accidentally discovered a molecule called staurosporine, a large molecule shaped like a lopsided Maltese cross that bound to a pocket present in most kinases. Staurosporine inhibited dozens of kinases. It was an exquisite poison, but a terrible drug—possessing virtually no ability to discriminate between any kinase, active or inactive, good or bad, in most cells.

The existence of staurosporine inspired Matter. If sea bacteria could synthesize a drug to block kinases nonspecifically, then surely a team of chemists could make a drug to block only certain kinases in cells. In 1986, Matter and Lydon found a critical lead. Having tested millions of potential molecules, they discovered a skeletal chemical that, like staurosporine, could also lodge itself into a kinase protein's cleft and inhibit its function. Unlike staurosporine, though, this skeletal structure was a much simpler chemical. Matter and Lydon could make dozens of variants of this chemical to determine if some might bind better to certain kinases. It was a self-conscious emulation of Paul Ehrlich, who had, in the 1890s, gradually coaxed specificity from his aniline dyes and thus created a universe of novel medicines. History repeats itself, but chemistry, Matter and Lydon knew, repeats itself more insistently.

It was a painstaking, iterative game—chemistry by trial and error. Jürg Zimmermann, a talented chemist on Matter's team, created thousands of variants of the parent molecule and handed them off to a cell biologist, Elisabeth Buchdunger. Buchdunger tested these new molecules on cells, weeding out those that were insoluble or toxic, then bounced them back to Zimmermann for resynthesis, resetting the relay race toward more and more specific and nontoxic chemicals. "[It was] what a locksmith does when he has to make a key fit," Zimmermann said. "You change the shape of the key and test it. Does it fit? If not, you change it again."

By the early nineties, this fitting and refitting had created dozens of new molecules that were structurally related to Matter's original kinase inhibitor. When Lydon tested this panel of inhibitors on various kinases found in cells, he discovered that these molecules possessed specificity: one molecule might inhibit *src* and spare every other kinase, while another might block *abl* and spare *src*. What Matter and Lydon now needed was a disease in which to apply this collection of chemicals—a form of cancer driven by a locked, overexuberant kinase that they could kill using a specific kinase inhibitor.

❦

In the late 1980s, Nick Lydon traveled to the Dana-Farber Cancer Institute in Boston to investigate whether one of the kinase inhibitors synthesized in Basel might inhibit the growth of a particular form of cancer. Lydon met Brian Druker, a young faculty member at the institute fresh from his oncology fellowship and about to launch an independent laboratory in Boston. Druker was particularly interested in chronic myelogenous leukemia—the cancer driven by the *Bcr-abl* kinase.

Druker heard of Lydon's collection of kinase-specific inhibitors, and he was quick to make the logical leap. "I was drawn to oncology as a medical student because I had read Farber's original paper on aminopterin and it had had a deep influence on me," he recalled. "Farber's generation had tried to target cancer cells empirically, but had failed because the mechanistic understanding of cancer was so poor. Farber had had the right idea, but at the wrong time."

Druker had the right idea at the right time. Once again, as with Slamon and Ullrich, two halves of a puzzle came together. Druker had a cohort of CML patients afflicted by a tumor driven by a specific hyperactive kinase. Lydon and Matter had synthesized an entire collection of kinase inhibitors now stocked in Ciba-Geigy's freezer in Basel. Somewhere in that Ciba collection, Druker reasoned, was lurking his fantasy drug—a chemical kinase inhibitor with specific affinity for *Bcr-abl*. Druker proposed an ambitious collaboration between Ciba-Geigy and the Dana-Farber Cancer Institute to test the kinase inhibitors in patients. But the agreement fell apart; the legal teams in Basel and Boston could not find agreeable terms. Drugs could recognize and bind kinases specifically, but scientists and lawyers could not partner with each other to bring these drugs to patients. The project, having generated an interminable trail of legal memos, was quietly tabled.

But Druker was persistent. In 1993, he left Boston to start his own laboratory at the Oregon Health and Science University (OHSU) in Portland. Unyoked, at last, from the institution that had forestalled his collaboration, he immediately called Lydon to reestablish a connection. Lydon informed him that the Ciba-Geigy team had synthesized an even larger collection of inhibitors and had found a molecule that might bind *Bcr-abl* with high specificity and selectivity. The molecule was called CGP57148. Summoning all the nonchalance that he could muster—having learned his lessons in Boston—Druker walked over to the legal department at OHSU and, revealing little about the potential of the chemicals, watched as the lawyers absentmindedly signed on the dotted line. "Everyone just humored me," he recalled. "No one thought even faintly that this drug might work." In two weeks, he received a package from Basel with a small collection of kinase inhibitors to test in his lab.

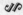

The clinical world of CML was, meanwhile, reeling from disappointment to disappointment. In October 1992, just a few months before CGP57148 crossed the Atlantic from Lydon's Basel lab into Druker's hands in Oregon, a fleet of leukemia experts descended on the historic town of Bologna in Italy for an international conference on CML. The location was resplendent and evocative—Vesalius had once lectured and taught in these quadrangles and amphitheaters, dismantling Galen's theory of cancer piece by piece. But the news at the meeting was uninspiring. The principal treatment for CML in 1993 was allogeneic bone marrow transplantation, the protocol pioneered in Seattle by Donnall Thomas in the sixties. Allo-transplantation, in which a foreign bone marrow was transplanted into a patient's body, could increase the survival of CML patients, but the gains were often so modest that massive trials were needed to detect them. At Bologna, even transplanters glumly acknowledged the meager benefits: "Although freedom from leukemia could be obtained only with BMT," one study concluded, "a beneficial effect of BMT on overall survival could be detected only in a patients' subset, and . . . many hundreds of cases and a decade could be necessary to evaluate the effect on survival."

Like most leukemia experts, Druker was all too familiar with this dismal literature. "Cancer is complicated, everyone kept telling me patronizingly—as if I had suggested that it was not complicated." The growing dogma, he knew, was that CML was perhaps intrinsically a chemotherapy-resistant disease. Even if the leukemia was initiated by that single translocation of the *Bcr-abl* gene, by the time the disease was identified in full bloom in real patients, it had accumulated a host of additional mutations, creating a genetic tornado so chaotic that even transplantation, the chemotherapist's bluntest weapon, was of no consequence. The inciting *Bcr-abl* kinase had likely long been overwhelmed by more powerful driver mutations. Using a kinase inhibitor to try to control the disease, Druker feared, would be like blowing hard on a matchstick long after it had ignited a forest fire.

In the summer of 1993, when Lydon's drug arrived in Druker's hands, he added it to CML cells in a petri dish, hoping, at best, for a small effect. But the cell lines responded briskly. Overnight, the drug-treated CML cells died, and the tissue-culture flasks filled up with floating husks of involuted leukemia cells. Druker was amazed. He implanted CML cells into mice to form real, living tumors and treated the mice with the drug. As with the first experiment, the tumors regressed in days. The response suggested specificity as well: normal mouse blood cells were left untouched. Druker performed a third experiment. He drew out samples of bone marrow from a few human patients with CML and applied CGP57148 to the cells in a petri dish. The leukemia cells in the marrow died immediately. The only cells remaining in the dish were normal blood cells. He had cured leukemia in the dish.

Druker described the findings in the journal *Nature Medicine*. It was a punchy, compact study—just five clean, well-built experiments—driving relentlessly toward a simple conclusion: "This compound may be useful in the treatment of *Bcr-abl* positive leukemias." Druker was the first author and Lydon the senior author, with Buchdunger and Zimmermann as key contributors.

❧

Druker expected Ciba-Geigy to be ecstatic about these results. This, after all, was the ultimate dream child of oncology—a drug with exquisite specificity for an oncogene in a cancer cell. But in Basel, Ciba-Geigy was in internal disarray. The company had fused with its archrival across the river, the pharma giant Sandoz, into a pharmaceutical behemoth called Novartis. For Novartis, it was the exquisite specificity of CGP57148 that was precisely its fatal undoing. Developing CGP57148 into a clinical drug for human use would involve further testing—animal studies and clinical trials that would cost $100 to $200 million. CML afflicts a few thousand patients every year in America. The prospect of spending millions on a molecule to benefit thousands gave Novartis cold feet.

Druker now found himself inhabiting an inverted world in which an academic researcher had to beg a pharmaceutical company to push its own products into clinical trials. Novartis had a plethora of predictable excuses: "The drug . . . would never work, would be too toxic, would never make any money." Between 1995 and 1997 Druker flew back and forth between Basel and Portland trying to convince Novartis to continue the clinical development of its drug. "Either get [the drug] into clinical trials or license it to me. Make a decision," Druker insisted. If Novartis would not make the drug, Druker thought he could have another chemist take it on. "In the worst case," he recalled, "I thought I would make it in my own basement."

Planning ahead, he assembled a team of other physicians to run a potential clinical trial of the drug on CML patients: Charles Sawyers from UCLA, Moshe Talpaz, a hematologist from Houston, and John Goldman from the Hammersmith Hospital in London, all highly regarded authorities on CML. Druker said, "I had patients in my clinic with CML with no effective treatment options remaining. Every day, I would come home from the clinic and promise to push Novartis a little."

In early 1998, Novartis finally relented. It would synthesize and release a few grams of CGP57148, just about enough to run a trial on about a hundred patients. Druker would have a shot—but only one shot. To Novartis, CGP57148, the product of its most ambitious drug-discovery program to date, was already a failure.

❧

I first heard of Druker's drug in the fall of 2002. I was a medical resident triaging patients in the emergency room at Mass General when an intern called me about a middle-aged man with a history of CML who had come in with a rash. I heard the story almost instinctively, drawing quick conclusions. The patient, I surmised, had been transplanted with foreign bone marrow, and the rash was the first blush of a cataclysm to come. The immune cells in the foreign marrow were attacking his own body—graft-versus-host disease. His prognosis was grim. He would need steroids, immunosuppressives, and immediate admission to the transplant floor.

But I was wrong. Glancing at the chart in the red folder, I saw no mention of a transplant. Under the stark neon light of the examining room when he held out his hand to be examined, the rash was just a few scattered, harmless-looking papules—nothing like the dusky, mottled haze that is often the harbinger of a graft reaction. Searching for an alternative explanation, I quickly ran my eye through his list of medicines. Only one drug was listed: Gleevec, the new name for Druker's drug, CGP57148.*

The rash was a minor side effect of the drug. The major effect of the drug, though, was less visible but far more dramatic. Smeared under the microscope in the pathology lab on the second floor, his blood cells looked extraordinarily ordinary—"normal red cells, normal platelets, normal white blood cells," I whispered under my breath as I ran my eyes slowly over the three lineages. It was hard to reconcile this field of blood cells in front of my eyes with the diagnosis; not a single leukemic blast was to be seen. If this man had CML, he was in a remission so deep that the disease had virtually vanished from sight.

By the winter of 1998, Druker, Sawyers, and Talpaz had witnessed dozens of such remissions. Druker's first patient to be treated with Gleevec was a sixty-year-old retired train conductor from the Oregon coast. The patient had read about the drug in an article about Druker in a local newspaper. He had called Druker immediately and offered to be a "guinea pig." Druker gave him a small dose of the drug, then stood by his bedside for the rest of the afternoon, nervously awaiting any signs of toxicity. By the end of the day there were no adverse effects; the man was still alive. "It was the first time that the molecule had entered a human body, and it could

---

* Gleevec, the commercial name, is used here because it is more familiar to patients. The scientific name for CGP57148 is imatinib. The drug was also called STI571.

easily have created havoc, but it didn't," Druker recalled. "The sense of relief was incredible."

Druker edged into higher and higher doses—25, 50, 85, and 140 mg. His cohort of patients grew as well. As the dose was escalated in patients, Gleevec's effect became even more evident. One patient, a Portland woman, had come to his clinic with a blood count that had risen to nearly thirtyfold the normal number; her blood vessels were engorged with leukemia, her spleen virtually heaving with leukemic cells. After a few doses of the drug, Druker found her counts dropping precipitously, then normalizing within one week. Other patients, treated by Sawyers at UCLA and Talpaz in Houston, responded similarly, with blood counts normalizing within a few weeks.

News of the drug spread quickly. The development of Gleevec paralleled the birth of the patient chat room on the Internet; by 1999, patients were exchanging information about trials online. In many cases, it was patients who informed their doctors about Druker's drug and then, finding their own doctors poorly informed and incredulous, flew to Oregon or Los Angeles to enroll themselves in the Gleevec trial.

Of the fifty-four patients who received high doses of the drug in the initial phase I study, fifty-three showed a complete response within days of starting Gleevec. Patients continued the medicine for weeks, then months, and the malignant cells did not visibly return in the bone marrow. Left untreated, chronic myeloid leukemia is only "chronic" by the standards of leukemia: as the disease accelerates, the symptoms run on a tighter, faster arc and most patients live only three to five years. Patients on Gleevec experienced a palpable deceleration of their disease. The balance between normal and malignant cells was restored. It was an *unsuppuration* of blood.

By June 1999, with many of the original patients still in deep remissions, Gleevec was evidently a success. This success continues; Gleevec has become the standard of care for patients with CML. Oncologists now use the phrases "pre-Gleevec era" and "post-Gleevec era" when discussing this once-fatal disease. Hagop Kantarjian, the leukemia physician at the MD Anderson Cancer Center in Texas, recently summarized the impact of the drug on CML: "Before the year 2000, when we saw patients with chronic myeloid leukemia, we told them that they had a very bad disease, that their course was fatal, their prognosis was poor with a median survival of maybe three to six years, frontline therapy was allogeneic transplant . . . and there was no second-line treatment. . . . Today when I see a patient with CML, I tell them that the disease is an indolent leukemia with an excellent prognosis, that they will usually live their functional life span provided they take an oral medicine, Gleevec, for the rest of their lives."

⹋

CML, as Novartis noted, is hardly a scourge on public health, but cancer is a disease of symbols. Seminal ideas begin in the far peripheries of cancer biology, then ricochet back into more common forms of the disease. And leukemia, of all forms of cancer, is often the seed of new paradigms. This story began with leukemia in Sidney Farber's clinic in 1948, and it must return to leukemia. If cancer is in our blood, as Varmus reminded us, then it seems only appropriate that we keep returning, in ever-widening circles, to cancer *of* the blood.

The success of Druker's drug left a deep impression on the field of oncology. "When I was a youngster in Illinois in the 1950s," Bruce Chabner wrote in an editorial, "the world of sport was shocked by the feat of Roger Bannister. . . . On May 6, 1954, he broke the four-minute barrier in the mile. While improving upon the world record by only a few seconds, he changed the complexion of distance running in a single afternoon. . . . Track records fell like ripe apples in the late 50s and 60s. Will the same happen in the field of cancer treatment?"

Chabner's analogy was carefully chosen. Bannister's mile remains a touchstone in the history of athletics not because Bannister set an unbreachable record—currently, the fastest mile is a good fifteen seconds under Bannister's. For generations, four minutes was thought to represent an intrinsic physiological limit, as if muscles could inherently not be made to move any faster or lungs breathe any deeper. What Bannister proved was that such notions about intrinsic boundaries are mythical. What he broke permanently was not a limit, but the idea of limits.

So it was with Gleevec. "It proves a principle. It justifies an approach," Chabner continued. "It demonstrates that highly specific, non-toxic therapy is possible." Gleevec opened a new door for cancer therapeutics. The rational synthesis of a molecule to kill cancer cells—a drug designed to specifically inactivate an oncogene—validated Ehrlich's fantasy of "specific affinity." Targeted molecular therapy for cancer was possible; one only needed to hunt for it by studying the deep biology of cancer cells.

A final note: I said CML was a "rare" disease, and that was true in the era before Gleevec. The incidence of CML remains unchanged from the past: only a few thousand patients are diagnosed with this form of leukemia every year. But the *prevalence* of CML—the number of patients presently alive with the disease—has dramatically changed with the introduction of Gleevec. As of 2009, CML patients treated with Gleevec are expected to survive an average of thirty years after their diagnosis. Based on that survival figure, Hagop Kantarjian estimates that within the next decade, 250,000 people will be living with CML in America, all of them on targeted therapy. Druker's drug will alter the national physiognomy of cancer, converting a once-rare disease into a relatively common one. (Druker jokes that he has achieved the perfect inversion of the goals of cancer medicine: his drug has increased the prevalence of cancer in the world.) Given that most of our social networks typically extend to about one thousand individuals, each of us, on average, will know one person with this leukemia who is being kept alive by a targeted anticancer drug.

The Red Queen's Race

In August 2000, Jerry Mayfield, a forty-one-year-old Louisiana policeman diagnosed with CML, began treatment with Gleevec. Mayfield's cancer responded briskly at first. The fraction of leukemic cells in his bone marrow dropped over six months. His blood count normalized and his symptoms improved; he felt rejuvenated—"like a new man [on] a wonderful drug." But the response was short-lived. In the winter of 2003, Mayfield's CML stopped responding. Moshe Talpaz, the oncologist treating Mayfield in Houston, increased the dose of Gleevec, then increased it again, hoping to outpace the leukemia. But by October of that year, there was no response. Leukemia cells had fully recolonized his bone marrow and blood and invaded his spleen. Mayfield's cancer had become resistant to targeted therapy.

Now in the fifth year of their Gleevec trial, Talpaz and Sawyers had seen several cases like Mayfield's. They were rare. The vast proportion of CML patients maintained deep, striking remissions on the drug, requiring no other therapy. But occasionally, a patient's leukemia stopped responding to Gleevec, and Gleevec-resistant leukemia cells grew back. Sawyers, having just entered the world of targeted therapy, swiftly entered a molecular world beyond targeted therapy: how might a cancer cell become resistant to a drug that directly inhibits its driving oncogene?

In the era of nontargeted drugs, cancer cells were known to become drug-resistant through a variety of ingenious mechanisms. Some cells acquire mutations that activate molecular pumps. In normal cells, these pumps extrude natural poisons and waste products from a cell's interior. In cancer cells, these activated pumps push chemotherapy drugs out from the interior of the cell. Spared by chemotherapy, the drug-resistant cells outgrow other cancer cells. Other cancer cells activate proteins that destroy or neutralize drugs. Yet other cancers escape drugs by migrating into reservoirs of the body where drugs cannot penetrate—as in lymphoblastic leukemia relapsing in the brain.

CML cells, Sawyers discovered, become Gleevec-resistant through an even wilier mechanism: the cells acquire mutations that specifically alter the structure of *Bcr-abl,* creating a protein still able to drive the growth of the leukemia but no longer capable of binding to the drug. Normally, Gleevec slips into a narrow, wedgelike cleft in the center of *Bcr-abl*—like "an arrow pierced through the center of the protein's heart," as one chemist described it. Gleevec-resistant mutations in *Bcr-abl* change the molecular "heart" of the *Bcr-abl* protein so that the drug can no longer access the critical cleft in the protein, thus rendering the drug ineffective. In Mayfield's case, a single alteration in the *Bcr-abl* protein had rendered it fully resistant to Gleevec, resulting in the sudden relapse of leukemia. To escape targeted therapy, cancer had changed the target.

To Sawyers, these observations suggested that overcoming Gleevec resistance with a second-generation drug would require a very different kind of attack. Increasing the dose of Gleevec, or inventing closely related molecular variants of the drug, would be useless. Since the mutations changed the structure of *Bcr-abl,* a second-generation drug would need to block the protein through an independent mechanism, perhaps by gaining another entry point into its crucial central cleft.

In 2005, working with chemists at Bristol-Myers Squibb, Sawyers's team generated another kinase inhibitor to target Gleevec-resistant *Bcr-abl.* As predicted, this new drug, dasatinib, was not a simple structural analogue of Gleevec; it accessed *Bcr-abl's* "heart" through a separate molecular crevice on the protein's surface. When Sawyers and Talpaz tested dasatinib on Gleevec-resistant patients, the effect was remarkable: the leukemia cells involuted again. Mayfield's leukemia, fully resistant to Gleevec, was forced back into remission in 2005. His blood count normalized again. Leukemia cells dissipated out of his bone marrow gradually. In 2009, Mayfield still remains in remission, now on dasatinib.

Even targeted therapy, then, was a cat-and-mouse game. One could direct endless arrows at the Achilles' heel of cancer, but the disease might simply shift its foot, switching one vulnerability for another. We were locked in a perpetual battle with a volatile combatant. When CML cells kicked Gleevec away, only a different molecular variant would drive them down, and when they outgrew that drug, then we would need the next-generation drug. If the vigilance was dropped, even for a moment, then the weight of the battle would shift. In Lewis Carroll's *Through the Looking-Glass,* the Red Queen tells Alice that the world keeps shifting so quickly under her feet that she has to keep running just to keep her position. This is our predicament with cancer: we are forced to keep running merely to keep still.

৵৸

In the decade since the discovery of Gleevec, twenty-four novel drugs have been listed by the National Cancer Institute as cancer-targeted therapies. Dozens more are in development. The twenty-four drugs have been shown to be effective against lung, breast, colon, and prostate cancers, sarcomas, lymphomas, and leukemias. Some, such as dasatinib, directly inactivate oncogenes. Others target oncogene-activated pathways—the "hallmarks of cancer" codified by Weinberg. The drug Avastin interrupts tumor angiogenesis by attacking the capacity of cancer cells to incite blood-vessel growth. Bortezomib, or Velcade, blocks an internal waste-dispensing mechanism for proteins that is particularly hyperactive in cancer cells.

More than nearly any other form of cancer, multiple myeloma, a cancer of immune-system cells, epitomizes the impact of these newly discovered targeted therapies. In the 1980s, multiple myeloma was treated by high doses of standard chemotherapy—old, hard-bitten drugs that typically ended up decimating patients about as quickly as they decimated the cancer. Over a decade, three novel targeted therapies have emerged for myeloma—Velcade, thalidomide, and Revlimid—all of which interrupt activated pathways in myeloma cells. Treatment of multiple myeloma today involves mixing and matching these drugs with standard chemotherapies, switching drugs when the tumor relapses, and switching again when the tumor relapses again. No single drug or treatment cures myeloma outright; myeloma is still a fatal disease. But as with CML, the cat-and-mouse game with cancer has extended the survival of myeloma patients—strikingly in some cases. In 1971, about half the patients diagnosed with multiple myeloma died within twenty-four months of diagnosis; the other half died by the tenth year. In 2008, about half of all myeloma patients treated with the shifting armamentarium of new drugs will still be alive at five years. If the survival trends continue, the other half will continue to be alive well beyond ten years.

In 2005, a man diagnosed with multiple myeloma asked me if he would be alive to watch his daughter graduate from high school in a few months. In 2009, bound to a wheelchair, he watched his daughter graduate from college. The wheelchair had nothing to do with his cancer. The man had fallen down while coaching his youngest son's baseball team.

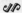

In a broader sense, the Red Queen syndrome—moving incessantly just to keep in place—applies equally to every aspect of the battle against cancer, including cancer screening and cancer prevention. In the early winter of 2007, I traveled to Framingham in Massachusetts to visit a study site that will likely alter the way we imagine cancer prevention. A small, nondescript Northeastern town bound by a chain of frozen lakes in midwinter, Framingham is nonetheless an iconic place writ large in the history of medicine. In 1948, epidemiologists identified a cohort of about five thousand men and women living in Framingham. The behavior of this cohort, its habits, its interrelationships, and its illnesses, has been documented year after year in exquisite detail, creating an invaluable longitudinal corpus of data for hundreds of epidemiological studies. The English mystery writer Agatha Christie often used a fictional village, St. Mary Mead, as a microcosm of all mankind. Framingham is the American epidemiologist's English village. Under sharp statistical lenses, its captive cohort has lived, reproduced, aged, and died, affording a rare glimpse of the natural history of life, disease, and death.

The Framingham data set has spawned a host of studies on risk and illness. The link between cholesterol and heart attacks was formally established here, as was the association of stroke and high blood pressure. But recently, a conceptual transformation in epidemiological thinking has also been spearheaded here. Epidemiologists typically measure the risk factors for chronic, noninfectious illnesses by studying the behavior of individuals. But recently, they have asked a very different question: what if the real locus of risk lies not in the behaviors of individual actors, but in social *networks*?

In May 2008, two Harvard epidemiologists, Nicholas Christakis and James Fowler, used this notion to examine the dynamics of cigarette smoking. First, Fowler and Christakis plotted a diagram of all known relationships in Framingham—friends, neighbors, and relatives, siblings, ex-wives, uncles, aunts—as a densely interconnected web. Viewed abstractly, the network began to assume familiar and intuitive patterns. A few men and women (call them "socializers") stood at the epicenter of these networks, densely connected to each other through multiple ties. In contrast, others lingered on the outskirts of the social web—"loners"—with few and fleeting contacts.

When the epidemiologists juxtaposed smoking behavior onto this network and followed the pattern of smoking over decades, a notable phenomenon emerged: circles of relationships were found to be more powerful predictors of the dynamics of smoking than nearly any other factor. Entire networks stopped smoking concordantly, like whole circuits flickering off. A family that dined together was also a family that quit together. When highly connected "socializers" stopped smoking, the dense social circle circumscribed around them also slowly stopped as a group. As a result, smoking gradually became locked into the far peripheries of all networks, confined to the "loners" with few social contacts, puffing away quietly in the distant and isolated corners of the town.

The smoking-network study offers, to my mind, a formidable challenge to simplistic models of cancer prevention. Smoking, this model argues, is entwined into our social DNA just as densely and as inextricably as oncogenes are entwined into our genetic material. The cigarette epidemic, we might recall, originated as a form of metastatic behavior—one site seeding another site seeding another. Soldiers brought smoking back to postwar Europe; women persuaded women to smoke; the tobacco industry, sensing opportunity, advertised cigarettes as a form of social glue that would "stick" individuals into cohesive groups. The capacity of metastasis is thus built into smoking. If entire networks of smokers can flicker off with catalytic speed, then they can also flicker on with catalytic speed. Sever the ties that bind the nonsmokers of Framingham (or worse, nucleate a large social network with a proselytizing smoker), and then, cataclysmically, the network might alter as a whole.

This is why even the most successful cancer-prevention strategies can lapse so swiftly. When the Red Queen's feet stop spinning even temporarily, she does not maintain her position; the world around her, counter-spinning, pushes her off-balance. So it is with cancer prevention. When antitobacco campaigns lose their effectiveness or penetrance—as has recently happened among teens in America or in Asia—smoking often returns like an old plague. Social behavior metastasizes, eddying out from its center toward the peripheries of social networks. Mini-epidemics of smoking-related cancers are sure to follow.

The landscape of carcinogens is not static either. We are chemical apes: having discovered the capacity to extract, purify, and react molecules to produce new and wondrous molecules, we have begun to spin a new chemical universe around ourselves. Our bodies, our cells, our genes are thus being immersed and reimmersed in a changing flux of molecules—pesticides, pharmaceutical drugs, plastics, cosmetics, estrogens, food products, hormones, even novel forms of physical impulses, such as radiation and magnetism. Some of these, inevitably, will be carcinogenic. We cannot wish this world away; our task, then, is to sift through it vigilantly to discriminate bona fide carcinogens from innocent and useful bystanders.

This is easier said than done. In 2004, a rash of early scientific reports suggested that cell phones, which produce radio frequency energy, might cause a fatal form of brain cancer called a glioma. Gliomas appeared on the same side of the brain that the phone was predominantly held, further tightening the link. An avalanche of panic ensued in the media. But was this a falsely perceived confluence of a common phenomenon and a rare disease—phone usage and glioma? Or had epidemiologists missed the "nylon stockings" of the digital age?

In 2004, an enormous British study was launched to confirm these ominous early reports. "Cases"—patients with gliomas—were compared to "controls"—men and women with no gliomas—in terms of cell phone usage. The study, reported in 2006, appeared initially to confirm an increased risk of right-sided brain cancers in men and women who held their phone on their right ear. But when researchers evaluated the data meticulously, a puzzling pattern emerged: right-sided cell phone use *reduced* the risk of *left-sided* brain cancer. The simplest logical explanation for this phenomenon was "recall bias": patients diagnosed with tumors unconsciously exaggerated the use of cell phones on the same side of their head, and selectively forgot the use on the other side. When the authors corrected for this bias, there was no detectable association between gliomas and cell phone use overall. Prevention experts, and phone-addicted teenagers, may have rejoiced—but only briefly. By the time the study was completed, new phones had entered the market and swapped out old phones—making even the negative results questionable.

The cell phone case is a sobering reminder of the methodological rigor needed to evaluate new carcinogens. It is easy to fan anxiety about cancer. Identifying a true preventable carcinogen, estimating the magnitude of risk at reasonable doses and at reasonable exposures, and reducing exposure through scientific and legislative intervention—keeping the legacy of Percivall Pott alive—is far more complex.

"Cancer at the *fin de siècle*," as the oncologist Harold Burstein described it, "resides at the interface between society and science." It poses not one but two challenges. The first, the "biological challenge" of cancer, involves "harnessing the fantastic rise in scientific knowledge . . . to conquer this ancient and terrible illness." But the second, the "social challenge," is just as acute: it involves forcing ourselves to confront our customs, rituals, and behaviors. These, unfortunately, are not customs or behaviors that lie at the peripheries of our society or selves, but ones that lie at their definitional cores: what we eat and drink, what we produce and exude into our environments, when we choose to reproduce, and how we age.

Thirteen Mountains

*"Every sickness
is a musical problem,"
so said Novalis,
"and every cure
a musical solution."*
—W. H. Auden

*The revolution in cancer research can be summed up in a
single sentence: cancer is, in essence, a genetic disease.*
—Bert Vogelstein

When I began writing this book, in the early summer of 2004, I was often asked how I intended to end it. Typically, I would dodge the question or brush it away. I did not know, I would cautiously say. Or I was not sure. In truth, I was sure, although I did not have the courage to admit it to myself. I was sure that it would end with Carla's relapse and death.

I was wrong. In July 2009, exactly five years after I had looked down the microscope into Carla's bone marrow and confirmed her first remission, I drove to her house in Ipswich, Massachusetts, with a bouquet of flowers. It was an overcast morning, excruciatingly muggy, with a dun-colored sky that threatened rain but would not deliver any. Just before I left the hospital, I glanced quickly at the first note that I had written on Carla's admission to the hospital in 2004. As I had written that note, I recalled with embarrassment, I had guessed that Carla would not even survive the induction phase of chemotherapy.

But she had made it; a charring, private war had just ended. In acute leukemia, the passage of five years without a relapse is nearly synonymous with a cure. I handed her the azaleas and she stood looking at them speechlessly, almost numb to the enormity of her victory. Once, earlier this year, preoccupied with clinical work, I had waited two days before calling her about a negative bone marrow biopsy. She had heard from a nurse that the results were in, and my delay had sent her into a terrifying spiral of depression: in twenty-four hours she had convinced herself that the leukemia had crept back and my hesitation was a signal of impending doom.

Oncologists and their patients are bound, it seems, by an intense subatomic force. So, albeit in a much smaller sense, this was a victory for me as well. I sat at Carla's table and watched her pour a glass of water for herself, unpurified and straight from the sink. She glowed radiantly, her eyes half-closed, as if the compressed autobiography of the last five years were flashing through a private and internal cinema screen. Her children played with their Scottish terrier in the next room, blissfully oblivious of the landmark date that had just passed for their mother. All of this was for the best. "The purpose of my book," Susan Sontag concluded in *Illness as Metaphor*, "was to calm the imagination, not to incite it." So it was with my visit. Its purpose was to declare her illness over, to normalize her life—to sever the force that had locked us together for five years.

I asked Carla how she thought she had survived her nightmare. The drive to her house from the hospital that morning had taken me an hour and a half through a boil of heavy traffic. How had she managed, through the long days of that dismal summer, to drive to the hospital, wait in the room for hours as her blood tests were run, and then, told that her blood counts were too low for her to be given chemotherapy safely, turn back and return the next day for the same pattern to be repeated?

"There was no choice," she said, motioning almost unconsciously to the room where her children were playing. "My friends often asked me whether I felt as if my life was somehow made abnormal by my disease. I would tell them the same thing: for someone who is sick, this *is* their new normal."

&

Until 2003, scientists knew that the principal distinction between the "normalcy" of a cell and the "abnormalcy" of a cancer cell lay in the accumulation of genetic mutations—*ras, myc, Rb, neu,* and so forth—that unleashed the hallmark behaviors of cancer cells. But this description of cancer was incomplete. It provoked an inevitable question: how many such mutations does a real cancer possess in total? Individual oncogenes and tumor suppressors had been isolated, but what was the comprehensive set of such mutated genes that exists in any true human cancer?

The Human Genome Project, the full sequence of the normal human genome, was completed in 2003. In its wake comes a far less publicized but vastly more complex project: fully sequencing the genomes of several human cancer cells. Once completed, this effort, called the Cancer Genome Atlas, will dwarf the Human Genome Project in its scope. The sequencing effort involves dozens of teams of researchers across the world. The initial list of cancers to be sequenced includes brain, lung, pancreatic, and ovarian cancer. The Human Genome Project will provide the normal genome, against which cancer's abnormal genome can be juxtaposed and contrasted.

The result, as Francis Collins, the leader of the Human Genome Project describes it, will be a "colossal atlas" of cancer—a compendium of every gene mutated in the most common forms of cancer: "When applied to the 50 most common types of cancer, this effort could ultimately prove to be the equivalent of more than 10,000 Human Genome Projects in terms of the sheer volume of DNA to be sequenced. The dream must therefore be matched with an ambitious but realistic assessment of the emerging scientific opportunities for waging a smarter war." The only metaphor that can appropriately describe this project is geological. Rather than understand cancer gene by gene, the Cancer Genome Atlas will chart the entire territory of cancer: by sequencing the entire genome of several tumor types, *every* single mutated gene will be identified. It will represent the beginnings of the comprehensive "map" so hauntingly presaged by Maggie Jencks in her last essay.

Two teams have forged ahead in their efforts to sequence the cancer genome. One, called the Cancer Genome Atlas consortium, has multiple interconnected teams spanning several labs in several nations. The second is Bert Vogelstein's group at Johns Hopkins, which has assembled its own cancer genome sequencing facility, raised private funding for the effort, and raced ahead to sequence the genomes of breast, colon, and pancreatic tumors. In 2006, the Vogelstein team revealed the first landmark sequencing effort by analyzing thirteen thousand genes in eleven breast and colon cancers. (Although the human genome contains about twenty thousand genes in total, Vogelstein's team initially had tools to assess only thirteen thousand.) In 2008, both Vogelstein's group and the Cancer Genome Atlas consortium extended this effort by sequencing hundreds of genes of several dozen specimens of brain tumors. As of 2009, the genomes of ovarian cancer, pancreatic cancer, melanoma, lung cancer, and several forms of leukemia have been sequenced, revealing the full catalog of mutations in each tumor type.

Perhaps no one has studied the emerging cancer genome as meticulously or as devotionally as Bert Vogelstein. A wry, lively, irreverent man in blue jeans and a rumpled blazer, Vogelstein recently began a lecture on the cancer genome in a packed auditorium at Mass General Hospital by attempting to distill the enormous array of discoveries in a few slides. Vogelstein's challenge was that of the landscape artist: How does one convey the gestalt of a territory (in this case, the "territory" of a genome) in a few broad strokes of a brush? How can a picture describe the essence of a place?

Vogelstein's answer to these questions borrows beautifully from an insight long familiar to classical landscape artists: negative space can be used to convey expanse, while positive space conveys detail. To view the landscape of the cancer genome panoramically, Vogelstein splayed out the entire human genome as if it were a piece of thread zigzagging across a square sheet of paper. (Science keeps eddying into its past: the word *mitosis*—Greek for "thread"—is resonant here again.) In Vogelstein's diagram, the first gene on chromosome one of the human genome occupies the top left corner of the sheet of paper, the second gene is below it, and so forth, zigzagging through the page, until the last gene of chromosome twenty-three occupies the bottom right corner of the page. This is the normal, unmutated human genome stretched out in its enormity—the "background" out of which cancer arises.

Against the background of this negative space, Vogelstein placed mutations. Every time a gene mutation was encountered in a cancer, the mutated gene was demarcated as a dot on the sheet. As the frequency of mutations in any given gene increased, the dots grew in height into ridges and hills and then mountains. The most commonly mutated genes in breast cancer samples were thus represented by towering peaks, while genes rarely mutated were denoted by small hills or flat dots.

Viewed thus, the cancer genome is at first glance a depressing place. Mutations litter the chromosomes. In individual specimens of breast and colon cancer, between fifty to eighty genes are mutated; in pancreatic cancers, about fifty to sixty. Even brain cancers, which often develop at earlier ages and hence may be expected to accumulate fewer mutations, possess about forty to fifty mutated genes.

Only a few cancers are notable exceptions to this rule, possessing relatively few mutations across the genome. One of these is an old culprit, acute lymphoblastic leukemia: only five or ten genetic alterations cross its otherwise pristine genomic landscape.* Indeed, the relative paucity of genetic aberrancy in this leukemia may be one reason that this tumor is so easily felled by cytotoxic chemotherapy. Scientists speculate that genetically simple tumors (i.e., those carrying few mutations) might inherently be more susceptible to drugs, and thus intrinsically more curable. If so, the strange discrepancy between the success of high-dose chemotherapy in curing leukemia and its failure to cure most other cancers has a deep biological explanation. The search for a "universal cure" for cancer was predicated on a tumor that, genetically speaking, is far from universal.

In contrast to leukemia, the genomes of the more common forms of cancer, Vogelstein finds, are filled with genetic bedlam—mutations piled upon mutations upon mutations. In one breast cancer sample from a forty-three-year-old woman, 127 genes were mutated—nearly one in every two hundred genes in the human genome. Even within a single type of tumor, the heterogeneity of mutations is daunting. If one compares two breast cancer specimens, the set of mutated genes is far from identical. "In the end," as Vogelstein put it, "cancer genome sequencing validates a hundred years of clinical observations. Every patient's cancer is unique because every cancer genome is unique. Physiological heterogeneity is genetic heterogeneity." Normal cells are identically normal; malignant cells become unhappily malignant in unique ways.

Yet, characteristically, where others see only daunting chaos in the littered genetic landscape, Vogelstein sees patterns coalescing out of the mess. Mutations in the cancer genome, he believes, come in two forms. Some are passive. As cancer cells divide, they accumulate mutations due to accidents in the copying of DNA, but these mutations have no impact on the biology of cancer. They stick to the genome and are passively carried along as the cell divides, identifiable but inconsequential. These are "bystander" mutations or "passenger" mutations. ("They hop along for the ride," as Vogelstein put it.)

---

* Thus far, the full sequencing of ALL genomes has not been completed. The alterations described are deletions or amplifications of genes. Detailed sequencing may reveal an increase in the number of mutated genes.

Other mutations are not passive players. Unlike the passenger mutations, these altered genes directly goad the growth and the biological behavior of cancer cells. These are "driver" mutations, mutations that play a crucial role in the biology of a cancer cell.

Every cancer cell possesses some set of driver and passenger mutations. In the breast cancer sample from the forty-three-year-old woman with 127 mutations, only about ten might directly be contributing to the actual growth and survival of her tumor, while the rest may have been acquired due to gene-copying errors in cancer cells. But while functionally different, these two forms of mutations cannot easily be distinguished. Scientists can identify some driver genes that directly goad cancer's growth using the cancer genome. Since passenger mutations occur randomly, they are randomly spread throughout the genome. Driver mutations, on the other hand, strike key oncogenes and tumor suppressors, and only a limited number of such genes exist in the genome. These mutations—in genes such as *ras, myc,* and *Rb*—recur in sample upon sample. They stand out as tall mountains in Vogelstein's map, while passenger mutations are typically represented by the valleys. But when a mutation occurs in a previously unknown gene, it is impossible to predict whether that mutation is consequential or inconsequential—driver or passenger, barnacle or engine.

The "mountains" in the cancer genome—i.e., genes most frequently mutated in a particular form of cancer—have another property. They can be organized into key cancer pathways. In a recent series of studies, Vogelstein's team at Hopkins reanalyzed the mutations present in the cancer genome using yet another strategy. Rather than focusing on individual genes mutated in cancers, they enumerated the number of *pathways* mutated in cancer cells. Each time a gene was mutated in any component of the Ras-Mek-Erk pathway, it was classified as a "Ras pathway" mutation. Similarly, if a cell carried a mutation in any component of the *Rb* signaling pathway, it was classified as "Rb pathway mutant," and so forth, until all driver mutations had been organized into pathways.

How many pathways are typically dysregulated in a cancer cell? Typically, Vogelstein found, between eleven and fifteen, with an average of thirteen. The mutational complexity on a gene-by-gene level was still enormous. Any one tumor bore scores of mutations pockmarked throughout the genome. But the same core pathways were characteristically dysregulated in any tumor type, even if the specific genes responsible for each broken pathway differed from one tumor to the next. *Ras* may be activated in one sample of bladder cancer; *Mek* in another; *Erk* in the third—but in each case, some vital piece of the Ras-Mek-Erk cascade was dysregulated.

The bedlam of the cancer genome, in short, is deceptive. If one listens closely, there are organizational principles. The language of cancer is grammatical, methodical, and even—I hesitate to write—quite beautiful. Genes talk to genes and pathways to pathways in perfect pitch, producing a familiar yet foreign music that rolls faster and faster into a lethal rhythm. Underneath what might seem like overwhelming diversity is a deep genetic unity. Cancers that look vastly unlike each other superficially often have the same or similar pathways unhinged. "Cancer," as one scientist recently put it, "really is a pathway disease."

❧

This is either very good news or very bad news. The cancer pessimist looks at the ominous number thirteen and finds himself disheartened. The dysregulation of eleven to fifteen core pathways poses an enormous challenge for cancer therapeutics. Will oncologists need thirteen independent drugs to attack thirteen independent pathways to "normalize" a cancer cell? Given the slipperiness of cancer cells, when a cell becomes resistant to one combination of thirteen drugs, will we need an additional thirteen?

The cancer optimist, however, argues that thirteen is a finite number. It is a relief: until Vogelstein identified these core pathways, the mutational complexity of cancers seemed nearly infinite. In fact, the hierarchical organization of genes into pathways in any given tumor type suggests that even deeper hierarchies might exist. Perhaps not all thirteen need to be targeted to attack complex cancers such as breast or pancreatic cancer. Perhaps some of the core pathways may be particularly responsive to therapy. The best example of this might be Barbara Bradfield's tumor, a cancer so hypnotically addicted to *Her-2* that targeting this key oncogene melted the tumor away and forced a decades-long remission.

❧

Gene by gene, and now pathway by pathway, we have an extraordinary glimpse into the biology of cancer. The complete maps of mutations in many tumor types (with their hills, valleys, and mountains) will soon be complete, and the core pathways that are mutated fully defined. But as the old proverb runs, there are mountains beyond mountains. Once the mutations have been identified, the mutant genes will need to be assigned functions in cellular physiology. We will need to move through a renewed cycle of knowledge that recapitulates a past cycle—from anatomy to physiology to therapeutics. The sequencing of the cancer genome represents the genetic anatomy of cancer. And just as Virchow made the crucial leap from Vesalian anatomy to the physiology of cancer in the nineteenth century, science must make a leap from the molecular anatomy to the molecular physiology of cancer. We will soon know what the mutant genes *are*. The real challenge is to understand what the mutant genes *do*.

This seminal transition from descriptive biology to the functional biology of cancer will provoke three new directions for cancer medicine.

The first is a direction for cancer therapeutics. Once the crucial driver mutations in any given cancer have been identified, we will need to launch a hunt for targeted therapies against these genes. This is not an entirely fantastical hope: targeted inhibitors of some of the core thirteen pathways mutated in many cancers have already entered the clinical realm. As individual drugs, some of these inhibitors have thus far had only moderate response rates. The challenge now is to determine which combinations of such drugs might inhibit cancer growth without killing normal cells.

In a piece published in the *New York Times* in the summer of 2009, James Watson, the codiscoverer of the structure of DNA, made a remarkable turnabout in opinion. Testifying before Congress in 1969, Watson had lambasted the War on Cancer as ludicrously premature. Forty years later, he was far less critical: "We shall soon know all the genetic changes that underlie the major cancers that plague us. We already know most, if not all, of the major pathways through which cancer-inducing signals move through cells. Some 20 signal-blocking drugs are now in clinical testing after first being shown to block cancer in mice. A few, such as Herceptin and Tarceva, have Food and Drug Administration approval and are in widespread use."

જ્જ

The second new direction is for cancer prevention. To date, cancer prevention has relied on two disparate and polarized methodologies to try to identify preventable carcinogens. There have been intensive, often massive, human studies that have connected a particular form of cancer with a risk factor, such as Doll and Hill's study identifying smoking as a risk factor for lung cancer. And there have been laboratory studies to identify carcinogens based on their ability to cause mutations in bacteria or incite precancer in animals and humans, such as Bruce Ames's experiment to capture chemical mutagens, or Marshall and Warren's identification of *H. pylori* as a cause for stomach cancer.

But important preventable carcinogens might escape detection by either strategy. Subtle risk factors for cancer require enormous population studies; the subtler the effect, the larger the population needed. Such vast, unwieldy, and methodologically challenging studies are difficult to fund and launch. Conversely, several important cancer-inciting agents are not easily captured by laboratory experiments. As Evarts Graham discovered to his dismay, even tobacco smoke, the most common human carcinogen, does not easily induce lung cancer in mice. Bruce Ames's bacterial test does not register asbestos as a mutagen.*

Two recent controversies have starkly highlighted such blind spots in epidemiology. In 2000, the so-called Million Women Study in the United Kingdom identified estrogen and progesterone, prescribed in hormone-replacement therapy to women to ease menopausal symptoms, as major risk factors for the incidence and fatality from estrogen-positive breast cancer. Scientifically speaking, this is an embarrassment. Estrogen is not identified as a mutagen in Bruce Ames's test; nor does it cause cancer in animals at low doses. But the two hormones have been known as pathological activators of the ER-positive subtype of breast cancer since the *1960s*. Beatson's surgery and tamoxifen induce remissions in breast cancer by blocking estrogen, and so it stands to reason that exogenous estrogen might incite breast cancer. A more integrated approach to cancer prevention, incorporating the prior insights of cancer biology, might have predicted this cancer-inducing activity, preempted the need for a million-person association study, and potentially saved the lives of thousands of women.

The second controversy also has its antecedents in the 1960s. Since the publication of Rachel Carson's *Silent Spring* in 1962, environmental activists have stridently argued that the indiscriminate overuse of pesticides is partially responsible for the rising incidence of cancer in America. This theory has spawned intense controversy, activism, and public campaigns over the decades. But although the hypothesis is credible, large-scale human-cohort experiments directly implicating particular pesticides as carcinogens have emerged slowly, and animal studies have been incon-

---

* Mice filter out many of the carcinogenic components of tar. Asbestos incites cancer by inducing a scar-forming, inflammatory reaction in the body. Bacteria don't generate this reaction and are thus "immune" to asbestos.

clusive. DDT and aminotriazole have been shown to cause cancer in animals at high doses, but thousands of chemicals proposed as carcinogens remain untested. Again, an integrated approach is needed. The identification of key activated pathways in cancer cells might provide a more sensitive detection method to discover carcinogens in animal studies. A chemical may not cause overt cancer in animal studies, but may be shown to activate cancer-linked genes and pathways, thus shifting the burden of proof of its potential carcinogenicity. Similarly, we now know there is a link between nutrition and the risk of particular forms of cancer, but this field remains in its infancy. Low fiber, red meat rich diets increase the risks of colon cancer, and obesity is linked to breast cancer, but much more about these links remain unknown, especially in molecular terms.

In 2005, the Harvard epidemiologist David Hunter argued that the integration of traditional epidemiology, molecular biology, and cancer genetics will generate a resurgent form of epidemiology that is vastly more empowered in its ability to prevent cancer. "Traditional epidemiology," Hunter reasoned, "is concerned with correlating exposures with cancer outcomes, and everything between the cause (exposure) and the outcome (a cancer) is treated as a 'black box.' . . . In molecular epidemiology, the epidemiologist [will] open up the 'black box' by examining the events intermediate between exposure and disease occurrence or progression."

Like cancer prevention, cancer screening will also be reinvigorated by the molecular understanding of cancer. Indeed, it has already been. The discovery of the BRCA genes for breast cancer epitomizes the integration of cancer screening and cancer genetics. In the mid-1990s, building on the prior decade's advances, researchers isolated two related genes, BRCA-1 and BRCA-2, that vastly increase the risk of developing breast cancer. A woman with an inherited mutation in BRCA-1 has a 50 to 80 percent chance of developing breast cancer in her lifetime (the gene also increases the risk for ovarian cancer), about three to five times the normal risk. Today, testing for this gene mutation has been integrated into prevention efforts. Women found positive for a mutation in the two genes are screened more intensively using more sensitive imaging techniques such as breast MRI. Women with BRCA mutations might choose to take the drug tamoxifen to prevent breast cancer, a strategy shown effective in clinical trials. Or, perhaps most radically, women with BRCA mutations might choose a prophylactic mastectomy of both breasts and ovaries before cancer develops, another strategy that dramatically decreases the chances of developing breast cancer. An Israeli woman with a BRCA-1 mutation who chose this strategy after developing cancer in one breast told me that at least part of her choice was symbolic. "I am rejecting cancer from my body," she said. "My breasts had become no more to me than a site for my cancer. They were of no more use to me. They harmed my body, my survival. I went to the surgeon and asked him to remove them."

⚮

The third, and arguably most complex, new direction for cancer medicine is to integrate our understanding of aberrant genes and pathways to explain the *behavior* of cancer as a whole, thereby renewing the cycle of knowledge, discovery, and therapeutic intervention.

One of the most provocative examples of a cancer cell's behavior, inexplicable by the activation of any single gene or pathway, is its immortality. Rapid cellular proliferation, or the insensitivity to growth-arresting signals, or tumor angiogenesis, can all largely be explained by aberrantly activated and inactivated pathways such as *ras, Rb,* or *myc* in cancer cells. But scientists cannot explain how cancers continue to proliferate endlessly. Most normal cells, even rapidly growing normal cells, will proliferate over several generations and then exhaust their capacity to keep dividing. What allows a cancer cell to keep dividing endlessly without exhaustion or depletion generation upon generation?

An emerging, although highly controversial, answer to this question is that cancer's immortality, too, is borrowed from normal physiology. The human embryo and many of our adult organs possess a tiny population of stem cells that are capable of immortal regeneration. Stem cells are the body's reservoir of renewal. The entirety of human blood, for instance, can arise from a single, highly potent blood-forming stem cell (called a hematopoietic stem cell), which typically lives buried inside the bone marrow. Under normal conditions, only a fraction of these blood-forming stem cells are active; the rest are deeply quiescent—asleep. But if blood is suddenly depleted, by injury or chemotherapy, say, then the stem cells awaken and begin to divide with awe-inspiring fecundity, generating cells that generate thousands upon thousands of blood cells. In weeks, a single hematopoietic stem cell can replenish the entire human organism with new blood—and then, through yet unknown mechanisms, lull itself back to sleep.

Something akin to this process, a few researchers believe, is constantly occurring in cancer—or at least in leukemia. In the mid-1990s, John Dick, a Canadian biologist working in Toronto, postulated that a small population of cells in human leukemias also possess this infinite self-renewing behavior. These "cancer stem cells" act as the persistent reservoir of cancer—generating and regenerating cancer infinitely. When chemotherapy kills the bulk of cancer cells, a small remnant population of these stem cells, thought to be intrinsically more resistant to death, regenerate and renew the cancer, thus precipitating the common relapses of cancer after chemotherapy. Indeed, cancer stem cells have acquired the behavior of normal stem cells by activating the same genes and pathways that make normal stem cells immortal—except, unlike normal stem cells, they cannot be lulled back into physiological sleep. Cancer, then, is quite literally trying to emulate a regenerating organ—or perhaps, more disturbingly, the regenerating *organism*. Its quest for immortality mirrors our own quest, a quest buried in our embryos and in the renewal of our organs. Someday, if a cancer succeeds, it will produce a far more perfect being than its host—imbued with both immortality and the drive to proliferate. One might argue that the leukemia cells growing in my laboratory derived from the woman who died three decades earlier have already achieved this form of "perfection."

Taken to its logical extreme, the cancer cell's capacity to consistently imitate, corrupt, and pervert normal physiology thus raises the ominous question of what "normalcy" *is*. "Cancer," Carla said, "is my new normal," and quite possibly cancer is *our* normalcy as well, that we are inherently destined to slouch towards a malignant end. Indeed, as the fraction of those affected by cancer creeps inexorably in some nations from one in four to one in three to one in *two,* cancer will, indeed, be the new normal—an inevitability. The question then will not be *if* we will encounter this immortal illness in our lives, but *when.*

Atossa's War

We aged a hundred years and this descended
In just one hour, as at a stroke
   —Anna Akhmatova,
      "In Memoriam, July 19, 1914"

It is time, it is time for me too to depart. Like an old man
who has outlived his contemporaries and feels a sad inner
emptiness, Kostoglotov felt that evening that the ward was
no longer his home, even though . . . there were the same
old patients asking the same old questions again and
again as though they had never been asked before: . . . Will
they cure me or won't they? What other remedies are there
that might help?
                  —Aleksandr Solzhenitsyn, *Cancer Ward*

On May 17, 1973, seven weeks after Sidney Farber's death in Boston, Hiram Gans, an old friend, stood up at the memorial service to read some lines from Swinburne's "A Forsaken Garden":

Here now in his triumph where all things falter,
Stretched out on the spoils that his own hand spread,
As a god self-slain on his own strange altar,
Death lies dead.

It was—careful listeners might have noted—a peculiar and deliberate inversion of the moment. It was *cancer* that was soon to be dead—its corpus outstretched and spread-eagled ceremonially on the altar—death lying dead.

The image belongs very much to Farber and his era, but its essence still haunts us today. In the end, every biography must also confront the death of its subject. Is the end of cancer conceivable in the future? Is it possible to eradicate this disease from our bodies and our societies forever?

The answers to these questions are embedded in the biology of this incredible disease. Cancer, we have discovered, is stitched into our genome. Oncogenes arise from mutations in essential genes that regulate the growth of cells. Mutations accumulate in these genes when DNA is damaged by carcinogens, but also by seemingly random errors in copying genes when cells divide. The former might be preventable, but the latter is endogenous. Cancer is a flaw in our growth, but this flaw is deeply entrenched in ourselves. We can rid ourselves of cancer, then, only as much as we can rid ourselves of the processes in our physiology that depend on growth—aging, regeneration, healing, reproduction.

Science embodies the human desire to understand nature; technology couples that desire with the ambition to control nature. These are related impulses—one might seek to understand nature in order to control it—but the drive to intervene is unique to technology. Medicine, then, is fundamentally a technological art; at its core lies a desire to improve human lives by intervening on life itself. Conceptually, the battle against cancer pushes the idea of technology to its far edge, for the object being intervened upon is our genome. It is unclear whether an intervention that discriminates between malignant and normal growth is even possible. Perhaps cancer, the scrappy, fecund, invasive, adaptable twin to our own scrappy, fecund, invasive, adaptable cells and genes, is impossible to disconnect from our bodies. Perhaps cancer defines the inherent outer limit of our survival. As our cells divide and our bodies age, and as mutations accumulate inexorably upon mutations, cancer might well be the final terminus in our development as organisms.

But our goals could be more modest. Above the door to Richard Peto's office in Oxford hangs one of Doll's favorite aphorisms: "Death in old age is inevitable, but death before old age is not." Doll's idea represents a far more reasonable proximal goal to define success in the War on Cancer. It is possible that we are fatally conjoined to this ancient illness, forced to play its cat-and-mouse game for the foreseeable future of our species. But if cancer deaths can be prevented before old age, if the terrifying game of treatment, resistance, recurrence, and more treatment can be stretched out longer and longer, then it will transform the way we imagine this ancient illness. Given what we know about cancer, even this would represent a technological victory unlike any other in our history. It would be a victory over our own inevitability—a victory over our genomes.

৶৶

To envision what such a victory might look like, permit a thought experiment. Recall Atossa, the Persian queen who likely had breast cancer in 500 BC.* Imagine her traveling through time—appearing and reappearing in one age after the next. She is cancer's Dorian Gray: as she moves through the arc of history, her tumor, frozen in its stage and behavior, remains the same. Atossa's case allows us to recapitulate past advances in cancer therapy and to consider its future. How has her treatment and prognosis shifted in the last four thousand years, and what happens to Atossa later in the new millennium?

First, pitch Atossa backward in time to Imhotep's clinic in Egypt in 2500 BC. Imhotep has a name for her illness, a hieroglyph that we cannot pronounce. He provides a diagnosis, but "there is no treatment," he says humbly, closing the case.

In 500 BC, in her own court, Atossa self-prescribes the most primitive form of a mastectomy, which is performed by her Greek slave. Two hundred years later, in Thrace, Hippocrates identifies her tumor as a *karkinos,* thus giving her illness a name that will ring through its future. Claudius Galen, in AD 168, hypothesizes a universal cause: a systemic overdose of black bile—trapped melancholia boiling out as a tumor.

A thousand years flash by; Atossa's entrapped black bile is purged from her body, yet the tumor keeps growing, relapsing, invading, and metastasizing. Medieval surgeons understand little about Atossa's disease, but they chisel away at her cancer with knives and scalpels. Some offer frog's blood, lead plates, goat dung, holy water, crab paste, and caustic chemicals as treatments. In 1778, in John Hunter's clinic in London, her cancer is assigned a stage—early, localized breast cancer or late, advanced, invasive cancer. For the former, Hunter recommends a local operation; for the latter, "remote sympathy."

When Atossa reemerges in the nineteenth century, she encounters a new world of surgery. In Halsted's Baltimore clinic in 1890, Atossa's breast

---

* As described earlier, there is uncertainty about Atossa's diagnosis since "cancer" was neither understood nor characterized in 500 BC.

cancer is treated with the boldest and most definitive therapy thus far—radical mastectomy with a large excision of the tumor and removal of the deep chest muscles and lymph nodes under the armpit and the collarbone. In the early twentieth century, radiation oncologists try to obliterate the tumor locally using X-rays. By the 1950s, yet another generation of surgeons learns to combine the two strategies, although tempered by moderation. Atossa's cancer is treated locally with a simple mastectomy, or a lumpectomy followed by radiation.

In the 1970s, new therapeutic strategies emerge. Atossa's surgery is followed by adjuvant combination chemotherapy to diminish the chance of a relapse. Her tumor tests positive for the estrogen receptor. Tamoxifen, the antiestrogen, is also added to prevent a relapse. In 1986, her tumor is further discovered to be *Her-2* amplified. In addition to surgery, radiation, adjuvant chemotherapy, and tamoxifen, she is treated with targeted therapy using Herceptin.

It is impossible to enumerate the precise impact of these interventions on Atossa's survival. The shifting landscape of trials does not allow a direct comparison between Atossa's fate in 500 BC and her fate in 1989. But surgery, chemotherapy, radiation, hormonal therapy, and targeted therapy have likely added anywhere between seventeen and thirty years to her survival. Diagnosed at forty, say, Atossa can reasonably be expected to celebrate her sixtieth birthday.

In the mid-1990s, the management of Atossa's breast cancer takes another turn. Her diagnosis at an early age and her Achaemenid ancestry raise the question of whether she carries a mutation in BRCA-1 or BRCA-2. Atossa's genome is sequenced, and indeed, a mutation is found. She enters an intensive screening program to detect the appearance of a tumor in her unaffected breast. Her two daughters are also tested. Found positive for BRCA-1, they are offered either intensive screening, prophylactic bilateral mastectomy, or tamoxifen to prevent the development of invasive breast cancer. For Atossa's daughters, the impacts of screening and prophylaxis are dramatic. A breast MRI identifies a small lump in one daughter. It is found to be breast cancer and surgically removed in its early, preinvasive stage. The other daughter chooses to undergo a prophylactic bilateral mastectomy. Having excised her breasts preemptively, she will live out her life free of breast cancer.

Move Atossa into the future now. In 2050, Atossa will arrive at her breast oncologist's clinic with a thumb-size flash drive containing the entire sequence of her cancer's genome, identifying every mutation in every gene. The mutations will be organized into key pathways. An algorithm might identify the pathways that are contributing to the growth and survival of her cancer. Therapies will be targeted against these pathways to prevent a relapse of the tumor after surgery. She will begin with one combination of targeted drugs, expect to switch to a second cocktail when her cancer mutates, and switch again when the cancer mutates again. She will likely take some form of medicine, whether to prevent, cure, or palliate her illness, for the rest of her life.

This, indubitably, is progress. But before we become too dazzled by Atossa's survival, it is worthwhile putting it into perspective. Give Atossa metastatic pancreatic cancer in 500 BC and her prognosis is unlikely to change by more than a few months over twenty-five hundred years. If Atossa develops gallbladder cancer that is not amenable to surgery, her survival changes only marginally over centuries. Even breast cancer shows a marked heterogeneity in outcome. If Atossa's tumor has metastasized, or is estrogen-receptor negative, *Her-2* negative, and unresponsive to standard chemotherapy, then her chances of survival will have barely changed since the time of Hunter's clinic. Give Atossa CML or Hodgkin's disease, in contrast, and her life span may have increased by thirty or forty years.

Part of the unpredictability about the trajectory of cancer in the future is that we do not know the biological basis for this heterogeneity. We cannot yet fathom, for instance, what makes pancreatic cancer or gallbladder cancer so markedly different from CML or Atossa's breast cancer. What is certain, however, is that even the knowledge of cancer's biology is unlikely to eradicate cancer fully from our lives. As Doll suggests, and as Atossa epitomizes, we might as well focus on prolonging life rather than eliminating death. This War on Cancer may best be "won" by redefining victory.

⁂

Atossa's tortuous journey also raises a question implicit in this book: if our understanding and treatment of cancer keep morphing so radically in time, then how can cancer's past be used to predict its future?

In 1997, the NCI director, Richard Klausner, responding to reports that cancer mortality had remained disappointingly static through the nineties, argued that the medical realities of one decade had little bearing on the realities of the next. "There are far more good historians than there are good prophets," Klausner wrote. "It is extraordinarily difficult to predict scientific discovery, which is often propelled by seminal insights coming from unexpected directions. The classic example—Fleming's discovery of penicillin on moldy bread and the monumental impact of that accidental finding—could not easily have been predicted, nor could the sudden demise of iron-lung technology when evolving techniques in virology allowed the growth of poliovirus and the preparation of vaccine. Any extrapolation of history into the future presupposes an environment of static discovery—an oxymoron."

In a limited sense, Klausner is right. When truly radical discoveries appear, their impact is often not incremental but cataclysmic and paradigm-shifting. Technology dissolves its own past. The speculator who bought stock options in an iron-lung company before the discovery of the polio vaccine, or the scientist who deemed bacterial pneumonias incurable just as penicillin was being discovered, were soon shown to be history's fools.

But with cancer, where no simple, universal, or definitive cure is in sight—and is never likely to be—the past is constantly conversing with the future. Old observations crystallize into new theories; time past is always contained in time future. Rous's virus was reincarnated, decades later, in the form of endogenous oncogenes; George Beatson's observation that removing ovaries might slow the growth of breast cancer, inspired by a Scottish shepherds' tale, roars back in the form of a billion-dollar drug named tamoxifen; Bennett's "suppuration of blood," the cancer that launches this book, is also the cancer that ends this book.

And there is a subtler reason to remember this story: while the content of medicine is constantly changing, its *form*, I suspect, remains astonishingly the same. History repeats, but science reverberates. The tools that we will use to battle cancer in the future will doubtless alter so dramatically in fifty years that the geography of cancer prevention and therapy might be unrecognizable. Future physicians may laugh at our mixing of primitive cocktails of poisons to kill the most elemental and magisterial disease known to our species. But much about this battle will remain the same: the relentlessness, the inventiveness, the resilience, the queasy pivoting between defeatism and hope, the hypnotic drive for universal solutions, the disappointment of defeat, the arrogance and the hubris.

The Greeks used an evocative word to describe tumors, *onkos,* meaning "mass" or "burden." The word was more prescient than they might have imagined. Cancer is indeed the load built into our genome, the leaden counterweight to our aspirations for immortality. But if one looks back even further behind the Greek to the ancestral Indo-European language, the etymology of the word *onkos* changes. *Onkos* arises from the ancient word *nek*. And *nek,* unlike the static *onkos,* is the active form of the word *load*. It means to carry, to move the burden from one place to the next, to bear something across a long distance and bring it to a new place. It is an image that captures not just the cancer cell's capacity to travel—metastasis—but also Atossa's journey, the long arc of scientific discovery—and embedded in that journey, the animus, so inextricably human, to outwit, to outlive and survive.

༄

Late one evening in the spring of 2005, toward the end of the first year of my fellowship, I sat in a room on the tenth floor of the hospital with a dying woman, Germaine Berne. She was a vivacious psychologist from Alabama. In 1999, she had been struck by nausea, a queasiness so sudden and violent that it felt as if it had been released from a catapult. Even more unsettling, the nausea had been accompanied by a vague sense of fullness, as if she were perpetually stuck devouring a large meal. Germaine had driven herself to the Baptist Hospital in Montgomery, where she had undergone a barrage of tests until a CAT scan had revealed a twelve-centimeter solid mass pushing into her stomach. On January 4, 2000, a radiologist had biopsied the mass. Under the microscope, the biopsy had revealed sheets of spindlelike cells dividing rapidly. The tumor, which had invaded blood vessels and bucked the normal planes of tissue, was a rare kind of cancer called a gastrointestinal stromal tumor, or simply, a GIST.

The news quickly became worse. Her scans showed spots in her liver, swellings in her lymph nodes, and a spray of masses peppering the left lung. The cancer had metastasized all over her body. A surgical cure was impossible, and in 2000, no chemotherapy was known to be effective against her kind of sarcoma. Her doctors in Alabama cobbled together a combination of chemotherapeutic drugs, but they were essentially biding their time. "I signed my letters, paid my bills, and made my will," she recalled. "There was no doubt about the verdict. I was told to go home to die."

In the winter of 2000, handed her death sentence, Germaine stumbled into a virtual community of cosufferers—GIST patients who spoke to each other through a website. The site, like most of its bloggers, was a strange and moribund affair, with desperate folks seeking desperate remedies. But in late April, news of a novel drug began to spread like wildfire through this community. The new drug was none other than Gleevec—imatinib—

the same chemical that Druker had found to be active against chronic myelogenous leukemia. Gleevec binds and inactivates the *Bcr-abl* protein. But serendipitously, the chemical inactivates another tyrosine kinase, called *c-kit*. Just as activated *Bcr-abl* drives cancer cells to divide and grow in CML, *c-kit* is a driver gene in GIST. In early trials, Gleevec had turned out to be remarkably clinically active against *c-kit*, and hence against GIST.

Germaine pulled strings to get enrolled in one of these trials. She was, by nature, effortlessly persuasive, able to cajole, badger, wheedle, pester, beg, and demand—and her illness had made her bold. ("Cure me, Doc, and I'll send you to Europe," she told me once—an offer that I politely declined.) She worked her way into a teaching hospital where patients were being given the drug on trial. Just as she was being enrolled, Gleevec had turned out to be so effective that doctors could no longer justify treating GIST patients with a placebo pill. Germaine started on the drug in August 2001. A month later, her tumors began to recede at an astonishing rate. Her energy returned; her nausea vanished. She was resurrected from the dead.

Germaine's recovery was a medical miracle. Newspapers in Montgomery picked up the story. She doled out advice to other cancer victims. Medicine was catching up on cancer, she wrote; there was reason for hope. Even if no cure was in sight, a new generation of drugs would control cancer, and another generation would round the bend just as the first one failed. In the summer of 2004, as she was celebrating the fourth anniversary of her unexpected recovery, the cells of Germaine's tumor suddenly grew resistant to Gleevec. Her lumps, having remained dormant for four years, sprouted vengefully back. In months, masses appeared in her stomach, lymph nodes, lungs, liver, spleen. The nausea returned, just as powerfully as the first time. Malignant fluid poured into the cisterns of her abdomen.

Resourceful as usual, Germaine scoured the Web, returning to her makeshift community of GIST patients for advice. She discovered that other drugs—second-generation analogues of Gleevec—were in trial in Boston and in other cities. In 2004, on a telephone halfway across the country, she enrolled in a trial of one such analogue called SU11248 that had just opened up at the Farber.

The new drug produced a temporary response, but did not work for long. By February 2005, Germaine's cancer had spiraled out of control, growing so fast that she could record its weight, in pounds, as she stood on the scales every week. Eventually her pain made it impossible for her to walk even from her bed to the door and she had to be hospitalized. My meeting with

Germaine that evening was not to discuss drugs and therapies, but to try to make an honest reconciliation between her and her medical condition.

As usual, she had already beaten me to it. When I entered her room to talk about next steps, she waved her hand in the air with a withering look and cut me off. Her goals were now simple, she told me. No more trials. No more drugs. The six years of survival that she had eked out between 1999 and 2005 had not been static, frozen years; they had sharpened, clarified, and cleansed her. She had severed her relationship with her husband and intensified her bond with her brother, an oncologist. Her daughter, a teenager in 1999 and now a preternaturally mature sophomore at a Boston college, had grown into her ally, her confidante, her sometime nurse, and her closest friend. ("Cancer breaks some families and makes some," Germaine said. "In my case, it did both.") Germaine realized that her reprieve had finally come to an end. She wanted to get to Alabama, to her own home, to die the death that she had expected in 1999.

☙

When I recall that final conversation with Germaine, embarrassingly enough, the objects seem to stand out more vividly than the words: a hospital room, with its sharp smell of disinfectant and hand soap; the steely, unflattering overhead light; a wooden side table on wheels, piled with pills, books, newspaper clippings, nail polish, jewelry, postcards. Her room, wallpapered with pictures of her beautiful house in Montgomery and of her daughter holding some fruit picked from her garden; a standard-issue plastic hospital pitcher filled with a bunch of sunflowers perched on a table by her side. Germaine, as I remember her, was sitting by the bed, one leg dangling casually down, wearing her usual eccentric and arresting combination of clothes and some large and unusual pieces of jewelry. Her hair was carefully arranged. She looked formal, frozen and perfect, like a photograph of someone in a hospital waiting to die. She seemed content; she laughed and joked. She made wearing a nasogastric tube seem effortless and dignified.

Only years later, in writing this book, could I finally put into words why that meeting left me so uneasy and humbled; why the gestures in that room seemed larger-than-life; why the objects seemed like symbols; why Germaine herself seemed like an actor playing a part. Nothing, I realized, was incidental. The characteristics of Germaine's personality that had once seemed spontaneous and impulsive were, in fact, calculated and almost reflexive responses to her illness. Her clothes were loose and vivid because they were decoys against the growing outline of the tumor in her abdomen. Her necklace was distractingly large so as to pull attention away from her cancer. Her room was topsy-turvy with baubles and pictures—the hospital pitcher filled with flowers, the cards tacked to the wall—because without them it would devolve into the cold anonymity of any other room in any other hospital. She had dangled her leg at that precise, posed angle because the tumor had invaded her spine and begun to paralyze her other leg, making it impossible to sit any other way. Her casualness was studied, the jokes rehearsed. Her illness had tried to humiliate her. It had made her anonymous and seemingly humorless; it had sentenced her to die an unsightly death in a freezing hospital room thousands of miles away from home. She had responded with vengeance, moving to be always one step ahead, trying to outwit it.

It was like watching someone locked in a chess game. Every time Germaine's disease moved, imposing yet another terrifying constraint on her, she made an equally assertive move in return. The illness acted; she reacted. It was a morbid, hypnotic game—a game that had taken over her life. She dodged one blow only to be caught by another. She, too, was like Carroll's Red Queen, stuck pedaling furiously just to keep still in one place.

Germaine seemed, that evening, to have captured something essential about our struggle against cancer: that, to keep pace with this malady, you needed to keep inventing and reinventing, learning and unlearning strategies. Germaine fought cancer obsessively, cannily, desperately, fiercely, madly, brilliantly, and zealously—as if channeling all the fierce, inventive energy of generations of men and women who had fought cancer in the past and would fight it in the future. Her quest for a cure had taken her on a strange and limitless journey, through Internet blogs and teaching hospitals, chemotherapy and clinical trials halfway across the country, through a landscape more desolate, desperate, and disquieting than she had ever imagined. She had deployed every morsel of energy to the quest, mobilizing and remobilizing the last dregs of her courage, summoning her will and wit and imagination, until, that final evening, she had stared into the vault of her resourcefulness and resilience and found it empty. In that haunted last night, hanging on to her life by no more than a tenuous thread, summoning all her strength and dignity as she wheeled herself to the privacy of her bathroom, it was as if she had encapsulated the essence of a four-thousand-year-old war.

—S.M., June 2010

Acknowledgments

I have many people to thank. My wife, Sarah Sze, whose unfailing faith, love, and patience sustained this book. My daughters Leela and Aria, for whom this book was often a rival sibling; who fell asleep on many nights to the mechanical lullaby of my furious typing and then woke the next morning to find me typing again. My agent Sarah Chalfant, who read and annotated draft upon draft of my proposals; my editor Nan Graham, with whom I began to communicate with "mental telepathy" and whose thoughts are stitched into every page. My early readers: Nell Breyer, Amy Waldman, Neel Mukherjee, Ashok Rai, Kim Gutschow, David Seo, Robert Brustein, Prasant Atluri, Erez Kalir, Yariv Houvras, Mitzi Angel, Diana Beinart, Daniel Menaker, and many mentors and interviewees, particularly Robert Mayer, who were crucial in the development of this book. My parents, Sibeswar and Chandana Mukherjee and my sister, Ranu Bhattacharyya and her family, who found vacations and family gatherings swallowed up by an interminable manuscript and Chia-Ming and Judy Sze who provided sustenance and help during my frequent visits to Boston.

As with any such book, this work also rests on the prior work of others: Susan Sontag's masterful and moving *Illness as Metaphor,* Richard Rhodes's *The Making of the Atomic Bomb,* Richard Rettig's *Cancer Crusade,* Barron Lerner's *The Breast Cancer Wars,* Natalie Angier's *Natural Obsessions,* Lewis Thomas's *The Lives of a Cell,* George Crile's *The Way It Was,* Adam Wishart's *One in Three,* Aleksandr Solzhenitsyn's *Cancer Ward,* David Rieff's devastating memoir *Swimming in a Sea of Death,* Robert Bazell's *Her-2,* Robert Weinberg's *Racing to the Beginning of the Road,* John Lazlo's *The Cure of Childhood Leukemia: Into the Age of Miracles,* Harold Varmus's *The Art and Politics of Science,* Michael Bishop's *How to Win the Nobel Prize,* David Nathan's *The Cancer Treatment Revolution,* James Patterson's *The Dread Disease,* and Tony Judt's *Postwar.* Many archives and libraries were accessed as primary sources for the book: Mary Lasker's papers, Benno Schmidt's papers, George Papanicolaou's papers, Arthur

Aufderheide's papers and specimen collection, William Halsted's papers, Rose Kushner's papers, the tobacco documents at UCSF, Evarts Graham's papers, Richard Doll's papers, Joshua Lederberg's papers, Harold Varmus's papers, the Boston Public Library, the Countway Library of Medicine, Columbia University libraries, and Sidney Farber's personal photographs and correspondence, shared by several sources, including Thomas Farber, his son. The manuscript was also read by Robert Mayer, George Canellos, Donald Berry, Emil Freireich, Al Knudson, Harold Varmus, Dennis Slamon, Brian Druker, Thomas Lynch, Charles Sawyers, Bert Vogelstein, Robert Weinberg, and Ed Gelmann, who provided corrections and alterations to the text.

Harold Varmus, in particular, provided astonishingly detailed and insightful commentary and annotations—emblematic of the extraordinary generosity that I received from scientists, writers, and doctors.

David Scadden and Gary Gilliland provided a fostering laboratory environment at Harvard. Ed Gelmann, Riccardo Dalla-Favera, and Cory and Michael Shen gave me a new academic "home" at Columbia University, where this book was finished. Tony Judt's Remarque Institute Forum (where I was a fellow) provided an inimitable environment for historical discussions; indeed, this book was conceived in its current form on a crystalline lake in Sweden during one such forum. Jason Rothauser, Paul Whitlatch, and Jaime Wolf read, edited, and checked the facts and figures in the manuscript. Alexandra Truitt and Jerry Marshall researched and cleared copyrights for the pictures.

Notes

vii Susan Sontag, *Illness as Metaphor and AIDS and Its Metaphors* (New York: Picador, 1990), 3.

PROLOGUE

1 *Diseases desperate grown:* William Shakespeare, *Hamlet,* Act IV, Scene III.

1 *Cancer begins and ends with people:* June Goodfield, *The Siege of Cancer* (New York: Random House, 1975), 219.

4 *In Aleksandr Solzhenitsyn's novel:* Aleksandr Solzhenitsyn, *Cancer Ward* (New York: Farrar, Straus and Giroux, 1968).

5 *Atossa, the Persian queen:* Herodotus, *The Histories* (Oxford: Oxford University Press, 1998), 223.

6 *"The universe," the twentieth-century biologist:* John Burdon Sanderson Haldane, *Possible Worlds and Other Papers* (New York: Harper & Brothers, 1928), 286.

PART ONE:
"OF BLACKE CHOLOR, WITHOUT BOYLING"

9 *In solving a problem of this sort:* Arthur Conan Doyle, *A Study in Scarlet* (Whitefish, MT: Kessinger Publishing, 2004), 107.

"A suppuration of blood"

11 *Physicians of the Utmost Fame:* Hilaire Belloc, *Cautionary Tales for Children* (New York: Alfred A. Knopf, 1922), 18–19.

11 *Its palliation is a daily task:* William B. Castle, "Advances in Knowledge concerning Diseases of the Blood, 1949–1950," in *The 1950 Year Book of Medicine: May 1949–May 1950* (Chicago: Year Book Publishers, 1950), 313–26.

11 *In a damp:* Details concerning aminopterin and its arrival in Farber's clinic are from several sources. Sidney Farber et al., "The Action of Pteroylglutamic Conjugates on Man," *Science,* 106, no. 2764 (1947): 619–21; S. P. K. Gupta, interview with author, February 2006; and S. P. K. Gupta, "An Indian Scientist in America: The Story of Dr. Yellapragada SubbaRow," *Bulletin of the Indian Institute of History of Medicine* (Hyderabad) 6, no. 2 (1976): 128–43; S. P. K. Gupta and Edgar L. Milford, *In Quest of Panacea* (New Delhi: Evelyn Publishers, 1987).

11 *Farber's specialty was pediatric pathology:* John Craig, "Sidney Farber (1903–1973)," *Journal of Pediatrics* 128, no. 1 (1996): 160–62. Also see "Looking Back: Sidney Farber and the First Remission of Acute Pediatric Leukemia," Children's Hospital, Boston, http://www.childrenshospital.org/gallery/index.cfm?G=49&page=2 (accessed January 4, 2010); H. R. Wiedemann, "Sidney Farber (1903–1973)," *European Journal of Pediatrics,* 153 (1994): 223.

12 *"It gave physicians plenty to wrangle over":* John Laszlo, *The Cure of Childhood Leukemia: Into the Age of Miracles* (New Brunswick, NJ: Rutgers University Press, 1995), 19.

12 *"diagnosed, transfused—and sent home to die":* Medical World News, November 11, 1966.

13 *"He is of dark complexion":* John Hughes Bennett, "Case of Hypertrophy of the Spleen and Liver in Which Death Took Place from Suppuration of the Blood," *Edinburgh Medical and Surgical Journal* 64 (October 1, 1845): 413–23. Also see John Hughes Bennett, *Clinical Lectures on the Principles and Practice of Medicine,* 3rd ed. (New York: William Wood & Company, 1866), 620.

13 *"A suppuration of blood":* Bennett, "Case of Hypertrophy of the Spleen." Also see Bennett, *Clinical Lectures,* 896.

13 *Rudolf Virchow, independently published:* Rudolf Ludwig Karl Virchow, *Cellular Pathology: As Based upon Physiological and Pathological Histology,* trans. Frank Chance (London: John Churchill, 1860), 169–71, 220. Also see Bennett, *Clinical Lectures,* 896.

14 *seeking a name for this condition:* Charles J. Grant, "Weisses Blut," *Radiologic Technology* 73, no. 4 (2003): 373–76.

14 *in the early 1980s, another change in name:* Randy Shilts, *And the Band Played On* (New York: St. Martin's), 171.

14 *Virchow's approach to medicine:* "Virchow," *British Medical Journal,* 2, no. 3171 (1921): 573–74. Also see Virchow, *Cellular Pathology*.

16 *Bennett's earlier fantasy:* William Seaman Bainbridge, *The Cancer Problem* (New York: Macmillan Company, 1914), 117.

17 *Michael Anton Biermer, described:* Laszlo, *Cure of Childhood Leukemia,* 7–9, 15.

17 *From its first symptom to diagnosis to death:* Biermer, "Ein Fall von Leukämie," *Virchow's Archives,* 1861, S. 552, cited in Suchannek, "Case of Leukaemia," 255–69.

19 *Farber completed his advanced training:* Denis R. Miller, "A Tribute to Sidney Farber— the Father of Modern Chemotherapy," *British Journal of Haematology* 134 (2006): 4, 20–26.

20 *What is true for* E. coli: This remark, attributed to Monod (perhaps apocryphally), appears several times in the history of molecular biology, although its precise origins remain unknown. See, for instance, Theresa M. Wizemann and Mary-Lou Pardue, eds., *Exploring the Biological Contributions to Human Health: Does Sex Matter?* (Washington, DC: National Academy Press, 2001), 32; Herbert Claus Friedmann, "From Butyribacterium to *E. coli*: An Essay on Unity in Biochemistry," *Perspectives in Biology and Medicine* 47, no. 1 (2004): 47–66.

"A monster more insatiable than the guillotine"

21 *The medical importance of leukemia:* Jonathan B. Tucker, *Ellie: A Child's Fight Against Leukemia* (New York: Holt, Rinehart, and Winston, 1982), 46.

21 *There were few successes in the treatment:* John Laszlo, *The Cure of Childhood Leukemia: Into the Age of Miracles* (New Brunswick, NJ: Rutgers University Press, 1995), 162.

21 *a cornucopia of pharmaceutical discoveries:* Michael B. Shimkin, "As Memory Serves—an Informal History of the National Cancer Institute, 1937–57," *Journal of the National Cancer Institute* 59 (suppl. 2) (1977): 559–600.

21 *the drug was reextracted:* Eric Lax, *The Mold in Dr. Florey's Coat: The Story of the Penicillin Miracle* (New York: Henry Holt and Co., 2004), 67.

21 *In 1942, when Merck had shipped:* "Milestone Moments in Merck History," http://www.merck.com/about/feature_story/01062003_penicillin.html (site is no longer available but can be accessed through http://www.archive.org/web/web.php).

21 *A decade later, penicillin:* E. K. Marshall, "Historical Perspectives in Chemotherapy," *Advances in Chemotherapy* 13 (1974): 1–8. Also see *Science News Letter* 41 (1942).

22 *chloramphenicol in 1947:* John Ehrlich et al., "Chloromycetin, a New Antibiotic from a Soil Actinomycete," *Science* 106, no. 2757 (1947): 417.

22 *tetracycline in 1948:* B. M. Duggar, "Aureomycin: A Product of the Continuing Search for New Antibiotics," *Annals of the New York Academy of Science* 51 (1948): 177–81.

22 *"The remedies are in our own backyard":* Time, November 7, 1949.

22 *In a brick building on the far corner:* John F. Enders, Thomas H. Weller, and Frederick C. Robbins, "Cultivation of the Lansing Strain of Poliomyelitis Virus in Cultures of Various Human Embryonic Tissues," *Science* 49 (1949): 85–87; Fred S. Rosen, "Isolation of Poliovirus—John Enders and the Nobel Prize," *New England Journal of Medicine* 351 (2004): 1481–83.

22 *by 1950, more than half the medicines:* A. N. Richards, "The Production of Penicillin in the United States: Extracts and Editorial Comment," *Annals of Internal Medicine,* suppl. 8 (1969): 71–73. Also see Austin Smith and Arthur Herrick, *Drug Research and Development* (New York: Revere Publishing Co., 1948).

22 *Typhoid fever:* Anand Karnad, *Intrinsic Factors: William Bosworth Castle and the Development of Hematology and Clinical Investigation at Boston City Hospital* (Boston: Harvard Medical School, 1997).

22 *Even tuberculosis:* Edgar Sydenstricker, "Health in the New Deal," *Annals of the American Academy of Political and Social Science* 176, Social Welfare in the National Recovery Program (1934): 131–37.

22 *The life expectancy of Americans:* Lester Breslow, *A Life in Public Health: An Insider's Retrospective* (New York: Springer, 2004), 69. Also see Nicholas D. Kristof, "Access, Access, Access," *New York Times,* March 17, 2010.

22 *Hospitals proliferated:* Rosemary Stevens, *In Sickness and in Wealth* (New York: Basic Books, 1989), 204, 229.

22 *As one student observed:* Temple Burling, Edith Lentz, and Robert N. Wilson, *The Give and Take in Hospitals* (New York: Putnam, 1956), 9.

22 *Lulled by the idea of the durability:* From *Newsweek* and *Time* advertisements, 1946–48. Also see Ruth P. Mack, "Trends in American Consumption," *American Economic Review* 46, no. 2, (1956):55–68.

23 *"illness" now ranked third:* Herbert J. Gans, *The Levittowners: Ways of Life and Politics in a New Suburban Community* (New York: Alfred A. Knopf), 234.

23 *Fertility rose steadily:* Paul S. Boyer et al., *The Enduring Vision: A History of the American People* (Florence, KY: Cengage Learning, 2008), 980.

23 *The "affluent society":* John Kenneth Galbraith, *The Affluent Society* (New York: Houghton Mifflin, 1958).

23 *In May 1937:* "Cancer: The Great Darkness," *Fortune,* May 1937.

24 *In 1899, when Roswell Park:* Robert Proctor, *Cancer Wars: How Politics Shapes What We Know and Don't Know About Cancer* (New York: Basic Books, 1995), 20.

24 *Smallpox was on the decline:* K. A. Sepkowitz, "The 1947 Smallpox Vaccination Campaign in New York City, Revisited," *Emerging Infectious Diseases* 10, no. 5 (2004): 960–61. Also see D. E. Hammerschmidt, "Hands: The Last Great Smallpox Outbreak in Minnesota (1924–25)," *Journal of Laboratory and Clinical Medicine* 142, no. 4 (2003): 278.

24 *Between 1900 and 1916:* Lucius Duncan Bulkley, *Cancer and Its Non-Surgical Treatment* (New York: W. Wood & Co., 1921).

24 *By 1926, cancer:* Proctor, *Cancer Wars,* 66.

24 *In May that year,* Life: "U.S. Science Wars against an Unknown Enemy: Cancer," *Life,* March 1, 1937.

24 *When cancer appeared:* "Medicine: Millions for Cancer," *Time,* July 5, 1937; "Medicine: After Syphilis, Cancer," *Time,* July 19, 1937.

24 American Association for Cancer Research: "AACR: A Brief History," http://www.aacr.org/home/about-us/centennial/aacr-history.aspx (accessed January 4, 2010).

25 *from 70,000 men and women in 1911:* "A Cancer Commission," *Los Angeles Times,* March 4, 1927.

25 *Neely asked Congress:* 69th Cong., 2nd sess., *Congressional Record,* 68 (1927): p3 2922.

25 *Within a few weeks:* Richard A. Rettig, *Cancer Crusade: The Story of the National Cancer Act of 1971* (Lincoln, NE: Author's Choice Press, 1977), 44.

25 *In June, a joint Senate-House conference:* "National Cancer Act of 1937," Office of Government and Congressional Relations, Legislative History, http://legislative.cancer.gov/history/1937 (accessed November 8, 2009).

25 *An advisory council of scientists:* Shimkin, "As Memory Serves," 559–600.

26 *"The nation is marshaling its forces": Congressional Record,* appendix 84:2991 (June 30, 1939); Margot J. Fromer, "How, After a Decade of Public & Private Wrangling, FDR Signed NCI into Law in 1937," *Oncology Times* 28 (19): 65–67.

26 *The U.S. Marine Hospital:* Ora Marashino, "Administration of the National Cancer Institute Act, August 5, 1937, to June 30, 1943," *Journal of the National Cancer Institute* 4: 429–43.

26 *"mostly silent":* Shimkin, "As Memory Serves," 599–600.

26 *"programmatic response to cancer":* Ibid.

26 *"a nice quiet place out here in the country":* Ibid.

26 *In the early 1950s, Fanny Rosenow:* Jimmie C. Holland and Sheldon Lewis, *The Human Side of Cancer* (New York: Harper Collins, 2001).

26 *In 1946–47, Neely and Senator Claude Pepper:* See House Foreign Affairs Committee, House Report 2565, 79th Cong., 2nd sess. Also see Report 1743 to the 79th Cong., 2nd sess., July 18, 1946; "Could a 'Manhattan Project' Conquer Cancer?" *Washington Post,* August 4, 1946.

27 *"Leukemia," as one physician put it:* J. V. Pickstone, "Contested Cumulations: Configurations of Cancer Treatments through the Twentieth Century," *Bulletin of the History of Medicine* 81, no. 1 (2007): 164–96.

27 *If leukemia "belonged" anywhere:* Grant Taylor, *Pioneers in Pediatric Oncology* (Houston: University of Texas M. D. Anderson Cancer Center, 1990).

28 *half a pound of chicken liver:* George Washington Corner, *George Hoyt Whipple and*

His Friends: The Life-Story of a Nobel Prize Pathologist (Philadelphia: Lippincott, 1963), 187.

28 *regurgitated gastric juices:* Taylor, *Pioneers in Pediatric Oncology,* 29; George R. Minot, "Nobel Lecture: The Development of Liver Therapy in Pernicious Anemia," *Nobel Lectures, Physiology or Medicine, 1922–1941* (Amsterdam: Elsevier Publishing Company, 1965).

28 *spiced up with butter, lemon, and parsley:* Francis Minot Rackemann, *The Inquisitive Physician: The Life and Times of George Richards Minot* (Cambridge: Harvard University Press, 1956), 151.

28 *Minot and his team of researchers:* George R. Minot and William P. Murphy, "Treatment of Pernicious Anemia by a Special Diet," *Journal of the American Medical Association,* 87 (7): 470–76.

28 *conclusively demonstrated in 1926:* Minot, "Nobel Lecture."

28 *In 1934, Minot and two of his colleagues:* Ibid.

28 *in the cloth mills of Bombay:* Lucy Wills, "A Biographical Sketch," *Journal of Nutrition* 108 (1978), 1379–83.

28 *In 1928, a young English physician named Lucy Willis:* H. Bastian, "Lucy Wills (1888–1964): The Life and Research of an Adventurous Independent Woman," *Journal of the Royal College of Physicians of Edinburgh* 38:89–91.

28 *Wills factor:* Janet Watson and William B. Castle, "Nutritional Macrocytic Anemia, Especially in Pregnancy: Response to a Substance in Liver Other Than That Effective in Pernicious Anemia," *American Journal of the Medical Sciences* 211, no. 5 (1946): 513–30; Lucy Wills, "Treatment of 'Pernicious Anaemia' of Pregnancy and 'Tropical Anaemia,' with Special Reference to Yeast Extract as a Curative Agent," *British Medical Journal* 1, no. 3676 (1931): 1059–64.

29 *He called this phenomenon acceleration:* Sidney Farber et al., "The Action of Pteroylglutamic Conjugates on Man," *Science* 106, no. 2764 (1947): 619–21. Also see Mills et al., "Observations on Acute Leukemia in Children Treated with 4-Aminopteroylglutamic Acid," *Pediatrics* 5, no. 1 (1950): 52–56.

30 *In his long walks from his laboratory:* Thomas Farber, interview with author, November 2007.

30 *He had arrived in Boston in 1923:* S. P. K. Gupta, "An Indian Scientist in America: The Story of Dr. Yellapragada SubbaRow," *Bulletin of the Indian Institute of History of Medicine* (Hyderabad), 6, no. 2 (1976): 128–43.

31 *In the 1920s, another drug company:* Corner, *George Hoyt Whipple,* 188.

31 *But in 1946, after many failed attempts:* Gupta, "Indian Scientist in America."

Farber's Gauntlet

32 *Throughout the centuries:* William Seaman Bainbridge, *The Cancer Problem* (New York: Macmillan Company, 1914), 2.

32 *The search for a way to eradicate this scourge:* "Cancer Ignored," *Washington Post,* August 5, 1946.

33 *Robert Sandler:* Biographical details were taken from an article in the *Boston Herald,* April 9, 1948, referred to in S. P. K. Gupta, "An Indian Scientist in America: The Story of Dr. Yellapragada SubbaRow," *Bulletin of the Indian Institute of History of Medicine* (Hyderabad), 6, no. 2 (1976): 128–43; and S. P. K. Gupta, interview with author,

February 2006. Sandler's address in Dorchester and his father's profession are from the Boston directory for 1946, obtained from the Boston Public Library. Sandler's case (R.S.) is described in detail in Sidney Farber's paper below.

33 Farber's treatment of Robert Sandler: Sidney Farber, "Temporary Remissions in Acute Leukemia in Children Produced by Folic Acid Antagonist, 4-Aminopteroyl-Glutamic Acid (Aminopterin)," *New England Journal of Medicine* 238 (1948): 787–93.

34 *The hospital staff voted:* Robert Cooke, *Dr. Folkman's War: Angiogenesis and the Struggle to Defeat Cancer* (New York: Random House, 2001), 113.

34 *"tucked in the farthest recesses":* Joseph E. Murray, *Surgery of the Soul: Reflections on a Curious Career* (Sagamore Beach, MA: Science History Publications, 2001), 127.

34 *"let them die in peace":* Robert D. Mercer, "The Team," in "Chronicle," *Medical and Pediatric Oncology* 33 (1999): 405–10.

34 *"By that time, the only chemical":* Thomas Farber, interview with author.

35 *His small staff was housed:* Taylor, *Pioneers in Pediatric Oncology,* 88.

35 *Farber's assistants sharpened their own:* Mercer, "The Team."

35 *Two boys treated with aminopterin:* Farber, "Temporary Remissions in Acute Leukemia," 787–93.

35 *Another child, a two-and-a-half-year-old:* Ibid.

35 *By April 1948, there was just enough data:* Ibid

36 *"with skepticism, disbelief, and outrage":* Denis R. Miller, "A Tribute to Sidney Farber—the Father of Modern Chemotherapy," *British Journal of Haematology* 134 (2006): 20–26.

36 *"The bone marrow looked so normal":* Mercer, "The Team."

A Private Plague

37 *We reveal ourselves:* Stephen Jay Gould, *Full House: The Spread of Excellence from Plato to Darwin* (New York: Three Rivers Press, 1996), 7.

37 *Thus, for 3,000 years and more:* "Cancer: The Great Darkness," *Fortune,* May 1937.

37 *Now it is cancer's turn:* Susan Sontag, *Illness as Metaphor and AIDS and Its Metaphors* (New York: Picador, 1990), 5.

38 *John Keats involuting silently:* "John Keats," *Annals of Medical History* 2, no. 5 (1930): 530.

38 *"Death and disease are often beautiful":* Sontag, *Illness as Metaphor,* 20.

38 *"in every possible sense, a nonconformist":* Sherwin Nuland, *How We Die: Reflections on Life's Final Chapter* (New York: Vintage Books, 1995), 202.

39 Edwin Smith papyrus: James Henry Breasted, *The Edwin Smith Papyrus:* Some Preliminary Observations (Paris: Librairie Ancienne Honoré Champion, Edward Champion, 1922); also available online at http://www.touregypt.net/edwinsmithsurgical.htm (accessed November 8, 2009).

40 Imhotep case forty-five: Breasted, *Edwin Smith Papyrus.* Also see F. S. Boulos. "Oncology in Egyptian Papyri," in *Paleo-oncology: The Antiquity of Cancer,* 5th ed., ed. Spyros Retsas (London: Farrand Press, 1986), 36; and Edward Lewison, *Breast Cancer and Its Diagnosis and Treatment* (Baltimore: Williams and Walkins, 1955), 3.

41 *A furious febrile plague:* Siro I. Trevisanato, "Did an Epidemic of Tularemia in Ancient Egypt Affect the Course of World History?" *Medical Hypotheses* 63, no. 5 (2004): 905–10.

41 *leaving its telltale pockmarks:* Sergio Donadoni, ed., *The Egyptians* (Chicago: University of Chicago Press, 1997), 292.

41 *Tuberculosis rose and ebbed:* Reddy D. V. Subba, "Tuberculosis in Ancient India," *Bulletin of the Institute of Medicine* (Hyderabad) 2 (1972): 156–61.

41 *In his sprawling* Histories: Herodotus, *The Histories* (Oxford: Oxford University Press, 1998), pt. VIII.

43 *At the Chiribaya site:* Arthur Aufderheide, *The Scientific Study of Mummies* (Cambridge: Cambridge University Press, 2003), 117; Arthur Aufderheide, interview with author, March 2009. Also see *Cambridge Encyclopedia of Paleopathology* (Cambridge: Cambridge University Press, 1998), 300

43 *In 1914, a team:* J. L. Miller, "Some Diseases of Ancient Man," *Annals of Medical History* 1 (1929): 394–402.

43 *Louis Leakey, the archaeologist:* Mel Greaves, *Cancer: The Evolutionary Legacy* (Oxford: Oxford University Press, 2000).

44 *"The early history of cancer":* Aufderheide, interview with author, 2009.

44 *A leprosy-like illness:* Boris S. Ostrer, "Leprosy: Medical Views of Leviticus Rabba," *Early Science and Medicine* 7, no. 2 (2002): 138–54.

44 *The risk of breast cancer:* See, for instance, "Risk Factors You Can't Control," Breastcancer.org, www.breastcancer.org/risk/everyone/cant_control.jsp (accessed January 4, 2010). Also see Report No. 1743, International Cancer Research Act, 79th Cong., 2nd Sess.; and "U.S. Science Wars against an Unknown Enemy: Cancer," *Life*, March 1, 1937.

45 *"captain of the men of death":* William Osler and Thomas McCrae, *The Principles and Practice of Medicine: Designed for the Use of Practitioners and Students of Medicine,* 9th ed. (New York: D. Appleton and Company, 1921), 156.

45 *Cancer still lagged:* Report No. 1743, International Cancer Research Act.

45 *By the early 1940s, cancer:* Life, March 1, 1937, 11.

45 *life expectancy among Americans:* Shrestha et al., "Life Expectancy in the United States," CRS Report for Congress, 2006. Also see Lewison, *Breast Cancer.*

Onkos

46 *Black bile without boiling:* Jeremiah Reedy, "Galen on Cancer and Related Diseases," *Clio Medica* 10, no. 3 (1975): 227.

46 *We have learned nothing:* Francis Carter Wood, "Surgery Is Sole Cure for Bad Varieties of Cancer," *New York Times,* April 19, 1914.

46 *It's bad bile:* Mel Greaves, *Cancer: The Evolutionary Legacy* (Oxford: Oxford University Press, 2000), 5.

46 *In some ways disease:* Charles E. Rosenberg, "Disease in History: Frames and Framers," *Milbank Quarterly* 67 (1989) (suppl. 1, *Framing Disease: The Creation and Negotiation of Explanatory Schemes*): 1–2.

47 *Later writers, both doctors and patients:* See, for instance, Henry E. Sigerist, "The Historical Development of the Pathology and Therapy of Cancer," *Bulletin of the New York Academy of Medicine* 8, no. 11 (1932): 642–53; James A. Tobey, *Cancer: What Everyone Should Know about It* (New York: Alfred A. Knopf, 1932).

48 *"Of blacke cholor":* Claudius Galen, *Methodus Medendi, with a Brief Declaration of the Worthie Art of Medicine, the Office of a Chirgion, and an Epitome of the Third*

Booke of Galen, of Naturall Faculties, trans. T. Gale (London: Thomas East, 1586), 180–82.

49 *"best left untreated":* Emile Littré's translation of the Hippocratic oath, *Oeuvres complètes d'Hippocrate,* bk. VI, aphorism 38. Von Boenninghausen, *Homeopathic Recorder,* vol. 58, nos. 10, 11, 12 (1943). Also see http://classics.mit.edu/Hippocrates/aphorisms.6.vi.html and http://julianwinston.com/archives/periodicals/vb_aphorisms6.php.

49 *"Do not be led away and offer":* George Parker, *The Early History of Surgery in Great Britain: Its Organization and Development* (London: Black, 1920), 44.

49 *"Those who pretend":* Joseph-François Malgaigne, *Surgery and Ambroise Paré* (Norman: University of Oklahoma Press, 1965), 73.

49 *Ambroise Paré described charring tumors:* See, for instance, "The History of Hemostasis," *Annals of Medical History* 1 (1): 137; Malgaigne, *Surgery and Ambroise Paré,* 73, 181.

49 *"Many females can stand the operation":* See Lorenz Heister, "Van de Kanker der boorsten," in H. T. Ulhoorn, ed., *Heelkundige onderwijzingen* (Amsterdam, 1718), 2: 845–856; also quoted in James S. Olson, *Bathsheba's Breast: Women, Cancer, and History* (Baltimore: Johns Hopkins University Press, 2002), 50.

50 *The apothecary:* See, for instance, William Seaman Bainbridge, *The Cancer Problem* (New York: Macmillan Company, 1914).

Vanishing Humors

51 *Rack't carcasses:* John Donne, "Love's Exchange," *Poems of John Donne,* vol. 1, ed. E. K. Chambers (London: Lawrence & Bullen, 1896), 35–36.

51 *"Aside from the eight muscles":* Andreas Vesalius, *The Fabric of the Human Body* [*De Fabrica Humani Corporis*], trans. W. P. Hotchkiss, preface. See *Sourcebook of Medical History* (Mineola, NY: Dover, 1960), 134; and *The Illustrations from the Works of Andreas Vesalius of Brussels* (Mineola, NY: Dover, 1950), 11–13.

51 *He needed his own specimens:* Charles Donald O'Malley, *Andreas Vesalius of Brussels, 1514–1564* (Berkeley: University of California Press, 1964).

52 *"In the course of explaining the opinion":* "Andreas Vesalius of Brussels Sends Greetings to His Master and Patron, the Most Eminent and Illustrious Doctor Narcissus Parthenopeus, First Physician to His Imperial Majesty," *The Illustrations from the Works of Andreas Vesalius of Brussels,* with annotations and translations by J. B. de C. M. Saunders and Charles D. O'Malley (Cleveland, OH: World Publishing Company, 1950), 233.

53 *"as large as an orange":* Matthew Baillie, *The Morbid Anatomy of Some of the Most Important Parts of the Human Body,* 2nd American ed. (Walpole, NH: 1808), 54.

53 *"a fungous appearance":* Ibid., 93.

53 *"a foul deep ulcer":* Ibid., 209.

"Remote sympathy"

55 *In treating of cancer:* Samuel Cooper, *A Dictionary of Practical Surgery* vol. 1 (New York: Harper & Brothers, 1836), 49.

55 *"If a tumor is not only movable"*: John Hunter, *Lectures on the Principles of Surgery* (Philadelphia: Haswell, Barrington, and Haswell, 1839).

56 *"I did not experience pain"*: See a history of ether at http://www.anesthesia-nursing.com/ether.html (accessed January 5, 2010).

56 *"It must be some subtle principle"*: M. Percy, "On the Dangers of Dissection," *New Journal of Medicine and Surgery, and Collateral Branches of Science* 8, no. 2 (1819): 192–96.

57 It *"occurred to me"*: Joseph Lister, "On the Antiseptic Principle in the Practice of Surgery," *British Medical Journal* 2, no. 351 (1867): 246.

57 *In August 1867, a thirteen-year-old*: Ibid., 247.

58 *In 1869, Lister removed a breast tumor*: James S. Olson, *Bathsheba's Breast* (Baltimore: Johns Hopkins University Press, 2002), 67.

58 *Lister performed an extensive amputation*: Edward Lewison, *Breast Cancer and Its Diagnosis and Treatment* (Baltimore: Williams and Walkins, 1955), 17.

58 *"The course so far is already"*: Harold Ellis, *A History of Surgery* (Cambridge: Cambridge University Press, 2001), 104.

59 Billroth's gastrectomy: See Theodor Billroth, Offenes schreiben an Herrn Dr. L. Wittelshöfer, Wien Med Wschr (1881), 31: 161–65; also see Owen Wangensteen and Sarah Wangensteen, *The Rise of Surgery* (Minneapolis: University of Minnesota Press, 1978), 149.

59 *Surgeons returned to the operating table*: Owen Pritchard, "Notes and Remarks on Upwards of Forty Operations for Cancer with Escharotics," *Lancet* 136, no. 3504 (1890): 864.

A Radical Idea

60 *The professor who blesses the occasion*: Mary Lou McCarthy McDonough, *Poet Physicians: An Anthology of Medical Poetry Written by Physicians* (Springfield, IL: Charles C. Thomas, 1945).

60 *It is over*: John Brown, *Rab and His Friends* (Edinburgh: David Douglas, 1885), 20.

60 *William Stewart Halsted*: W. G. MacCallum, *William Stewart Halsted, Surgeon* (Kessinger Publishing, 2008), 106. Also see Michael Osborne, "William Stewart Halsted: His Life and Contributions to Surgery"; and S. J. Crowe, *Halsted of Johns Hopkins: The Man and His Men* (Springfield, IL: Charles C. Thomas).

61 *"I opened a large orifice"*: W. H. Witt, "The Progress of Internal Medicine since 1830," in *The Centennial History of the Tennessee State Medical Association, 1830–1930,* ed. Philip M. Hammer (Nashville: Tennessee State Medical Association, 1930), 265.

61 *"Small bleedings give temporary relief"*: Walter Hayle Walshe, *A Practical Treatise on the Diseases of the Lungs including the Principles of Physical Diagnosis,* 3rd ed. (Philadelphia: Blanchard and Lea, 1860), 416.

61 *"pus-pails"*: Lois N. Magner, *A History of Medicine* (New York: Marcel Dekker, 1992), 296.

62 *In October 1877, leaving behind*: MacCallum, *William Stewart Halsted*. Also see D. W. Cathell, *The Physician Himself* (1905), 2.

62 merely an *"audacious step"* away: Karel B. Absolon, *The Surgeon's Surgeon: Theodor Billroth: 1829–1894,* (Kansas: Coronado Press, 1979).

62 *In 1882, he removed an infected gallbladder*: John L. Cameron, "William Stewart Halsted: Our Surgical Heritage," *Annals of Surgery* 225, no. 5 (1996): 445–58.

63 *"clearer and clearer, with no sense of fatigue"*: Donald Fleming, *William H. Welch and the Rise of Modern Medicine* (Baltimore: Johns Hopkins University Press, 1987).

63 *"cold as stone and most unlivable"*: Harvey Cushing, letter to his mother, 1898, Harvey Cushing papers at Yale University.

64 *"Mammary cancer requires"*: Charles H. Moore, "On the Influence of Inadequate Operations on the Theory of Cancer," *Medico-Chirurgical Transactions* 50, no. 245 (1867): 277.

64 *"mistaken kindness"*: Edward Lewison. *Breast Cancer and Its Diagnosis and Treatment* (Baltimore: Williams and Walkins, 1955), 16.

65 *"We clean out or strip"*: William S. Halsted, "A Clinical and Histological Study of Certain Adenocarcinomata of the Breast: And a Brief Consideration of the Supraclavicular Operation and of the Results of Operations for Cancer of the Breast from 1889 to 1898 at the Johns Hopkins Hospital," *Annals of Surgery* 28: 557–76.

65 *At Hopkins, Halsted's diligent students:* W. M. Barclay, "Progress of the Medical Sciences: Surgery," *Bristol Medical-Chirurgical Journal* 17, no. 1 (1899): 334–36.

65 *"It is likely"*: Halsted, "Clinical and Histological Study."

65 *In Europe, one surgeon evacuated three ribs:* See Westerman, "Thoraxexcisie bij recidief can carcinoma mammae," *Ned Tijdschr Geneeskd* (1910): 1686.

65 *"surgical elephantiasis," "Good use of arm," "Married, Four Children"*: from William Stewart Halsted, *Surgical Papers* (Baltimore: Johns Hopkins, 1924), 2:17, 22, 24.

66 *"performance of an artist"*: Matas, "William Stewart Halsted, an appreciation," *Bulletin of the Johns Hopkins Hospital* 36, no. 2 (1925).

66 *"I find myself inclined"*: Halsted, "Clinical and Histological Study of Certain Adenocarcinomata of the Breast," *Annals of Surgery* 28: 560.

67 *"cancer storehouse"*: Ibid., 557.

67 *On April 19, 1898:* Ibid., 557–76.

68 *A surgeon should "operate on the neck"*: Ibid., 572.

68 Halsted's 1907 report to the American Surgical Association: William Stewart Halsted, "The Results of Radical Operations for the Cure of Carcinoma of the Breast," *Annals of Surgery* 46, no. 1 (1907): 1–19.

68 *"If the disease was so advanced"*: "A Vote for Partial Mastectomy: Radical Surgery Is Not the Best Treatment for Breast Cancer, He Says," *Chicago Tribune*, October 2, 1973.

68 *"But even without the proof"*: Halsted, "Results of Radical Operations," 7. Also see Halsted, "The Results of Radical Operations for the Cure of Cancer of the Breast," *Transactions of the American Surgical Association* 25: 66.

68 *"It is especially true of mammary cancer"*: Ibid., 61.

70 *"With no protest from any other quarter"*: Ellen Leopold, *A Darker Ribbon: Breast Cancer, Women, and Their Doctors in the Twentieth Century* (Boston: Beacon Press, 1999), 88.

70 *"Undoubtedly, if operated upon properly"*: *Transactions of the American Surgical Association* 49.

70 *"the more radical the better"*: "Breast Cancer, New Choices," *Washington Post*, December 22, 1974.

70 *Alexander Brunschwig devised an operation:* Alexander Brunschwig and Virginia K. Pierce, "Partial and Complete Pelvic Exenteration: A Progress Report Based upon the First 100 Operations," *Cancer* 3 (1950): 927–74; Alexander Brunschwig, "Complete Excision of Pelvic Viscera for Advanced Carcinoma: A One-Stage Abdominoperineal

Operation with End Colostomy and Bilateral Ureteral Implantation into the Colon above the Colostomy," *Cancer* 1 (1948): 177–83.

70 *Pack the Knife:* From George T. Pack's papers, quoted in Barron Lerner, *The Breast Cancer Wars: Hope, Fear, and the Pursuit of a Cure in Twentieth-Century America* (Oxford: Oxford University Press, 2003), 73.

70 *"Even in its widest sense":* Stanford Cade, *Radium Treatment of Cancer* (New York: William Wood, 1929), 1.

70 *"There is an old Arabian proverb":* Urban Maes, "The Tragedy of Gastric Carcinoma: A Study of 200 Surgical Cases," *Annals of Surgery* 98, no. 4 (1933): 629.

71 *"I know you didn't know anything":* Hugh H. Young, *Hugh Young: A Surgeon's Autobiography* (New York: Harcourt, Brace and Company, 1940), 76.

71 *In 1904, with Halsted as his assistant:* Bertram M. Bernheim, *The Story of the Johns Hopkins* (Surrey: World's Work, 1949); A. McGehee Harvey et al., *A Model of Its Kind,* vol. 1, *A Centennial History of Medicine at Johns Hopkins University* (Baltimore: Johns Hopkins University Press, 1989); Leonard Murphy, *The History of Urology* (Springfield, IL: Charles C. Thomas, 1972), 132.

71 *"the slow separation of brain from tumor":* Harvey Cushing, "Original Memoirs: The Control of Bleeding in Operations for Brain Tumors. With the Description of Silver 'Clips' for the Occlusion of Vessels Inaccessible to the Ligature," *Annals of Surgery* 49, no. 1 (1911): 14–15.

72 *In 1933, at the Barnes hospital:* Evarts G. Graham, "The First Total Pneumonectomy," *Texas Cancer Bulletin* 2 (1949): 2–4.

72 *A surgical procedure:* Alton Ochsner and M. DeBakey, "Primary Pulmonary Malignancy: Treatment by Total Pneumonectomy—Analysis of 79 Collected Cases and Presentation of 7 Personal Cases," *Surgery, Gynecology, and Obstetrics* 68 (1939): 435–51.

The Hard Tube and the Weak Light

73 *We have found in [X-rays]:* "X-ray in Cancer Cure," *Los Angeles Times,* April 6, 1902.

73 *By way of illustration:* "Last Judgment," *Washington Post,* August 26, 1945.

73 Röntgen's discovery of X-rays: Wilhelm C. Röntgen, "On a New Kind of Rays," *Nature* 53, no. 1369 (1896): 274–76; John Maddox, "The Sensational Discovery of X-rays," *Nature* 375 (1995): 183.

75 *One man who gave "magical" demonstrations:* Robert William Reid, *Marie Curie* (New York: Collins, 1974), 122.

75 *In 1896, barely a year after Röntgen:* Emil H. Grubbe, "Priority in Therapeutic Use of X-rays," *Radiology* 21 (1933): 156–62; Emil H. Grubbe, *X-ray Treatment: Its Origin, Birth and Early History* (St. Paul: Bruce Publishing, 1949).

76 *"I believe this treatment is an absolute cure":* "X-rays Used as a Remedy for Cancer," *New York Times,* November 2, 1901.

76 *advertised for sale to laypeople:* "Mining: Surplus of Radium," *Time,* May 24, 1943.

76 *"millions of tiny bullets of energy":* Oscar Carl Simonton, Stephanie Simonton, and James Creighton, *Getting Well Again: A Step-by-Step, Self-Help Guide to Overcoming Cancer for Patients and Their Families* (Los Angeles: J. P. Tarcher, 1978), 7.

76 *"The patient is put on a stretcher":* "Medicine: Advancing Radiotherapy," *Time,* October 6, 1961.

77 *One woman with a brain tumor:* "Atomic Medicine: The Great Search for Cures on the New Frontier," *Time*, April 7, 1952.

77 Undark and the "Radium girls": Claudia Clark, *Radium Girls: Women and Industrial Health Reform, 1910–1935* (Chapel Hill: University of North Carolina Press, 1997); Ross Mullner, *Deadly Glow: The Radium Dial Worker Tragedy* (Washington, DC: American Public Health Association, 1999).

78 *Marie Curie died of leukemia:* Curie's disease was diagnosed as "aplastic anemia" of rapid, feverish development, but is widely considered to have been a variant of myelodysplasia, a preleukemic syndrome that resembles aplastic anemia and progresses to a fatal leukemia.

78 *Grubbe's fingers had been amputated:* Otha Linton, "Radiation Dangers," *Academic Radiology* 13, no. 3 (2006): 404.

78 Willy Meyer's posthumous address: Willy Meyer, "Inoperable and Malignant Tumors," *Annals of Surgery* 96, no. 5 (1932): 891–92.

Dyeing and Dying

80 *Those who have not been trained in chemistry:* Michael B. Shimkin, "As Memory Serves—an Informal History of the National Cancer Institute, 1937–57," *Journal of the National Cancer Institute* 59 (suppl. 2) (1977): 559–600.

80 *Life is . . . a chemical incident:* Martha Marquardt, *Paul Ehrlich* (New York: Schuman, 1951), 11. Also see Frederick H. Kasten, "Paul Ehrlich: Pathfinder in Cell Biology," *Biotechnic & Histochemistry* 71, no. 1 (1996).

81 *Between 1851 and 1857:* Phyllis Deane and William Alan Cole, *British Economic Growth, 1688–1959: Trends and Structure* (Cambridge: Cambridge University Press, 1969), 210.

81 *By the 1850s, that proportion had peaked:* Stanley D. Chapman, *The Cotton Industry: Its Growth and Impact, 1600–1935* (Bristol: Thoemmes, 1999), v–xviii.

81 *Cloth dyes had to be extracted:* A. S. Travis, *The Rainbow Makers: The Origins of the Synthetic Dyestuffs Industry in Western Europe* (Bethlehem, PA: Lehigh University Press, 1993), 13.

81 *ever-popular calico prints:* Ibid.

81 *"half of a small but long-shaped room":* William Cliffe, "The Dyemaking Works of Perkin and Sons, Some Hitherto Unrecorded Details," *Journal of the Society of Dyers and Colorists* 73 (1957): 313–14.

82 *In 1883, the German output of alizarin:* Travis, *Rainbow Makers,* 195.

83 *"most impudent, ignorant, flatulent, fleshy":* H. A. Colwell, "Gideon Harvey: Sidelights on Medical Life from the Restoration to the End of the XVII Century," *Annals of Medical History* 3, no. 3 (1921): 205–37.

83 *"None of these compounds have, as yet":* "Researches Conducted in the Laboratories of the Royal College of Chemistry," *Reports of the Royal College of Chemistry and Researches Conducted in the Laboratories in the Years 1845-6-7* (London: Royal College of Chemistry, 1849), liv; Travis, *Rainbow Makers,* 35.

83 *In 1828, a Berlin scientist named Friedrich Wöhler:* Friedrich Wöhler, "Ueber künstliche Bildung des Harnstoffs," *Annalen der Physik und Chemie* 87, no. 2 (1828): 253–56.

84 *In 1878, in Leipzig, a twenty-four-year-old:* Paul Ehrlich, "Über das Methylenblau und

Seine Klinisch-Bakterioskopische Verwerthung," *Zeitschrift für Klinische Medizin* 2 (1882): 710–13.

84 *In 1882, working with Robert Koch:* Paul Ehrlich, "Über die Färbung der Tuberkelbazillen," *Deutsche Medizinische Wochenschrift* 8 (1882): 269.

85 *"It has occurred to me":* Marquardt, *Paul Ehrlich*, 91.

85 *His laboratory was now physically situated:* Travis, *Rainbow Makers*, 97.

86 *On April 19, 1910, at the densely packed:* See Felix Bosch and Laia Rosich, "The Contributions of Paul Ehrlich to Pharmacology," *Pharmacology* (2008): 82, 171–79.

86 *"syphilis—the "secret malady":* Linda E. Merians, ed., *The Secret Malady: Venereal Disease in Eighteenth-Century Britain and France* (Lexington: The University Press of Kentucky, 1996). Also see Ehrlich, "A Lecture on Chemotherapeutics," *Lancet*, ii, 445.

87 Ehrlich and Kaiser Wilhelm: M. Lawrence Podolsky, *Cures out of Chaos: How Unexpected Discoveries Led to Breakthroughs in Medicine and Health* (Amsterdam: Overseas Publishers Association, 1997), 273.

88 *"thick, yellowish green cloud":* Richard Lodoïs Thoumin, *The First World War* (New York: Putnam, 1963), 175.

88 *In 1919, a pair of American pathologists:* E. B. Krumbhaar and Helen D. Krumbhaar, "The Blood and Bone Marrow in Yellow Cross Gas (Mustard Gas) Poisoning: Changes Produced in the Bone Marrow of Fatal Cases," *Journal of Medical Research* 40, no. 3 (1919): 497–508.

Poisoning the Atmosphere

89 *"What if this mixture do not work at all?:* William Shakespeare, *Romeo and Juliet*, act 4, scene 3 (Philadelphia: J. B. Lippincott, 1913), 229.

89 *We shall so poison the atmosphere:* Robert Nisbet, "Knowledge Dethroned: Only a Few Years Ago, Scientists, Scholars and Intellectuals Had Suddenly Become the New Aristocracy. What Happened?" *New York Times*, September 28, 1975.

89 *Every drug, the sixteenth-century:* W. Pagel, *Paracelsus: An Introduction to Philosophical Medicine in the Era of the Renaissance*, 2nd ed. (New York: Karger, 1982), 129–30.

89 *On December 2, 1943:* D. M. Saunders, "The Bari Incident," *United States Naval Institute Proceedings* (Annapolis: United States Naval Institute, 1967).

89 *Of the 617 men rescued:* Guy B. Faguet, *The War on Cancer: An Anatomy of Failure, A Blueprint for the Future* (New York: Springer, 2005), 71.

90 *Goodman and Gilman weren't interested:* Alfred Gilman, "Therapeutic Applications of Chemical Warfare Agents," *Federation Proceedings* 5 (1946): 285–92; Alfred Gilman and Frederick S. Philips, "The Biological Actions and Therapeutic Applications of the B-Chloroethyl Amines and Sulfides," *Science* 103, no. 2675 (1946): 409–15; Louis Goodman et al., "Nitrogen Mustard Therapy: Use of Methyl-Bis(Beta-Chlorethyl)amine Hydrochloride and Tris(Beta-Chloroethyl)amine Hydrochloride for Hodgkin's Disease, Lymphosarcoma, Leukemia and Certain Allied and Miscellaneous Disorders," *Journal of the American Medical Association* 132, no. 3 (1946): 126–32.

91 *George Hitchings had also:* Grant Taylor, *Pioneers in Pediatric Oncology* (Houston: University of Texas M. D. Anderson Cancer Center, 1990), 137. Also see Tonse N. K. Raju, "The Nobel Chronicles," *Lancet* 355, no. 9208 (1999): 1022; Len Goodwin, "George Hitchings and Gertrude Elion—Nobel Prizewinners," *Parasitology Today* 5, no. 2 (1989): 33.

91 *"Scientists in academia stood disdainfully"*: John Laszlo, *The Cure of Childhood Leukemia* (New Brunswick, NJ: Rutgers University Press, 1995), 65.

92 *Instead of sifting through mounds:* Gertrude B. Elion, "Nobel Lecture in Physiology or Medicine—1988. The Purine Path to Chemotherapy," *In Vitro Cellular and Developmental Biology* 25, no. 4 (1989): 321–30; Gertrude B. Elion, George H. Hitchings, and Henry Vanderwerff, "Antagonists of Nucleic Acid Derivatives: VI. Purines," *Journal of Biological Chemistry* 192 (1951): 505. Also see Tom Brokaw, *The Greatest Generation* (1998; reprint, 2004), 304.

92 *In the early 1950s, two physician-scientists:* Joseph Burchenal, Mary L. Murphy, et al., "Clinical Evaluation of a New Antimetabolite, 6-Mercaptopurine, in the Treatment of Leukemia and Allied Diseases," *Blood* 8 no. 11 (1953): 965–99.

The Goodness of Show Business

93 *The name "Jimmy" is a household word in New England:* George E. Foley, *The Children's Cancer Research Foundation: The House That "Jimmy" Built: The First Quarter-Century* (Boston: Sidney Farber Cancer Institute, 1982).

93 *I've made a long voyage:* Maxwell E. Perkins, "The Last Letter of Thomas Wolfe and the Reply to It," *Harvard Library Bulletin,* Autumn 1947, 278.

94 *artificial respirator known as the iron lung:* Philip Drinker and Charles F. McKhann III, "The Use of a New Apparatus for the Prolonged Administration of Artificial Respiration: I. A Fatal Case of Poliomyelitis," *Journal of the American Medical Association* 92: 1658–60.

94 *Polio research was shaken out of its torpor:* For a discussion of the early history of polio, see Naomi Rogers, *Dirt and Disease: Polio before FDR* (Rutgers: Rutgers University Press, 1992). Also see Tony Gould, *A Summer Plague: Polio and Its Survivors* (New Haven: Yale University Press, 1995).

94 *Within a few weeks, 2,680,000 dimes:* Kathryn Black, *In the Shadow of Polio: A Personal and Social History* (New York: Perseus Books, 307), 25; Paul A. Offit, *The Cutter Incident: How America's First Polio Vaccine Led to the Growing Vaccine Crisis* (New Haven: Yale University Press, 2005); *History of the National Foundation for Infantile Paralysis Records; Volume II: Raising Funds to Fight Infantile Paralysis, Book 2* (March of Dimes Archives, 1957), 256–60.

95 *Please take care of my baby. Her name is Catherine:* Variety, the Children's Charity, "Our History," http://www.usvariety.org/about_history.html (accessed November 11, 2009).

96 *"Well, I need a new microscope"*: Robert Cooke, *Dr. Folkman's War: Angiogenesis and the Struggle to Defeat Cancer* (New York: Random House, 2001), 115.

96 *money and netted $45,456:* Foley, *Children's Cancer Research Foundation* (Boston: Sidney Farber Cancer Institute, 1982).

96 *Gustafson was quiet:* Phyllis Clauson, interview with author, July 2009; Karen Cummins, interview with author, July 2009. Also see Foley, *Children's Cancer Research Foundation.*

97 *On May 22, 1948, on a warm Saturday night in the Northeast:* The original broadcast recording can be accessed on the Jimmy Fund website at http://www.jimmyfund.org/abo/broad/jimmybroadcast.asp. Also see Saul Wisnia, *Images of America: The Jimmy Fund of the Dana-Farber Cancer Institute* (Charleston, SC: Arcadia, 2002), 18–19.

99 *Jimmy's mailbox was inundated:* Foley, *Children's Cancer Research Foundation.*

99 *the Manhattan Project spent:* See "The Manhattan Project, An Interactive History," U.S. Department of Energy, Office of History, 2008.

99 *In 1948, Americans spent more than $126 million:* Mark Pendergrast, *For God, Country and Coca-Cola: The Definitive History of the Great American Soft Drink and the Company That Makes It* (New York: Basic Books, 2000), 212.

The House That Jimmy Built

101 *Etymologically, patient means sufferer:* Susan Sontag, *Illness as Metaphor and AIDS and Its Metaphors* (New York: Picador, 1990), 125.

101 *Sidney Farber's entire purpose: Medical World News,* November 25, 1966.

101 *"One assistant and ten thousand mice":* George E. Foley, *The Children's Cancer Research Foundation: The House That "Jimmy" Built: The First Quarter-Century* (Boston: Sidney Farber Cancer Institute, 1982).

101 *"Most of the doctors":* Name withheld, a hospital volunteer in the 1950s to 1960s, interview with author, May 2001.

102 *In 1953, when the Braves franchise left:* "Braves Move to Milwaukee; Majors' First Shift since '03," *New York Times,* March 19, 1953.

102 *the Jimmy Fund planned a "Welcome Home, Ted" party:* "Dinner Honors Williams: Cancer Fund Receives $150,000 from $100-Plate Affair," *New York Times,* August 18, 1953.

102 *Funds poured in from:* Foley, *Children's Cancer Research Foundation.*

102 *"You can take the child out of the Depression":* Robin Pogrebin and Timothy L. O'Brien, "A Museum of One's Own," *New York Times,* December 5, 2004.

103 *"If a little girl got attached to a doll":* "Medicine: On the Track," *Time,* January 21, 1952.

103 *"Once I discover that almost all":* Jeremiah Goldstein, "Preface to My Mother's Diary," *Journal of Pediatric Hematology/Oncology* 30, no. 7 (2008): 481–504.

104 *"Acute leukemia," he wrote:* Sidney Farber, "Malignant Tumors of Childhood," *CA: A Cancer Journal for Clinicians* (1953): 3, 106–7.

104 *The money that he had raised:* Sidney Farber letter to Mary Lasker, August 19, 1955.

PART TWO:
AN IMPATIENT WAR

105 *Perhaps there is only one cardinal sin:* Franz Kafka, *The Great Wall of China and Other Pieces* (London: Secker and Warburg, 1946), 142.

105 *The 325,000 patients with cancer:* Sidney Farber, quoted in Guy B. Faguet, *The War on Cancer: An Anatomy of Failure, a Blueprint for the Future* (New York: Springer, 2005), 97.

"They form a society"

107 *All of this demonstrates why:* Michael B. Shimkin, "As Memory Serves—an Informal History of the National Cancer Institute, 1937–57," *Journal of the National Cancer Institute* 59 (suppl. 2) (1977): 559–600.

107 *I am aware of some alarm:* Senator Lister Hill, "A Strong Independent Cancer Agency," October 5, 1971, Mary Lasker Papers.

107 *"Americans of all ages":* Alexis de Tocqueville, *Democracy in America* (New York, Penguin), 296.

108 *a woman who "could sell":* Mary Lasker Oral History Project, Part 1, Session 1, p. 3, http://www.columbia.edu/cu/lweb/digital/collections/nny/laskerm/transcripts/laskerm_1_1_3.html.

109 *In 1939, Mary Woodard met Albert Lasker:* Ibid., p. 56.

109 *"salesmanship in print":* Stephen R. Fox, *The Mirror Makers: A History of American Advertising and Its Creators* (New York: William Morrow, 1984), 51.

109 *they were married just fifteen months after:* Mary Lasker Oral History Project, Part 1, Session 3, p. 80.

110 *"I am opposed to heart attacks and cancer":* J. Michael Bishop, "Mary Lasker and Her Prizes: An Appreciation," *Journal of the American Medical Association* 294, no. 11 (2005): 1418–19.

111 *"If a toothpaste":* Mary Lasker Oral History Project, Part 1, Session 7.

111 *"the fairy godmother of medical research":* "The Fairy Godmother of Medical Research," *Business Week,* July 14, 1986.

111 *In April 1943, Mary Lasker visited:* Mary Lasker Oral History Project, Part 1, Session 5, p. 136, and Session 16, pp. 477–79.

111 *The visit left her cold:* Ibid., Session 16, pp. 477–79.

111 *Of its small annual budget of:* Ibid. Also see Mary Lasker interview, October 23, 1984, in Walter Ross, *Crusade, the Official History of the American Cancer Society* (Westminster, MD: Arbor House, 1987), 33.

111 *"Doctors," she wrote, "are not administrators":* Mary Lasker Oral History Project, Part 1, Session 7, p. 183.

112 *In October 1943, Lasker persuaded a friend: Reader's Digest,* October 1945.

112 *"My mother died from cancer":* Letter from a soldier to Mary Lasker, 1949.

112 *Over the next months:* Richard A. Rettig, *Cancer Crusade: The Story of the National Cancer Act of 1971* (Lincoln, NE: Author's Choice Press, 1977), 21.

112 *"A two-pronged attack":* Letter from Cornelius A. Wood to Mary Lasker, January 6, 1949, Mary Lasker Papers, Box 210.

112 *Albert Lasker . . . recruited Emerson Foote:* Ibid.

112 *The "Lay Group":* Letter from Mary Lasker to Jim Adams, May 13, 1945, Mary Lasker Papers.

112 *In a single year, it printed 9 million:* these numbers are culled from letters and receipts found in the Mary Lasker Papers.

113 *"Ladies' Garden Club":* Charles Cameron, *Cancer Control,* vol. 3, 1972.

113 *"unjustified, troublesome and aggressive":* James T. Patterson, *The Dread Disease: Cancer and Modern American Culture* (Cambridge, MA: Harvard University Press, 1987), 173. Also see Rettig, *Cancer Crusade,* 22.

113 *The society's bylaws and constitution were rewritten:* Letter from Frank Adair to ACS members, October 23, 1945.

113 *"The Committee should not include":* Telegram from Jim Adams to Mary Lasker, 1947, Mary Lasker Papers.

113 *"You were probably the first person":* Letter from Rose Kushner to Mary Lasker, July 22, 1988, Rose Kushner Papers, Harvard University.

114 *"a penicillin for cancer"*: "Doctor Foresees Cancer Penicillin," *New York Times*, October 3, 1953.

114 *By the early 1950s, she was regularly*: See, for instance, letter from John R. Heller to Mary Lasker, October 15, 1948, Mary Lasker Papers, Box 119; and Memorandum on Conversation with Dr. Farber, February 24, 1952, Mary Lasker Papers, Box 76.

114 *"scientific treatises"*: Letter from Sidney Farber to Mary Lasker, August 19, 1955, Mary Lasker Papers, Box 170.

114 *"An organizational pattern is developing"*: Ibid.

115 *a "regular on the Hill"*: Robert Mayer, interview with author, July 2008.

115 *"Put a tambourine in [his] hands"*: Rettig, *Cancer Crusade*, 26.

115 *"I have written to you so many times"*: Letter from Sidney Farber to Mary Lasker, September 5, 1958.

"These new friends of chemotherapy"

116 *The death of a man*: Czeslaw Milosz, *New and Collected Poems: 1931–2001* (New York: Ecco, 2001), 431.

116 *I had recently begun to notice*: K. E. Studer and Daryl E. Chubin, *The Cancer Mission: Social Contexts of Biomedical Research* (Newbury Park, CA: Sage Publications, 1980).

116 *By February 1952, Albert was confined*: Mary Lasker Oral History Project, Part 1, Session 9, p. 260.

116 *"It seems a little unfair"*: Letter from Lowel Cogeshall to Mary Lasker, March 11, 1952, Mary Lasker Papers, Box 76.

117 *Albert Lasker died at eight o'clock*: "A. D. Lasker Dies; Philanthropist, 72," *New York Times*, May 31, 1952.

117 *"We are at war with an insidious"*: Senator Lister Hill, "A Strong Independent Cancer Agency," October 5, 1971, Mary Lasker Papers, Columbia University.

119 *"University professors who are opposed"*: "Science and the Bomb," *New York Times*, August 7, 1945.

120 *Science the Endless Frontier*: Vannevar Bush, *Science the Endless Frontier: A Report to the President by Vannevar Bush, Director of the Office of Scientific Research and Development, July 1945* (Washington, DC: United States Government Printing Office, 1945).

121 *The National Science Foundation (NSF), founded in 1950*: Daniel S. Greenberg, *Science, Money, and Politics: Political Triumph and Ethical Erosion* (Chicago: University of Chicago Press, 2001), 167.

121 *"long term, basic scientific research"*: Ibid., 419.

121 *"so great a co-ordination of medical scientific labor"*: Stephen Parks Strickland, *Politics, Science, and the Dread Disease: A Short History of the United States Medical Research Policy* (Cambridge, MA: Harvard University Press, 1972), 16.

121 *"Should I refuse my dinner"*: Ernest E. Sellers, "Early Pragmatists," *Science* 154, no. 3757 (1996): 1604.

121 *The outspoken Philadelphia pathologist Stanley Reimann*: Stanley Reimann, "The Cancer Problem as It Stands Today," *Transactions and Studies of the College of Physicians of Philadelphia* 13 (1945): 21.

NOTES

122 *the Cancer Chemotherapy National Service Center:* C. G. Zubrod et al., "The Chemotherapy Program of the National Cancer Center Institute: History, Analysis, and Plans," *Cancer Chemotherapy Reports* 50 (1966): 349–540; V. T. DeVita, "The Evolution of Therapeutic Research in Cancer," *New England Journal of Medicine* 298 (1978): 907–10.

122 *Farber was ecstatic, but impatient:* Letter from Sidney Farber to Mary Lasker, August 19, 1955, Mary Lasker Papers, Box 170.

122 *One such antibiotic came from a rod-shaped microbe:* Selman Waksman and H. B. Woodruff, "Bacteriostatic and Bacteriocidal Substances Produced by a Soil Actinomyces," *Proceedings of the Society for Experimental Biology and Medicine* 45 (1940): 609.

122 Farber and actinomycin D: Sidney Farber, Giulio D'Angio, Audrey Evans, and Anna Mitus, "Clinical Studies of Actinomycin D with Special Reference to Wilms' Tumor in Children," *Annals of the New York Academy of Science* 89 (1960): 421–25.

123 *"In about three weeks lungs previously riddled with":* Giulio D'Angio, "Pediatric Oncology Refracted through the Prism of Wilms' Tumor: A Discourse," *Journal of Urology* 164 (2000): 2073–77.

124 Sonja Goldstein's recollections: Jeremiah Goldstein, "Preface to My Mother's Diary," *Journal of Pediatric Hematology/Oncology* 30, no. 7 (2008): 481–504.

"The butcher shop"

128 *Randomised screening trials are bothersome:* H. J. de Koning, "Mammographic Screening: Evidence from Randomised Controlled Trials," *Annals of Oncology* 14 (2003): 1185–89.

128 *The best [doctors] seem to have a sixth sense:* Michael LaCombe, "What Is Internal Medicine?" *Annals of Internal Medicine* 118, no. 5 (1993): 384–88.

128 Emil Freireich and Emil Frei: John Laszlo, *The Cure of Childhood Leukemia: Into the Age of Miracles* (New Brunswick, NJ: Rutgers University Press, 1995), 118–20.

129 *"I have never seen Freireich in a moderate mood":* Emil Frei III, "Confrontation, Passion, and Personalization," *Clinical Cancer Research* 3 (1999): 2558.

129 *Gordon Zubrod, the new director:* Emil Frei III, "Gordon Zubrod, MD," *Journal of Clinical Oncology* 17 (1999): 1331. Also see Taylor, *Pioneers in Pediatric Oncology,* 117.

130 *Freireich came just a few weeks later:* Grant Taylor, *Pioneers in Pediatric Oncology* (Houston: University of Texas M. D. Anderson Cancer Center, 1990), 117.

130 *"Frei's job," one researcher recalled:* Edward Shorter, *The Health Century* (New York: Doubleday, 1987), 192.

130 *To avert conflicts:* Andrew M. Kelahan, Robert Catalano, and Donna Marinucci, "The History, Structure, and Achievements of the Cancer Cooperative Groups," (May/June 2000): 28–33.

131 *"For the first time":* Robert Mayer, interview with author, July 2008. Also see Frei, "Gordon Zubrod," 1331; and Taylor, *Pioneers in Pediatric Oncology,* 117.

131 Hill and randomized trials: Austin Bradford Hill, *Principles of Medical Statistics* (Oxford: Oxford University Press, 1966); A. Bradford Hill, "The Clinical Trial," *British Medical Bulletin* 7, no. 4 (1951): 278–82.

132 *"The analogy of drug resistance":* Emil Freireich, interview with author, September 2009.

490

132 *The first protocol was launched:* Emil Frei III et al., "A Comparative Study of Two Regimens of Combination Chemotherapy in Acute Leukemia," *Blood* 13, no. 12 (1958): 1126–48; Richard Schilsky et al., "A Concise History of the Cancer and Leukemia Group B," *Clinical Cancer Research* 12, no. 11, pt. 2 (2006): 3553s–55s.

133 *"This work is one of the first comparative studies":* Frei et al., "Comparative Study of Two Regimens."

134 *"The resistance would be fierce":* Emil Freireich, personal interview.

134 *a "butcher shop":* Vincent T DeVita, Jr. and Edward Chu, "A History of Cancer Chemotherapy," *Cancer Research* 68, no. 21 (2008): 8643.

An Early Victory

135 *But I do subscribe to the view:* Brian Vastag, "Samuel Broder, MD, Reflects on the 30th Anniversary of the National Cancer Act," *Journal of the American Medical Association* 286 (2001): 2929–31.

135 Min Chiu Li: Emil J. Freireich, "Min Chiu Li: A Perspective in Cancer Therapy," *Clinical Cancer Research* 8 (2002): 2764–65.

136 Li and Ethel Longoria: Mickey Goulian, interview with author, September 2007.

136 *"She was bleeding so rapidly":* Ibid.

137 *Li and Hertz rushed to publish:* M. C. Li, R. Hertz, and D. M. Bergenstal, "Therapy of Choriocarcinoma and Related Trophoblastic Tumors with Folic Acid and Purine Antagonists," *New England Journal of Medicine* 259, no. 2 (1958): 66–74.

137 *Li's use of hcg level in chemotherapy:* John Laszlo, *The Cure of Childhood Leukemia: Into the Age of Miracles* (New Brunswick, NJ: Rutgers University Press, 1995), 145–47.

137 *In mid-July, the board summoned:* Ibid.

137 *"Li was accused of experimenting on people":* Emil Freireich, interview with author, September 2009.

138 *When Freireich heard about Li's dismissal:* Laszlo, *Cure of Childhood Leukemia,* 145.

Mice and Men

139 *A model is a lie that helps:* Margie Patlak, "Targeting Leukemia: From Bench to Bedside," *FASEB Journal* 16 (2002): 273E.

139 *"Clinical research is a matter of urgency":* John Laszlo, *The Cure of Childhood Leukemia: Into the Age of Miracles* (New Brunswick, NJ: Rutgers University Press, 1995).

139 *To test three drugs, the group insisted:* Ibid., 142.

139 *"The wards were filling up with these terribly sick children":* Emil Freireich, interview, September 2009.

139 *Vincristine had been discovered in 1958:* Norman R. Farnsworth, "Screening Plants for New Medicines," in *Biodiversity,* ed. E. O. Wilson (Washington, DC: National Academy Press, 1988), 94; Normal R. Farnsworth, "Rational Approaches Applicable to the Search for and Discovery of New Drugs From Plants," in *Memorias del 1er Symposium Latinoamericano y del Caribe de Farmacos Naturales, La Habana, Cuba, 21 al 28 de Junio, 1980, 27–59* (Montevideo, Uruguay: UNESCO Regional Office Academia de Ciencias de Cuba y Comisión Nacional de Cuba ante la UNESCO).

140 *"Frei and Freireich were simply taking drugs"*: David Nathan, *The Cancer Treatment Revolution* (Hoboken, NJ: Wiley, 2007), 59.

140 *A scientist from Alabama, Howard Skipper*: Laszlo, *Cure of Childhood Leukemia*, 199–209.

141 *Skipper emerged with two pivotal findings*: See, for example, Howard E. Skipper, "Cellular Kinetics Associated with 'Curability' of Experimental Leukemias," in William Dameshek and Ray M. Dutcher, eds., *Perspectives in Leukemia* (New York: Grune & Stratton, 1968), 187–94.

141 *"Maximal, intermittent, intensive, up-front"*: Emil Frei, "Curative Cancer Chemotherapy," *Cancer Research* 45 (1985): 6523–37.

VAMP

143 *If we didn't kill the tumor*: William C. Moloney and Sharon Johnson, *Pioneering Hematology: The Research and Treatment of Malignant Blood Disorders—Reflections on a Life's Work* (Boston: Francis A. Countway Library of Medicine, 1997).

143 *"I wanted to treat them with full doses of vincristine"*: John Laszlo, *The Cure of Childhood Leukemia: Into the Age of Miracles* (New Brunswick, NJ: Rutgers University Press, 1995), 141.

143 *"poison of the month"*: Edward Shorter, *The Health Century* (New York: Doubleday, 1987), 189.

144 *Farber, for one, favored giving one drug at a time*: See David Nathan, *The Cancer Treatment Revolution* (Hoboken, NJ: Wiley, 2007), 63.

144 *"Oh, boy," Freireich recalled*: Emil Freireich, interview with author, September 2009.

145 *"You can imagine the tension"*: Laszlo, *Cure of Childhood Leukemia*, 143.

145 First VAMP trial: E. J. Freireich, M. Karon, and E. Frei III, "Quadruple Combination Therapy (VAMP) for Acute Lymphocytic Leukemia of Childhood," *Proceedings of the American Association for Cancer Research* 5 (1963): 20; E. Frei III, "Potential for Eliminating Leukemic Cells in Childhood Acute Leukemia," *Proceedings of the American Association for Cancer Research* 5 (1963): 20.

145 *"I did little things"*: Laszlo, *Cure of Childhood Leukemia*, 143–44.

145 *"like a drop from a cliff with a thread tied"*: Mickey Goulian, interview with author, September 2007.

145 *The patient "is amazingly recovered"*: Letter from a Boston physician to patient K.L. (name withheld). K.L., interview with author, September 2009.

146 *"The mood among pediatric oncologists changed"*: Jonathan B. Tucker, *Ellie: A Child's Fight against Leukemia* (New York: Holt, Rinehart, and Winston, 1982).

146 *In September 1963, not long after Frei and Freireich*: Freireich, interview with author.

146 *"Some of us didn't make much of it at first"*: Goulian, interview with author.

146 *By October, there were more children back at the clinic*: Freireich, interview with author.

147 *"I know the patients, I know their brothers and sisters"*: "Kids with Cancer," *Newsweek*, August 15, 1977.

147 *morale at the institute to the breaking point*: Freireich, interview with author.

148 *A few, a small handful*: Emil Frei, "Curative Cancer Chemotherapy," *Cancer Research* 45 (1985): 6523–37.

150 *he triumphantly brought photographs of a few*: Harold P. Rusch, "The Beginnings of Cancer Research Centers in the United States," 74 (1985): 391–403.

150 *further proof was "anticlimactic and unnecessary"*: Ibid.

150 *"We are attempting"*: Sidney Farber, letter to Etta Rosensohn, Mary Lasker Papers, Columbia University.

An Anatomist's Tumor

151 *It took plain old courage to be a chemotherapist*: Vincent T. DeVita Jr. and Edward Chu, "A History of Cancer Chemotherapy," *Cancer Research* 68, no. 21 (2008): 8643–53.

156 *Hodgkin was born in 1798 to a Quaker family*: Louis Rosenfeld, *Thomas Hodgkin: Morbid Anatomist & Social Activist* (Lanham, MD: Madison Books, 1993), 1. Also see Amalie M. Kass and Edward H. Kass, *Perfecting the World: The Life and Times of Dr. Thomas Hodgkin, 1798–1866* (Boston: Harcourt Brace Jovanovich, 1988).

157 *a series of cadavers, mostly of young men*: T. Hodgkin, "On Some Morbid Appearances of the Absorbent Glands and Spleen," *Medico-Chirurgical Transactions* 17 (1832): 68–114. The paper was read to the society by Robert Lee because Hodgkin was not a member of the society himself.

157 *"A pathological paper may perhaps be thought"*: Hodgkin, "On Some Morbid Appearances," 96.

157 *In 1837, after a rather vicious political spat*: Marvin J. Stone, "Thomas Hodgkin: Medical Immortal and Uncompromising Idealist," *Baylor University Medical Center Proceedings* 18 (2005): 368–75.

157 *In 1898, some thirty years after Hodgkin's death*: Carl Sternberg, "Über eine eigenartige unter dem Bilde der Pseudoleu Kamie Verlaufende Tuberkuloses des Lymphatischen Apparates," *Ztschr Heitt* 19 (1898): 21–91.

158 *more "capricious," as one oncologist put it*: A. Aisenberg, "Prophylactic Radiotherapy in Hodgkin's Disease," *New England Journal of Medicine* 278, no. 13 (1968): 740; A. Aisenberg, "Management of Hodgkin's Disease," *New England Journal of Medicine* 278, no. 13 (1968): 739; A. C. Aisenberg, "Primary Management of Hodgkin's Disease," *New England Journal of Medicine* 278, no. 2 (1968): 92–95.

158 *the plan to build a linear accelerator*: Z. Fuks and M. Feldman, "Henry S. Kaplan, 1918–1984: A Physician, a Scientist, a Friend," *Cancer Surveys* 4, no. 2 (1985): 294–311.

159 *In 1953, he persuaded a team*: Malcolm A. Bagshaw, Henry E. Jones, Robert F. Kallman, and Joseph P. Kriss, "Memorial Resolution: Henry S. Kaplan (1918–1984)," Stanford University Faculty Memorials, Stanford Historical Society, http://histsoc.stanford.edu/pdfmem/KaplanH.pdf (accessed November 22, 2009).

159 *The accelerator was installed:* Ibid.

159 *"Henry Kaplan was Hodgkin's disease"*: George Canellos, interview with author, March 2008.

159 *Rene Gilbert had shown*: R. Gilbert, "Radiology in Hodgkin's Disease [malignant granulomatosis]. Anatomic and Clinical Foundations," *American Journal of Roentgenology and Radium Therapy* 41 (1939): 198–241; D. H. Cowan, "Vera Peters and the Curability of Hodgkin's Disease," *Current Oncology* 15, no. 5 (2008): 206–10.

160 *Peters observed that broad-field radiation could*: M. V. Peters and K. C. Middlemiss, "A

Study of Hodgkin's Disease Treated by Irradiation," *American Journal of Roentgenology and Radium Therapy* 79 (1958): 114–21.

160 *The trials that Kaplan designed:* H. S. Kaplan, "The Radical Radiotherapy of Regionally Localized Hodgkin's Disease," *Radiology* 78 (1962): 553–61; Richard T. Hoppe, Peter T. Mauch, James O. Armitage, Volker Diehl, and Lawrence M. Weiss, *Hodgkin Lymphoma* (Philadelphia: Lippincott Williams & Wilkins, 2007), 178.

160 *"meticulous radiotherapy":* Aisenberg, "Primary Management of Hodgkin's Disease," 95.

160 *But Kaplan knew that a diminished relapse rate was not a cure:* H. S. Kaplan, "Radical Radiation for Hodgkin's Disease," *New England Journal of Medicine* 278, no. 25 (1968): 1404; H. S. Kaplan, "Clinical Evaluation and Radiotherapeutic Management of Hodgkin's Disease and the Malignant Lymphomas," *New England Journal of Medicine* 278, no. 16 (1968): 892–99.

161 *"Fundamental to all attempts at curative treatment":* Aisenberg, "Primary Management of Hodgkin's Disease," 93.

An Army on the March

162 *Now we are an army on the march:* "Looking Back: Sidney Farber and the First Remission of Acute Pediatric Leukemia," Children's Hospital Boston, http://www.childrenshospital.org/gallery/index.cfm?G=49&page=1 (accessed November 22, 2009).

162 *The next step—the complete cure:* Kenneth Endicott, quoted in the Mary Lasker Papers, "Cancer Wars," National Library of Medicine.

162 *The role of aggressive multiple drug therapy:* R. C. Stein et al., "Prognosis of Childhood Leukemia," *Pediatrics* 43, no. 6 (1969): 1056–58.

162 *George Canellos, then a senior fellow at the NCI:* George Canellos, interview with author, March 2008.

163 *"A new breed of cancer investigators in the 1960s":* V. T. DeVita Jr., *British Journal of Haematology* 122, no. 5 (2003): 718–27.

164 *"maniacs doing cancer research":* Ronald Piana, "ONI Sits Down with Dr. Vincent DeVita," *Oncology News International* 17, no. 2 (February 1, 2008), http://www.consultantlive.com/display/article/10165/1146581?pageNumber=2&verify=0 (accessed November 22, 2009).

164 *As expected:* See Vincent T. DeVita Jr. and Edward Chu, "A History of Cancer Chemotherapy," *Cancer Research* 21: 8643.

164 The MOPP trial: Vincent T. DeVita Jr. et al., "Combination Chemotherapy in the Treatment of Advanced Hodgkin's Disease," *Annals of Internal Medicine* 73, no. 6 (1970): 881–95.

166 *A twelve-year-old boy:* Bruce Chabner, interview with author, July 2009.

166 *"Some of the patients with advanced disease":* Henry Kaplan, *Hodgkin's Disease* (New York: Commonwealth Fund, 1972), 15, 458. Also see DeVita et al., "Combination Chemotherapy in the Treatment."

167 *"no track record, uncertain finances, an unfinished building":* Joseph V. Simone, "A History of St. Jude Children's Research Hospital," *British Journal of Haematology* 120 (2003): 549–55.

168 *"an all-out combat":* R. J. Aur and D. Pinkel, "Total Therapy of Acute Lymphocytic Leukemia," *Progress in Clinical Cancer* 5 (1973): 155–70.

168 *"in maximum tolerated doses":* Joseph Simone et al., "'Total Therapy' Studies of Acute

Lymphocytic Leukemia in Children: Current Results and Prospects for Cure," *Cancer* 30, no. 6 (1972): 1488–94.

168 *it was impossible to even dose it and monitor it correctly:* Aur and Pinkel, "Total Therapy of Acute Lymphocytic Leukemia."

168 *senior researchers, knowing its risks:* "This Week's Citations Classic: R. J. A. Aur et al., "Central Nervous System Therapy and Combination Chemotherapy of Childhood Lymphocytic Leukemia," *Citation Classics* 28 (July 14, 1986).

169 *"From the time of his diagnosis":* Jocelyn Demers, *Suffer the Little Children: The Battle against Childhood Cancer* (Fountain Valley, CA: Eden Press, 1986), 17.

170 *In July 1968, the St. Jude's team published:* Donald Pinkel et al., "Nine Years' Experience with 'Total Therapy' of Childhood Acute Lymphocytic Leukemia," *Pediatrics* 50, no. 2 (1972): 246–51.

170 *The longest remission was now in its sixth year:* S. L. George et al., "A Reappraisal of the Results of Stopping Therapy in Childhood Leukemia," *New England Journal of Medicine* 300, no. 6 (1979):269–73.

170 *In 1979, Pinkel's team revisited:* Donald Pinkel, "Treatment of Acute Lymphocytic Leukemia" *Cancer* 23 (1979): 25–33.

170 *"ALL in children cannot be considered an incurable disease":* Pinkel et al, "Nine Years' Experience with 'Total Therapy.' "

The Cart and the Horse

171 *I am not opposed to optimism:* P. T. Cole, "Cohorts and Conclusions," *New England Journal of Medicine* 278, no. 20 (1968): 1126–27.

171 *The iron is hot and this is the time:* Letter from Sidney Farber to Mary Lasker, September 4, 1965.

171 *In the late fifties, as DeVita recalled:* Vincent T. DeVita Jr. and Edward Chu, "A History of Cancer Chemotherapy," *Cancer Research* 68, no. 21 (2008): 8643–53.

171 *"A revolution [has been]":* Vincent T. DeVita Jr., "A Selective History of the Therapy of Hodgkin's Disease," *British Journal of Hemotology* 122 (2003): 718–27.

171 *The next step—the complete cure:* Kenneth Endicott, quoted in "Cancer Wars," Mary Lasker Papers, Profiles in Science, National Libraries of Medicine. Also see V. T. DeVita Jr., "A Perspective on the War on Cancer," *Cancer Journal* 8, no. 5 (2002): 352–56.

172 *"The chemical arsenal," one writer noted:* Ellen Leopold, *A Darker Ribbon: Breast Cancer, Women, and Their Doctors in the Twentieth Century* (Boston: Beacon Press, 1999), 269–70.

173 *"one cause, one mechanism and one cure":* "Fanfare Fades in the Fight against Cancer," *U.S. News and World Report,* June 19, 1978.

173 *Peyton Rous:* Heather L. Van Epps, "Peyton Rous: Father of the Tumor Virus," *Journal of Experimental Medicine* 201, no. 3 (2005): 320; Peter K. Vogt, "Peyton Rous: Homage and Appraisal," *Journal of the Federation of American Societies for Experimental Biology* 10 (1996): 1559–62.

173 Peyton Rous's work on sarcomas in chickens: Peyton Rous, "A Transmissible Avian Neoplasm (Sarcoma of the Common Fowl)," *Journal of Experimental Medicine* 12, no. 5 (1910): 696–705; Peyton Rous, "A Sarcoma of the Fowl Transmissible by an Agent Separable from the Tumor Cells," *Journal of Experimental Medicine* 13, no. 4 (1911): 397–411.

174 *"I have propagated a spindle-cell sarcoma"*: Rous, "A Transmissible Avian Neoplasm."

174 *Richard Schope reported a papillomavirus:* Richard E. Shope, "A Change in Rabbit Fibroma Virus Suggesting Mutation: II. Behavior of the Varient Virus in Cottontail Rabbits," *Journal of Experimental Medicine* 63, no. 2 (1936): 173–78; Richard E. Shope, "A Change in Rabbit Fibroma Virus Suggesting Mutation: III. Interpretation of Findings," *Journal of Experimental Medicine* 63, no. 2 (1936): 179–84.

174 *Denis Burkitt, discovered an aggressive form of lymphoma:* Denis Burkitt, "A Sarcoma Involving the Jaws in African Children," *British Journal of Surgery* 46, no. 197 (1958): 218–23.

175 *"Cancer may be infectious":* "New Evidence That Cancer May Be Infectious," *Life,* June 22, 1962. Also see "Virus Link Found," *Los Angeles Times,* November 30, 1964.

175 *"Is there something I can do to kill the cancer germ?":* Letter from Mary Kirkpatrick to Peyton Rous, June 23, 1962, Peyton Rous papers, the American Philosophical Society, quoted in James T. Patterson, *The Dread Disease: Cancer and Modern American Culture* (Cambridge, MA: Harvard University Press, 1987), 237.

175 *the NCI inaugurated a Special Virus Cancer Program:* Nicholas Wade, "Special Virus Cancer Program: Travails of a Biological Moonshot," *Science* 174, no. 4016(1971): 1306–11.

175 *the cancer virus program siphoned away more than 10 percent:* Ibid.

176 *"Relatively few viruses":* Peyton Rous, "The Challenge to Man of the Neoplastic Cell," Nobel lecture, December 13, 1966, *Nobel Lectures, Physiology or Medicine, 1963–1970* (Amsterdam: Elsevier, 1972).

176 *"Relatively few viruses":* Peyton Rous, "Surmise and Fact on the Nature of Cancer," *Nature* 183, no. 4672 (1959): 1357–61.

177 *"The program directed by the National Cancer Institute":* "Hunt Continues for Cancer Drug," *New York Times,* October 13, 1963.

177 *"The iron is hot and this is the time":* Letter from Sidney Farber to Mary Lasker, September 4, 1965, Mary Lasker Papers, Box 171.

177 *"No large mission or goal-directed effort":* Mary Lasker, "Need for a Commission on the Conquest of Cancer as a National Goal by 1976," Mary Lasker Papers, Box 111.

177 *Solomon Garb, a little-known professor of pharmacology:* Solomon Garb, *Cure for Cancer: A National Goal* (New York: Springer, 1968).

177 *"A major hindrance to the cancer effort":* Ibid.

178 *At 4:17 p.m. EDT on July 20, 1969:* "The Moon: A Giant Leap for Mankind," *Time,* July 25, 1969.

178 *"magnificent desolation":* Buzz Aldrin, *Magnificent Desolation: The Long Journey Home from the Moon* (New York: Harmony Books, 2009).

178 *"It suddenly struck me":* "Space: The Greening of the Astronauts," *Time,* December 11, 1972.

178 *"It was a stunning scientific and intellectual accomplishment":* "The Moon," *Time.*

178 *When Max Faget, the famously taciturn engineer:* Glen E. Swanson, *Before This Decade Is Out: Personal Reflections on the Apollo Program* (Washington, DC: NASA History Office, 1999), 374.

179 *In her letters, Mary Lasker began:* Lasker, "Need for a Commission."

179 *Lister Hill, the Alabama senator:* "Two Candidates in Primary in Alabama Count Ways They Love Wallace," *New York Times,* May 27, 1968.

179 *Edward Kennedy, Farber's ally from Boston:* "Conflicted Ambitions, Then, Chappaquiddick," *Boston Globe,* February 17, 2009.

179 *"We're in the worst," Lasker recalled:* Mary Lasker Oral History Project, Part II, Session 5, p. 125.

"A moon shot for cancer"

180 *The relationship of government:* William Carey, "Research Development and the Federal Budget," Seventeenth National Conference on the Administration of Research, September 11, 1963.

180 *What has Santa Nixon:* Robert Semple, *New York Times,* December 26, 1971.

180 *On December 9, 1969, on a chilly Sunday:* Advertisement from the American Cancer Society, *New York Times,* December 17, 1971.

181 *in Aleksandr Solzhenitsyn's* Cancer Ward: Aleksandr Solzhenitsyn, *Cancer Ward* (New York: Farrar, Straus and Giroux, 1968).

181 *in* Love Story: Erich Segal, *Love Story,* DVD, directed by Arthur Hiller, 2001.

181 Bang the Drum Slowly, *a 1973 release:* Mark Harris, *Bang the Drum Slowly,* DVD, directed by John D. Hancock, 2003.

181 Brian's Song, *the story of the Chicago Bears star:* Al Silverman, Gale Sayers, and William Blinn, *Brian's Song,* DVD, directed by Buzz Kulik, 2000.

181 *"plunged into numb agony":* Richard A. Rettig, *Cancer Crusade: The Story of the National Cancer Act of 1971* (Lincoln, NE: Author's Choice Press, 1977), 175.

181 *"Cancer changes your life," a patient wrote:* "My Fight against Cancer," *Chicago Tribune,* May 6, 1973.

182 *"A radical change happened to the perception":* Renata Salecl, *On Anxiety* (London: Routledge, 2004), 4. Also Renata Salecl, interview with author, April 2006.

182 *The "Big Bomb," a columnist wrote:* Ellen Goodman, "A Fear That Fits the Times," September 14, 1978.

183 *"To oppose big spending against cancer":* James T. Patterson, *The Dread Disease: Cancer and Modern American Culture* (Cambridge, MA: Harvard University Press, 1987), 149.

183 *Nixon often groused:* For Nixon's comments, see National Archives and Records Administration, Nixon Presidential Materials Project, 513–14, June 7, 1971, transcribed by Daniel Greenberg. See I. I. Rabi, quoted in Daniel S. Greenberg, *The Politics of Pure Science* (Chicago: University of Chicago Press, 1999), 3.

184 *Mary Lasker proposed that a "neutral" committee:* Rettig, *Cancer Crusade,* 82.

184 *The commission, she wrote, should "include space scientists":* Mary Lasker, "Need for a Commission on the Conquest of Cancer as a National Goal by 1976," Mary Lasker Papers, Box 111.

184 *Sidney Farber was selected as the cochairman:* Rettig, *Cancer Crusade,* 74–89.

184 *Yarborough wrote to Mary Lasker in the summer of 1970:* Letter from Ralph W. Yarborough to Mary Lasker, June 2, 1970, Mary Lasker Papers, Box 112.

184 *The panel's final report:* The report was published in two documents in November 1970 and reprinted in December 1970 and April 1971. See Senate Document 92–99, 1st sess., April 14, 1971. Also see Rettig, *Cancer Crusade,* 105.

185 *"Not only can we afford the effort":* Benno Schmidt, quoted by Alan C. Davis (interview with Richard Rettig) in Rettig, *Cancer Crusade,* 109.

185 *On March 9, 1971, acting on the panel's recommendations:* Ibid.

185 *she persuaded her close friend Ann Landers:* "Mary Woodard Lasker: First Lady of

Medical Research," presentation by Neen Hunt at the National Library of Medicine, http://profiles.nlm.nih.gov/TL/B/B/M/P/ (accessed January 6, 2010).

185 *Landers's column appeared on April 20, 1971:* Ask Ann Landers, *Chicago Sun-Times,* April 20, 1971.

186 *"I saw trucks arriving at the Senate":* Rick Kogan, *America's Mom: The Life, Lessons, and Legacy of Ann Landers* (New York: Harper Collins, 2003), 104.

186 *An exasperated secretary charged with sorting:* "Ann Landers," *Washington Post,* May 18, 1971.

186 *Stuart Symington, the senator from Missouri:* Ann Landers and Margo Howard, A Life in Letters (New York: Warner Books, 2003), 255.

186 *"Cancer is not simply an island":* Philip Lee. Also see Committee on Labor and Public Welfare Report No. 92–247, June 28, 1971, p. 43. S. 1828, 92nd Cong., 1st sess.

186 *"An all-out effort at this time":* Patterson, *Dread Disease,* 152.

186 *James Watson, who had discovered the structure of DNA:* See James Watson, "To Fight Cancer, Know the Enemy," *New York Times,* August 5, 2009.

186 *"Doing 'relevant' research":* James Watson, "The Growing Up of Cancer Research," *Science Year: The Book World Science Annual, 1973;* Mary Lasker Papers.

187 *"In a nutshell":* "Washington Rounds," *Medical World News,* March 31, 1972.

187 *"I suspect there is trouble ahead":* Irvine H. Page, "The Cure of Cancer 1976," *Journal of Laboratory and Clinical Medicine* 77, no. 3 (1971): 357–60.

187 *"If Richard Milhous Nixon":* "Tower Ticker," *Chicago Tribune,* January 28, 1971.

187 *"Don't worry about it":* Benno Schmidt, oral history and memoir (gift and property of Elizabeth Smith, New York).

187 *In November 1971, Paul Rogers:* For details of Representative Rogers's bill, see Rettig, *Cancer Crusade,* 250–75.

188 *In December 1971, the House finally:* Iwan W. Morgan, *Nixon* (London: Arnold, 2002), 72.

188 *On December 23, 1971, on a cold, windswept afternoon:* "Nixon Signs Cancer Bill; Cites Commitment to Cure," *New York Times,* December 24, 1971.

188 *$400 million for 1972:* "The National Cancer Act of 1971," Senate Bill 1828, enacted December 23, 1871 (P.L. 92–218), National Cancer Institute, http://legislative.cancer. gov/history/phsa/1971 (accessed December 2, 2009). Frank Rauscher, the director of the National Cancer Program, estimated the real numbers to have been $233 million in 1971, $378 million in 1972, $432 million in 1973, and $500 million in 1974. Frank Rauscher, "Budget and the National Cancer Program (NCP)," *Cancer Research* 34, no. 7 (1974): 1743–48.

188 *If money was "frozen energy":* Mary Lasker Oral History Project, Part 1, Session 7, p. 185.

188 *The new bill, she told a reporter, "contained nothing":* Ibid., Part 2, Session 10, p. 334.

188 *Lasker and Sidney Farber withdrew:* Ibid., Part 1, Session 7, p. 185; and Thomas Farber, interview with author, December 2007.

189 *"Powerful? I don't know":* "Mary Lasker: Still Determined to Beautify the City and Nation," *New York Times,* April 28, 1974.

189 *"A crash program can produce only one result":* Chicago Tribune, June 23, 1971, p. 16.

189 *On March 30, 1973, in the late afternoon:* Denis R. Miller, "A Tribute to Sidney Farber—the Father of Modern Chemotherapy," *British Journal of Haematology* 134 (2006): 20–26; "Dr. Sidney Farber, a Pioneer in Children's Cancer Research; Won

Lasker Award," *New York Times,* March 31, 1973. Also see Mary Lasker, "A Personal Tribute to Sidney Farber, M.D. (1903–1973)," *CA: A Cancer Journal for Clinicians* 23, no. 4 (1973): 256–57.

190 *"Surely," she wrote, "the world will never be the same":* Lasker, "A Personal Tribute."

PART THREE:
"WILL YOU TURN ME OUT IF I CAN'T GET BETTER?"

191 *Oft expectation fails:* William Shakespeare, *All's Well That Ends Well* (New York: Macmillan, 1912), act 2, scene 1, lines 145–47, p. 34.

191 *I have seen the moment of my greatness flicker:* T. S. Eliot, "The Love Song of J. Alfred Prufrock," lines 84–86, *The Norton Anthology of Poetry,* 4th ed. (New York: Norton, 1996), 1232.

191 *You are absolutely correct:* Frank Rauscher, letter to Mary Lasker, March 18, 1974, Mary Lasker Papers, Box 118.

"In God we trust. All others [must] have data"

193 *In science, ideology tends to corrupt:* "Knowledge Dethroned," *New York Times,* September 28, 1975.

193 *Orthodoxy in surgery is like orthodoxy in other departments:* G. Keynes, "Carcinoma of the Breast, the Unorthodox View," *Proceedings of the Cardiff Medical Society,* April 1954, 40–49.

193 *You mean I had a mastectomy for nothing?:* Untitled document, 1981, Rose Kushner Papers, 1953–90, Box 43, Harvard University.

194 *"In my own surgical attack on carcinoma":* Cushman Davis Haagensen, *Diseases of the Breast* (New York: Saunders, 1971), 674.

194 Halsted's "centrifugal theory": W. S. Halsted, "The Results of Operations for the Cure of the Cancer of Breast Performed at the Johns Hopkins Hospital from June 1889 to January 1894," *Johns Hopkins Hospital Bulletin* 4 (1894): 497–555.

194 *"To some extent," he wrote:* Haagensen, *Diseases of the Breast,* 674.

194 *"operated on cancer of the breast solely":* D. Hayes Agnew, *The Principles and Practice of Surgery, Being a Treatise on Surgical Diseases and Injuries,* 2nd ed. (Philadelphia: J. B. Lippincott Company, 1889), 3: 711.

194 *"I do not despair of carcinoma being cured":* Ibid.

195 *at St. Bartholomew's Hospital in London:* G. Keynes, "The Treatment of Primary Carcinoma of the Breast with Radium," *Acta Radiologica* 10 (1929): 393–401; G. Keynes, "The Place of Radium in the Treatment of Cancer of the Breast," *Annals of Surgery* 106 (1937): 619–30. For biographical details, see W. LeFanu, "Sir Geoffrey Keynes (1887–1982)," *Bulletin of the History of Medicine* 56, no. 4 (1982): 571–73.

195 *In August 1924, Keynes examined a patient:* "The Radiation Treatment of Carcinoma of the Breast," *St. Bartholomew's Hospital Reports,* vol. 60, ed. W. McAdam Eccles et al. (London: John Murray, 1927), 91–93.

195 *"The ulcer rapidly heal[ed]":* Ibid.

195 *"extension of [the] operation beyond a local removal":* Ibid., 94.

196 *the lumpectomy:* Roger S. Foster Jr., "Breast Cancer Detection and Treatment: A Personal and Historical Perspective," *Archives of Surgery* 138, no. 4 (2003): 397–408.

196 George Barney Crile: Ibid.; G. Crile Jr., "The Evolution of the Treatment of Breast Cancer," *Breast Cancer: Controversies in Management,* ed. L. Wise and H. Johnson Jr. (Armonk, NY: Futura Publishing Co., 1994).

196 *Crile's father. George Crile Sr.:* Narendra Nathoo, Frederick K. Lautzenheiser, and Gene H. Barnett, "The First Direct Human Blood Transfusion: the Forgotten Legacy of George W. Crile," *Neurosurgery* 64 (2009): 20–26; G. W. Crile, *Hemorrhage and Transfusion: An Experimental and Clinical Research* (New York: D. Appleton, 1909).

196 *Political revolutions, the writer Amitav Ghosh writes:* Amitav Ghosh, *Dancing in Cambodia, at Large in Burma* (New Delhi: Ravi Dayal, 1998), 25.

196 *Crile Jr. was beginning to have his own doubts:* Foster, "Breast Cancer Detection and Treatment"; George Crile, *The Way It Was: Sex, Surgery, Treasure and Travel* (Kent, OH: Kent University Press, 1992), 391–400.

197 *Crile soon gave up on the radical mastectomy:* George Crile Jr., "Treatment of Breast Cancer by Local Excision," *American Journal of Surgery* 109 (1965): 400–403; George Crile Jr., "The Smaller the Cancer the Bigger the Operation? Rational of Small Operations for Small Tumors and Large Operations for Large Tumors," *Journal of the American Medical Association* 199 (1967): 736–38; George Crile Jr., *A Biologic Consideration of Treatment of Breast Cancer* (Springfield, IL: Charles C. Thomas, 1967); G. Crile Jr. and S. O. Hoerr, "Results of Treatment of Carcinoma of the Breast by Local Excision," *Surgery, Gynecology, and Obstetrics* 132 (1971): 780–82.

197 *two statisticians, Jerzy Neyman and Egon Pearson:* J. Neyman and E. S. Pearson, "On the Use and Interpretation of Certain Test Criteria for Purposes of Statistical Inference. Part I," *Biometrika* 20A, nos. 1–2 (1928): 175–240; J. Neyman and E. S. Pearson, "On the Use and Interpretation of Certain Test Criteria for Purposes of Statistical Inference. Part II," *Biometrika* 20A, nos. 3–4 (1928): 263–94.

198 *"Go thou and do likewise":* Haagensen, *Diseases of the Breast,* 674.

198 *It took a Philadelphia surgeon:* Kate Travis, "Bernard Fisher Reflects on a Half-Century's Worth of Breast Cancer Research," *Journal of the National Cancer Institute* 97, no. 22 (2005): 1636–37.

199 *"It has become apparent":* Bernard Fisher, Karnosfky Memorial Lecture transcript, Rose Kushner papers, Box 4, File 62, Harvard University.

199 *Thalidomide, prescribed widely to control:* Phillip Knightley, *Suffer the Children: The Story of Thalidomide* (New York: Viking Press, 1979).

199 *In Texas, Jane Roe: Roe v. Wade,* 410 U.S. 113 (1973).

199 *"Refuse to submit to a radical mastectomy":* "Breast Cancer: Beware of These Danger Signals," *Chicago Tribune,* October 3, 1973.

199 *Rachel Carson, the author of* Silent Spring: Ellen Leopold, *A Darker Ribbon: Breast Cancer, Women, and Their Doctors in the Twentieth Century* (Boston: Beacon Press, 1999), 199.

200 *Betty Rollin and Rose Kushner:* Betty Rollin, *First, You Cry* (New York: Harper, 2000); Rose Kushner, *Why Me?* (Philadelphia: Saunders Press, 1982).

200 *"Happily for women," Kushner wrote:* Rose Kushner papers, Box 2, File 22; Kushner, *Why Me?*

200 *In 1967, bolstered by the activism:* See Fisher's NSABP biography at http://www .nsabp.pitt.edu/BCPT_Speakers_Biographies.asp (accessed January 11, 2010).

200 *"The clinician, no matter how venerable":* Bernard Fisher, "A Commentary on the Role

of the Surgeon in Primary Breast Cancer," *Breast Cancer Research and Treatment* 1 (1981): 17–26.

200 *"In God we trust"*: "Treating Breast Cancer: Findings Question Need for Removal," *Washington Post,* October 29, 1979.

200 *"To get a woman to participate in a clinical trial"*: "Bernard Fisher in Conversation," *Pitt Med Magazine* (University of Pittsburgh School of Medicine magazine), July 2002.

200 Fisher's NSABP mastectomy trial: Bernard Fisher et al., "Findings from NSABP Protocol No. B-04: Comparison of Radical Mastectomy with Alternative Treatments. II. The Clinical and Biological Significance of Medial-Central Breast Cancers," *Cancer* 48, no. 8 (1981): 1863–72.

"The smiling oncologist"

202 *Few doctors in this country*: Rose Kushner, "Is Aggressive Adjuvant Chemotherapy the Halsted Radical of the '80s?" *CA: A Cancer Journal for Clinicians* 34, no. 6 (1984): 345–51.

202 *And it is solely by risking life*: Georg Wilhelm Friedrich Hegel, *The Phenomenology of Mind* (New York: Humanities Press, 1971), 232.

202 *"large-scale chemotherapeutic attack"*: James D. Hardy, *The World of Surgery, 1945–1985: Memoirs of One Participant* (Philadelphia: University of Pennsylvania Press, 1986), 216.

202 *"our trench and our bunker"*: Mickey Goulian, interview with author, December 2005.

202 *"Wandering about the NIH clinical center"*: Stewart Alsop, *Stay of Execution: A Sort of Memoir* (New York: Lippincott, 1973), 218.

203 *"Although this was a cancer ward"*: Kathleen R. Gilbert, ed. *The Emotional Nature of Qualitative Research* (Boca Raton, FL: CRC Press, 2001).

203 *"accepted roles, a predetermined outcome, constant stimuli"*: Gerda Lerner, *A Death of One's Own* (New York: Simon and Schuster, 1978), 71.

203 *"yellow and orange walls in the corridors"*: "Cancer Ward Nurses: Where 'C' Means Cheerful," *Los Angeles Times,* July 25, 1975.

203 *the nurses wore uniforms with plastic yellow buttons*: Alsop, *Stay of Execution,* 52.

203 *"Saving the individual patient"*: Ibid., 84.

204 *In 1965, at Michigan State University*: Barnett Rosenberg, Loretta Van Camp, and Thomas Krigas, "Inhibition of Cell Division in *Escherichia coli* by Electrolysis Products from a Platinum Electrode," *Nature* 205, no. 4972 (1965): 698–99.

205 John Cleland: Larry Einhorn, interview with author, November 2009; also see *Cure,* Winter 2004; Craig A. Almeida and Sheila A. Barry, *Cancer: Basic Science and Clinical Aspects* (Hoboken, NJ: Wiley-Blackwell, 2010), 259; "Survivor Milks Life for All It's Worth," *Purdue Agriculture Connections,* Spring 2006; "John Cleland Carried the Olympic Torch in 2000 When the Relay Came through Indiana," Friends 4 Cures, http://www.friends4cures.org/cure_mag_article.shtml (accessed January 9, 2010).

205 *"I cannot remember what I said"*: John Cleland, *Cure,* Winter 2004.

205 *By 1975, Einhorn had treated*: Einhorn, interview with author, December 2009.

205 *"Walking up to that podium"*: Ibid.

205 *"It was unforgettable"*: Ibid. Also see "Triumph of the Cure," *Salon,* July 29, 1999, http://www.salon.com/health/feature/1999/07/29/lance/index.html (accessed November 30, 2009).

205 *Margaret Edson's play* Wit: Margaret Edson, *Wit* (New York: Dramatists Play Service, 1999).

205 *"You may think my vocabulary"*: Ibid., 28.

206 *"We want and need and seek better guidance"*: Howard E. Skipper, "Cancer Chemotherapy Is Many Things: G.H.A. Clowes Memorial Lecture," *Cancer Research* 31, no. 9 (1971): 1173–80.

206 *There was Taxol:* Monroe E. Wall and Mansukh C. Wani, "Camptothecin and Taxol: Discovery to Clinic—Thirteenth Bruce F. Cain Memorial Award Lecture," *Cancer Research* 55 (1995): 753–60; Jordan Goodman and Vivien Walsh, *The Story of Taxol: Nature and Politics in the Pursuit of an Anti-Cancer Drug* (Cambridge, England: Cambridge University Press, 2001).

206 *Adriamycin, discovered in 1969:* F. Arcamone et al., "Adriamycin, 14-hydroxydaimo-mycin, a New Antitumor Antibiotic from *S. Peucetius* var. *caesius,"* *Biotechnology and Bioengineering* 11, no. 6 (1969): 1101–10.

206 *could irreversibly damage the heart:* C. A. J. Brouwer et al., "Long-Term Cardiac Follow-Up in Survivors of a Malignant Bone Tumor," *Annals of Oncology* 17, no. 10 (2006): 1586–91.

206 *Etoposide came from the fruit:* A. M. Arnold and J. M. A. Whitehouse, "Etoposide: A New Anti-cancer Agent," *Lancet* 318, no. 8252 (1981): 912–15.

206 *Bleomycin, which could scar lungs without warning:* H. Umezawa et al., "New Antibiotics, Bleomycin A and B," *Journal of Antibiotics* (Tokyo) 19, no. 5 (1966): 200–209; Nuno R. Grande et al., "Lung Fibrosis Induced by Bleomycin: Structural Changes and Overview of Recent Advances," *Scanning Microscopy* 12, no. 3 (1996): 487–94; R. S Thrall et al., "The Development of Bleomycin-Induced Pulmonary Fibrosis in Neutrophil-Depleted and Complement-Depleted Rats," *American Journal of Pathology* 105 (1981): 76–81.

207 *"Did we believe we were going to cure cancer"*: George Canellos, interview with author.

207 *In the mid-1970s:* J. Ziegler, I. T. McGrath, and C. L. Olweny, "Cure of Burkitt's Lymphoma—Ten-Year Follow-Up of 157 Ugandan Patients," *Lancet* 3, no. 2 (8149) (1979): 936–38. Also see Ziegler et al., "Combined Modality Treatment of Burkitt's Lymphoma," *Cancer Treatment Report* 62, no. 12 (1978): 2031–34.

207 *"Our applications skyrocketed"*: Ibid.

207 *"There is no cancer that is not potentially curable"*: "Cancer: The Chill Is Still There," *Los Angeles Times,* March 20, 1979.

208 *the eight-in-one study:* J. Russel Geyer et al., "Eight Drugs in One Day Chemotherapy in Children with Brain Tumors: A Critical Toxicity Appraisal," *Journal of Clinical Oncology* 6, no. 6 (1988): 996–1000.

209 *"When doctors say that the side effects are tolerable"*: "Some Chemotherapy Fails against Cancer," *New York Times,* August 6, 1985.

209 *"The smiling oncologist"*: Rose Kushner, "Is Aggressive Adjuvant Chemotherapy the Halsted Radical of the '80s?" 1984, draft 9, Rose Kushner papers. The phrase was deleted in the final text that appeared in 1984.

209 *"Hexamethophosphacil with Vinplatin to potentiate"*: Edson, *Wit,* 31.

Knowing the Enemy

210 *It is said that if you know your enemies:* Sun Tzu, *The Art of War* (Boston: Shambhala, 1988), 82.

210 *a urological surgeon, Charles Huggins:* Luis H. Toledo-Pereyra, "Discovery in Surgical Investigation: The Essence of Charles Brenton Huggins," *Journal of Investigative Surgery* 14 (2001): 251–52; Robert E. Forster II, "Charles Brenton Huggins (22 September 1901–12 January 1997)," *Proceedings of the American Philosophical Society* 143, no. 2 (1999): 327–31.

211 Huggins's studies of prostatic fluid: C. Huggins et al., "Quantitative Studies of Prostatic Secretion: I. Characteristics of the Normal Secretion; the Influence of Thyroid, Suprarenal, and Testis Extirpation and Androgen Substitution on the Prostatic Output," *Journal of Experimental Medicine* 70, no. 6 (1939): 543–56; Charles Huggins, "Endocrine-Induced Regression of Cancers." *Science* 156, no. 3778 (1967): 1050–54; Tonse N. K. Raju, "The Nobel Chronicles. 1966: Francis Peyton Rous (1879–1970) and Charles Brenton Huggins (1901–1997), *Lancet* 354, no. 9177 (1999): 520.

212 *"It was vexatious to encounter a dog":* Huggins, "Endocrine-Induced Regression."

213 *"Cancer is not necessarily autonomous":* Ibid.

213 *"Its growth can be sustained and propagated":* Ibid.

213 *In 1929, Edward Doisy, a biochemist:* Edward A. Doisy, "An Autobiography," *Annual Review of Biochemistry* 45 (1976): 1–12.

213 *diethylstilbestrol (or DES):* E. C. Dodds et al., "Synthetic Oestrogenic Compounds Related to Stilbene and Diphenylethane. Part I," *Proceedings of the Royal Society of London, Series B, Biological Sciences* 127, no. 847 (1939): 140–67; E. C. Dodds et al., "Estrogenic Activity of Certain Synthetic Compounds," *Nature* 141, no. 3562 (1938): 247–48; Edward Charles Dodds, *Biochemical Contributions to Endocrinology: Experiments in Hormonal Research* (Palo Alto, CA: Stanford University Press, 1957); Robert Meyers, *D.E.S., the Bitter Pill* (New York: Seaview/Putnam, 1983).

213 *Premarin, natural estrogen purified:* Barbara Seaman, *The Greatest Experiment Ever Performed on Women: Exploding the Estrogen Myth* (New York: Hyperion, 2004), 20–21.

213 *he could inject them to "feminize" the male body:* Huggins, "Endocrine-Induced Regression"; Charles Huggins et al., "Studies on Prostatic Cancer: II. The Effects of Castration on Advanced Carcinoma of the Prostate Gland," *Archives of Surgery* 43 (1941): 209–23.

214 George Beatson and breast cancer: George Thomas Beatson, "On the Treatment of Inoperable Cases of Carcinoma of the Mamma: Suggestions for a New Method of Treatment, with Illustrative Cases," *Lancet* 2 (1896): 104–7; Serena Stockwell, "George Thomas Beatson, M.D. (1848–1933)," *CA: A Cancer Journal for Clinicians* 33 (1983): 105–7.

214 *only about two-thirds of all women:* Alexis Thomson, "Analysis of Cases in Which Oophorectomy was Performed for Inoperable Carcinoma of the Breast," *British Medical Journal* 2, no. 2184 (1902): 1538–41.

214 *"It is impossible to tell beforehand":* Ibid.

215 *a young chemist in Chicago:* E. R. DeSombre, "Estrogens, Receptors and Cancer: The Scientific Contributions of Elwood Jensen," *Progress in Clinical and Biological*

Research 322 (1990): 17–29; E. V. Jensen and V. C. Jordan, "The Estrogen Receptor: A Model for Molecular Medicine," *Clinical Cancer Research* 9, no. 6 (2003): 1980–89.

215 *Ovarian removal produced many other severe side effects:* R. Sainsbury, "Ovarian Ablation as a Treatment for Breast Cancer," *Surgical Oncology* 12, no. 4 (2003): 241–50.

216 *"there was little enthusiasm":* Jensen and Jordan, "The Estrogen Receptor."

216 Tamoxifen: Walter Sneader, *Drug Discovery: A History* (New York: John Wiley and Sons, 2005), 198–99; G. R. Bedford and D. N. Richardson, "Preparation and Identification of *cis* and *trans* Isomers of a Substituted Triarylethylene," *Nature* 212 (1966): 733–34.

216 *Originally invented as a birth control pill:* M. J. Harper and A. L. Walpole, "Mode of Action of I.C.I. 46,474 in Preventing Implantation in Rats," *Journal of Endocrinology* 37, no. 1 (1967): 83–92.

216 *tamoxifen had turned out to have exactly the opposite effect:* A. Klopper and M. Hall, "New Synthetic Agent for Induction of Ovulation: Preliminary Trials in Women," *British Medical Journal* 1, no. 5741 (1971): 152–54.

216 Arthur Walpole and breast cancer: V. C. Jordan, "The Development of Tamoxifen for Breast Cancer Therapy: A Tribute to the Late Arthur L. Walpole," *Breast Cancer Research and Treatment* 11, no. 3 (1988): 197–209.

216 Mary Cole's tamoxifen trial: M. P. Cole et al., "A New Anti-oestrogenic Agent in Late Breast Cancer: An Early Clinical Appraisal of ICI46474," *British Journal of Cancer* 25, no. 2 (1971): 270–75; Sneader, *Drug Discovery,* 199.

217 *In 1973, V. Craig Jordan:* See V. C. Jordan, *Tamoxifen: A Guide for Clinicians and Patients* (Huntington, NY: PRR, 1996). Also see V. C. Jordan, "Effects of Tamoxifen in Relation to Breast Cancer," *British Medical Journal* 6075 (June 11, 1977): 1534–35.

Halsted's Ashes

218 *I would rather be ashes:* Jack London, *Tales of Adventure* (Fayetteville, AR: Hannover House, 1956), vii.

218 *Will you turn me out:* Cicely Saunders, *Selected Writings, 1958–2004,* 1st ed. (Oxford: Oxford University Press, 2006), 71.

219 *at the NCI, Paul Carbone, had launched a trial:* Vincent T. DeVita, "Paul Carbone: 1931–2002," *Oncologist* 7, no. 2 (2002): 92–93.

219 *"Except for an occasional woman":* Paul Carbone, "Adjuvant Therapy of Breast Cancer 1971–1981," *Breast Cancer Research and Treatment* 2 (1985): 75–84.

220 *With his own trial, the NSABP-04:* B. Fisher et al., "Comparison of Radical Mastectomy with Alternative Treatments for Primary Breast Cancer. A First Report of Results from a Prospective Randomized Clinical Trial," *Cancer* 39 (1977): 2827–39.

220 *In 1972, as the NCI was scouring the nation:* G. Bonadonna et al., "Combination Chemotherapy as an Adjuvant Treatment in Operable Breast Cancer," *New England Journal of Medicine* 294, no. 8 (1976): 405–10; Vincent T. DeVita Jr. and Edward Chu, "A History of Cancer Chemotherapy," *Cancer Research* 68, no. 21 (2008): 8643–53.

220 *"The surgeons were not just skeptical":* Springer, *European Oncology Leaders* (Berlin, 2005), 159–65.

221 Fisher's tamoxifen trial: B. Fisher et al., "Adjuvant Chemotherapy with and without Tamoxifen in the Treatment of Primary Breast Cancer: 5-Year Results from

the National Surgical Adjuvant Breast and Bowel Project Trial," *Journal of Clinical Oncology* 4, no. 4 (1986): 459–71.

223 *"We were all more naive a decade ago"*: "Some Chemotherapy Fails against Cancer," *New York Times,* August 6, 1985.

223 *"We shall so poison the atmosphere of the first act"*: James Watson, *New York Times,* May 6, 1975.

225 *"If there is persistent pain"*: J. C. White, "Neurosurgical Treatment of Persistent Pain," *Lancet* 2, no. 5 (1950): 161–64.

225 *"a window in [her] home"*: Saunders, *Selected Writings,* xiv.

225 care, *she wrote, "is a soft word"*: ibid., 255.

225 *"The resistance to providing palliative care to patients"*: Nurse J. N. (name withheld), interview with author, June 2007.

226 *"The provision of . . . terminal care:* Saunders, *Selected Writings,* 71.

Counting Cancer

227 *We must learn to count the living:* Audre Lourde, *The Cancer Journals,* 2nd ed. (San Francisco: Aunt Lute, 1980), 54.

227 *Counting is the religion of this generation:* Gertrude Stein, *Everybody's Autobiography* (New York: Random House, 1937), 120.

227 *"These registries," Cairns wrote in an article:* John Cairns, "Treatment of Diseases and the War against Cancer," *Scientific American* 253, no. 5 (1985): 51–59.

229 John Bailar and Elaine Smith's analysis: J. C. Bailar III and E. M. Smith, "Progress against Cancer?" *New England Journal of Medicine* 314, no. 19 (1986): 1226–32.

231 *cancer mortality was not declining:* This was not unique to the United States; the statistics were similarly grim across Europe. In 1985, a separate analysis of age-adjusted cancer mortality across twenty-eight developed countries revealed an increase in cancer mortality of about 15 percent.

231 *There is "no evidence"*: Bailar and Smith, "Progress against Cancer?"

231 *"a thorn in the side of the National Cancer Institute"*: Gina Kolata, "Cancer Progress Data Challenged," *Science* 232, no. 4753 (1986): 932–33.

232 *As evidence, they pointed to a survey:* See E. M. Greenspan, "Commentary on September 1985 NIH Consensus Development Conference on Adjuvant Chemotherapy for Breast Cancer," *Cancer Investigation* 4, no. 5 (1986): 471–75. Also see Ezra M. Greenspan, letter to the editor, *New England Journal of Medicine* 315, no. 15 (1986): 964.

232 *"The problem with reliance on a single measure"*: Lester Breslow and William G. Cumberland, "Progress and Objectives in Cancer Control," *Journal of the American Medical Association* 259, no. 11 (1988): 1690–94.

233 *"Our purpose in making these calculations"*: Ibid. The order of the quotation has been inverted for the purpose of this narrative.

234 *prevention research received:* John Bailar interviewed by Elizabeth Farnsworth, "Treatment versus Prevention" (transcript), *NewsHour with Jim Leher,* PBS, May 29, 1997; Richard M. Scheffler and Lynn Paringer, "A Review of the Economic Evidence on Prevention," *Medical Care* 18, no. 5 (1980): 473–84.

234 *By 1992, this number had increased:* Samuel S. Epstein, *Cancer-Gate: How to Win the Losing Cancer War* (Amityville, NY: Baywood Publishing Company, 2005), 59.

234 *In 1974, describing to Mary Lasker:* Letter from Frank Rauscher to Mary Lasker, March 18, 1974, Mary Lasker Papers, Box 118, Columbia University.

234 *At Memorial Sloan-Kettering in New York:* Ralph W. Moss, *The Cancer Syndrome* (New York: Grove Press, 1980), 221.

234 *"not one" was able to suggest an "idea":* Edmund Cowdry, *Etiology and Prevention of Cancer in Man* (New York: Appleton-Century, 1968), xvii.

234 *Prevention, he noted drily:* Moss, *The Cancer Syndrome,* 221.

234 *"A shift in research emphasis":* Bailar and Smith, "Progress against Cancer?"

PART FOUR:
PREVENTION IS THE CURE

235 *It should first be noted:* David Cantor, "Introduction: Cancer Control and Prevention in the Twentieth Century," *Bulletin of the History of Medicine* 81 (2007): 1–38.

235 *The idea of preventive medicine:* "False Front in War on Cancer," *Chicago Tribune,* February 13, 1975.

235 *The same correlation could be drawn:* Ernest L. Wynder letter to Evarts A. Graham, June 20, 1950, Evarts Graham papers.

"Coffins of black"

237 *When my mother died I was very young:* "The Chimney Sweeper," William Blake, *The Complete Poetry and Prose of William Blake,* ed. David V. Erdman (New York: Random House, 1982), 10.

237 *It is a disease, he wrote:* Percivall Pott and James Earles, *The Chirurgical Works of Percivall Pott, F.R.S. Surgeon to St. Bartholomew's Hospital, a New Edition, with His Last Corrections, to Which Are Added, a Short Account of the Life of the Author, a Method of Curing the Hydrocele by Injection, and Occasional Notes and Observations, by Sir James Earle, F.R.S. Surgeon Extraordinary to the King* (London: Wood and Innes, 1808), 3: 177.

238 *"Syphilis," as the saying ran:* Michael J. O'Dowd and Elliot E. Philipp, *The History of Obstetrics & Gynaecology* (New York: Parthenon Publishing Group, 2000), 228.

238 *In 1713, Ramazzini had published:* Bernardino Ramazzini, *De Morbis Artificum Diatriba* (Apud Josephum Corona, 1743).

238 *"All this makes it (at first) a very different case":* Pott and Earles, *Chirurgical Works,* 3: 177.

239 *Eighteenth-century England:* See Peter Kirby, *Child Labor in Britain, 1750–1870* (Hampshire, UK: Palgrave Macmillan, 2003). For details on chimney sweeps, see ibid., 9; and *Parliamentary Papers* 1852–52, 88, pt. 1, tables 25, 26.

239 *"I wants a 'prentis":* Charles Dickens, *Oliver Twist, or The Parish Boy's Progress* (London: J. M. Dent & Sons, 1920), 16.

239 *In 1788, the Chimney Sweepers Act:* Joel H. Wiener, *Great Britain: The Lion at Home: A Documentary History of Domestic Policy, 1689–1973* (New York: Chelsea House Publishers, 1974), 800.

239 *In 1761, more than a decade before:* John Hill, *Cautions against the Immoderate Use of Snuff* (London: R. Baldwin and J. Jackson, 1761).

240 *a self-professed "Bottanist, apothecary, poet":* G. S. Rousseau, ed. *The Letters and Papers of Sir John Hill, 1714–1775* (New York: AMS Press, 1982), 4.

240 *"close, clouded, hot, narcotic rooms":* George Crabbe, *The Poetical Works of the Rev. George Crabbe: With his Letters and Journals, and His Life* (London: John Murray, 1834), 3: 180.

240 *By the mid-1700s, the state of Virginia:* See Paul G. E. Clemens, "From Tobacco to Grain," *Journal of Economic History* 35, no. 1: 256–59.

240 *In England the import of tobacco:* Kenneth Morgan, *Bristol and the Atlantic Trade in the Eighteenth Century* (Cambridge University Press, 1993), 152.

240 *In 1855, legend runs, a Turkish soldier:* See Richard Klein, *Cigarettes Are Sublime* (Durham, NC: Duke University Press, 1993), 134–35.

240 *In 1870, the per capita consumption in America:* Jack Gottsegen, *Tobacco: A Study of Its Consumption in the United States* (New York: Pittman, 1940).

241 *A mere thirty years later, Americans:* Ibid.

241 *On average, an adult American smoked ten cigarettes:* Harold F. Dorn, "The Relationship of Cancer of the Lung and the Use of Tobacco," *American Statistician* 8, no. 5 (1954): 7–13.

241 *By the early twentieth century, four out of five:* Richard Peto, interview with author, September 2008.

241 *"By the early 1940s, asking about a connection":* Ibid.

242 *"So has the use of nylon stockings":* John Wilds and Ira Harkey, *Alton Ochsner, Surgeon of the South* (Baton Rouge: Louisiana State University Press, 1990), 180.

242 *"the cigarette century":* Allan M. Brandt, *The Cigarette Century: The Rise, Fall, and Deadly Persistence of the Product That Defined America* (New York: Basic Books, 2007).

The Emperor's Nylon Stockings

243 *Whether epidemiology alone can:* Sir Richard Doll, "Proof of Causality: Deduction from Epidemiological Observation," *Perspectives in Biology and Medicine* 45 (2002): 499–515.

243 *lung cancer morbidity had risen nearly fifteenfold:* Richard Doll and A. Bradford Hill, "Smoking and Carcinoma of the Lung," *British Medical Journal* 2, no. 4682 (1950): 739–48.

243 *"matter that ought to be studied":* Richard Peto, "Smoking and Death: The Past 40 Years and the Next 40," *British Medical Journal* 309 (1994): 937–39.

243 *In February 1947, in the midst of a bitterly cold:* Ibid.

243 *One expert, having noted parenthetically:* British Public Records Office, file FD. 1, 1989, as quoted by David Pollock, *Denial and Delay* (Washington, DC: Action on Smoking and Health, 1989); full text available through Action on Smoking and Health, www.ash.org.

243 *Yet the resources committed for the study:* Medical Research Council 1947/366 and Ibid.

244 *In the summer of 1948:* Pollock, *Denial and Delay,* prologue. Also see Sir Richard Doll, "The First Report on Smoking and Lung Cancer," in *Ashes to Ashes: The History of Smoking and Health*, Stephen Lock, Lois A. Reynolds, and E. M. Tansey, eds. (Amsterdam: Editions Rodopi B.V., 1998), 129–37.

244 *"The same correlation could be drawn to the intake of milk":* Ernst L. Wynder, letter to Evarts A. Graham, June 20, 1950, Evarts Graham papers.

245 *Wynder and Graham's trial:* Ernst L. Wynder and Evarts A. Graham, "Tobacco Smoking as a Possible Etiologic Factor in Bronchiogenic Carcinoma: A Study of Six Hundred and Eighty-Four Proved Cases," *Journal of the American Medical Association* 143 (1950): 329–38.

245 *When Wynder presented his preliminary ideas:* Ernst L. Wynder, "Tobacco as a Cause of Lung Cancer: Some Reflections," *American Journal of Epidemiology* 146 (1997), 687–94. Also see Jon Harkness, "The U.S. Public Health Service and Smoking in the 1950s: The Tale of Two More Statements," *Journal of the History of Medicine and Allied Sciences* 62, no. 2 (2007): 171–212.

245 Doll and Hill's study: Doll and Hill, "Smoking and Carcinoma of the Lung."

246 *When the price of cigarettes was increased:* Richard Peto, personal interview. Also see Virginia Berridge, *Marketing Health: Smoking and the Discourse of Public Health in Britain* (Oxford: Oxford University Press, 2007), 45.

246 *By May 1, 1948, 156 interviews:* David Pollock, "Denial and Delay," collections from the public record office files deposited in the Action on Smoking and Health archives, UK. Also see the Action on Smoking and Health Tobacco Chronology, http://www.ash.org.uk/ash_669pax88_archive.htm (accessed January 21, 2010).

247 *In the early 1940s, a similar notion had gripped:* R. A. Fisher and E. B. Ford, "The Spread of a Gene in Natural Conditions in a Colony of the Moth *Panaxia diminula* L.," *Heredity* 1 (1947): 143–74.

248 *And the notion of using a similar cohort:* Stephen Lock, Lois A. Reynolds, and E. M. Tansey, eds., *Ashes to Ashes* (Amsterdam: Editions Rodopi B.V., 1998), 137.

249 Doll and Hill's study of smoking habits and lung cancer in doctors: Richard Doll and A. Bradford Hill, "The Mortality of Doctors in Relation to Their Smoking Habits: A Preliminary Report," *British Medical Journal* 1, no. 4877 (1954): 1451–55.

"A thief in the night"

250 *By the way, [my cancer]:* Evarts Graham, letter to Ernst Wynder, February 6, 1957, Evarts Graham papers.

250 *We believe the products that we make:* "A Frank Statement to Cigarette Smokers," *New York Times,* January 4, 1954.

250 *Cigarette sales had climbed:* See, for instance, Richard Kluger, *Ashes to Ashes* (New York: Vintage Books, 1997), 104–6, 123, 125. Also see Verner Grise, *U.S. Cigarette Consumption: Past, Present and Future,* conference paper, 30th Tobacco Workers Conference, Williamsburg, VA, 1983 (archived at http://tobaccodocuments.org).

250 *cigarette industry poured tens, then hundreds:* For a succinct history of postwar advertising campaigns of cigarette makers see Kluger, *Ashes to Ashes,* 80–298.

251 *"More doctors smoke Camels":* See, for example, *Life,* October 6, 1952, back cover.

251 *At the annual conferences of the American Medical Association:* See Martha N. Gardner and Allan M. Brandt, "'The Doctors' Choice Is America's Choice': The Physician in US Cigarette Advertisements, 1930–1953," *American Journal of Public Health* 96, no. 2 (2006): 222–32.

251 *In 1955, when Philip Morris:* Katherine M. West, "The Marlboro Man: The Making of

an American Image," American Studies at the University of Virginia website, http://xroads.virginia.edu/~CLASS/marlboro/mman.html (accessed December 23, 2009).

251 *"Man-sized taste of honest tobacco"*: Ibid.

251 *By the early 1960s, the gross annual sale:* Estimated from U.S. Surgeon General's report on per capita consumption rates for 1960–1970.

251 *On average, Americans were consuming:* Jeffrey E. Harris, "Patterns of Cigarette Smoking," *The Health Consequences of Smoking for Women: A Report of the Surgeon General* (Washington, DC: U.S. Department of Health and Human Services, 1980), 15–342. Also see Allan Brandt, *The Cigarette Century,* 97.

251 *On December 28, 1953, three years before:* "Notes on Minutes of the Tobacco Industry Research Committee Meeting—December 28, 1953," John W. Hill papers, "Selected and Related Documents on the Topic of the Hill & Knowlton Public Relations Campaign Formulated on Behalf of the Tobacco Industry Research Committee," State Historical Society of Wisconsin, http://www.ttlaonline.com/HKWIS/12307.pdf (accessed December 23, 2009).

252 *The centerpiece of that counterattack:* "Frank Statement," *New York Times.*

253 *In January 1954, after a protracted search:* Brandt, *Cigarette Century,* 178.

254 *In a guest editorial written for the journal:* C. C. Little, "Smoking and Lung Cancer," *Cancer Research* 16, no. 3 (1956): 183–84.

254 *In a stinging rebuttal written to the editor:* Evarts A. Graham, "To the Editor of *Cancer Research,*" *Cancer Research* 16 (1956): 816–17.

254 *"We may subject mice, or other laboratory animals"*: Sir Austin Bradford Hill, *Statistical Methods in Clinical and Preventative Medicine* (London: Livingstone, 1962), 378.

254 *Graham had invented a "smoking machine"*: Ernst L. Wynder, Evarts A. Graham, and Adele B. Croninger, "Experimental Production of Carcinoma with Cigarette Tar," *Cancer Research* 13 (1953): 855–64.

255 Forbes *magazine had famously spoofed the research:* Forbes 72 (1953): 20.

255 *Bradford Hill's nine criteria for epidemiology:* Sir Austin Bradford Hill, "The Environment and Disease: Association or Causation?" *Proceedings of the Royal Society of Medicine* 58, no. 5 (1965): 295–300.

256 *"Perhaps you have heard that"*: Letter from Evarts Graham to Alton Ochsner, February 14, 1957, Evarts Graham papers.

257 *In the winter of 1954, three years before:* Alton Ochsner, *Smoking and Cancer: A Doctor's Report* (New York: J. Messner, 1954).

"A statement of warning"

258 *Our credulity would indeed be strained: Eva Cooper v. R. J. Reynolds Tobacco Company,* 256 F.2d 464 (1st Cir., 1958).

258 *Certainly, living in America in the last half:* Burson Marsteller (PR firm) internal document, January 1, 1988. Cipollone postverdict document available at the UCSF Legacy Tobacco Documents Library.

258 *In the summer of 1963, seven years after:* See Richard Kluger, *Ashes to Ashes,* 254–55.

258 *Auerbach's paper describing the lesions:* O. Auerbach and A. P. Stout, "The Role of Carcinogens, Especially Those in Cigarette Smoke, in the Production of Precancerous Lesions," *Proceedings of the National Cancer Conference* 4 (1960): 297–304.

259 *Auerbach's three visitors that morning:* See Kluger, *Ashes to Ashes,* 254.

259 *In 1961, the American Cancer Society:* "The 1964 Report on Smoking and Health," Reports of the Surgeon General, Profiles in Science: National Library of Medicine, http://profiles.nlm.nih.gov/NN/Views/Exhibit/narrative/smoking.html (accessed December 26, 2009); U.S. Surgeon General. "Smoking and Health," *Report of the Advisory Committee to the Surgeon General of the Public Health Service,* Public Health Service publication no. 1103 (Washington, DC: U.S. Department of Health, Education, and Welfare, Public Health Service, 1964).

260 *"a reluctant dragon":* Lester Breslow, *A History of Cancer Control in the United States, 1946–1971* (Bethesda, MD: U.S. National Cancer Institute, 1979), 4: 24.

260 *he announced that he would appoint an advisory committee:* U.S. Surgeon General's report: *Smoking and Health,* 1964.

261 *Data, interviews, opinions, and testimonies:* Ibid.

261 *Each member of the committee:* Ibid. Also see Kluger, *Ashes to Ashes,* 243–45.

262 *"The word 'cause,'" the report read:* U.S. Surgeon General's report: *Smoking and Health.*

262 *Luther Terry's report, a leatherbound, 387-page:* "1964 Report on Smoking and Health."

262 *"While the propaganda blast was tremendous":* George Weissman memo to Joseph Cullman III, January 11, 1964, Tobacco Documents Online, http://tobaccodocuments.org/landman/1005038559–8561.html (accessed December 26, 2009).

263 *the commission's shining piece of lawmaking: Annual Report of the Federal Trade Commission* (Washington DC: United States Printing Office, 1950), 65.

263 *In 1957, John Blatnik, a Minnesota chemistry teacher:* "Making Cigarette Ads Tell the Truth," *Harper's,* August 1958.

263 *The FTC had been revamped:* "Government: The Old Lady's New Look," *Time,* April 16, 1965.

264 *A week later, in January 1964:* Federal Trade Commission, "Advertising and Labeling of Cigarettes. Notice of Rule-Making Proceeding for Establishment of Trade Regulation Rules," *Federal Register,* January 22, 1964, 29:530–32.

264 *they voluntarily requested regulation by Congress:* "The Quiet Victory of the Cigarette Lobby: How It Found the Best Filter Yet—Congress," *Atlantic,* September 1965.

264 *Entitled the Federal Cigarette Labeling and Advertising Act:* Cigarette Labeling and Advertising Act, Title 15, chap. 36, 1965; "Quiet Victory of the Cigarette Lobby."

265 *In the early summer of 1967, Banzhaf: John F. Banzhaf III v. Federal Communications Commission et al.,* 405 F.2d 1082 (D.C. Cir. 1968).

266 *"The advertisements in question":* Ibid.

266 *"a squadron of the best-paid lawyers in the country":* John Banzhaf, interview with author, June 2008.

266 *"Doubt is our product":* "Smoking and Health Proposal,"1969, Brown & Williamson Collection, Legacy Tobacco Documents Library, University of California, San Francisco.

266 *In 1968, a worn and skeletal-looking William Talman:* A video of the ad is available at http://www.classictvads.com/smoke_1.shtml (accessed December 26, 2009).

267 *The last cigarette commercial:* See Brandt, *Cigarette Century,* 271.

267 *He had already died:* "William Hopper, Actor, Dies; Detective in 'Perry Mason,' 54," *New York Times,* March 7, 1970.

267 *cigarette consumption in America plateaued:* U.S. Department of Agriculture, *Tobacco Situation and Outlook Report,* publication no. TBS-226 (Washington, DC: U.S. Department of Agriculture, Economic Research Service, Commodity Economics

Division, April 1994) table 2; G. A. Glovino, "Surveillance for Selected Tobacco-Use Behaviors—United States, 1900–1994," *Morbidity and Mortality Weekly Report CDC Surveillance Summaries* 43, no. 3 (1994): 1–43.

267 *"Statistics," the journalist Paul Brodeur once wrote:* Paul Brodeur, *Outrageous Misconduct: The Asbestos Industry on Trial* (New York: Pantheon Books, 1985).

267 *She represented the midpoint:* See "Women and Smoking," Report of the U.S. Surgeon General 2001, and prior report from 1980.

268 *"[It's] a game only for steady nerves":* See, for example, *Popular Mechanics,* November 1942, back cover.

268 *"never twittery, nervous or jittery":* Redd Evans and John Jacob Loeb, "Rosie the Riveter" (New York: Paramount Music Corp., 1942).

269 *Marc Edell, a New Jersey attorney:* For details of Cipollone's case see *Cipollone v. Liggett Group, Inc.,* 505 U.S. 504 (1992).

269 *"deaf, dumb and blind":* Ibid.

269 *In the three decades between 1954 and 1984:* Burson Marsteller (PR firm), Position Paper, *History of Tobacco Litigation Third Draft,* May 10, 1988.

270 *"Plaintiff attorneys can read the writing":* Burson Marsteller (PR firm), internal document, Cipollone postverdict communication plan, January 1, 1988.

270 *In one letter, Fred Panzer:* David Michaels, *Doubt Is Their Product: How Industry's Assault on Science Threatens Your Health* (Oxford: Oxford University Press, 2008), 11. Also see Brown and Williamson (B & W), "Smoking and Health Proposal," B & W document no. 680561778-1786, 1969, available at http://legacy.library.ucsf.edu/tid/nvs40f00.

270 *"In a sense, the tobacco industry may be thought":* "Research Planning Memorandum on the Nature of the Tobacco Business and the Crucial Role of Nicotine Therein," April 14, 1972, Anne Landman's Collection, Tobacco Documents Online, http://tobacco documents.org/landman/501877121–7129.html (accessed December 26, 2009).

271 *"Think of the cigarette pack as a storage container":* "Motives and Incentives in Cigarette Smoking," 1972, Anne Landman's Collection, Tobacco Documents Online, http://tobaccodocuments.org/landman/2024273959–3975.html (accessed December 26, 2009).

271 *Edell quizzed Liggett's president:* Cipollone v. Liggett Group, Inc., et al., transcript of proceedings [excerpt], *Tobacco Products Litigation Reporter* 3, no. 3 (1988): 3.2261–3.268.

271 *the Cipollone cancer trial appeared before the court in 1987:* See *Cipollone v. Liggett Group, Inc., et al.,* 893 F.2d 541 (1990); *Cipollone v. Liggett Group, Inc., et al.,* 505 U.S. 504 (1992).

272 *By 1994, the per capita consumption of cigarettes in America:* "Trends in Tobacco Use," American Lung Association Research and Program Services Epidemiology and Statistics Unit, July 2008, http://www.lungusa.org/finding-cures/for-professionals/epidemiology-and-statistics-rpts.html (accessed December 27, 2009).

272 *Among men, the age-adjusted incidence:* "Trends in Lung Cancer Morbidity and Mortality," American Lung Association Epidemiology and Statistics Unit, Research and Program Services Division, September 2008, http://www.lungusa.org/finding-cures/for-professionals/epidemiology-and-statistics-rpts.html (accessed December 27, 2009).

272 *In 1994, in yet another landmark case:* "Mississippi Seeks Damages from Tobacco Companies," *New York Times,* May 24, 1994.

272 *"You caused the health crisis":* Ibid.

273 *Several other states then followed:* "Tobacco Settlement Nets Florida $11.3B," *USA Today,* August 25, 1997; "Texas Tobacco Deal Is Approved," *New York Times,* January 17, 1998.

273 *In June 1997, facing a barrage:* The Master Settlement Agreement is available online from the Office of the Attorney General of California, http://www.ag.ca.gov/tobacco/msa.php (accessed December 27, 2009).

273 *Tobacco smoking is now a major preventable cause:* Gu et al., "Mortality Attributable to Smoking in China," *New England Journal of Medicine* 360, no. 2 (2009): 150–59; P. Jha et al., "A Nationally Representative Case-Control Study of Smoking and Death in India," *New England Journal of Medicine* 358, no. 11 (2008): 1137–47.

273 *Richard Peto, an epidemiologist at Oxford:* Ibid.

274 *In China, lung cancer is already:* Gu et al., "Mortality Attributable to Smoking in China."

274 *In 2004, tobacco companies signed:* Samet et al., "Mexico and the Tobacco Industry," *BMJ* 3 (2006): 353–55.

274 *In the early 1990s, a study noted, British American Tobacco:* Gilmore et al., "American Tobacco's Erosion of Health Legislation in Uzbekistan," *BMJ* 332 (2006): 355–58.

274 *Cigarette smoking grew by about 8 percent:* Ibid.

274 *In a recent editorial in the* British Medical Journal: Ernesto Sebrié and Stanton A. Glantz, "The Tobacco Industry in Developing Countries," *British Medical Journal* 332, no. 7537 (2006): 313–14.

"Curiouser and curiouser"

276 *You're under a lot of stress:* Transcript of interview with Barry Marshall and an anonymous interviewer, National Health and Medical Research Council archives, Australia.

276 *In the early 1970s, for instance, a series of studies:* J. S. Harrington, "Asbestos and Mesothelioma in Man," *Nature* 232, no. 5305 (1971): 54–55; P. Enterline, P. DeCoufle, and V. Henderson, "Mortality in Relation to Occupational Exposure in the Asbestos Industry," *Journal of Occupational Medicine* 14, no. 12 (1972): 897–903; "Asbestos, the Saver of Lives, Has a Deadly Side," New York Times, January 21, 1973; "New Rules Urged For Asbestos Risk," *New York Times,* October 5, 1975.

277 *In 1971, yet another such study identified:* Arthur L. Herbst, Howard Ulfelder, and David C. Poskanzer, *New England Journal of Medicine* 284, no. 15 (1971): 878–81.

277 *In the late 1960s, a bacteriologist named Bruce Ames:* Bruce N. Ames et al., "Carcinogens Are Mutagens: A Simple Test System Combining Liver Homogenates for Activation and Bacteria for Detection," *Proceedings of the National Academy of Sciences of the United States of America* 70, no. 8 (1973): 2281–85; Bruce N. Ames, "An Improved Bacterial Test System for the Detection and Classification of Mutagens and Carcinogens," *Proceedings of the National Academy of Sciences of the United States of America* 70, no. 3 (1973): 82–786.

278 *So did X-rays, benzene compounds, and nitrosoguanidine*: "Carcinogens as Frameshift Mutagens: Metabolites and Derivatives of 2-Acetylaminofluorene and Other Aromatic Amine Carcinogens," *Proceedings of the National Academy of Sciences of the United States of America* 69, no. 11 (1972): 3128–32.

278 *Not every known carcinogen scored on the test:* For DES, see Ishikawa et al., "Lack of Mutagenicity of Diethylstilbestrol Metabolite and Analog, (±)-Indenestrols A and B, in Bacterial Assays," *Mutation Research/Genetic Toxicology* 368, nos. 3–4 (1996): 261–65; for asbestos, see K. Szyba and A. Lange, "Presentation of Benzo(a)pyrene to Microsomal Enzymes by Asbestos Fibers in the Salmonella/Mammalian Microsome Mutagenicity Test," *Environmental Health Perspectives* 51 (1983): 337–41.

278 *A biochemistry student at Oxford:* Marc A. Shampo and Robert A. Kyle, "Baruch Blumberg—Work on Hepatitis B Virus," *Mayo Clinic Proceedings* 78, no. 9 (2003): 1186.

279 *The work of Baruch Blumberg:* Baruch S. Blumberg, "Australia Antigen and the Biology of Hepatitis B," *Science* 197, no. 4298 (1977): 17–25; Rolf Zetterström, "Nobel Prize to Baruch Blumberg for the Discovery of the Aetiology of Hepatitis B," *Acta Paediatrica* 97, no. 3 (2008): 384–87; Shampo and Kyle, "Baruch Blumberg," 1186.

279 *Blumberg began to scour far-flung places:* A. C. Allison et al., "Haptoglobin Types in British, Spanish, Basque and Nigerian African Populations," *Nature* 181 (1958): 824–25.

279 *In 1964, after a brief tenure at the NIH:* Zetterström, "Nobel Prize to Baruch Blumberg."

279 *One blood antigen that intrigued him:* Baruch S. Blumberg, Harvey J. Alter, and Sam Visnich, "A 'New' Antigen in Leukemia Sera," *Journal of the American Medical Association* 191, no. 7 (1965): 541–46.

279 *In 1966, Blumberg's lab set out to characterize:* Baruch S. Blumberg et al., "A Serum Antigen (Australia Antigen) in Down's Syndrome, Leukemia, and Hepatitis," *Annals of Internal Medicine* 66, no. 5 (1967): 924–31.

279 *Au and hepatitis:* Blumberg, "Australia Antigen and the Biology of Hepatitis B."

280 *"roughly circular . . . about forty-two nanometers":* Baruch Blumberg, *Hepatitis B: The Hunt for a Killer Virus* (Princeton: Princeton University Press, 2002), 115.

280 *By 1969, Japanese researchers:* Baruch S. Blumberg, "Australia Antigen and the Biology of Hepatitis B."; K. Okochi and S. Murakami, "Observations on Australia Antigen in Japanese," *Vox Sanguinis* 15, no. 5 (1968): 374–85.

280 *But another illness soon stood out:* Blumberg, *Hepatitis B*, 155.

281 *"discipline-determined rigidity of the constituent institutes":* Ibid., 72.

281 *By 1979, his group had devised one:* Ibid., 134–46.

282 *"Since the early days of medical bacteriology":* J. Robin Warren, "Helicobacter: The Ease and Difficulty of a New Discovery (Nobel Lecture)," *ChemMedChem* 1, no. 7 (2006): 672–85.

282 Barry Marshall and Robin Warren's discovery of ulcer-causing bacteria: J. R. Warren, "Unidentified Curved Bacteria on Gastric Epithelium in Active Chronic Gastritis," *Lancet* 321, no. 8336 (1983): 1273–75; Barry J. Marshall and J. Robin Warren, "Unidentified Curved Bacilli in the Stomach of Patients with Gastritis and Peptic Ulceration," *Lancet* 323, no. 8390 (1984): 1311–15; Barry Marshall, *Helicobacter Pioneers: Firsthand Accounts from the Scientists Who Discovered Helicobacters, 1892–1982* (Hoboken, NJ: Wiley-Blackwell, 2002); Warren, "Helicobacter: The Ease and Difficulty"; Barry J. Marshall, "Heliobacter Connections," *ChemMedChem* 1, no. 8 (2006): 783–802.

283 *"On the morning of the experiment":* Marshall, "Heliobacter Connections."

284 *The effect of antibiotic therapy on cancer:* Johannes G. Kusters, Arnoud H. M. van Vliet, and Ernst J. Kuipers, "Pathogenesis of *Helicobacter pylori* Infection," *Clinical Microbiology Reviews* 19, no. 3 (2006): 449–90.

"A spider's web"

286 *It is to earlier diagnosis that we must look:* J. P. Lockhart-Mummery, "Two Hundred Cases of Cancer of the Rectum Treated by Perineal Excision," *British Journal of Surgery* 14 (1926–27): 110–24.

286 *The greatest need we have today:* Sidney Farber, letter to Etta Rosensohn, November 1962.

286 *Lady, have you been "Paptized"?:* "Lady, Have You Been 'Paptized'?" *New York Amsterdam News,* April 13, 1957.

286 George Papanicolaou: For an overview, see George A. Vilos, "After Office Hours: The History of the Papanicolaou Smear and the Odyssey of George and Andromache Papanicolaou," *Obstetrics and Gynecology* 91, no. 3 (1998): 479–83; S. Zachariadou-Veneti, "A Tribute to George Papanicolaou (1883–1962)," *Cytopathology* 11, no. 3 (2000): 152–57.

287 *By the late 1920s:* Zachariadou-Veneti, "Tribute to George Papanicolaou."

287 *As one gynecologist archly remarked:* Edgar Allen, "Abstract of Discussion on Ovarian Follicle Hormone," *Journal of the American Medical Association* 85 (1925): 405.

287 *Papanicolaou thus began to venture:* George N. Papanicolaou, "The Cancer-Diagnostic Potential of Uterine Exfoliative Cytology," *CA: A Cancer Journal for Clinicians* 7 (1957): 124–35.

288 *"aberrant and bizarre forms":* Ibid.

288 *Papanicolaou published his method:* G. N. Papanicolaou, "New Cancer Diagnosis," *Proceedings of the Third Race Betterment Conference* (1928): 528.

288 *"I think this work will be carried":* Ibid.

288 *Between 1928 and 1950:* George A. Vilos, "After Office Hours," *Obstetrics and Gynecology* 91 (March 1998): 3.

288 *A Japanese fish and bird painter:* George N. Papanicolaou, "The Cell Smear Method of Diagnosing Cancer," *American Journal of Public Health and the Nation's Health* 38, no. 2 (1948): 202–5.

289 *At a Christmas party in the winter of 1950:* Irena Koprowska, *A Woman Wanders through Life and Science* (Albany: State University of New York Press, 1997), 167–68.

289 *"It was a revelation":* Ibid.

289 *In 1952, Papanicolaou convinced the National Cancer Institute:* Cyrus C. Erickson, "Exfoliative Cytology in Mass Screening for Uterine Cancer: Memphis and Shelby County, Tennessee," *CA: A Cancer Journal for Clinicians* 5 (1955): 63–64.

289 *In the initial cohort of about 150,000:* Harold Speert, "Memorable Medical Mentors: VI. Thomas S. Cullen (1868–1953)," *Obstetrical and Gynecological Survey* 59, no. 8 (2004): 557–63.

289 *557 women were found to have preinvasive cancers:* Ibid.

290 *In 1913, a Berlin surgeon named Albert Salomon:* D. J. Dronkers et al., eds., *The Practice of Mammography: Pathology, Technique, Interpretation, Adjunct Modalities* (New York: Thieme, 2001), 256.

291 *"trabeculae as thin as a spider's web":* H. J. Burhenne, J. E. Youker, and R. H. Gold, eds., *Mammography* (symposium given on August 24, 1968, at the University of California School of Medicine, San Francisco) (New York: S. Karger, 1969), 109.

294 *In the winter of 1963, three men set out:* Sam Shapiro, Philip Strax, and Louis Venet, "Evaluation of Periodic Breast Cancer Screening with Mammography: Methodology

and Early Observations," *Journal of the American Medical Association* 195, no. 9 (1966): 731–38.

294 *By the mid-1950s, a triad of forces:* Thomas A. Hirschl and Tim B. Heaton, eds., *New York State in the 21ˢᵗ Century* (Santa Barbara, CA: Greenwood Publishing Group, 1999), 144.

294 *By the early 1960s, the plan had enrolled:* See, for instance, Philip Strax, "Screening for breast cancer," *Clinical Obstetrics and Gynecology* 20, no. 4 (1977): 781–802.

295 *Strax and Venet eventually outfitted a mobile van:* Philip Strax, "Female Cancer Detection Mobile Unit," *Preventive Medicine* 1, no. 3 (1972): 422–25.

295 *"Interview . . . 5 stations X 12 women":* Abraham Schiff quoted in Philip Strax, *Control of Breast Cancer through Mass Screening* (Philadelphia: Mosby, 1979), 148.

296 *In 1971, eight years after the study:* S. Shapiro et al., "Proceedings: Changes in 5-Year Breast Cancer Mortality in a Breast Cancer Screening Program," *Proceedings of the National Cancer Conference* 7 (1972): 663–78.

296 *"The radiologist," he wrote:* Philip Strax, "Radiologist's Role in Screening Mammography," unpublished document quoted in Barron H. Lerner, "'To See Today with the Eyes of Tomorrow': A History of Screening Mammography," *Canadian Bulletin of Medical History* 20, no. 2 (2003): 299–321.

296 *"Within 5 years, mammography has moved":* G. Melvin Stevens and John F. Weigen, "Mammography Survey for Breast Cancer Detection. A 2-Year Study of 1,223 Clinically Negative Asymptomatic Women over 40," *Cancer* 19, no. 1 (2006): 51–59.

296 *"The time has come":* Arthur I. Holleb, "Toward Better Control of Breast Cancer," American Cancer Society press release, October 4, 1971 (New York: ACS Media Division), Folder: Breast Cancer Facts, quoted in Lerner, " 'To See Today with the Eyes of Tomorrow.' "

296 *the Breast Cancer Detection and Demonstration Project:* Myles P. Cunningham, "The Breast Cancer Detection Demonstration Project 25 Years Later," *CA: A Cancer Journal for Clinicians* 47, no. 3 (1997): 131–33.

298 *Between 1976 and 1992, enormous parallel trials:* See below for particular studies. Also see Madelon Finkel, ed., *Understanding the Mammography Controversy* (Westport, CT: Praeger, 2005), 101–5.

298 *In Canada, meanwhile, researchers lurched:* A. B. Miller, G. R. Howe, and C. Wall, "The National Study of Breast Cancer Screening Protocol for a Canadian Randomized Controlled Trial of Screening for Breast Cancer in Women," *Clinical Investigative Medicine* 4, nos. 3–4 (1981): 227–58.

298 *Edinburgh was a disaster:* A. Huggins et al., "Edinburgh Trial of Screening for Breast Cancer: Mortality at Seven Years," *Lancet* 335, no. 8684 (1990): 241–46; Denise Donovan et al., "Edinburgh Trial of Screening for Breast Cancer," *Lancet* 335, no. 8695 (1990): 968–69.

298 *The Canadian trial, meanwhile:* Miller, Howe, and Wall, "National Study of Breast Cancer Screening Protocol."

298 For a critical evaluation of the CNBSS, HIP, and Swedish studies, see David Freedman et al., "On the Efficacy of Screening for Breast Cancer," *International Journal of Epidemiology* 33, no. 1 (2004): 43–5.

298 Randomization problems in the Canadian National Breast Screening Study: Curtis J. Mettlin and Charles R. Smart, "The Canadian National Breast Screening Study: An Appraisal and Implications for Early Detection Policy," *Cancer* 72, no. S4 (1993): 1461–65; John C. Bailar III and Brian MacMahon, "Randomization in the Canadian

National Breast Screening Study: A Review for Evidence of Subversion," *Canadian Medical Association Journal* 156, no. 2 (1997): 193–99.

299 *"Suspicion, like beauty"*: Cornelia Baines, *Canadian Medical Association Journal* 157 (August 1, 1997): 249.

299 *"One lesson is clear"*: Norman F. Boyd, "The Review of Randomization in the Canadian National Breast Screening Study: Is the Debate Over?" *Canadian Medical Association Journal* 156, no. 2 (1997): 207–9.

300 *Migration into and out of the city*: See, for instance, *Scandinavian Journal of Gastroenterology* 30 (1995): 33–43.

300 *In 1976, forty-two thousand women enrolled:* Ingvar Andersson et al., "Mammographic Screening and Mortality from Breast Cancer: The Malmö Mammographic Screening Trial," *British Medical Journal* 297, no. 6654 (1988): 943–48.

300 *"There was only one"*: Ingvar Andersson, interview with author, March 2010.

300 *In 1988, at the end of its twelfth year*: Andersson et al., "Mammographic Screening and Mortality." Also Andersson, interview with author.

300 *When the groups were analyzed by age:* Ibid.

301 *In 2002, twenty-six years after the launch of the original*: Lennarth Nyström et al., "Long-Term Effects of Mammography Screening: Updated Overview of the Swedish Randomised Trials," *Lancet* 359, no. 9310 (2002): 909–19.

301 *Its effects, as the statistician Donald Berry describes it*: Donald Berry, interview with author, November 2009.

301 *Berry wrote, "Screening is a lottery"*: "Mammograms Before 50 a Waste of Time," *Science a Go Go,* October 12, 1998, http://www.scienceagogo.com/news/ 19980912094305data_trunc_sys.shtml (accessed December 29, 2009).

302 *"This is a textbook example"*: Malcolm Gladwell, "The Picture Problem: Mammography, Air Power, and the Limits of Looking," *New Yorker,* December 13, 2004.

303 *"All photographs are accurate"*: Richard Avedon, *An Autobiography* (New York: Random House, 1993); Richard Avedon, *Evidence, 1944–1994* (New York: Random House, 1994).

304 *"As the decade ended," Bruce Chabner*: Bruce Chabner, interview with author, August 2009.

STAMP

305 *Then did I beat them:* 2 Samuel 22:43 (King James Version).

306 *Cancer therapy is like beating the dog*: Anna Deveare Smith, *Let Me Down Easy,* script and monologue, December 2009.

306 *"If a man die"*: William Carlos Williams, *The Collected Poems of William Carlos Williams: 1939–1962* (New York: New Directions Publishing, 1991), 2: 334.

306 *In his poignant memoir of his mother's illness:* David Rieff, *Swimming in a Sea of Death: A Son's Memoir* (New York: Simon & Schuster, 2008), 6–10.

306 *"Like so many doctors"*: Ibid., 8.

308 *"To say this was a time of unreal"*: Abraham Verghese, *My Own Country: A Doctor's Story of a Town and Its People in the Age of AIDS* (New York: Simon & Schuster, 1994), 24.

308 *"There seemed to be little that medicine could not do"*: Ibid., 24.

309 *E. Donnall Thomas, had shown that bone marrow:* E. Donnall Thomas, "Bone Marrow

Transplantation from the Personal Viewpoint," *International Journal of Hematology* 81 (2005): 89–93.

309 *In Thomas's initial trial at Seattle*: E. Thomas et al., "Bone Marrow Transplantation," *New England Journal of Medicine* 292, no. 16 (1975): 832–43.

310 *"We have a cure for breast cancer"*: Craig Henderson, interview with Richard Rettig, quoted in Richard Rettig et al., *False Hope: Bone Marrow Transplantation for Breast Cancer* (Oxford: Oxford University Press, 2007), 29.

311 *"It was an intensely competitive place"*: Robert Mayer, interview with author, July 2008.

311 *In 1982, Frei recruited William Peters*: Shannon Brownlee, "Bad Science and Breast Cancer," *Discover*, August 2002.

311 *In the fall of 1983, he invited Howard Skipper*: William Peters, interview with author, May 2009.

312 *a "seminal event"*: Ibid.

312 *George Canellos, for one, was wary*: George Canellos, interview with author, March 2008.

312 *"We were going to swing and go for the ring"*: Brownlee, "Bad Science and Breast Cancer."

312 *The first patient to "change history" with STAMP*: Ibid., and Peters, interview with author.

313 *"The ultimate trial of chemotherapeutic intensification"*: Peters, interview with author.

314 *"Suddenly, everything broke loose"*: Ibid.

314 *The woman was thirty-six years old*: Ibid.

314 *"the most beautiful remission you could have imagined"*: Ibid.

315 *In March 1981, in the journal* Lancet: Kenneth B. Hymes et al., "Kaposi's Sarcoma in Homosexual Men—a Report of Eight Cases," *Lancet* 318, no. 8247 (1981): 598–600.

316 *"gay compromise syndrome"*: Robert O. Brennan and David T. Durack, "Gay Compromise Syndrome," *Lancet* 318, no. 8259 (1981): 1338–39.

316 *In July 1982, with an understanding of the cause*: "July 27, 1982: A Name for the Plague," *Time*, March 30, 2003.

316 *In a trenchant essay written as a reply*: Susan Sontag, *Illness as Metaphor and AIDS and Its Metaphors* (New York: Picador, 1990).

317 *For Volberding, and for many of his earliest*: See ACT UP Oral History Project, http://www.actuporalhistory.org/.

317 *Volberding borrowed something more ineffable*: Arthur J. Amman et al., *The AIDS Epidemic in San Francisco: The Medical Response, 1981–1884*, vol. 3 (Berkeley: Regional Oral History Office, the Bancroft Library, University of California, Berkeley, 1997).

317 *"What we did here"*: Ibid.

318 *In January 1982, as AIDS cases boomed*: "Building Blocks in the Battle on AIDS," *New York Times*, March 30, 1997; Randy Shilts, *And the Band Played On* (New York: St. Martin's Press).

318 *In January 1983, Luc Montagnier's group*: Shilts, *And the Band Played On*, 219; F. Barré-Sinoussi et al. "Isolation of a T-Lymphotropic Retrovirus from a Patient at Risk for Acquired Immune Deficiency Syndrome (AIDS)," *Science* 220, no. 4599 (1983): 868–71.

318 *Gallo also found a retrovirus*: Mikulas Popovic et al., "Detection, Isolation, and Continuous Production of Cytopathic Retroviruses (HTLV-III) from Patients with AIDS and Pre-AIDS," *Science* 224, no. 4648 (1984): 497–500; Robert C. Gallo et

al., "Frequent Detection and Isolation of Cytopathic Retroviruses (HTLV-III) from Patients with AIDS and at Risk for AIDS," *Science* 224, no. 4648 (1984): 500–503.

318 *On April 23, 1984, Margaret Heckler:* James Kinsella, *Covering the Plague: AIDS and the American Media* (Piscataway, NJ: Rutgers University Press, 1992), 84.

318 *In the spring of 1987:* Steven Epstein, *Impure Science: AIDS, Activism, and the Politics of Knowledge* (Berkeley: University of California Press, 1998), 219.

318 *"genocide by neglect":* Ibid., 221.

318 *"Many of us who live in daily terror":* "The F.D.A.'s Callous Response to AIDS," *New York Times,* March 23, 1987.

318 *"Drugs into bodies":* Raymond A. Smith and Patricia D. Siplon, *Drugs into Bodies: Global AIDS Treatment Activism* (Santa Barbara, CA: Greenwood Publishing Group, 2006).

318 *"The FDA is fucked-up":* "Acting Up: March 10, 1987," *Ripples of Hope: Great American Civil Rights Speeches,* ed. Josh Gottheimer (New York: Basic Civitas Books, 2003), 392.

318 *"Double-blind studies":* "F.D.A.'s Callous Response to AIDS," *New York Times.*

318 *He concluded, "AIDS sufferers":* Ibid.

320 *By the winter of 1984, thirty-two women:* Peters, interview with author.

320 *"There was so much excitement within the cancer community":* Donald Berry, interview with author, November 2009.

320 *Peters flew up from Duke to Boston:* Peters, interview with author.

The Map and the Parachute

321 *Oedipus: What is the rite of purification?:* Sophocles, *Oedipus the King.*

321 *Transplanters, as one oncologist:* Craig Henderson, quoted in Brownlee, "Bad Science and Breast Cancer."

321 Nelene Fox and bone marrow transplantation: See Michael S. Lief and Harry M. Caldwell, *And the Walls Came Tumbling Down: Closing Arguments that Changed the Way We Live, from Protecting Free Speech to Winning Women's Suffrage to Defending the Right to Die* (New York: Simon & Schuster, 2004), 299–354; "$89 Million Awarded Family Who Sued H.M.O.," *New York Times,* December 30, 1993.

322 *On June 19, a retinue:* Lief and Caldwell, *And the Walls Came Tumbling Down,* 310.

322 *"You marketed this coverage to her":* Ibid., 307.

323 *In August 1992, Nelene Fox:* Ibid., 309.

323 *"The dose-limiting barrier":* S. Ariad and W. R. Bezwoda, "High-Dose Chemotherapy: Therapeutic Potential in the Age of Growth Factor Support," *Israel Journal of Medical Sciences* 28, no. 6 (1992): 377–85.

323 *In Johannesburg, more than 90 percent:* W. R. Bezwoda, L. Seymour, and R. D. Dansey, "High-Dose Chemotherapy with Hematopoietic Rescue as Primary Treatment for Metastatic Breast Cancer: A Randomized Trial," *Journal of Clinical Oncology* 13, no. 10 (1995): 2483–89.

324 *On April 22, eleven months after:* Lief and Caldwell, *And the Walls Came Tumbling Down,* 309.

324 *In 1993 alone:* Papers were assessed on www.pubmed.org.

324 *"If all you have is a cold or the flu":* Lief and Caldwell, *And the Walls Came Tumbling Down,* 234.

324 *On the morning of December 28, 1993:* Ibid.

324 *That evening, it returned a verdict:* "$89 Million Awarded Family," *New York Times.*

325 *In Massachusetts, Charlotte Turner:* "Cancer Patient's Kin Sues Fallon" and "Coverage Denied for Marrow Transplant," *Worcester (MA) Telegram & Gazette,* December 7, 1995; Erin Dominique Williams and Leo Van Der Reis, *Health Care at the Abyss: Managed Care vs. the Goals of Medicine* (Buffalo, NY: William S. Hein Publishing, 1997), 3.

325 *Between 1988 and 2002:* See Richard Rettig et al., eds., *False Hope: Bone Marrow Transplantation for Breast Cancer* (New York: Oxford University Press, 2007), 85, and Table 3.2.

325 *"complicated, costly and potentially dangerous":* Bruce E. Brockstein and Stephanie F. Williams, "High-Dose Chemotherapy with Autologous Stem Cell Rescue for Breast Cancer: Yesterday, Today and Tomorrow," *Stem Cells* 14, no. 1 (1996): 79–89.

325 *Between 1991 and 1999, roughly forty thousand:* JoAnne Zujewski, Anita Nelson, and Jeffrey Abrams, "Much Ado about Not . . . Enough Data," *Journal of the National Cancer Institute* 90 (1998): 200–209. Also see Rettig et al., *False Hope,* 137.

326 *"Transplants, transplants, everywhere":* Robert Mayer, interview with author, July 2008.

326 *As Bezwoda presented the data:* W. R. Bezwoda, "High Dose Chemotherapy with Haematopoietic Rescue in Breast Cancer," *Hematology and Cell Therapy* 41, no. 2 (1999): 58–65. Also see Werner Bezwoda, plenary session, American Society of Clinical Oncology meeting, 1999 (video recordings available at www.asco.org).

326 *three other trials presented that afternoon:* Ibid.

326 *At Duke, embarrassingly enough:* Ibid.

326 *"even a modest improvement":* Ibid.

326 *A complex and tangled trial from Sweden:* Ibid.

326 *"My goal here," one discussant began:* Ibid.

327 *"People who like to transplant will continue to transplant":* "Conference Divided over High-Dose Breast Cancer Treatment," *New York Times,* May 19, 1999.

327 Investigation of Bezwoda's breast cancer study: Raymond B. Weiss et al., "High-Dose Chemotherapy for High-Risk Primary Breast Cancer: An On-Site Review of the Bezwoda Study," *Lancet* 355, no. 9208 (2000): 999–1003.

328 *Another patient record, tracked back to its origin:* "Bezwoda," Kate Barry (producer), archived in video format at http://beta.mnet.co.za/Carteblanche, M-Net TV Africa (March 19, 2000).

328 *"I have committed a serious breach of scientific honesty":* "Breast Cancer Study Results on High-Dose Chemotherapy Falsified," Imaginis, February 9, 2000, http://www .imaginis.com/breasthealth/news/news2.09.00.asp (accessed January 2, 2010).

328 *"By the late 1990s, the romance was already over":* Robert Mayer, interview with author.

328 *Maggie Keswick Jencks:* Maggie Keswick Jencks, *A View from the Front Line* (London, 1995).

329 *"There you are, the future patient":* Ibid., 9.

330 *In May 1997, exactly eleven years after:* John C. Bailar and Heather L. Gornik, "Cancer Undefeated," *New England Journal of Medicine* 336, no. 22 (1997): 1569–74.

332 *Pressed on public television, he begrudgingly conceded:* "Treatment vs. Prevention," *NewsHour with Jim Lehrer,* May 29, 1997, PBS, transcript available at http://www.pbs .org/newshour/bb/health/may97/cancer_5-29.html (accessed January 2, 2010).

332 *"Cancer' is, in truth, a variety of diseases"*: Barnett S. Kramer and Richard D. Klausner, "Grappling with Cancer—Defeatism versus the Reality of Progress," *New England Journal of Medicine* 337, no. 13 (1997): 931–35.

PART FIVE:
"A DISTORTED VERSION OF OUR NORMAL SELVES"

335 *It is vain to speak of cures:* Robert Burton, *The Anatomy of Melancholy* (: C. Armstrong and Son, 1893), 235.

335 *You can't do experiments to see:* Samuel S. Epstein, *Cancer-Gate: How to Win the Losing Cancer War* (Amityville, NY: Baywood Publishing Company, 2005), 57.

335 *What can be the "why" of these happenings?:* Peyton Rous, "The Challenge to Man of the Neoplastic Cell," *Nobel Lectures, Physiology or Medicine, 1963–1970* (Amsterdam: Elsevier Publishing Company, 1972).

"A unitary cause"

340 *As early as 1858:* Rudolf Virchow, *Lecture XX, Cellular Pathology as Based upon Physiological and Pathological Histology,* trans. Frank Chance (London: Churchill, 1860). The passage on irritation appears on page 488 of the translated version: "A pathological tumor in man forms . . . where any pathological irritation occurs . . . all of them depend upon a proliferation of cells."

340 *Walther Flemming, a biologist working in Prague:* Neidhard Paweletz, "Walther Flemming: Pioneer of Mitosis Research," *Nature Reviews Molecular Cell Biology* 2 (2001): 72–75.

340 *It was Virchow's former assistant David Paul von Hansemann:* Leon P. Bignold, Brian L. D. Coghlan, and Hubertus P. A. Jersmann, eds., *Contributions to Oncology: Context, Comments and Translations* (Basel: Birkhauser Verlag, 2007), 83–90.

341 *Boveri devised a highly unnatural experiment*: Theodor Boveri, *Concerning the Origin of Malignant Tumours by Theodor Boveri,* translated and annotated by Henry Harris (New York: Cold Spring Harbor Press, 2006). This is a reprint and new translation of the original text.

342 *"unitary cause of carcinoma"*: Ibid., 56.

342 *not "an unnatural group of different maladies"*: Ibid., 56.

342 *In 1910, four years before Boveri had published his theory:* Peyton Rous, "A Transmissible Avian Neoplasm (Sarcoma of the Common Fowl)," *Journal of Experimental Medicine* 12, no. 5 (1910): 696–705; Peyton Rous, "A Sarcoma of the Fowl Transmissible by an Agent Separable from the Tumor Cells," *Journal of Experimental Medicine* 13, no. 4 (1911): 397–411.

342 *In 1909, a year before:* Karl Landsteiner et al., "La transmission de la paralysie infantile aux singes," *Compt. Rend. Soc. Biologie* 67 (1909).

343 *In the early 1860s, working alone:* Gregor Mendel, "Versuche über Plfanzenhybriden," *Verhandlungen des Naturforschenden Vereines in Brünn. IV für das Jahr 1865, Abhandlungen* (1866): 3–47. English translation available at http://www.esp.org/foundations/genetics/classical/gm-65.pdf (accessed January 2, 2010). Also see Robin

Marantz Henig, *The Monk in the Garden: The Lost and Found Genius of Gregor Mendel, the Father of Genetics* (Boston: Mariner Books, 2001), 142.

343 *decades later, in 1909, botanists:* Wilhelm Ludwig Johannsen, *Elemente der Exakten Erblichkeitlehre* (1913), http://caliban.mpiz-koeln.mpg.de/johannsen/elemente/index.html (accessed January 2, 2010).

344 *In 1910, Thomas Hunt Morgan:* See T. H. Morgan, "Chromosomes and Heredity," *American Naturalist* 44 (1910): 449–96. Also see Muriel Lederman, "Research Note: Genes on Chromosomes: the Conversion of Thomas Hunt Morgan," *Journal of the History of Biology* 22, no. 1 (1989): 163–76.

344 *The third vision of the "gene":* Oswald T. Avery et al., "Studies on the Chemical Nature of the Substance Inducing Transformation of Pneumococcal Types: Induction of Transformation by a Deoxyribonucleic Acid Fraction Isolated from Pneumococcus Type III," *Journal of Experimental Medicine* 79 (1944): 137–58.

345 *George Beadle, Thomas Morgan's student:* See George Beadle, "Genes and Chemical Reactions in Neurospora," *Nobel Lectures, Physiology or Medicine, 1942–1962* (Amsterdam: Elsevier Publishing Company, 1964), 587–99.

346 *In the mid-1950s, biologists termed:* See for instance Francis Crick, "Ideas on Protein Synthesis," October 1956, Francis Crick Papers, National Library of Medicine. Crick's statement of the central dogma proposed that RNA could be back converted as a special case, but that proteins could never be back converted into DNA or RNA. Reverse transcription was thus left as a possibility.

347 *In 1872, Hilário de Gouvêa:* A. N. Monteiro and R. Waizbort, "The Accidental Cancer Geneticist: Hilário de Gouvêa and Hereditary Retinoblastoma," *Cancer Biology and Therapy* 6, no. 5 (2007): 811–13.

348 *In 1928, Hermann Joseph Muller:* See Hermann Muller, "The Production of Mutations," *Nobel Lectures, Physiology or Medicine, 1942–1962* (Amsterdam: Elsevier Publishing Company, 1964).

348 *"the doctor may then want to call in his geneticist friends for consultation!":* Thomas Morgan, "The Relation of Genetics to Physiology and Medicine," *Nobel Lectures, Physiology or Medicine 1922–1941* (Amsterdam: Elsevier Publishing Company, 1965).

Under the Lamps of Viruses

349 *Unidentified flying objects, abominable snowmen: Medical World News*, January 11, 1974.

349 *The biochemist Arthur Kornberg once joked:* Arthur Kornberg, "Ten Commandments: Lessons from the Enzymology of DNA Replication," *Journal of Bacteriology* 182, no. 13 (2000): 3613–18.

351 *Temin was cooking up an unusual experiment:* See Howard Temin and Harry Rubin, "Characteristics of an Assay for Rous Sarcoma Virus," *Virology* 6 (1958): 669–83.

351 *"The virus, in some structural as well as functional sense":* Howard Temin, quoted in Howard M. Temin et al., *The DNA Provirus: Howard Temin's Scientific Legacy* (Washington, DC: ASM Press, 1995), xviii.

352 *"Temin had an inkling":* J. Michael Bishop, interview with author, August 2009.

352 *"The hypothesis":* J. Michael Bishop in Temin et al., *DNA Provirus*, 81.

353 *Mizutani was a catastrophe:* See Robert Weinberg, *Racing to the Beginning of the Road* (New York: Bantam, 1997), 61.

353 *At MIT, in Boston:* Ibid., 61–65.

353 *"It was all very dry biochemistry":* Ibid., 64.

354 *In their respective papers:* David Baltimore, "RNA-Dependent DNA Polymerase in Virions of RNA Tumor Viruses," *Nature* 226, no. 5252 (1970): 1209–11; and H. M Temin and S. Mizutani, "RNA-Dependent DNA Polymerase in Virions of Rous Sarcoma Virus," *Nature* 226, no. 5252 (1970): 1211–13.

355 *Spiegelman raced off to prove:* Weinberg, *Racing to the Beginning,* 70.

355 *"It became his single-minded preoccupation":* Robert Weinberg, interview with author, January 2009.

356 *"The hoped-for human virus":* Weinberg, *Racing to the Beginning,* 83.

"The hunting of the sarc"

357 *For the Snark* was *a Boojum, you see:* Lewis Carroll, *The Hunting of the Snark: An Agony in Eight Fits* (New York: Macmillan, 1914), 53.

358 *By analyzing the genes altered in these mutant viruses:* For a review of Duesberg's and Vogt's contributions, see G. Steven Martin, "The Hunting of the Src," *Nature Reviews Molecular Cell Biology* 2, no. 6 (2001): 467–75.

358 *A chance discovery in Ray Erikson's laboratory:* J. S. Brugge and R. L. Erikson, "Identification of a Transformation-Specific Antigen Induced by an Avian Sarcoma Virus," *Nature* 269, no. 5626 (1977): 346–48.

360 *other scientists nicknamed the project:* See, for instance, Martin, "The Hunting of the Src."

361 *"Src," Varmus wrote in a letter:* Harold Varmus to Dominique Stehelin, February 3, 1976, Harold Varmus papers, National Library of Medicine archives. Also see Stehelin et al., "DNA Related to the Transforming Genes of Avian Sarcoma Viruses Is Present in Normal DNA," *Nature* 260, no. 5547 (March 1976): 170–73.

362 *"Nature," Rous wrote in 1966:* Peyton Rous, "The Challenge to Man of the Neoplastic Cell," *Nobel Lectures, Physiology or Medicine, 1963–1970* (Amsterdam: Elsevier Publishing Company, 1972).

363 *"We have not slain our enemy":* Harold Varmus, "Retroviruses and Oncogenes I," *Nobel Lectures, Physiology or Medicine, 1981–1990,* ed. Jan Lindsten (Singapore: World Scientific Publishing Co., 1993).

The Wind in the Trees

364 *The fine, fine wind:* D. H. Lawrence, "The Song of a Man Who Has Come Through," *Penguin Book of First World War Poetry,* ed. John Silkin (New York: Penguin Classics, 1996), 213.

365 *Rowley's specialty was studying:* Janet Rowley, "Chromosomes in Leukemia and Lymphoma," *Seminars in Hematology* 15, no. 3 (1978): 301–19.

365 *In the late 1950s, Peter Nowell:* P. C. Nowell and D. Hungerford, *Science* 142 (1960): 1497.

366 *In 1969, Knudson moved:* Al Knudson, interview with author, July 2009.

367 *"The number two," he recalled:* Ibid.

368 *Knudson's two-hit theory:* A. Knudson, "Mutation and Cancer: Statistical Study of Retinoblastoma," *Proceedings of the National Academy of Sciences of the United States of America* 68, no. 4 (1971): 820–23.

368 *"Two classes of genes are apparently critical":* A. Knudson, "The Genetics of Childhood Cancer," *Bulletin du Cancer* 75, no. 1 (1988): 135–38.

369 *"jammed accelerators" and "missing brakes":* J. Michael Bishop, in Howard M. Temin et al., *The DNA Provirus: Howard Temin's Scientific Legacy* (Washington, DC: ASM Press, 1995), 89.

A Risky Prediction

370 *They see only their:* Plato, *The Republic of Plato,* Benjamin Jowett, trans. (Oxford: Clarendon Press, 1908), 220.

370 *"Isolating such a gene":* Robert Weinberg, interview with author, January 2009.

371 *"The chair of the department":* Ibid.

371 *Clarity came to him one morning:* Ibid.

373 *In the summer of 1979, Chiaho Shih:* Ibid.

374 *"If we were going to trap a real oncogene":* Ibid. Also, Cliff Tabin, interview with author, December 2009.

374 *In 1982, Weinberg:* C. Shih and R. A. Weinberg (1982), "Isolation of a Transforming Sequence from a Human Bladder Carcinoma Cell Line," *Cell* 29: 161–169. Also see M. Goldfarb, K. Shimizu, M. Perucho, and M. Wigler, "Isolation and Preliminary Characterization of a Human Transforming Gene from T24 Bladder Carcinoma Cells," *Nature* 296 (1982): 404–9. Also see S. Pulciani et al., "Oncogenes in Human Tumor Cell Lines: Molecular Cloning of a Transforming Gene from Human Bladder Carcinoma Cells," *Proceedings of the National Academy of Sciences. USA* 79: 2845–49.

375 *"Once we had cloned":* Robert Weinberg, *Racing to the Beginning of the Road* (New York: Bantam, 1997), 165.

375 *Ray Erikson traveled to Washington:* Ray Erikson, interview with author, October 2009.

375 *"I don't remember any enthusiasm":* Ibid.

376 *"How can one capture genes":* Robert Weinberg, *One Renegade Cell* (New York: Basic Books, 1999), 74.

376 *"We knew where Rb lived":* Weinberg, interview with author.

377 *Dryja began his hunt for Rb:* Thaddeus Dryja, interview with author, November 2008.

378 *"I stored the tumors obsessively":* Ibid.

378 *"It was at that moment":* Ibid.

380 *"We have isolated [a human gene]":* Stephen H. Friend et al., "A Human DNA Segment with Properties of the Gene that Predisposes to Retinoblastoma and Osteosarcoma," *Nature* 323, no. 6089 (1986): 643–46.

380 *When scientists tested the gene isolated by Dryja:* D. W. Yandell et al., "Oncogenic Point Mutations in the Human Retinoblastoma Gene: Their Application to Genetic Counseling," *New England Journal of Medicine* 321, no. 25 (1989): 1689–95.

380 *Its chief function is to bind to several other proteins:* See for instance James A. DeCaprio, "How the Rb Tumor Suppressor Structure and Function was Revealed by the Study of Adenovirus and SV40," *Virology* 384, no. 2 (2009): 274–84.

380 *a horde of other oncogenes and anti-oncogenes:* George Klein, "The Approaching Era of the Tumor Suppressor Genes," *Science* 238, no. 4833 (1987): 1539–45.

382 *Philip Leder's team at Harvard engineered:* Timothy A. Stewart, Paul K. Pattengale, and Philip Leder, "Spontaneous Mammary Adenocarcinomas in Transgenic Mice That Carry and Express MTV/myc Fusion Genes," *Cell* 38 (1984): 627–37.

382 *In 1988, he successfully applied for a patent:* Daniel J. Kevles, "Of Mice & Money: The Story of the World's First Animal Patent," *Daedalus* 131, no. 2 (2002): 78.

382 *"The active* myc *gene does not appear to be sufficient":* Stewart, Pattengale, and Leder, "Spontaneous Mammary Adenocarcinomas," 627–37.

383 *Leder created a second OncoMouse:* E. Sinn et al., "Coexpression of MMTV/v-Ha-ras and MMTV/c-myc Genes in Transgenic Mice: Synergistic Action of Oncogenes in Vivo," *Cell* 49, no. 4 (1987): 465–75.

383 *"Cancer genetics," as the geneticist Cliff Tabin:* Tabin, interview with author, November 2009.

The Hallmarks of Cancer

384 *I do not wish to achieve immortality:* Eric Lax, *Woody Allen and His Comedy* (London: Elm Tree Books, 1976).

385 *"The four molecular alterations accumulated":* B. Vogelstein et al., "Genetic Alterations During Colorectal-Tumor Development," *New England Journal of Medicine* 319, no. 9 (1988): 525–32.

387 *A tumor could thus "acquire" its own blood supply:* Judah Folkman, "Angiogenesis," *Annual Review of Medicine* 57 (2006): 1–18.

387 *Folkman's Harvard colleague Stan Korsmeyer:* W. B. Graninger et al., "Expression of Bcl-2 and Bcl-2-Ig Fusion Transcripts in Normal and Neoplastic Cells," *Journal of Clinical Investigation* 80, no. 5 (1987): 1512–15. Also see Stanley J. Korsemeyer, "Regulators of Cell Death," 11, no. 3 (1995): 101–5.

390 *In the fall of 1999, Robert Weinberg attended:* Robert Weinberg, interview with author, January 2009.

390 *In January 2000, a few months after their walk:* Douglas Hanahan and Robert A. Weinberg, "The Hallmarks of Cancer," *Cell* 100, no. 1 (2000): 57–70.

390 *"We discuss . . . rules that govern":* Ibid.

392 *"With holistic clarity of mechanism":* Ibid. Also see Bruce Chabner, "Biological Basis for Cancer Treatment," *Annals of Internal Medicine* 118, no. 8 (1993): 633–37.

PART SIX:
THE FRUITS OF LONG ENDEAVORS

393 *We are really reaping the fruits:* Mike Gorman, letter to Mary Lasker, September 6, 1985, Mary Lasker Papers.

393 *The National Cancer Institute, which has overseen:* "To Fight Cancer, Know the Enemy," *New York Times,* August 5, 2009.

393 *The more perfect a power is:* See for instance St. Aquinas, *Commentary on the Book of Causes,* trans. Vincent Guagliardo et al. (CUA Press, 1996), 9.

"No one had labored in vain"

395 *Have you met Jimmy?:* Jimmy Fund solicitation pamphlet, 1963.

395 *In the summer of 1997:* "Einar Gustafson, 65, 'Jimmy' of Child Cancer Fund, Dies," *New York Times,* January 24, 2001; "Jimmy Found," *People,* June 8, 1998.

395 *Only Sidney Farber had known:* Phyllis Clauson, interview with author, 2009.

395 *"Jimmy's story," she recalled:* Ibid.

396 *A few weeks later, in January 1998:* Karen Cummings, interview with author, 2009.

396 *And so it was in May 1998:* Ibid.

397 *"Everything has changed":* Clauson, interview with author.

398 *"How to overcome him became":* Max Lerner, *Wrestling with the Angel: A Memoir of My Triumph over Illness* (New York: Touchstone, 1990), 26.

398 *The poet Jason Shinder wrote, "Cancer":* "The Lure of Death," *New York Times,* December 24, 2008.

400 *"I've made a long voyage":* Maxwell E. Perkins, "The Last Letter of Thomas Wolfe and the Reply to It," *Harvard Library Bulletin,* Autumn 1947, 278.

401 *In 2005, an avalanche of papers:* See, for example, Peter Boyle and Jacques Ferlay, "Mortality and Survival in Breast and Colorectal Cancer," *Nature Reviews and Clinical Oncology* 2 (2005): 424–25; Itsuro Yoshimi and S. Kaneko, "Comparison of Cancer Mortality (All Malignant Neoplasms) in Five Countries: France, Italy, Japan, UK and USA from the WHO Mortality Database (1960–2000)," *Japanese Journal of Clinical Oncology* 35, no. 1 (2005): 48–51; Alison L. Jones, "Reduction in Mortality from Breast Cancer," *British Medical Journal* 330, no. 7485 (2005): 205–6.

401 *The mortality for nearly every major:* Eric J. Kort et al., "The Decline in U.S. Cancer Mortality in People Born Since 1925," *Cancer Research* 69 (2009): 6500–6505.

401 *mortality had declined by about 1 percent:* Ibid. Also see Ahmedin Jemal et al., "Cancer Statistics, 2005," *CA: A Cancer Journal for Clinicians* 55 (2005): 10–30; "Annual Report to the Nation on the Status of Cancer, 1975–2002," *Journal of the National Cancer Institute,* October 5, 2005.

401 *between 1990 and 2005, the cancer-specific:* Ibid.

401 *more than half a million American men and women:* American Cancer Society, *Cancer Facts & Figures 2008* (Atlanta: American Cancer Society, 2008), 6.

402 *Donald Berry, a statistician in Houston:* Donald A. Berry, "Effect of Screening and Adjuvant Therapy on Mortality from Breast Cancer," *New England Journal of Medicine* 353, no. 17 (2005): 1784–92.

402 *"No one," as Berry said:* Donald Berry, interview with author, November 2009.

403 *Mary Lasker died of heart failure:* "Mary W. Lasker, Philanthropist for Medical Research, Dies at 93," *New York Times,* February 23, 1994.

403 *the cancer geneticist Ed Harlow captured:* Ed Harlow, "An Introduction to the Puzzle," *Cold Spring Harbor Symposia on Quantitative Biology* 59 (1994): 709–23.

404 *In the winter of 1945, Vannevar Bush:* Vannevar Bush, *Science the Endless Frontier: A Report to the President by Vannevar Bush, Director of the Office of Scientific Research and Development, July 1945* (Washington, D.C.: U.S. Government Printing Office, 1945).

NOTES

New Drugs for Old Cancers

405 *In the story of Patroclus:* Louise Gluck, *The Triumph of Achilles* (New York: Ecco Press, 1985), 16.

405 *The perfect therapy has not been developed:* Bruce Chabner letter to Rose Kushner, Rose Kushner Papers, Box 50.

408 *In the summer of 1985:* Laurent Degos, "The History of Acute Promyelocytic Leukaemia," *British Journal of Haematology* 122, no. 4 (2003): 539–53; Raymond P. Warrell et al., "Acute Promyelocytic Leukemia," *New England Journal of Medicine* 329, no. 3 (1993): 177–89; Huang Meng-er et al., "Use of All-*Trans* Retinoic Acid in the Treatment of Acute Promyelocytic Leukemia," *Blood* 72 (1988): 567–72.

409 *"The nucleus became larger":* Meng-er et al., "Use of All-*Trans* Retinoic Acid."

410 *In 1982, a postdoctoral scientist:* Robert Bazell, *Her-2: The Making of Herceptin, a Revolutionary Treatment for Breast Cancer* (New York: Random House, 1998), 17.

411 *"It would have been an overnight test":* Ibid.

411 *although Padhy's discovery was published:* Lakshmi Charon Padhy et al., "Identification of a Phosphoprotein Specifically Induced by the Transforming DNA of Rat Neuroblastomas," *Cell* 28, no. 4 (1982): 865–71.

A City of Strings

412 *In Ersilia, to establish the relationships:* Italo Calvino, *Invisible Cities* (Boston: Houghton Mifflin Harcourt, 1978), 76.

412 *In his book* Invisible Cities: Ibid.

413 *In the summer of 1984:* Robert Bazell, *Her-2: The Making of Herceptin, a Revolutionary Treatment for Breast Cancer* (New York: Random House, 1998).

414 *In 1982, Genentech unveiled the first:* "A New Insulin Given Approval for Use in U.S.," *New York Times,* October 30, 1982.

414 *in 1984, it produced a clotting factor:* "Genentech Corporate Chronology," http://www .gene.com/gene/about/corporate/history/timeline.html (accessed January 30, 2010).

414 *in 1985, it created a recombinant version:* Ibid.

414 *It was under the aegis:* L. Coussens et al., "3 Groups Discovered the Neu Homolog (Her-2, Also Called Erb-b2)," *Science* 230 (1985): 1132–39. Also see T. Yamamoto et al., *Nature* 319 (1986): 230–34, and C. King et al., *Science* 229 (1985): 974–76.

415 *In the summer of 1986:* Bazell, *Her-2,* and Dennis Slamon, interview with author, April 2010.

415 *Dennis Slamon, a UCLA oncologist:* Ibid.

415 *a "velvet jackhammer":* Eli Dansky, "Dennis Slamon: From New Castle to New Science," *SU2C Mag,* http://www.standup2cancer.org/node/194 (accessed January 24, 2010).

415 *"a murderous resolve":* Ibid.

415 *In Chicago, Slamon had performed a series:* See, for example, I. S. Chen et al., "The x Gene Is Essential for HTLV Replication," *Science* 229, no. 4708 (1985): 54–58; W. Wachsman et al., "HTLV x Gene Mutants Exhibit Novel Transcription Regulatory Phenotypes," *Science* 235, no. 4789 (1987): 647–77; C. T. Fang et al., "Detection of Antibodies to Human T-Lymphotropic Virus Type 1 (HTLV-1)," *Transfusion* 28, no. 2 (1988): 179–83.

415 *If Ullrich sent him the DNA probes:* Details of the Ullrich and Slamon collaboration are outlined in Bazell, *Her-2,* and from Slamon, interview with author.

416 *In a few months:* D. Slamon et al., "Human Breast Cancer: Correlation of Relapse and Survival with Amplification of the Her-2/Neu Oncogene," *Science* 235 (1987): 177–82.

417 *In the mid-1970s, two immunologists at Cambridge University:* See *Nobel Lectures, Physiology or Medicine, 1981–1990,* ed. Jan Lindsten (Singapore: World Scientific Publishing, 1993).

418 *"allergic to cancer":* Merrill Goozner, *The $800 Million Pill: The Truth Behind the Cost of New Drugs* (Berkeley: University of California Press, 2004), 195.

418 *Drained and dejected:* Ibid.

418 *"Nobody gave a shit":* Bazell, *Her-2,* 49.

419 *"When I was finished with all that":* Ibid. Also Barbara Bradfield, interview with author, July 2008.

419 *But there was more river to ford:* Ibid.

420 *"His tone changed," she recalled:* Ibid.

420 *"I was at the end of my road":* Ibid

420 *"Survivors look back and see omens":* Joan Didion, *The Year of Magical Thinking* (New York: Vintage, 2006), 152.

420 *On a warm August morning in 1992:* Bradfield, interview with author. Details of the trial and the treatment are from Bradfield's interview, from Bazell's *Her-2,* and from Slamon, interview with author, April 2010.

Drugs, Bodies, and Proof

423 *Dying people don't have time or energy:* "Dying for Compassion," *Breast Cancer Action Newsletter* 31 (August 1995).

423 *It seemed as if we had:* Musa Mayer, *Breast Cancer Action Newsletter* 80 (February/ March 2004).

423 *"True success happens":* *Breast Cancer Action Newsletter* 32 (October 1995).

424 *The number of women enrolled in these trials:* Robert Bazell, *Her-2: The Making of Herceptin, a Revolutionary Treatment for Breast Cancer* (New York: Random House, 1998), 160–80.

424 *"We do not provide . . . compassionate use":* Ibid., 117.

424 *"If you start making exceptions":* Ibid., 127.

424 *"Why do women dying of breast cancer":* "Dying for Compassion," *Breast Cancer Action Newsletter.*

424 *"Scientific uncertainty is no excuse":* Charlotte Brody et al., "Rachel's Daughters, Searching for the Causes of Breast Cancer: A Light-Saraf-Evans Production Community Action & Resource Guide," http://www.wmm.com/filmCatalog/study/ rachelsdaughters.pdf (accessed January 31, 2010).

424 *Marti Nelson, for one, certainly could not:* Marti Nelson's case and its aftermath are described in Bazell, *Her-2.*

427 *On Sunday, May 17:* Bruce A. Chabner, "ASCO 1998: A Commentary," *Oncologist* 3, no. 4 (1998): 263–66; D. J. Slamon et al., "Addition of Herceptin to First-Line Chemotherapy for HER-2 Overexpressing Metastatic Breast Cancer Markedly Increases Anti-Cancer Activity: A Randomized, Multinational Controlled Phase

III Trial (abstract 377)," *Proceedings of the American Society of Clinical Oncology 16* (1998): 377.

427 *In the pivotal 648 study:* Slamon et al., "Addition of Herceptin to First-Line Chemotherapy," 377.

428 *In 2003, two enormous multinational studies:* Romond et al. and Piccart-Gebhart et al., *New England Journal of Medicine* 353 (2005): 1659–84.

428 *"The results," one oncologist wrote:* Gabriel Hortobagyi, "Trastuzumab in the treatment of breast cancer," editorial, *New England Journal of Medicine,* 353, no. 16 (2005): 1734.

428 *"The company," Robert Bazell, the journalist:* Bazell, *Her-2,* 180–82.

A Four-Minute Mile

430 *The nontoxic curative compound:* James F. Holland, "Hopes for Tomorrow versus Realities of Today: Therapy and Prognosis in Acute Lymphocytic Leukemia of Childhood," *Pediatrics* 45:191–93.

430 *Why, it is asked, does the supply of new miracle drugs:* Lewis Thomas, *The Lives of a Cell* (New York: Penguin, 1978), 115.

430 *This abnormality, the so-called Philadelphia chromosome:* John M. Goldman and Junia V. Melo, "Targeting the BCR-ABL Tyrosine Kinase in Chronic Myeloid Leukemia," *New England Journal of Medicine* 344, no. 14 (2001): 1084–86.

431 *The identity of the gene:* Annelies de Klein et al., "A Cellular Oncogene Is Translocated to the Philadelphia Chromosome in Chronic Myelocitic Leukemia," *Nature* 300, no. 5894 (1982): 765–67.

431 *The mouse developed the fatal spleen-choking:* E. Fainstein et al., "A New Fused Transcript in Philadelphia Chromosome Positive Acute Lymphocytic Leukaemia," *Nature* 330, no. 6146 (1987): 386–88; Nora Heisterkamp et al., "Structural Organization of the Bcr Gene and Its Role in the Ph' Translocation," *Nature* 315, no. 6022 (1985): 758–61; de Klein et al., "Cellular Oncogene Is Translocated"; Nora Heisterkamp et al., "Chromosomal Localization of Human Cellular Homologues of Two Viral Oncogenes," *Nature* 299, no. 5885 (1982): 747–49.

431 *In the mid-1980s:* Daniel Vasella and Robert Slater, *Magic Cancer Bullet: How a Tiny Orange Pill Is Rewriting Medical History* (New York: HarperCollins, 2003), 40–48; Elisabeth Buchdunger and Jürg Zimmermann, "The Story of Gleevec," innovation. org, http://www.innovation.org/index.cfm/StoriesofInnovation/InnovatorStories/The_Story_of_Gleevec (accessed January 31, 2010).

433 *Jürg Zimmermann, a talented chemist:* Howard Brody, *Hooked: Ethics, the Medical Profession, and the Pharmaceutical Industry* (Lanham, MD: Rowman & Littlefield, 2007), 14–15; Buchdunger and Zimmermann, "Story of Gleevec."

433 *"[It was] what a locksmith does":* Buchdunger and Zimmermann, "Story of Gleevec."

433 *"I was drawn to oncology as a medical student":* Brian Druker, interview with author, November 2009.

434 *In 1993, he left Boston:* Ibid.

434 *"Everyone just humored me":* Ibid.

434 *In October 1992, just a few months:* Ibid.

435 *"Although freedom from leukemia":* S. Tura et al., "Evaluating Survival After Allogeneic Bone Marrow Transplant for Chronic Myeloid Leukaemia in Chronic Phase: A

Comparison of Transplant Versus No-Transplant in a Cohort of 258 Patients First Seen in Italy Between 1984 and 1986," *British Journal of Haematology* 85 (1993): 292–99.

435 *"Cancer is complicated"*: Druker, interview with author.

435 *In the summer of 1993, when Lydon's drug:* Ibid.

435 *Druker described the findings in the journal:* Brian J. Druker, "Effects of a Selective Inhibitor of the Abl Tyrosine Kinase on the Growth of Bcr-Abl Positive Cells," *Nature Medicine* 2, no. 5 (1996): 561–66.

436 *"The drug . . . would never work":* The story of Gleevec's development is from Druker, interview with author.

436 *In early 1998, Novartis finally relented:* Lauren Sompayrac, *How Cancer Works* (Sudbury, MA: Jones and Bartlett, 2004), 21.

438 *Druker edged into higher and higher:* Brian J. Druker et al., "Efficacy and Safety of a Specific Inhibitor of the BCR-ABL Tyrosine Kinase in Chronic Myeloid Leukemia," *New England Journal of Medicine* 344, no. 14 (2001): 1031–37.

438 *Of the fifty-four patients:* Ibid.

438 *"Before the year 2000":* Hagop Kantarjian, Georgetown Oncology Board Review Lectures, 2008.

439 *"When I was a youngster in Illinois":* Bruce A. Chabner, "The Oncologic Four-Minute Mile," *Oncologist* 6, no. 3 (2001): 230–32.

439 *"It proves a principle":* Ibid.

The Red Queen's Race

441 *"Well, in our country," said Alice:* Lewis Carroll, *Alice in Wonderland and Through the Looking Glass* (Boston: Lothrop, 1898), 125.

441 *In August 2000:* Details of Jerry Mayfield's case are from the CML blog newcmldrug .com. This website is run by Mayfield to provide information to patients about CML and targeted therapy.

442 *CML cells, Sawyers discovered:* See for instance M. E. Gorre et al., "Clinical Resistance to STI-571 Cancer Therapy Caused by BCR-ABL Gene Mutation or Amplification," *Science* 293, no. 5531 (2001): 876–80; Neil P. Shah et al., "Multiple *BCR-ABL* Kinase Domain Mutations Confer Polyclonal Resistance to the Tyrosine Kinase Inhibitor Imatinib (STI571) in Chronic Phase and Blast Crisis Chronic Myeloid Leukemia," *Cancer Cell* 2, no. 2 (2002): 117–25.

442 *"an arrow pierced through the center of the protein's heart":* Attributed to John Kuriyan; quoted by George Dmitri to the author at a Columbia University seminar, November 2009.

442 *In 2005, working with chemists:* Jagabandhu Das et al., "2-Aminothiazole as a Novel Kinase Inhibitor Template. Structure-Activity Relationship Studies toward the Discovery of N-(2-Chloro-6-methylphenyl)-2-[[6-[4-(2-hydroxyethyl)-1-(piperazinyl)]-2-methyl-4-pyrimidinyl](amino)]-1,3-thiazole-5-carboxamide (Dasatinib, BMS-354825) as a Potent *pan*-Src Kinase Inhibitor," *Journal of Medicinal Chemistry* 49, no. 23 (2006): 6819–32; Neil P. Shah et al., "Overriding Imatinib Resistance with a Novel ABL Kinase Inhibitor," *Science* 305, no. 5682 (2004): 399–401; Moshe Talpaz et al., "Dasatinib in Imatinib-Resistant Philadelphia Chromosome–Positive Leukemias," *New England Journal of Medicine* 354, no. 24 (2006): 2531–41.

443 *twenty-four novel drugs:* For a full list, see National Cancer Institute, targeted ther-

apies list, http://www.cancer.gov/cancertopics/factsheet/Therapy/targeted (accessed February 23, 2010). This website also details the role of such drugs as Avastin and bortezomib.

443 *Over a decade:* "Velcade (Bortezomib) Is Approved for Initial Treatment of Patients with Multiple Myeloma," U.S. Food and Drug Administration, http://www.fda.gov/AboutFDA/CentersOffices/CDER/ucm094633.htm (accessed January 31, 2010); "FDA Approval for Lenalidomide," National Cancer Institute, U.S. National Institutes of Health, http://www.cancer.gov/cancertopics/druginfo/fda-lenalidomide (accessed January 31, 2010).

444 *In 1948, epidemiologists identified a cohort:* Framingham Heart Study, the National Heart, Lung and Blood Institute and Boston University, http://www.framingham-heartstudy.org/ (accessed January 31, 2010).

445 *In May 2008, two Harvard epidemiologists:* Nicholas A. Christakis, "The Collective Dynamics of Smoking in a Large Social Network," *New England Journal of Medicine* 358, no. 21 (2008): 2249–58.

447 *"Cancer at the* fin de siècle*":* Harold J. Burstein, "Cancer at the *Fin de Siècle,*" *Medscape Today,* February 1, 2000, http://www.medscape.com/viewarticle/408448 (accessed January 31, 2010).

Thirteen Mountains

448 *"Every sickness is a musical problem":* W. H. Auden, "The Art of Healing (*In Memoriam David Protetch, M.D.*)," *New Yorker,* September 27, 1969.

448 *The revolution in cancer research:* Bert Vogelstein and Kenneth Kinzler, "Cancer Genes and the Pathways They Control," *Nature Medicine* 10, no. 8 (2004): 789–99.

449 *"The purpose of my book":* Susan Sontag, *Illness as Metaphor and AIDS and Its Metaphors* (New York: Picador, 1990), 102.

450 *The Human Genome Project:* "Once Again, Scientists Say Human Genome Is Complete," *New York Times,* April 15, 2003.

450 *the Cancer Genome Atlas:* "New Genome Project to Focus on Genetic Links in Cancer," *New York Times,* December 14, 2005.

450 *"When applied to the 50 most common":* "Mapping the Cancer Genome," *Scientific American,* March 2007.

450 *In 2006, the Vogelstein team revealed:* Tobias Sjöblom et al., "The Consensus Coding Sequences of Human Breast and Colorectal Cancers," *Science* 314, no. 5797 (2006): 268–74.

450 *In 2008, both Vogelstein's group and the Cancer Genome Atlas:* Roger McLendon et al., "Comprehensive Genomic Characterization Defines Human Glioblastoma Genes and Core Pathways," *Nature* 455, no. 7216 (2008): 1061–68. Also see D. Williams Parsons et al., "An Integrated Genomic Analysis of Human Glioblastoma Multiforme," *Science* 321, no. 5897 (2008): 1807–12; and Roger McLendon et al., "Comprehensive Genomic Characterization."

452 *Only a few cancers are notable exceptions:* C. G. Mullighan et al., "Genome-Wide Analysis of Genetic Alterations in Acute Lymphoblastic Leukemia," *Nature* 446, no. 7137 (2007): 758–64.

452 *"In the end," as Vogelstein put it:* Bert Vogelstein, comments on lecture at Massachusetts

General Hospital, 2009; also see Vogelstein and Kinzler, "Cancer Genes and the Pathways They Control."

453 *Other mutations are not passive players:* The distinction between passenger and driver mutations has generated an enormous debate in cancer genetics. Many scientists suspect that the initial analysis of the breast cancer genome may have overestimated the number of driver mutations. Currently, this remains an open question in cancer genetics. See, for instance, Getz et al., Rubin et al., and Forrest et al., *Science* 317, no 5844: 1500, comments on Sjöblom article above.

453 *In a recent series of studies, Vogelstein's team:* See, for example, Rebecca J. Leary, "Integrated Analysis of Homozygous Deletions, Focal Amplifications, and Sequence Alterations in Breast and Colorectal Cancers," *Proceedings of the National Academy of Sciences of the United States of America* 105, no. 42 (2008): 16224–29; Siân Jones et al., "Core Signaling Pathways in Human Pancreatic Cancer Revealed by Global Genomic Analyses," *Science* 321, no. 5897 (2008): 1801–6.

454 *"Cancer," as one scientist recently put it:* Emmanuel Petricoin, quoted in Dan Jones, "Pathways to Cancer Therapy," *Nature Reviews Drug Discovery* 7 (2008): 875–76.

455 *In a piece published in the* New York Times: "To Fight Cancer, Know the Enemy," *New York Times,* August 5, 2009.

456 *In 2000, the so-called Million Women Study:* Valerie Beral et al., "Breast Cancer and Hormone-Replacement Therapy in the Million Women Study," *Lancet* 362, no. 9382 (2003): 419–27.

456 *The second controversy also has its antecedents:* See, for instance, F. J. Roe and M. C. Lancaster et al., "Natural, Metallic and Other Substances, as Carcinogens," *British Medical Bulletin* 20 (1964): 127–33; and Jan Dich et al., "Pesticides and Cancer," *Cancer Causes & Control* 8, no. 3 (1997): 420–43.

457 *In 2005, the Harvard epidemiologist David Hunter:* Yen-Ching Chen and David J. Hunter, "Molecular Epidemiology of Cancer," *CA: A Cancer Journal for Clinicians* 55 (2005): 45–54.

457 *In the mid-1990s, building on the prior decade's advances:* Yoshio Miki et al., "A Strong Candidate for the Breast and Ovarian Cancer Susceptibility Gene BRCA1," *Science* 266, no. 5182 (1994): 66–71; R. Wooster et al., "Localization of a Breast Cancer Susceptibility Gene, BRCA2, to Chromosome 13q12–13," *Science* 265, no. 5181 (1994): 2088–90; J. M. Hall et al., "Linkage of Early-Onset Familial Breast Cancer to Chromosome 17q21," *Science* 250, no. 4988 (1990): 1684–89; Michael R. Stratton et al., "Familial Male Breast Cancer Is Not Linked to the *BRCA1* Locus on Chromosome 17q," *Nature Genetics* 7, no. 1 (1994): 103–7.

457 *An Israeli woman:* Breast cancer patient O. B-L. (name withheld), interview with author, December 2008.

458 *In the mid-1990s, John Dick:* Tsvee Lapidot et al., "A Cell Initiating Human Acute Myeloid Leukaemia After Transplantation into SCID Mice," *Nature* 367, no. 6464 (1994): 645–58.

459 *Indeed, as the fraction of those affected by cancer creeps:* "One in three" is from the recent evaluation by the National Cancer Institute. See http://www.cancer.gov/news-center/tip-sheet-cancer-health-disparities. The number "one in two" comes from the NCI seer statistics, http://seer.cancer.gov/statfacts/html/all.html, but includes all cancer sites, summarized in Matthew Hayat et al., "Cancer Statistics, Trends and Multiple Primary Cancer Analyses," *Oncologist* 12 (2007): 20–37.

ATOSSA'S WAR

461 *We aged a hundred years:* Anna Akhmatova, "In Memoriam, July 19, 1914," in *The Complete Poems of Anna Akhmatova,* vol. 1 (Chicago: Zephyr Press, 1990), 449.

461 *It is time, it is time for me too to depart:* Aleksandr Solzhenitsyn, *Cancer Ward* (New York: Farrar, Straus and Giroux, 1974), 476.

461 *On May 17, 1973:* "A Memorial Tribute in Honor of Dr. Sidney Farber, 1903–1973," Thursday, May 17, 1973. Gift of Thomas Farber to the author.

464 *It is impossible to enumerate:* Atossa's case and her survival numbers are speculative, but based on several sources. See, for instance, "Effects of chemotherapy and hormonal therapy for early breast cancer on recurrence and 15-year survival: An overview of the randomised trials," *Lancet,* 365, no. 9472: 1687–1717.

465 *In 1997, the NCI director, Richard Klausner:* See Barnett S. Kramer and Richard D. Klausner, "Grappling with Cancer—Defeatism Versus the Reality of Progress," *New England Journal of Medicine* 337, no. 13 (1997): 931–35.

467 *The new drug was none other than Gleevec:* See, for example, H. Joensuu, "Treatment of Inoperable Gastrointestinal Stromal Tumors (GIST) with Imatinib (Glivec, Gleevec)," *Medizinische Klinik* (Munich) 97, suppl. 1 (2002): 28–30; M. V. Chandu de Silva and Robin Reid, "Gastrointestinal Stromal Tumors (GIST): C-kit Mutations, CD117 Expression, Differential Diagnosis and Targeted Cancer Therapy with Imatinib," *Pathology Oncology Research* 9, no. 1 (2003): 13–19.

Glossary

Acute lymphoblastic leukemia: a variant of white blood cell cancer that affects the lymphoid lineage of blood cells.

Acute myeloid leukemia: a variant of white blood cell cancer that affects the myeloid lineage of blood cells.

Apoptosis: the regulated process of cell death that occurs in most cells, involving specific cascades of genes and proteins.

Carcinogen: a cancer-causing or cancer-inciting agent.

Chimeric gene: A gene created by the mixing together of two genes. A chimeric gene might be the product of a natural translocation, or might be engineered in the lab.

Chromosome: a structure within a cell comprised of DNA and proteins that stores genetic information.

Cytotoxic: Cell-killing. Usually refers to chemotherapy that works by killing cells, particularly rapidly dividing cells.

DNA: Deoxyribonucleic acid, a chemical that carries genetic information in all cellular organisms. It is usually present in the cell as two paired, complementary strands. Each strand is a chemical chain made up of four chemical units—abbreviated A, C, T, and G. Genes are carried in the form of a genetic "code" in the strand and the sequence is converted (transcribed) into RNA (see p. 534) and then translated into proteins (see p.534).

Enzyme: a protein that accelerates a biochemical reaction.

Gene: a unit of inheritance, normally comprised of a stretch of DNA that codes for a protein or for an RNA chain (in special cases, genes might be carried in the RNA form).

Genetic engineering: the capacity to manipulate genes in organisms to create new genes, or introduce genes into heterologous organisms (e.g., a human gene in a bacterial cell).

Genome: the full complement of all genes within the organism.

Incidence: In epidemiology, the number (or fraction) of patients who are diagnosed with a disease in a given period of time. It differs from prevalence because incidence reflects the rate of new diagnosis.

Kinase: a protein enzyme that attaches phosphate groups to other proteins.

Metastatic: cancer that has spread beyond its local site of origin.

Mitosis: the division of one cell to form two cells that occurs in most adult tissues of the body (as opposed to meiosis, which generates germ cells in the ovary and the testes).

Mutation: An alteration in the chemical structure of DNA. Mutations can be silent—i.e., the change might not affect any function of the organism—or can result in a change in the function or structure of an organism.

Neoplasm, neoplasia: an alternative name for cancer.

Oncogene: A cancer-causing or cancer-promoting gene. Activation or overexpression of a proto-oncogene (see below) promotes the transformation of a cell from normal to a cancer cell.

Prevalence: in epidemiology, the number (or fraction) of affected patients in any given period of time.

Primary prevention: prevention aimed at avoiding the development of a disease, typically by attacking the cause of the disease.

Prospective trial: a trial in which a cohort of patients is followed forward in time (as opposed to retrospective, in which a cohort of patients is followed backward).

Protein: A chemical comprised, at its core, of a chain of amino acids that is created when a gene is translated. Proteins carry out the bulk of cellular functions, including relaying signals, providing structural support, and accelerating biochemical reactions. Genes usually "work" by providing the blueprint for proteins (see DNA, p. 533). Proteins can be modified chemically by the addition of small chemicals such as phosphates or sugars or lipids.

Proto-oncogene: A precursor to an oncogene. Typically, proto-oncogenes are normal cellular genes that, when activated by mutation or overexpression, promote cancer. Proto-oncogenes typically code for proteins that are associated with cell growth and differentiation. Examples of proto-oncogenes include *ras* and *myc*.

Randomized trial: a trial in which treatment and control groups are randomly assigned.

Retrovirus: an RNA virus that keeps its genes in the form of RNA and is capable, by virtue of an enzyme, reverse transcriptase, to convert its genes from the RNA form into a DNA form.

Reverse transcriptase: An enzyme that converts a chain of RNA into a chain of DNA. Reverse transcription is a property of retroviruses.

RNA: Ribonucleic acid, a chemical that performs several functions in the cells, including acting as an "intermediate" message for a gene to become a protein. Certain viruses also use RNA, not DNA, to maintain their genes (see Retrovirus, above).

Secondary prevention: Prevention strategies that are aimed at early detection of a disease, typically by screening asymptomatic men and women. Typically, secondary prevention strategies attack early, pre-symptomatic stages of the disease.

Transfection: the introduction of DNA into a cell.

Transgenic mice: mice in which a genetic change has been artificially introduced.

Translocation (of a gene): the physical reattachment of a gene from one chromosome to another.

Tumor suppressor gene (also called anti-oncogene): A gene that, when inactivated fully, promotes the progression of a cell into a cancer cell. Tumor suppressors usually protect a cell from one step on the progression toward cancer. When this gene is mutated to cause a loss or reduction in its function, the cell can progress to cancer. Typically, this occurs in combination with other genetic changes.

Two-hit hypothesis: the notion that for tumor suppressor genes, both functionally intact copies of the gene must be inactivated in order for a cell to progress toward cancer.

Virus: A microorganism that is incapable of reproducing by itself, but capable of creating progeny once it has infected a cell. Viruses come in diverse forms, including DNA viruses and RNA viruses. Viruses possess a core of either DNA or RNA, coated with proteins, and can be bound by an outer membrane made of lipids and proteins.

Selected Bibliography

Absolon, Karel B. *Surgeon's Surgeon: Theodor Billroth, 1829–1894*. Kansas: Coronado Press, 1979.

Airley, Rachel. *Cancer Chemotherapy: Basic Science to the Clinic*. Hoboken, N.J.: Wiley, 2009.

Alberts, Bruce. *Molecular Biology of the Cell*. London: Garland Science, 2008.

Alsop, Stewart. *Stay of Execution: A Sort of Memoir*. New York: Lippincott, 1973.

Altman, Roberta. *Waking Up, Fighting Back: The Politics of Breast Cancer*. New York: Little, Brown, 1996.

Angier, Natalie. *Natural Obsessions: Striving to Unlock the Deepest Secrets of the Cancer Cell*. New York: Mariner Books, 1999.

Archives Program of Children's Hospital Boston, *Children's Hospital Boston*. Chicago: Arcadia Publishing, 2005.

Aufderheide, Arthur. *The Scientific Study of Mummies*. Cambridge: Cambridge University Press, 2003.

Austoker, Joan. *A History of the Imperial Cancer Research Fund 1902–1986*. Oxford: Oxford University Press, 1988.

Baillie, Matthew. *The Morbid Anatomy of Some of the Most Important Parts of the Human Body*. Walpole, N.H.: Thomas & Thomas, 1808.

Baillie, Matthew, and James Wardrop, ed. *The Works of Matthew Baillie, M.D.: To Which Is Prefixed an Account of His Life*. Vol. 1. London: Longman, Hurst, Rees, Orme, Brown and Green, 1825.

Ballance, Charles Alfred. *A Glimpse into the History of the Surgery of the Brain*. New York: Macmillan, 1922.

Bazell, Robert. *Her-2: The Making of Herceptin, a Revolutionary Treatment for Breast Cancer*. New York: Random House, 1998.

Billings, John Shaw. *The History and Literature of Surgery*. Philadelphia: Lea Bros., 1885.

Bishop, J. Michael. *How to Win the Nobel Prize: An Unexpected Life in Science*. Cambridge: Harvard University Press, 2003.

Bliss, Michael. *Harvey Cushing: A Life in Surgery*. Oxford: Oxford University Press, 2005.

Blumberg, Baruch S. *Hepatitis B: The Hunt for a Killer Virus*. Princeton: Princeton University Press, 2002.

Boveri, Theodor. *Concerning the Origin of Malignant Tumours by Theodor Boveri*. New York: Cold Spring Harbor Press, 2006.

Brandt, Allan M., *The Cigarette Century: The Rise, Fall, and Deadly Persistence of the Product That Defined America*. New York: Basic Books, 2007.

Breasted, James Henry. *The Edwin Smith Papyrus: Some Preliminary Observations*. Paris: Librairie Ancienne Honoré Champion, Édouard Champion, 1922.

Broyard, Anatole. *Intoxicated by My Illness and Other Writings on Life and Death*. New York: C. Potter, 1992.

Bunz, Fred. *Principles of Cancer Genetics*. New York: Springer, 2008.

Burjet, W. C., ed. *Surgical Papers by William Stewart Halsted*. 2 Vols. Baltimore: Johns Hopkins, 1924.

Cairns, John. *Cancer: Science and Society*. New York: W. H. Freeman, 1979.

———. *Matters of Life and Death: Perspectives on Public Health, Molecular Biology, Cancer, and the Prospects for the Human Race*. Princeton: Princeton University Press, 1997.

Cantor, David. *Cancer in the Twentieth Century*. Baltimore: The Johns Hopkins University Press, 2008.

Carroll, Lewis. *Alice in Wonderland and Through the Looking-Glass*. Boston: Lothrop, 1898.

Carson, Rachel. *Silent Spring*. New York: Mariner Books, 2002.

Chung, Daniel C., and Daniel A. Haber. *Principles of Clinical Cancer Genetics: A Handbook from the Massachusetts General Hospital*. New York: Springer, 2010.

Cooper, Geoffrey M., Rayla Greenberg Temin, and Bill Sugden, eds. *The DNA Provirus: Howard Temin's Scientific Legacy*. Washington, D.C.: ASM Press, 1995.

Criles, George. *Cancer and Common Sense*. New York: Viking Press, 1955.

DeGregorio, Michael W., and Valerie J. Wiebe. *Tamoxifen and Breast Cancer*. New Haven: Yale University Press, 1999.

de Moulin, Daniel. *A Short History of Breast Cancer*. Boston: M. Nijhoff, 1983.

de Tocqueville, Alexis. *Democracy in America*. New York: Penguin, 2003.

Diamond, Louis Klein. *Reminiscences of Louis K. Diamond: Oral*. Interview transcript. New York: Columbia University, 1990.

Edson, Margaret. *Wit*. New York: Dramatists Play Service, 1999.

Ellis, Harold. *A History of Surgery*. Cambridge: Cambridge University Press, 2001.

Faguet, Guy. *The War on Cancer: An Anatomy of Failure*. Dordecht: Springer, 2008.

Farber, Sidney. *The Postmortem Examination*. Springfield, Ill.: C. C. Thomas, 1937.

Finkel, Madelon L. *Understanding the Mammography Controversy: Science, Politics, and Breast Cancer Screening*. Santa Barbara, Calif.: Praeger, 2005.

Fujimura, Joan H. *Crafting Science: A Sociohistory of the Quest for the Genetics of Cancer*. Cambridge: Harvard University Press, 1996.

Galen. *On Diseases and Symptoms*. Cambridge: Cambridge University Press, 2006.

———. *On the Natural Faculties*. Whitefish, Mont.: Kessinger Publishing, 2004.

———. *Selected Works*. Oxford: Oxford University Press, 2002.

Garb, Solomon. *Cure for Cancer: A National Goal*. New York: Springer, 1968.

Goodman, Jordan, and Vivien Walsh. *Story of Taxol: Nature and Politics in the Pursuit of an Anti-Cancer Drug*. New York: Cambridge University Press, 2001.

Gunther, John. *Taken at the Flood: The Story of Albert D. Lasker*. New York: Harper, 1960.

Haagenson, Cushman Davis. *Diseases of the Breast*. Philadelphia: W. B. Saunders Company, 1974.

Haddow, Alexander, Herman M. Kalckar, and Otto Warburg. *On Cancer and Hormones: Essays in Experimental Biology*. Chicago: University of Chicago Press, 1962.

Hall, Steven S. *Invisible Frontiers: The Race to Synthesize a Human Gene*. New York: Atlantic Monthly Press, 1987.

Henig, Robin Marantz. *The Monk in the Garden: The Lost and Found Genius of Gregor Mendel, the Father of Genetics*. New York: Mariner Books, 2001.

Hill, John. *Cautions against the Immoderate Use of Snuff*. London: R. Baldwin and J. Jackson, 1761.

Hilts, Philip J. *Protecting America's Health: The FDA, Business, and One Hundred Years of Regulation.* New York: Knopf, 2003.

Huggins, Charles. *Frontiers of Mammary Cancer.* Glasgow: Jackson, 1961.

ICON Health Publications. *Gleevec: A Medical Dictionary, Bibliography, and Annotated Research Guide.* Logan, Utah: ICON Health, 2004.

Imber, Gerald. *Genius on the Edge: The Bizarre Double Life of Dr. William Stewart Halsted.* New York: Kaplan, 2010.

Jencks, Maggie Keswick. *A View from the Front Line.* London, 1995.

Jordan, V. C. *Tamoxifen, a Guide for Clinicians and Patients.* Huntington, N.Y.: PRR, 1996.

Justman, Stewart. *Seeds of Mortality: The Public and Private Worlds of Cancer.* Chicago: Ivan R. Dee, 2003.

Kannel, William B., and Tavia Gordon. *The Framingham Study: An Epidemiological Investigation of Cardiovascular Disease.* Washington, D.C.: U.S. Department of Health, Education, and Welfare, National Institutes of Health, 1968.

Kaplan, Henry. *Hodgkin's Disease.* Cambridge: Harvard University Press, 1980.

Kleinman, Arthur. *The Illness Narratives: Suffering, Healing, and the Human Condition.* New York: Basic Books, 1988.

Kluger, Richard. *Ashes to Ashes.* New York: Vintage Books, 1997.

Knapp, Richard B. *Gift of Surgery to Mankind: A History of Modern Anesthesiology.* Springfield, Ill.: C. C. Thomas, 1983.

Knight, Nancy, and J. Frank Wilson. *The Early Years of Radiation Therapy: A History of the Radiological Sciences, Radiation Oncology.* Reston, Va.: Radiological Centennial, 1996.

Kushner, Rose. *Why Me?.* Philadelphia: Saunders Press, 1982.

Kyvig, David E. *Daily Life in the United States, 1920–1940: How Americans Lived Through the Roaring Twenties and the Great Depression.* Chicago: Ivan R. Dee, 2004.

Laszlo, John. *The Cure of Childhood Leukemia: Into the Age of Miracles.* New Brunswick, N.J.: Rutgers University Press, 1995.

Leopold, Ellen. *A Darker Ribbon: Breast Cancer, Women, and Their Doctors in the Twentieth Century.* Boston: Beacon Press, 1999.

Lerner, Barron H. *The Breast Cancer Wars: Hope, Fear, and the Pursuit of a Cure in Twentieth-Century America.* Oxford: Oxford University Press, 2001.

Levi, Primo. *Survival at Auschwitz: If This Is a Man.* Phoenix, Ariz.: Orion Press, 2008.

Lewison, Edward. *Breast Cancer: Its Diagnosis and Treatment.* Baltimore: Williams and Wilkins Company, 1955.

Lock, Stephen, Lois A. Reynolds, and E. M. Tansey, eds. *Ashes to Ashes.* Amsterdam: Editions Rodopi B.V., 1998.

Love, Susan M. *Dr. Susan Love's Breast Book.* New York: Random House, 1995.

MacCallum, W. G., and W. H. Welch. *William Stewart Halsted, Surgeon.* Whitefish, Mont.: Kessinger Publishing, 2008.

Marquardt, Martha. *Paul Ehrlich.* New York: Schuman, 1951.

McKelvey, Maureen D. *Evolutionary Innovations: The Business of Biotechnology.* Oxford: Oxford University Press, 1996.

Moss, Ralph W. *The Cancer Syndrome.* New York: Grove Press, 1980.

Mueller, Charles Barber. *Evarts A. Graham: The Life, Lives, and Times of the Surgical Spirit of St. Louis.* Hamilton, Ont., Can.: BC Decker, Inc., 2002.

Nathan, David G. *The Cancer Treatment Revolution: How Smart Drugs and Other New Therapies Are Renewing Our Hope and Changing the Face of Medicine.* Hoboken, N.J.: Wiley, 2007.

Nuland, Sherwin B. *Doctors: The Biography of Medicine*. New York: Knopf, 1988.

Olson, James S. *Bathsheba's Breast: Women, Cancer, and History*. Baltimore: Johns Hopkins University Press, 2002.

———. *History of Cancer: An Annotated Bibliography*. New York: Greenwood Press, 1989.

Oshinski, David M. *Polio: An American Story*. Oxford: Oxford University Press, 2005.

Parker, George. *The Early History of Surgery in Great Britain: Its Organization and Development*. London: Black, 1920.

Patterson, James T. *The Dread Disease: Cancer and Modern American Culture*. Cambridge: Harvard University Press, 1987.

Porter, Roy, ed. *The Cambridge Illustrated History of Medicine*. Cambridge: Cambridge University Press, 1996.

Pott, Percivall, and James Earle. *The Chirurgical Works of Percivall Pott, F.R.S., Surgeon to St. Bartholomew's Hospital, a New Edition, with His Last Corrections, to Which Are Added, a Short Account of the Life of the Author, a Method of Curing the Hydrocele by Injection, and Occasional Notes and Observations, by Sir James Earle, F.R.S., Surgeon Extraordinary to the King*. London: Wood and Innes, 1808.

Rather, L. J. *Genesis of Cancer: A Study in the History of Ideas*. Baltimore: Johns Hopkins University Press, 1978.

Reid, Robert William. *Marie Curie*. New York: Collins, 1974.

Resnik, Susan. *Blood Saga: Hemophilia, AIDS, and the Survival of a Community*. Berkeley: University of California Press, 1999.

Retsas, Spyros, ed. *Palaeo-oncology: The Antiquity of Cancer*. London: Farrand Press, 1986.

Rettig, Richard, Peter D. Jacobson, Cynthia M. Farquhar, and Wade M. Aubry. *False Hope: Bone Marrow Transplantation for Breast Cancer*. Oxford: Oxford University Press, 2007.

Rettig, Richard A. *Cancer Crusade: The Story of the National Cancer Act of 1971*. Lincoln, Neb.: Author's Choice Press, 1977.

Rhodes, Richard. *The Making of the Atomic Bomb*. New York: Simon & Schuster, 1995.

Robbins-Roth, Cynthia. *From Alchemy to IPO: The Business of Biotechnology*. Cambridge, Mass.: Perseus, 2000.

Rosenfeld, Louis. *Thomas Hodgkin: Morbid Anatomist & Social Activist*. Lanham, Md.: Madison Books, 1993.

Ross, Walter Sanford. *Crusade: The Official History of the American Cancer Society*. New York: Arbor House, 1987.

Rutkow, Ira M. *History of Surgery in the United States, 1775–1900*. San Francisco: Norman Publishers, 1988.

Salecl, Renata. *On Anxiety*. London: Routledge, 2004.

Saunders, Cicely. *Selected Writings, 1958–2004*. Oxford: Oxford University Press, 2006.

Saunders, J. B. deC. M., and Charles D. O'Malley. *The Illustrations from the Works of Andreas Vesalius of Brussels*. Mineola, N.Y.: Dover, 1973.

Seaman, Barbara. *The Greatest Experiment Ever Performed on Women: Exploding the Estrogen Myth*. New York: Hyperion, 2004.

Shilts, Randy. *And the Band Played On*. New York: St. Martin's, 2007.

Skipper, Howard E. *Cancer Chemotherapy*. University Microfilms International for American Society of Clinical Oncology, 1979.

Smith, Clement A. *Children's Hospital of Boston: "Built Better Than They Knew."* Boston: Little, Brown, 1983.

Solzhenitsyn, Aleksandr. *Cancer Ward*. New York: Farrar, Straus and Giroux, 1968.

Sontag, Susan. *Illness as Metaphor and AIDS and Its Metaphors*. New York: Picador, 1990.

Starr, Paul. *The Social Transformation of American Medicine*. New York: Basic Books, 1983.

Stevens, Rosemary. *In Sickness and in Wealth*. New York: Basic Books, 1989.

Stokes, Donald E. *Pasteur's Quadrant: Basic Science and Technological Innovation*. Washington, D.C.: Brookings Institution Press, 1997.

Stone, William Stephen. *Review of the History of Chemical Therapy in Cancer*. New York: Wood, 1916.

Strax, Phillip, ed. *Control of Breast Cancer Through Mass Screening*. Littleton, Mass.: PSG Publishing, 1979.

Strickland, Stephen Parks. *Politics, Science, and the Dread Disease: A Short History of the United States Medical Research Policy*. Cambridge: Harvard University Press, 1972.

Taylor, Grant, ed. *Pioneers in Pediatric Oncology*. Houston: University of Texas M. D. Anderson Cancer Center, 1990.

Taylor, Tanya. *The Cancer Monologue Project*. San Francisco: MacAdam/Cage, 2002.

Teitelman, Robert. *Gene Dreams: Wall Street, Academia and the Rise of Biotechnology*. New York: Basic Books, 1989.

Travis, Anthony S. *The Rainbow Makers: The Origins of the Synthetic Dyestuffs Industry in Western Europe*. Bethlehem, Pa.: Lehigh University Press, 1993.

U.S. Surgeon General. "Smoking and Health." *Report of the Advisory Committee to the Surgeon General of the Public Health Service,* Public Health Service publication no. 1103. Washington, D.C.: U.S. Department of Health, Education, and Welfare, Public Health Service, 1964.

Varmus, Harold. *The Art and Politics of Science*. New York: W. W. Norton & Company, 2009.

Vasella, Daniel, and Robert Slater. *Magic Cancer Bullet: How a Tiny Orange Pill Is Rewriting Medical History*. New York: HarperCollins, 2003.

Vesalius, Andreas. *On the Fabric of the Human Body: A Translation of De Humana Corporis Fabrica Libri Septem*. Novato, Calif.: Norman Publishers, 2003.

Wangensteen, Owen, and Sarah Wangensteen. *Rise of Surgery*. Minneapolis: University of Minnesota, 1978.

Weinberg, Robert. *The Biology of Cancer*. London: Garland Science, 2006.

———. *One Renegade Cell*. New York: Basic Books, 1999.

———. *Racing to the Beginning of the Road*. New York: Bantam, 1997.

Werth, Barry. *The Billion-Dollar Molecule: One Company's Quest for the Perfect Drug*. New York: Simon & Schuster, 1994.

Wishart, Adam. *One in Three: A Son's Journey into the History and Science of Cancer*. New York: Grove Press, 2007.

Wisnia, Saul. *The Jimmy Fund of Dana-Farber Cancer Institute*. Charleston, S.C.: Arcadia Publishing, 2002.

Zachary, Gregg Pascal. *Endless Frontier: Vannevar Bush, Engineer of the American Century*. New York: Free Press, 1997.

Photograph Credits

Index

An Interview with Siddhartha Mukherjee

Why did you decide to write a book about cancer?
The book is a very long answer to a question first posed to me by a patient I was treating in Boston, a woman with a very aggressive form of abdominal cancer. She had been treated with chemotherapy and had relapsed and been treated again. At one point, deep into her treatment, she said to me, "I'm willing to go on, but I need to know what it is I'm battling." My book is an attempt to answer her question by going back to the origin of the disease and showing its development through history. I called it "a biography of cancer," because it draws a portrait of an illness over time.

What exactly is cancer?
Cancer is not a disease but a whole family of diseases. These diseases are linked at a fundamental biological level. They're characterized by the pathological proliferation of cells—occasionally cells that don't know how to die, but certainly cells that don't know how to stop dividing. That abnormal, uncontrollable growth of cells is a process that typically starts in a single cell and the cell multiplies over and over, and every generation produces a little evolutionary cycle such that you get more and more evolved cells. But although there's a deep commonality between prostate cancer, breast cancer, leukemia, although they're connected as the cellular level, every cancer has a different face.

Did you have a particular audience in mind while writing the book?
Was the idea to write it for patients or for a layperson to understand?
The book is written entirely for a layperson to understand, but I wanted to treat this audience with the utmost seriousness. I wanted to address the desire of patients and families for a larger history, one that goes back to the origins and then takes us into the future. I wrote with patients and families in mind, but also with the scientist in mind, with the student in mind, with the reader of literature in mind.

The book drives home the amount of suffering patients experienced in the past that allowed us to get where we are today. What made you decide to focus so much on this aspect of cancer's story?

One of the many messages of the book is that there are other people who have given up their lives to help us understand more about this disease. I think we need to remember them and do their memory honor. That might mean understanding cancer culturally; that might mean understanding it socially; that might mean participating in clinical trials. It might mean spearheading prevention mechanisms. One of the points of the book is to say, "Let's make sure that these efforts weren't made in vain." There's a respect for history that I'd like to signal in this book.

A recent retrospective in the* New York Times *suggested that, because death rates had not declined monumentally since 1971, not much progress had been made against cancer. Would you say* The Emperor of All Maladies *attests to a lack of progress in oncology?

Absolutely not. There is a very clear place that lies between the nihilism that has been reported in the media lately and the over-optimism—or the hype that existed thirty years ago. To lean in one direction while neglecting the other does a disservice to the progress that has been made. There's kind of a pendulum quality about cancer research. One decade we're told that we are making such enormous progress on cancer, that the whole thing is going to be licked or cured in five months, and the next decade we're told that nothing has happened. And clearly, neither of those statements is true.

Do you think we need to change the way we educate patients and the public about cancer to move away from the mind-set that cancer is a single disease, to explain that it comprises many diseases?

Yes. Part of my attempt with this book is to allow the public to understand the level of complexity and thereby appreciate the ingenuity and the resilience of knowledge that has come about in terms of discovery. The sequencing of the cancer genome is a good example. It revealed deep complexities within cancer. If you sequence the genomes of multiple specimens of breast cancer, you find deep disparities between even truly identical-looking specimens. So, you might take a nihilistic approach to this and say, "Gosh, this is an unsolvable problem." Yet, if you look deeply, you find that within those wide differences there are organizational patterns.

In the book, I call it a kind of music behind the genes. Again, you have to go through additional cycles of knowledge and thinking before you can make the next discovery.

You described an almost unilateral focus early in the twentieth century by some prominent cancer researchers and virologists on viruses as the only cause of cancer, which was later disproved. Some of today's most prominent researchers—such as Robert Weinberg, whose fundamental discoveries on cancer genetics you discuss in the book—are now saying too much focus is placed on genetic mutation as the cause of cancer and too little research is being devoted to seeking other possible causes. Do you agree with Weinberg or do you feel keeping the focus on genetics offers the best opportunities for improving care?

Genetics is a vital part, but only a small part of it, one piece of a much larger puzzle. There's a line in the book about how every era casts illness in its own image. Well, every era casts cancer in its own image, and this happens to be the era of genetics. Therefore, we use genetics to understand cancer. There was a time when viruses were all the rage, and we had to use the lens of viruses to understand cancer. I think the next series of breakthroughs will involve something beyond cancer genetics. Just to name a few things, the role of the microenvironment in cancer is underappreciated—it's an expanding field. The understanding of epigenetics in cancer? Also an interesting, exploding field. The relationship between the biology of cancer and the stem cell? Also a deeply complex field that involves genetics and involves the microenvironment.

In The Emperor of All Maladies, *you talk about how some physicians become indifferent, not just to death but also to life. What do you mean?*

Anyone who has spent time in the oncology clinic understands that it can be—if you look at it in a certain way—a very depressing place. Perhaps the most striking sign of that is when young residents and fellows say, "I don't want to become an oncologist because everyone dies." It is absolutely not true.

To take care of cancer patients is an enormous privilege, but it also involves deploying everything in your toolbox: the emotional, the psychological, the scientific, the epidemiologic. There's laboratory science, history, clinical trials, and palliative medicine. Every aspect of medicine is involved, and the difference that you can make to a person's life as an oncologist is incredible. You're present at the most moving and terrifying times of a person's life, and the ability to help at that time is a powerful experience.

When you have to deliver bad news, how do you prepare for that?
What really helps is to listen to the person you're delivering bad news to. That's the first thing I've learned from my teachers. And by that, I mean that often bad news involves a crushing or a deflation of aspirations. Someone wants to attend their daughter's graduation, and that may be two months away; another person's goals might involve graduating from college herself. If you understand the patient's goals and how they may or may not be achieved—what is achievable and what is not achievable—it makes the conversation concrete. You can say, "Well, if it means a lot for you to watch your son reach this landmark moment in his life, we can probably get there." I think it really mitigates what bad news *means*.

The Emperor of All Maladies *appears to highlight how ego and distrust between professionals in the different disciplines, such as surgery and chemotherapy, hindered progress in cancer research. Has this gotten better?*
It's gotten vastly better because the prior years have been humbling, and the disciplines have become less isolated. These days, there is hardly a cancer center in which there are not collaborative groups between surgeons, chemotherapists, and radiation oncologists. I think that model evolved out of those humbling experiences—the idea that you can't just use one weapon to battle cancer but must instead deploy multiple ones. A cancer patient today has a team that works around him or her, including nurses, psychiatrists, psychologists, and, in some cases, pain and palliative medicine experts. When I was working in Boston, the one person whose judgment I trusted almost universally was the very first oncologist that the patient often saw, and this often was a community oncologist. They had a real sense of what was happening not only medically to the person, but also socially, emotionally, and so forth, and made a valuable ally in treating a patient.

Do you think community oncologists are reluctant to adopt new discoveries in practice?

No, I don't think so. I think community oncologists are really the frontline of cancer medicine. I have enormous respect for community oncologists because much more than oncologists at tertiary care centers, they see the full range and breadth of the disease.

Do you think the historical memory of those early experiences with basically unregulated clinical trials is at all responsible for the very negative regard many Americans today have of clinical trials and their reluctance to participate in clinical trials?

I think there's a lot of reluctance about clinical trials because we've done a very bad job of educating the public on what a clinical trial means and how important it is and how the only way to learn with this disease is to participate. If we don't partner with patients, then this discipline is lost. The partnership with patients is absolutely critical.

In the book, I talk about the famous Herceptin trials. Genentech and breast cancer activists really didn't see eye-to-eye until they figured out that the only way to move forward was to combine their efforts, such that Genentech—as I say in the book—decides not to perform experiments *on* breast cancer patients but instead performs experiments *with* breast cancer patients. That's the critical piece that is missing. Somehow, the American public still thinks medicine is performing experiments *on* it, but really, medicine should be performing experiments *with* patients.

You spend several pages discussing early advocacy efforts and how people like Mary and Albert Lasker and Farber convinced the public to pay attention to this disease and mobilized funding. Sometimes, things became political, and we see this today, with Avastin, for example. The science seems to suggest it might not be as effective in breast cancer as previously thought, yet some groups and politicians are pressuring the FDA not to rescind approval. We see the same thing with prostate and breast cancer screening, with researchers largely on one side and advocates pushing for something else. How do you reconcile the two?

You balance the issue through the tried-and-tested mechanisms of politics. You try to reach compromises between the desire to push forward with an experimental approach and the desire to stick with what's known.

That involves, again, a degree of education and a degree of diplomacy between patient advocates and, for instance, the FDA or hospitals.

The second way you approach this is by creating more data. To give you an example, there has been a lot of controversy about whether mammography should be performed between the ages of forty and fifty. The way to resolve this is either to perform an extremely detailed analysis of patients between forty and fifty years of age who have been screened with mammography and figure out whether this is a preventive mechanism that allows us to save lives; or to say, "This is not going to work because the technology does not have the resolution required to catch a small breast tumor in a woman between 40 and 50 [years of age]." Let's then find a mechanism to screen better, to risk stratify better, so that high-risk women, for instance, can be given mammographic exams, and determine whether that saves lives. Let's combine risk analysis with mammography, or even genetics with mammography. The answer almost always lies in thinking deeply about what the data show and making modifications in response until a compromise is reached between advocates and regulatory bodies. They all want the same thing, which is to try to get patients to live in the best possible manner for the longest possible time.

Cancer biology and medicine are enormous, complex, and constantly shifting fields. How did you choose what to include in the book and what to exclude?

Last year alone, more than 100,000 journal articles were published on cancer. It would have been impossible to address every scientific or medical advance in this book. Nor could I name every scientific luminary in this vast field. I used a few simple criteria to judge inclusion versus exclusion. If an area of cancer biology had a direct impact on human lives—in the treatment or prevention of cancer—I tried to address it. A discovery in cancer biology had to "transform" into a medical reality.

Some subjects were too esoteric to include, even if they fit that criteria. I left out, for example, the incredible research on cancer telomeres. Telomeres are stretches of DNA at the ends of chromosomes that protect the chromosomes (which house genes) from fraying and being corrupted—much like the plastic tips on shoelaces. As our cells divide, these telomeres get shorter—this is a bit like the shortening of a fuse on a bomb. Ultimately, a shortened telomere might act as an internal gauge of the number of cell divisions—i.e., aging.

Specific proteins maintain and repair these telomeres. Cancer cells—which divide uncontrollably—often have shortened telomeres, as expected. But they also have activated pathways that maintain and repair the telomeres. In effect, some cancer cells appear to have evolved so as to thwart the normal process of aging that exists in normal cells. It is a truly beautiful scientific story, but we are still awaiting the human impact of this theory—a drug that attacks these telomere-maintaining enzymes, for instance, or a mechanism to screen for cancer by measuring this activity. I did not include this research, even though it is so compelling.

I did not write about the mechanisms by which cancer cells metastasize, or the means by which some cancers, such as melanoma, appear to resist attack by the immune system, and the role of the cell cycle in normal cells and cancer cells. I did include BRCA1 and BRCA2, but not at length. These genes are worthy of a full book. I also had to exclude major non-scientific fields: the delivery of cancer care, the global impact of cancer, and the economics of cancer (though I do occasionally touch on issues of funding for research and of drug development by pharmaceutical companies).

Surgery is still the mainstay of cancer treatment for most localized forms of cancer and the surgeon's role in treatment remains crucial. But though I wrote extensively about the early years of cancer surgery—from Billroth to Halsted and Evarts Graham's seminal work—I did not dwell on more recent advances in surgery. I tried to cover some essential stories in relative depth and to create a narrative.

What are some particularly promising areas of cancer biology where laboratory advances are becoming clinical realities?

There are four significant areas. The first is the role of the immune system in certain kinds of cancer. For several decades, research on the immune system in the context of cancer biology was moribund. Clinicians knew that there were rare, spontaneous remissions of cancer—i.e. a malignant melanoma would go into remission without treatment. They suspected that this was because the immune system was attacking the tumor. But what was the precise mechanism of attack? Why were only certain cancers being attacked? Could such an immune activation be used as a therapeutic tool?

As my book was first being published, research in this field exploded. Immunologists have shown that reactivating the immune system can, indeed, have a therapeutic benefit in some cancers, such as melanoma. The role of the host immune system in cancer has emerged as a powerful new focus in cancer therapy.

The second area is cancer metabolism. In the 1920s, the German biologist Otto Warburg proposed that the way that some cancer cells generate energy from oxygen and glucose (a process termed "cellular respiration") is extremely unusual. Normal cells, regardless of their origin or function, use similar ways to generate energy from glucose and oxygen. Cancer cells use a variant of this process that more closely resembles fermentation—the way yeast cells generate energy when there is little or no oxygen. But cancer cells use this pathway even when there is abundant oxygen. Scientists now know that there are genes in certain cancers, such as leukemia and brain cancers, that specifically affect cell metabolism—how oxygen and glucose and energy are handled. These genes could represent new Achilles heels of these cancers.

The third area of interest is the role of gene regulation in cancer cells. Nearly every normal cell in an organism (except for sperm and egg cells) possesses the same set of genes. And yet a retina cell expresses genes to detect light or color, and a white blood cell expresses genes to fight infection. How can such different cells be created out the same genetic blueprint?

Part of the regulation appears to occur by making changes in DNA that do not directly change the genetic code. For instance, DNA can be chemically modified—and these chemical modifications can change the way genes are expressed in a retinal cell versus a white blood cell. Well, it turns out that certain cancer cells have disrupted or altered these DNA-modifying and gene expression pathways, and this allows them to function unlike normal cells. Once again, this is an emerging area of research that will doubtless lead to new therapies and understanding.

The final area of promising investigation is the role of the microenvironment of cancer cells, and its relationship with growth, invasion, and metastasis. Why do certain leukemias grow only within the bone marrow and spleen? Why does prostate cancer metastasize to the bone? What is the link between these unique environments and the growth of the tumor, or its ability to resist drugs? Are there specific "safe harbors" for certain cancer cells, and might disrupting these harbors allow for new therapies?

But what about the mounting costs of these new therapies? You mentioned a drug that activates the immune system in melanoma. The survival benefit of such a drug in metastatic melanoma is only a few months for a subset of patients, but a course of treatment might cost hundreds of thousands of dollars. As a society, can we justify and afford the escalating costs of cancer drugs?

There is a difference between the "cost" of a drug and the "price" of a drug. A pill of Gleevec—I mean, the *chemical* that we call Gleevec—can be synthesized for pennies. That is its real "cost." But the "price" of Gleevec is something else. It is set by a series of social arrangements, by our willingness or ability to pay this set "price" and, of course, by the profit motives of the pharmaceutical industry.

Pharmaceutical companies claim that they need to recoup their investments in research and development—and they do. But we must find a middle ground between the cost and the price, and we are nowhere close to it. As I illustrate in the story of Herceptin, we need to find a mechanism by which clinicians, patients, advocates and the pharmaceutical industry can work together in drug development.

The second point is not about cost, but about cost *effectiveness*: is spending $100,000 on a drug that extends lives by eight weeks worthwhile? To some extent, it depends on who is asking. As a society, our boundary for "effectiveness" is constantly shifting. There's a loose consensus in the field that spending $30,000 to $40,000 for a year of life extension is "worth it"—but of course, that is a highly context-specific decision is far from absolute. In another country, or another century, $40,000 per year of life extended might not be plausible. And then there's the question of *quality* of life. I address this—with the help of Lester Breslow and others—in the chapter "Counting Cancer."

We need a great degree of intelligence to judge the "cost effectiveness" of a drug. In lymphoblastic leukemia, every trial in the 1950s and 1960s typically added between six and ten weeks of survival benefit. By the late 1960s, a substantial fraction of patients, about sixty percent, were being cured. If we had judged the cost effectiveness of Aminopterin in Sidney Farber's trials—which showed a survival benefit of only a few weeks in only some children—we might have abandoned the drug altogether. Judge "cost effectiveness" too early and you might throw out powerful drugs that have not been adequately tested.

There's a similar problem in judging the cost effectiveness of a cancer medicine or prevention mechanism in the wrong *population* of patients. Tamoxifen is cost effective in women with estrogen-receptor positive breast cancer—and highly ineffective in women with estrogen receptor negative breast cancer. If a trial combined ER+ and ER- women in the same group, Tamoxifen would look vastly less effective. If you acted on those results, you would deny a good drug to a large population to whom it is extremely beneficial.

Your book focuses on cancer in the United States. What about cancer in the international context?
Stories in the book take us to Germany, Austria, Egypt, Greece, and the United Kingdom. The discovery of trans-retinoic acid that launches the search for targeted therapy for leukemia takes place in China and France.

That said, I was a Fellow in Boston and I chose Sidney Farber as one of the principal protagonists in the story I wanted to tell. Farber's use of anti-folates in leukemia was clearly path-breaking, but there are plenty of other innovators in this story. One can just as easily tell the entire story of cancer through the eyes of Evarts Graham, the surgeon, or through Richard Doll, the epidemiologist. What was truly distinctive about Farber was his role in the War on Cancer. He was Mary Lasker's collaborator and friend, and it was their convergence that altered the social and political landscape of this disease.

I've written elsewhere about how cancer is being tackled in other parts of the world, particularly in developing nations. One point is obvious: there are well-established mechanisms to prevent, treat and palliate cancer around the world that are practical and even affordable, and yet we are not deploying them. A powerful, international anti-tobacco campaign would prevent tens or hundreds of thousands of cases. Vaccination against viruses that cause cancer could reduce incidence. Cervical cancer, which can be caused by sexually transmitted human papillomavirus, could be drastically reduced through sexual education and vaccination. Yet, thousands of women, some in their thirties and forties, die of this preventable form of cancer. Even breast cancer prevention and treatment can be applied to the developing world. Mammographic screening in appropriate age groups, or even treatment in the form of estrogen modulation for ER positive cancers, should be more prevalent.

You talked about prevention. And yet, aside from tobacco, asbestos, radiation etc, you do not speak at length about other cancer prevention mechanisms. Why?

Cancer prevention is a complex issue, and I dedicated a section of the book to it. But despite its historical origins, it is a discipline in its relative infancy. Epidemiologists and biologists have identified powerful carcinogens that affect large human populations—tobacco among them. But there are likely many carcinogens we have not yet discovered. One of the surprising things about cancer epidemiology is that despite the growing global prevalence of cancer, finding preventable carcinogens that have a substantial magnitude of impact at a population level has been an enormous challenge.

We know some of the common culprits for some cancers: ultraviolet light for melanoma and other skin cancers; tobacco for lung cancer and cancers of the lip, throat, esophagus and pancreas; alcohol as a co-factor for liver and esophagus cancer; the NCI maintains an official list of "nasties," including arsenic, cadmium, beryllium, nickel, lead, benzene, vinyl chloride and asbestos, though the number of men and women with cancer due to benzene or beryllium exposure is small. There are also cancer-linked viruses, such as human papillomavirus, and hepatitis B and C viruses—and exposures to these are potentially preventable.

Pinpointing the role of diet for many cancers has been much more difficult. Diet clearly has a role in colon cancer, but for other cancers, the effect is much more subtle. There have been reports in the press recently that high fat diets cause breast cancer. But the role is difficult to assess. Indeed, very few scientific studies have definitively linked high fat diet to breast cancer, and other studies have not confirmed the link. In contrast to diet, obesity, which has both a dietary and genetic basis, has been much more clearly linked to certain cancers, including breast cancer.

We need rigorous studies to identify and define chemical carcinogens. In the book, I chose to highlight the methodological aspects of finding carcinogens—either in population studies or in the laboratory. This process is deeply informed by history, and is likely to influence how we identify carcinogens in the future.

Moving back to the science, you provide a framework for thinking about the role of genes in cancer—as "accelerators" and "brakes" in a car. Can you give us some more specifics about how such an accelerator or brake gene might work?

The list of oncogenes and tumor suppressor genes is huge—there are more than a hundred—and they are specific for every type of cancer. But let's take an example—a gene called p53, which is mutated in many different forms of cancer. The p53 gene encodes a protein that acts as a "guardian" of the genome. When the DNA of the cell is damaged—say by X-rays—the p53 gene may be activated and the protein may launch a signal to repair DNA. If the DNA is not adequately repaired, p53 initiates a signal for the cell to die. So p53 acts as a sensor of DNA-damage, and activates a cell division "brake" in DNA-damaged cells.

When this "guardian" gene is no longer functional, genes are not appropriately repaired, and cells do not die appropriately. But coordinating DNA damage repair and cellular death are only some functions of p53. There are many other functions, and there is cross-talk with other genetic pathways.

What about the role of the mind/brain in cancer?

There's little doubt that the mind/brain connection plays an important role in one's psychic response to any illness. But there is no "correct" response to a diagnosis of cancer. I am deeply offended when people say to a patient: "you are not healing properly because you aren't thinking positively" or "negative thoughts cause cancer—think positively."

This form of thinking is medieval—it blames the victim and increases the burden of illness. I know dozens of cancer patients who thought "positively"—but inevitably succumbed to a deadly variant of cancer. And I know dozens who had no "positive" response but are alive today. There is no archetypal cancer, so why should there be an archetypal patient? I am horrified by quacks who promise "psychic therapies" for the treatment of cancer. There can be treatment of cancer symptoms or cancer-related pain or anxiety. But the notion of psychic treatment for cancer is incredibly dangerous.

That said, there's growing scientific interest in the ability of hormones secreted by the brain to modify the biology of cancer cells. It's a field in its infancy, but perhaps we will learn much more in the next decade.

What about alternative medicine?

I think all medicine is "alternative" before it becomes mainstream—chemotherapy was "alternative" at some point—so I am eager to see where this field goes. Much of our pharmacopeia is derived from plant sources, and there are more chemicals in plants than we know of or know how to use. As yet, there have been few unbiased trials of these medicines in cancer treatment or prevention.

Is there a cancer prevention lifestyle?

Finding a cancer prevention lifestyle has turned out to be much more difficult than anyone initially imagined. There are some general principles. We should avoid the known toxins—radon, cadmium, asbestos. The number of people who have high exposure to these is small, but the exposure should cease. We should avoid exposure to tobacco and avoid or reduce our exposure to alcohol. We could eat low-meat, fiber-rich diets, we could avoid exposure to UV and to ionizing radiation. But these are rather obvious insights. I have yet to find a "cancer prevention lifestyle" that has been clinically tested in large-scale population studies.

As a practicing oncologist and a father, where did you find time to write a book so big and so complex?

I had to make time. What was important was to have a reason to do it. And the reason to do it was that I was trying to answer my patient's question. As long as I always kept that in mind, I felt as if the book sort of wrote itself. I would come back in the evening after rounds or from the laboratory and I would write. I kept writing until I had answered the question left over from the night before. For instance, when I was writing about mammography, the previous night's question might have been, "Where did this leave us in 1986?" And then the next day's writing would bring us from that period up to 1996, filling out the story in between. I think I was able to write because I was responding to a certain sense of urgency that this story had to be told.

Portions of this interview first appeared in OncNurse *magazine in February 2011. We are grateful to Christin Melton for her questions.*